LAM AND OTHER DISEASES CHARACTERIZED BY SMOOTH MUSCLE PROLIFERATION

LUNG BIOLOGY IN HEALTH AND DISEASE

Executive Editor

Claude Lenfant
Director, National Heart, Lung and Blood Institute
National Institutes of Health
Bethesda, Maryland

1. Immunologic and Infectious Reactions in the Lung, *edited by Charles H. Kirkpatrick and Herbert Y. Reynolds*
2. The Biochemical Basis of Pulmonary Function, *edited by Ronald G. Crystal*
3. Bioengineering Aspects of the Lung, *edited by John B. West*
4. Metabolic Functions of the Lung, *edited by Y. S. Bakhle and John R. Vane*
5. Respiratory Defense Mechanisms (in two parts), *edited by Joseph D. Brain, Donald F. Proctor, and Lynne M. Reid*
6. Development of the Lung, *edited by W. Alan Hodson*
7. Lung Water and Solute Exchange, *edited by Norman C. Staub*
8. Extrapulmonary Manifestations of Respiratory Disease, *edited by Eugene Debs Robin*
9. Chronic Obstructive Pulmonary Disease, *edited by Thomas L. Petty*
10. Pathogenesis and Therapy of Lung Cancer, *edited by Curtis C. Harris*
11. Genetic Determinants of Pulmonary Disease, *edited by Stephen D. Litwin*
12. The Lung in the Transition Between Health and Disease, *edited by Peter T. Macklem and Solbert Permutt*
13. Evolution of Respiratory Processes: A Comparative Approach, *edited by Stephen C. Wood and Claude Lenfant*
14. Pulmonary Vascular Diseases, *edited by Kenneth M. Moser*
15. Physiology and Pharmacology of the Airways, *edited by Jay A. Nadel*
16. Diagnostic Techniques in Pulmonary Disease (in two parts), *edited by Marvin A. Sackner*
17. Regulation of Breathing (in two parts), *edited by Thomas F. Hornbein*
18. Occupational Lung Diseases: Research Approaches and Methods, *edited by Hans Weill and Margaret Turner-Warwick*
19. Immunopharmacology of the Lung, *edited by Harold H. Newball*
20. Sarcoidosis and Other Granulomatous Diseases of the Lung, *edited by Barry L. Fanburg*
21. Sleep and Breathing, *edited by Nicholas A. Saunders and Colin E. Sullivan*
22. *Pneumocystis carinii* Pneumonia: Pathogenesis, Diagnosis, and Treatment, *edited by Lowell S. Young*

23. Pulmonary Nuclear Medicine: Techniques in Diagnosis of Lung Disease, *edited by Harold L. Atkins*
24. Acute Respiratory Failure, *edited by Warren M. Zapol and Konrad J. Falke*
25. Gas Mixing and Distribution in the Lung, *edited by Ludwig A. Engel and Manuel Paiva*
26. High-Frequency Ventilation in Intensive Care and During Surgery, *edited by Graziano Carlon and William S. Howland*
27. Pulmonary Development: Transition from Intrauterine to Extrauterine Life, *edited by George H. Nelson*
28. Chronic Obstructive Pulmonary Disease: Second Edition, Revised and Expanded, *edited by Thomas L. Petty*
29. The Thorax (in two parts), *edited by Charis Roussos and Peter T. Macklem*
30. The Pleura in Health and Disease, *edited by Jacques Chrétien, Jean Bignon, and Albert Hirsch*
31. Drug Therapy for Asthma: Research and Clinical Practice, *edited by John W. Jenne and Shirley Murphy*
32. Pulmonary Endothelium in Health and Disease, *edited by Una S. Ryan*
33. The Airways: Neural Control in Health and Disease, *edited by Michael A. Kaliner and Peter J. Barnes*
34. Pathophysiology and Treatment of Inhalation Injuries, *edited by Jacob Loke*
35. Respiratory Function of the Upper Airway, *edited by Oommen P. Mathew and Giuseppe Sant'Ambrogio*
36. Chronic Obstructive Pulmonary Disease: A Behavioral Perspective, *edited by A. John McSweeny and Igor Grant*
37. Biology of Lung Cancer: Diagnosis and Treatment, *edited by Steven T. Rosen, James L. Mulshine, Frank Cuttitta, and Paul G. Abrams*
38. Pulmonary Vascular Physiology and Pathophysiology, *edited by E. Kenneth Weir and John T. Reeves*
39. Comparative Pulmonary Physiology: Current Concepts, *edited by Stephen C. Wood*
40. Respiratory Physiology: an Analytical Approach, *edited by H. K. Chang and Manuel Paiva*
41. Lung Cell Biology, *edited by Donald Massaro*
42. Heart--Lung Interactions in Health and Disease, *edited by Steven M. Scharf and Sharon S. Cassidy*
43. Clinical Epidemiology of Chronic Obstructive Pulmonary Disease, *edited by Michael J. Hensley and Nicholas A. Saunders*
44. Surgical Pathology of Lung Neoplasms, *edited by Alberto M. Marchevsky*
45. The Lung in Rheumatic Diseases, *edited by Grant W. Cannon and Guy A. Zimmerman*
46. Diagnostic Imaging of the Lung, *edited by Charles E. Putman*
47. Models of Lung Disease: Microscopy and Structural Methods, *edited by Joan Gil*
48. Electron Microscopy of the Lung, *edited by Dean E. Schraufnagel*
49. Asthma: Its Pathology and Treatment, *edited by Michael A. Kaliner, Peter J. Barnes, and Carl G. A. Persson*
50. Acute Respiratory Failure: Second Edition, *edited by Warren M. Zapol and Francois Lemaire*
51. Lung Disease in the Tropics, *edited by Om P. Sharma*

52. Exercise: Pulmonary Physiology and Pathophysiology, *edited by Brian J. Whipp and Karlman Wasserman*
53. Developmental Neurobiology of Breathing, *edited by Gabriel G. Haddad and Jay P. Farber*
54. Mediators of Pulmonary Inflammation, *edited by Michael A. Bray and Wayne H. Anderson*
55. The Airway Epithelium, *edited by Stephen G. Farmer and Douglas Hay*
56. Physiological Adaptations in Vertebrates: Respiration, Circulation, and Metabolism, *edited by Stephen C. Wood, Roy E. Weber, Alan R. Hargens, and Ronald W. Millard*
57. The Bronchial Circulation, *edited by John Butler*
58. Lung Cancer Differentiation: Implications for Diagnosis and Treatment, *edited by Samuel D. Bernal and Paul J. Hesketh*
59. Pulmonary Complications of Systemic Disease, *edited by John F. Murray*
60. Lung Vascular Injury: Molecular and Cellular Response, *edited by Arnold Johnson and Thomas J. Ferro*
61. Cytokines of the Lung, *edited by Jason Kelley*
62. The Mast Cell in Health and Disease, *edited by Michael A. Kaliner and Dean D. Metcalfe*
63. Pulmonary Disease in the Elderly Patient, *edited by Donald A. Mahler*
64. Cystic Fibrosis, *edited by Pamela B. Davis*
65. Signal Transduction in Lung Cells, *edited by Jerome S. Brody, David M. Center, and Vsevolod A. Tkachuk*
66. Tuberculosis: A Comprehensive International Approach, *edited by Lee B. Reichman and Earl S. Hershfield*
67. Pharmacology of the Respiratory Tract: Experimental and Clinical Research, *edited by K. Fan Chung and Peter J. Barnes*
68. Prevention of Respiratory Diseases, *edited by Albert Hirsch, Marcel Goldberg, Jean-Pierre Martin, and Roland Masse*
69. *Pneumocystis carinii* Pneumonia: Second Edition, Revised and Expanded, *edited by Peter D. Walzer*
70. Fluid and Solute Transport in the Airspaces of the Lungs, *edited by Richard M. Effros and H. K. Chang*
71. Sleep and Breathing: Second Edition, Revised and Expanded, *edited by Nicholas A. Saunders and Colin E. Sullivan*
72. Airway Secretion: Physiological Bases for the Control of Mucous Hypersecretion, *edited by Tamotsu Takishima and Sanae Shimura*
73. Sarcoidosis and Other Granulomatous Disorders, *edited by D. Geraint James*
74. Epidemiology of Lung Cancer, *edited by Jonathan M. Samet*
75. Pulmonary Embolism, *edited by Mario Morpurgo*
76. Sports and Exercise Medicine, *edited by Stephen C. Wood and Robert C. Roach*
77. Endotoxin and the Lungs, *edited by Kenneth L. Brigham*
78. The Mesothelial Cell and Mesothelioma, *edited by Marie-Claude Jaurand and Jean Bignon*
79. Regulation of Breathing: Second Edition, Revised and Expanded, *edited by Jerome A. Dempsey and Allan I. Pack*
80. Pulmonary Fibrosis, *edited by Sem Hin Phan and Roger S. Thrall*

81. Long-Term Oxygen Therapy: Scientific Basis and Clinical Application, *edited by Walter J. O'Donohue, Jr.*
82. Ventral Brainstem Mechanisms and Control of Respiration and Blood Pressure, *edited by C. Ovid Trouth, Richard M. Millis, Heidrun F. Kiwull-Schöne, and Marianne E. Schläfke*
83. A History of Breathing Physiology, *edited by Donald F. Proctor*
84. Surfactant Therapy for Lung Disease, *edited by Bengt Robertson and H. William Taeusch*
85. The Thorax: Second Edition, Revised and Expanded (in three parts), *edited by Charis Roussos*
86. Severe Asthma: Pathogenesis and Clinical Management, *edited by Stanley J. Szefler and Donald Y. M. Leung*
87. *Mycobacterium avium*–Complex Infection: Progress in Research and Treatment, *edited by Joyce A. Korvick and Constance A. Benson*
88. Alpha 1–Antitrypsin Deficiency: Biology • Pathogenesis • Clinical Manifestations • Therapy, *edited by Ronald G. Crystal*
89. Adhesion Molecules and the Lung, *edited by Peter A. Ward and Joseph C. Fantone*
90. Respiratory Sensation, *edited by Lewis Adams and Abraham Guz*
91. Pulmonary Rehabilitation, *edited by Alfred P. Fishman*
92. Acute Respiratory Failure in Chronic Obstructive Pulmonary Disease, *edited by Jean-Philippe Derenne, William A. Whitelaw, and Thomas Similowski*
93. Environmental Impact on the Airways: From Injury to Repair, *edited by Jacques Chrétien and Daniel Dusser*
94. Inhalation Aerosols: Physical and Biological Basis for Therapy, *edited by Anthony J. Hickey*
95. Tissue Oxygen Deprivation: From Molecular to Integrated Function, *edited by Gabriel G. Haddad and George Lister*
96. The Genetics of Asthma, *edited by Stephen B. Liggett and Deborah A. Meyers*
97. Inhaled Glucocorticoids in Asthma: Mechanisms and Clinical Actions, *edited by Robert P. Schleimer, William W. Busse, and Paul M. O'Byrne*
98. Nitric Oxide and the Lung, *edited by Warren M. Zapol and Kenneth D. Bloch*
99. Primary Pulmonary Hypertension, *edited by Lewis J. Rubin and Stuart Rich*
100. Lung Growth and Development, *edited by John A. McDonald*
101. Parasitic Lung Diseases, *edited by Adel A. F. Mahmoud*
102. Lung Macrophages and Dendritic Cells in Health and Disease, *edited by Mary F. Lipscomb and Stephen W. Russell*
103. Pulmonary and Cardiac Imaging, *edited by Caroline Chiles and Charles E. Putman*
104. Gene Therapy for Diseases of the Lung, *edited by Kenneth L. Brigham*
105. Oxygen, Gene Expression, and Cellular Function, *edited by Linda Biadasz Clerch and Donald J. Massaro*
106. $Beta_2$-Agonists in Asthma Treatment, *edited by Romain Pauwels and Paul M. O'Byrne*
107. Inhalation Delivery of Therapeutic Peptides and Proteins, *edited by Akwete Lex Adjei and Pramod K. Gupta*
108. Asthma in the Elderly, *edited by Robert A. Barbee and John W. Bloom*

109. Treatment of the Hospitalized Cystic Fibrosis Patient, *edited by David M. Orenstein and Robert C. Stern*
110. Asthma and Immunological Diseases in Pregnancy and Early Infancy, *edited by Michael Schatz, Robert S. Zeiger, and Henry N. Claman*
111. Dyspnea, *edited by Donald A. Mahler*
112. Proinflammatory and Antiinflammatory Peptides, *edited by Sami I. Said*
113. Self-Management of Asthma, *edited by Harry Kotses and Andrew Harver*
114. Eicosanoids, Aspirin, and Asthma, *edited by Andrew Szczeklik, Ryszard J. Gryglewski, and John R. Vane*
115. Fatal Asthma, *edited by Albert L. Sheffer*
116. Pulmonary Edema, *edited by Michael A. Matthay and David H. Ingbar*
117. Inflammatory Mechanisms in Asthma, *edited by Stephen T. Holgate and William W. Busse*
118. Physiological Basis of Ventilatory Support, *edited by John J. Marini and Arthur S. Slutsky*
119. Human Immunodeficiency Virus and the Lung, *edited by Mark J. Rosen and James M. Beck*
120. Five-Lipoxygenase Products in Asthma, *edited by Jeffrey M. Drazen, Sven-Erik Dahlén, and Tak H. Lee*
121. Complexity in Structure and Function of the Lung, *edited by Michael P. Hlastala and H. Thomas Robertson*
122. Biology of Lung Cancer, *edited by Madeleine A. Kane and Paul A. Bunn, Jr.*
123. Rhinitis: Mechanisms and Management, *edited by Robert M. Naclerio, Stephen R. Durham, and Niels Mygind*
124. Lung Tumors: Fundamental Biology and Clinical Management, *edited by Christian Brambilla and Elisabeth Brambilla*
125. Interleukin-5: From Molecule to Drug Target for Asthma, *edited by Colin J. Sanderson*
126. Pediatric Asthma, *edited by Shirley Murphy and H. William Kelly*
127. Viral Infections of the Respiratory Tract, *edited by Raphael Dolin and Peter F. Wright*
128. Air Pollutants and the Respiratory Tract, *edited by David L. Swift and W. Michael Foster*
129. Gastroesophageal Reflux Disease and Airway Disease, *edited by Mark R. Stein*
130. Exercise-Induced Asthma, *edited by E. R. McFadden, Jr.*
131. LAM and Other Diseases Characterized by Smooth Muscle Proliferation, *edited by Joel Moss*

ADDITIONAL VOLUMES IN PREPARATION

The Lung at Depth, *edited by Claes Lundgren and John N. Miller*

Diagnostic Pulmonary Pathology, *edited by Philip T. Cagle*

Immunotherapy in Asthma, *edited by Jean Bousquet and Hans Yssel*

Regulation of Sleep and Circadian Rhythms, *edited by Fred W. Turek and Phyllis C. Zee*

Multimodality Treatment of Lung Cancer, *edited by Arthur T. Skarin*

Cytokines in Pulmonary Infectious Disease, *edited by Steven Nelson and Thomas Martin*

Asthma's Impact on Society: the Social and Economic Burden, *edited by Kevin B. Weiss, A. Sonia Buist, and Sean D. Sullivan*

Anticholinergic Agents in the Upper and Lower Airways, *edited by Sheldon L. Spector*

Asthma and Respiratory Infections, *edited by David P. Skoner*

New and Exploratory Therapeutic Agents for Asthma, *edited by Michael Yeadon and Zuzana Diamant*

Control of Breathing in Health and Disease, *edited by Murray D. Altose and Yoshikazu Kawakami*

Chronic Lung Disease of Early Infancy, *edited by Richard D. Bland and Jacqueline J. Coalson*

LAM AND OTHER DISEASES CHARACTERIZED BY SMOOTH MUSCLE PROLIFERATION

Edited by

Joel Moss

National Heart, Lung and Blood Institute
National Institutes of Health
Bethesda, Maryland

MARCEL DEKKER

MARCEL DEKKER, INC. NEW YORK • BASEL

ISBN: 0-8247-0214-X

This book is printed on acid-free paper.

Headquarters
Marcel Dekker, Inc.
270 Madison Avenue, New York, NY 10016
tel: 212-696-9000; fax: 212-685-4540

Eastern Hemisphere Distribution
Marcel Dekker AG
Hutgasse 4, Postfach 812, CH-4001 Basel, Switzerland
tel: 41-61-261-8482; fax: 41-61-261-8896

World Wide Web
http://www.dekker.com

The publisher offers discounts on this book when ordered in bulk quantities. For more information, write to Special Sales/Professional Marketing at the headquarters address above.

Current printing (last digit):
10 9 8 7 6 5 4 3 2 1

PRINTED IN THE UNITED STATES OF AMERICA

INTRODUCTION

Let's face it, lymphangioleiomyomatosis—or LAM for short—is a foreign word to many, even to pulmonary physicians. Why? Because it is a relatively rare condition.

Although the Japanese researchers Yamanaka and Saiki were the first to have reported a few cases in the contemporary literature in 1970 (1), in 1937 there were publications from Germany and England that described cellular differentiation in LAM patients. The authors of these articles wrote of leiomyosarcoma and muscular cirrhosis of the lung.

Subsequently, various observations were reported under different names, but it became apparent that all had a relatively common feature, namely, myomatosis of the lung, and that, in most instances, the patients were women. Today we know that lower airway smooth muscle proliferation is the cardinal anatomical feature of LAM, but otherwise little was learned about this disease until the last few years.

Proliferation of smooth muscle cells is not a rare occurrence: it appears in many pulmonary conditions and also in the vascular system, especially the coronary vessels. For obvious reasons, this process—including that which apparently occurs in LAM—is receiving much attention from the scientific community.

LAM, however, remains a condition on which very few investigators are working.

This volume, edited by Dr. Joel Moss, is about LAM and smooth muscle proliferation in the lower airways and elsewhere. As one looks at the list of contributors, it is easy to recognize the names of the leaders in these areas of research. To my knowledge, this volume is the very first published about LAM and the fundamental biological processes and changes that cause this disease.

The series of monographs, Lung Biology in Health and Disease, has introduced many firsts but this one is of special importance because it addresses a health problem with very grave consequences. I am grateful to Dr. Moss and to the authors for this pioneering contribution.

Claude Lenfant, M.D.
Bethesda, Maryland

Reference

1. Yamanaka A, Saiki A. Hamartoangiomyomatosis—for the differential diagnosis of chronic obstructive lung disease. Hai-to-Shin 1970; 17:171–181 (in Japanese).

PREFACE

Lymphangiomyomatosis (LAM) is a rare disease found exclusively in women of childbearing age. The rarity of LAM and the fact that the pathology is seemingly unique has made investigation into pathogenesis and therapy difficult. For these reasons, in the preparation of this volume, an attempt has been made to broaden the knowledge base; expert opinions were solicited from clinician-investigators and basic scientists worldwide. In the case of the clinician-investigators, we have tried to determine and compare the presentation of this disease and its treatment in Europe, North America, and the Far East. Similarly, diverse opinions were elicited when lung transplantation and LAM pathology were considered.

Only a few laboratories are focusing on understanding this perplexing disease. Research on LAM has been hampered by lack of appropriate in vitro cultured cell and animal models; investigation has, however, led to some intriguing findings. First, LAM is characterized by the proliferation of smooth muscle cells. LAM smooth muscle cells share characteristics with both primary and cultured melanoma cells, including the expression of melanoma proteins, yet they contain the expected smooth muscle cell antigens. Second, LAM is found disproportionately in some patients with a disease of known genetic etiology, tuberous sclerosis complex (TSC). At least in some cases, TSC results from defective signaling pathways involving guanine nucleotide-binding proteins. Third, high-resolution CT scan of the lung in LAM yields an almost pathognomonic picture of uniformly distributed cysts. Pathologically, it appears that the LAM cells may form the walls of some of the cysts and, hence, participate in lung destruction and cyst formation.

Each of these findings is dealt with in the text, with sections devoted to smooth muscle cells in disease, characterization of melanoma cells, tuberous sclerosis, guanine nucleotide-dependent signaling pathways, and mechanisms of lung destruction. In view of the apparent importance of smooth muscle cells to the pathogenesis of LAM and the obvious fact that smooth muscle abnormalities are found in a number of other, more common, and perhaps better understood diseases, the question was raised whether information from years of study of other conditions includes findings that might be applicable to LAM. Similarly, reports of studies in other areas (e.g., melanoma antigens, guanine nucleotide-dependent signaling, protease imbalance, lung destruction) have broadened the scope of the text to encompass these potential topics of future investigation.

I hope that this volume will serve as a reference for clinicians who might extract a clue to novel therapies and for investigators, who might find a key to pathogenesis. A fresh perspective might reveal what has been in the past obscured by dogma as well as insufficient knowledge.

My gratitude goes to the contributors, for their time and especially the extra effort needed to make their chapters relevant to this text, and to Dr. Claude Lenfant, Executive Editor of the Lung Biology in Health and Disease series, for his encouragement during the preparation of this volume and for his continued support of research on LAM.

Joel Moss

CONTRIBUTORS

Gosse J. Adema, Ph.D. Department of Tumor Immunology, University Hospital Nijmegen, Nijmegen, The Netherlands

Nilo A. Avila, M.D. Chief, Computed Tomography, Diagnostic Radiology Department, Clinical Center, National Institutes of Health, Bethesda, Maryland

Pauline Barnes, R.N. Clinical Center Nursing Department, Pulmonary-Critical Care Medicine Branch, National Heart, Lung and Blood Institute, National Institutes of Health, Bethesda, Maryland

Gerald J. Beck, Ph.D. Department of Biostatistics and Epidemiology, The Cleveland Clinic Foundation, Cleveland, Ohio

Gerald J. Berry, M.D. Assistant Professor of Pathology, Stanford University Medical Center, Stanford, California

David A. Bobak, M.D. Associate Professor, Departments of Medicine and Microbiology, University of Virginia School of Medicine, Charlottesville, Virginia

Annette Boehler, M.D. Assistant Professor, Respiratory Division, University Hospital Zurich, Zurich, Switzerland

Manfred Böhm University of Michigan Medical Center, Ann Arbor, Michigan

Mitchell D. Botney, M.D. Assistant Professor, Medicine, Respiratory and Critical Care Division, Washington University School of Medicine, St. Louis, Missouri

Richard O. Cannon, III, M.D. Acting Chief, Cardiology Branch, National Heart, Lung and Blood Institute, National Institutes of Health, Bethesda, Maryland

André M. Cantin, M.D., F.R.C.P.(C) Professor, Department of Medicine, Respiratory Division, University of Sherbrooke, Sherbrooke, Quebec, Canada

Clara C. Chen, M.D. Department of Nuclear Medicine, Clinical Center, National Institutes of Health, Bethesda, Maryland

Shan C. Chu, M.D. Pulmonary-Critical Care Medicine Branch, National Heart, Lung and Blood Institute, National Institutes of Health, Bethesda, Maryland

Ray Coakley, M.D. Division of Respiratory Medicine, Royal College of Surgeons in Ireland/Beaumont Hospital, Dublin, Ireland

Jean-François Cordier, M.D. Professor and Head, Department of Pulmonary Medicine–Hôpital Louis Pradel–Université Claude Bernard, Lyon, France

Robert S. Crausman, M.D., M.M.S. Director, Internal Medicine Residency Program, Memorial Hospital of Rhode Island, and Assistant Professor, Department of Medicine, Brown University School of Medicine, Providence, Rhode Island

Jeffrey E. DeClue, Ph.D. Investigator, Laboratory of Cellular Oncology, National Cancer Institute, National Institutes of Health, Bethesda, Maryland

Roland M. duBois, M.D., F.R.C.P. Department of Occupational and Environmental Medicine, Royal Brompton Hospital, London, England

Henricus J. Duckers University of Michigan Medical Center, Ann Arbor, Michigan

Raed A. Dweik, M.D. Department of Pulmonary and Critical Care Medicine, The Cleveland Clinic Foundation, Cleveland, Ohio

Mary Ehrmantraut, CRNP, M.S. Clinical Center Nursing Department, Pulmonary-Critical Care Medicine Branch, National Heart, Lung and Blood Institute, National Institutes of Health, Bethesda, Maryland

Serpil C. Erzurum, M.D. Division of Pulmonary and Critical Care Medicine, The Cleveland Clinic Foundation, Cleveland, Ohio

Victor J. Ferrans, M.D., Ph.D. Chief, Pathology Section, National Heart, Lung and Blood Institute, National Institutes of Health, Bethesda, Maryland

Carl G. Figdor, Ph.D. Professor, Department of Tumor Immunology, University Hospital Nijmegen, Nijmegen, The Netherlands

Yuh Fukuda, M.D., Ph.D. Associate Professor, Department of Pathology, Nippon Medical School, Tokyo, Japan

Kateri Gabriele, R.N. Clinical Center Nursing Department, Pulmonary-Critical Care Medicine Branch, National Heart, Lung and Blood Institute, National Institutes of Health, Bethesda, Maryland

Patricia Glynn, M.D. Division of Respiratory Medicine, Royal College of Surgeons in Ireland/Beaumont Hospital, Dublin, Ireland

Susan E. Hoegy National Cancer Institute, National Institutes of Health, Bethesda, Maryland

Koji Horiba, M.D., Ph.D. Pathology Section, National Heart, Lung and Blood Institute, National Institutes of Health, Bethesda, Maryland

Takateru Izumi, M.D., Ph.D. Professor, Department of Respiratory Medicine, Graduate School of Medicine, Kyoto University, Kyoto, Japan

Kenneth G. Kalassian, M.D. Division of Pulmonary and Critical Care Medicine, Stanford University Medical Center, Stanford, California

John A. Kelly, M.B. Pulmonary-Critical Care Medicine Branch, National Heart, Lung and Blood Institute, National Institutes of Health, Bethesda, Maryland

Talmadge E. King, Jr., M.D.* National Jewish Medical and Research Center and University of Colorado Health Sciences Center, Denver, Colorado

Masanori Kitaichi, M.D. Associate Professor, Laboratory of Anatomic Pathology, Kyoto University, Kyoto, Japan

David J. Kwiatkowski, M.D., Ph.D. Genetics Laboratory, Hematology Division, Brigham and Women's Hospital, Boston, Massachusetts

Romain Lazor, M.D. Fellow, Centre D'Etudes et de Recherche sur les Maladies "Orphelines" Pulmonaires, Hôpital Louis Pradel–Université Claude Bernard, Lyon, France

Stewart J. Levine, M.D. Pulmonary–Critical Care Medicine Branch, National Heart, Lung and Blood Institute, National Institutes of Health, Bethesda, Maryland

Marc C. I. Lipman, M.D., F.R.C.P. Royal Free Hospital School of Medicine, London, England

Francis X. McCormack, M.D. Assistant Professor, Department of Pulmonary and Critical Care Medicine, University of Cincinnati Medical Center, Cincinnati, Ohio

Noel G. McElvaney, M.D., F.R.C.P.I., F.R.C.P.C. Professor, Division of Respiratory Medicine, Department of Medicine, Royal College of Surgeons in Ireland/Beaumont Hospital, Dublin, Ireland

Anil G. Menon, Ph.D. Associate Professor, Department of Molecular Genetics, University of Cincinnati Medical Center, Cincinnati, Ohio

Jonathan Moorman, M.D. Assistant Professor, Department of Internal Medicine, University of Virginia School of Medicine, Charlottesville, Virginia

---

*Current affiliation: Chief, Medical Services, San Francisco General Hospital, and Professor and Vice-Chair, Department of Medicine, University of California School of Medicine, San Francisco, California.

Joel Moss, M.D., Ph.D. Chief, Pulmonary-Critical Care Medicine Branch, National Heart, Lung and Blood Institute, National Institutes of Health, Bethesda, Maryland

Elizabeth G. Nabel, M.D. Professor, Department of Internal Medicine, and Chief, Division of Cardiology, University of Michigan Medical Center, Ann Arbor, Michigan

Somoko Nagai, M.D. Associate Professor, Department of Respiratory Medicine, Kyoto University, Kyoto, Japan

Shane O'Neill Department of Respiratory Research, Royal College of Surgeons in Ireland/Beaumont Hospital, Dublin, Ireland

Benoit Paquette, Ph.D. Assistant Professor, Department of Nuclear Medicine and Radiobiology, University of Sherbrooke, Sherbrooke, Quebec, Canada

Walter A. Patton, Ph.D. Pulmonary-Critical Care Medicine Branch, National Heart, Lung and Blood Institute, National Institutes of Health, Bethesda, Maryland

Thomas A. Raffin, M.D. Professor and Chief, Division of Pulmonary and Critical Care Medicine, Stanford University Medical Center, Stanford, California

Stephen I. Rennard, M.D. Professor, Department of Internal Medicine, University of Nebraska Medical Center, Omaha, Nebraska

Erich W. Russi, M.D. Professor and Head, Respiratory Division, University Hospital Zurich, Zurich, Switzerland

Jay H. Ryu, M.D. Department of Pulmonary and Critical Care Medicine, Mayo Clinic, and Associate Professor, Mayo Medical School, Rochester, Minnesota

Marco W. J. Schreurs, M.Sc. Medical Biologist, Department of Tumor Immunology, University Hospital Nijmegen, Nijmegen, The Netherlands

James H. Shelhamer, M.D. Deputy Chief, Critical Care Medicine Department, Clinical Center, National Institutes of Health, Bethesda, Maryland

M. Priscilla Short, M.D. Assistant Professor, University of Chicago, Chicago, Illinois

Teresa A. Smolarek, Ph.D. Department of Molecular Genetics, University of Cincinnati Medical Center, Cincinnati, Ohio

George Sopko, M.D., M.P.H. Division of Heart and Vascular Diseases, National Heart, Lung and Blood Institute, National Institutes of Health, Bethesda, Maryland

Rudolf Speich, M.D. Associate Professor, Medicine, University Hospital Zurich, Zurich, Switzerland

Edith H. Speir Cardiology Branch, National Heart, Lung and Blood Institute, National Institutes of Health, Bethesda, Maryland

John R. Spurzem, M.D., M.S.P.H. Associate Professor, Department of Internal Medicine, University of Nebraska Medical Center, Omaha, Nebraska

William G. Stetler-Stevenson Extracellular Matrix Pathology Section, National Cancer Institute, National Institutes of Health, Bethesda, Maryland

James K. Stoller, M.D. Vice Chairman, Division of Medicine, and Head, Section of Respiratory Therapy, Department of Pulmonary and Critical Care, The Cleveland Clinic Foundation, Cleveland, Ohio

Eugene J. Sullivan, M.D., F.C.C.P. Department of Pulmonary and Critical Care Medicine, The Cleveland Clinic Foundation, Cleveland, Ohio

Clifford Taggart, Ph.D. Division of Respiratory Medicine, Royal College of Surgeons in Ireland/Beaumont Hospital, Dublin, Ireland

William D. Travis, M.D. Chief, Department of Pulmonary and Mediastinal Pathology, Armed Forces Institute of Pathology, Washington, D.C.

Elbert P. Trulock, M.D. Professor, Division of Pulmonary and Critical Care Medicine, Washington University School of Medicine, St. Louis, Missouri

Jiro Usuki, M.D., Ph.D. Pathology Section, National Heart, Lung and Blood Institute, National Institutes of Health, Bethesda, Maryland

Walter Weder, M.D. Head, Thoracic Unit, Department of Surgery, University Hospital Zurich, Zurich, Switzerland

Zhi Yong Yang University of Michigan Medical Center, Ann Arbor, Michigan

CONTENTS

LAM AND OTHER DISEASES CHARACTERIZED BY SMOOTH MUSCLE PROLIFERATION

1

Perspectives on Lymphangioleiomyomatosis in Japan

TAKATERU IZUMI, MASANORI KITAICHI, and SOMOKO NAGAI

Kyoto University
Kyoto, Japan

I. Introduction

Pulmonary lymphangioleiomyomatosis (LAM) is an uncommon chronic debilitating disorder of unknown etiology afflicting women of childbearing age, characterized histologically by proliferation of atypical smooth muscle cells in the lungs (1–5). The pulmonary lesions in tuberous sclerosis are considered to be similar as those of LAM (6–9). Patients with LAM have been reported in Japan since the 1970s. As almost 100% of Japanese citizens are covered by public health insurance and the country's abundant medical facilities tend to be better equipped with computed tomographic and other diagnostic equipment than those in other countries, more patients with LAM, as well as those with other diseases, are discovered at an early stage.

This chapter describes the status and clinical features of LAM in Japan in comparison with Europe and America. The discussion also extends to problems concerning the management and treatment of LAM.

II. Study of LAM in Japan

Yamanaka and Saiki were the first to report LAM in Japan when they published an account of three cases in 1970 (10). The first two cases, both 40-year-old females, were diagnosed at autopsy, and the third, a 28-year-old female, was diagnosed by open lung biopsy. All three cases showed findings of spontaneous pneumothorax. In their report, the disease was called hamartoangiomyomatosis (HAM), and the distinction from chronic obstructive lung disease was stressed. The term HAM was used to refer to the hematoma-like hypertrophy of smooth muscle tissue growing in areas where it is not normally found, distinguishing it from muscular hyperplasia with simple proliferation of collagen fibers.

Since this initial report, many cases of LAM have been reported in Japan. In 1986, Onodera et al. reviewed 36 cases, including their own, that had been reported in Japan, and summarized the clinicopathological findings (11). All 36 cases were encountered in females between 16 and 53 years of age (mean 33 years), most of whom were still in their reproductive years (11 in their twenties and 13 in their thirties). The most frequent initial symptoms were chest pain accompanied by dyspnea and pneumothorax (29 patients), and there were a few patients with bloody sputum (2 patients) and chylous effusion and ascites (4 patients). The chest radiograph findings were reticulonodular shadow in 19 patients, pulmonary emphysema in 6 patients, and other manifestations in 11 patients. Reticulonodular shadow, the initial finding in most of the cases, finally showed a honeycomb lung appearance. Onodera et al. (11) reported that, compared to the cases described in Corrin's report (2), more Japanese cases were accompanied by pneumothorax, and fewer Japanese cases were accompanied by chylous effusion, ascites, bloody sputum, and hemoptysis. In this review, eight LAM cases exhibited accompanying tuberous sclerosis.

Saiki and Ibata also published a review of Japanese LAM cases in 1991 (12). Their review covered 65 cases of LAM not accompanied by tuberous sclerosis and 21 cases with tuberous sclerosis. All of the former cases were encountered in females. Clinically, the most frequent initial symptom, spontaneous pneumothorax, which was sometimes simultaneously bilateral, was shown in 42 out of 65 cases (64.5%). Thirteen cases had chylous effusion, 32 cases did not, and no description was provided in 34 cases. The respiratory function tests showed obstructive dysfunction in 16 patients, restrictive dysfunction in 11 patients, combined restrictive and obstructive dysfunction in 2 patients, and normal findings in 6 patients, with no description in 30 patients. The chest radiograph revealed hyperinflation in 9 patients, reticulonodular shadows in 29 patients, lung cysts in 6 patients, pulmonary emphysema in 5 patients, and normal findings in 3 patients, with no description in 13 patients. The diagnostic procedure was autopsy in 9 cases, open lung biopsy in 19 patients, transbronchial lung biopsy in 14 patients, and biopsy during surgical procedure for pneumothorax or other procedure in 12 cases. The 21 LAM patients with accompanying tuberous sclerosis included two male patients 61 and 38 years of age. Ten of 17 patients (59%) in this group had pneumothorax findings.

On February 26, 1993, the clinical records, chest radiographs, CT films of the chest, and histopathological specimens obtained in 54 cases suspected as having lung lesions of LAM not accompanying tuberous sclerosis from 34 facilities in Japan, 5 facilities in Korea, and 1 facility in Taiwan were collected and reviewed at an international meeting on LAM in Kyoto. The following findings were summarized (5).

A. Pathologic Diagnosis

Histologically, 46 patients were diagnosed with LAM. Eight patients were excluded from the study because those patients were diagnosed pathologically as having pulmonary diseases other than LAM such as chronic interstitial pneumonia with honeycoming, bulla and benign metastasizing leiomyoma. The confirmative material for the diagnosis was from open lung biopsy (n = 37), transbronchial lung biopsy (n = 6), lymph node biopsy (n = 2), autopsy (n = 3), and/or postmortem needle necropsy of the lungs (n = 1).

B. Clinical Features

The 46 LAM patients were all females. Thirty-nine patients were Japanese, five were Korean, and two were Taiwanese. The mean age at onset was 32.0 ± 8.9 years (range, 20–63 years). The major symptoms at the time of onset were dyspnea (57%) and cough (33%), and pneumothorax was noted in 52% of the patients.

Examination of chest radiographs showed the presence of pneumothorax in 39% of the patients. Bilateral reticulonodular infiltrates (85%), cysts or bullae (56%), and hyperinflation (48%) were also noted (Table 1).

A review of the computed tomograms of the chest from 38 LAM patients showed diffuse small lung cysts in all patients, and ground glass opacities were noted in 22 (59%) of 37 patients (Table 2).

Twelve (29%) of 42 patients who underwent pulmonary function tests showed air flow limitation (VC > 80% of the predicted value and FEV_1/FVC < 70%), 11 (26%) showed a restrictive dysfunction (VC < 80% of the predicted value and FEV_1/FVC > 70%), and 15 (36%) showed a combined restrictive and obstructive dysfunction (VC < 80% of the predicted value and FEV_1/FVC < 70%) (Table 2).

Table 1 Summary of Clinical and Radiographic Findings from the Kyoto Congress on Lymphangioleiomyomatosis

Age					34.8 ± 9.1 yr (range, 21–65 yr)
Smoking history:	Nonsmokers	36	Smokers	3	
	Ex-smokers	5	Unknown	2	
Symptoms					
Dyspnea					
Resting					13/43 (30%)
Exertional					38/43 (88%)
Cough					25/41 (61%)
Chest pain					14/42 (33%)
Chyloptysis					0/40 (0%)
Hemoptysis					11/39 (28%)
Physical findings					
Clubbing					2/42 (5%)
Crackles					10/45 (22%)
Rhonchi					6/42 (14%)
Chylothorax					3/41 (7%)
Chylous ascites					2/41 (5%)
Chest radiography					
Normal					1/46 (2%)
Bilateral infiltrates					45/46 (98%)
Reticulonodular shadows					39/46 (85%)
Cysts or bullae					25/45 (56%)
Effusion					5/45 (11%)
Pneumothorax					18/46 (39%)
Hyperinflation					22/46 (48%)
Physiologic findings					
Normal range					4/42 (10%)
Obstructive (%VC ≥ 80% and FEV_1/FVC < 70%)					12/42 (29%)
Restrictive (%VC < 80% and FEV_1/FVC ≥ 70%)					11/42 (26%)
Combined restrictive and obstructive					15/42 (36%)
Increased %TLC (%TLC > 120% predicted)					7/23 (30%)
Decreased %TLC (%TLC < 80% predicted)					3/23 (13%)
Increased RV/TLC (RV/TLC > 45%)					19/35 (54%)
Decreased diffusing capacity					
(< 80% predicted)					30/31 (97%)
(< 45% predicted)					22/31 (71%)
Hypoxemia (Pa_{O_2}) < 80 mmHg)					35/43 (81%)

Source: Ref. 5.

Table 2 Findings of CT of the Chest in 36 Women with Lymphangioleiomyomatosis

Finding	No. of Women (%)
Bilateral lung cysts	38/38 (100)
Ground glass opacities	22/37 (59)
Linear densities	0/37 (0)
Nodular densities	2/37 (5)
Pneumothorax	6/38 (16)
Pleural effusion	5/38 (13)
Hilar or mediastinal lymphadenopathy	0/38 (0)

Source: Ref. 5.

C. Treatment and Prognosis

In addition to management for pneumothoraces and hypoxemia, several modalities of hormone therapy were conducted, including oophorectomy (n = 22) and/or administration of tamoxifen (n = 18), and progestogen (n = 34) and/or gonadotrophin-releasing hormone agonist (n = 9). Each treatment was evaluated by comparing the general conditions and the pulmonary function data, particularly FVC, FEV_1, and Pa_{O_2}, before and after the treatment. Improvements were observed only in one patient; the initial therapy of approximately 4 months of tamoxifen and cyclophosphamide (50 mg/day) did not show any improvement. When progesterone administration (medroxyprogesterone 400 mg/day) was added, the physiologic condition improved. After stopping cyclophosphamide, which did not seem to have beneficial effects for LAM, oophorectomy and progesterone administration resulted in additional improvements. Thirty-eight other treatments were assessed as showing either no change (n = 9) or a deterioration (n = 29).

The Kaplan-Meier plot of actuarial survival of patients with LAM from the onset of symptoms is shown in Figure 1 together with similar plots of the patients reported by Silverstein et al. (1) and Corrin et al. (2). Kaplan-Meier plots of patients reported in this study and those reported by Silverstein et al. were significantly different ($p < 0.01$). The Kaplan-Meier plot of patients reported by Corrin et al. was not significantly different from the plot of the patients reported by Silverstein et al. or the spots in this study.

D. Clinical Analysis of Prognostic Factors

Pulmonary function data at the first examination were tested in relation to survival. A reduction of the FEV_1/FVC ratio and an increase in percent predicted total lung capacity (%TLC) were associated with a tendency toward a poor prognosis from 2 to 5 years after the first examination. FEV_1/FVC correlated with

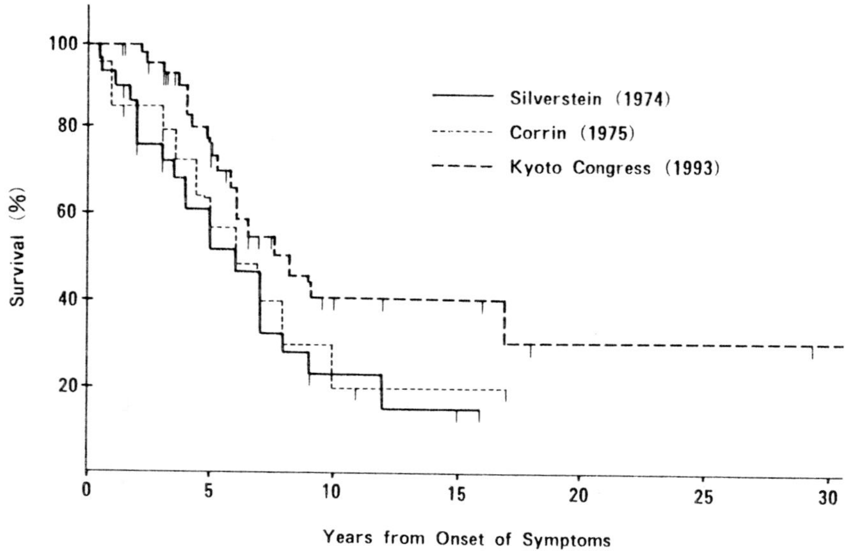

Figure 1 Kaplan-Meier plots of actual survival of patients with LAM from the onset of symptoms, including 46 patients reported in a study from the Kyoto Congress (1993), 31 patients summarized by Silverstein and coworkers in 1974, and 23 patients studied by Corrin and coworkers in 1975. (From Ref. 5.)

survival at 2 years after the first examination with a statistically significant difference ($p < 0.05$). An increase in the %TLC was inversely corrected with the survival at 2, 3, and 5 years after the first examination with statistically significant differences ($p < 0.05$).

E. Prognostic Factors of Open Lung Biopsy Findings

Histologically, two types of pulmonary lesions were observed among LAM patients who underwent open lung biopsy: a predominantly cystic type (11 patients) showing cystic lesions as the major pulmonary lesion, and a predominantly muscular type (21 patients) showing a marked proliferation of immature smooth muscle cells, some of which were surrounded the cystic lesions. Patients with predominantly cystic LAM lesions showed a tendency toward poor prognosis after the lung biopsy.

III. Summary and Future Problems of LAM

We reviewed the three major reports on LAM patients encountered in Japan, although some patients were summarized commonly in each report, and 7 of the

46 LAM patients in the 1993 Kyoto meeting were non-Japanese. In comparison with European and American LAM patients, clinical features appear less pronounced and the rate of survival appears higher in Japanese patients. These differences might be due to the earlier detection described above. Furthermore, since Japanese consider early discovery and early treatment important and CT is starting to be popularly employed as a tool for health examinations, there is a possibility that some symptomatic patients are being discovered.

However, the management and treatment of the LAM patients after diagnosis still poses significant problems. Since the patients were females of reproductive age, several modalities of hormone therapy were conducted, including oophorectomy and/or administration tamoxifen, and progestogen and/or gonadotrophin-releasing hormone agonist. However, reports from Europe, America, and Japan all clearly show that no effective method of treatment has been found for the prevention of the progression of lung lesions. At present, the therapy is centered on symptomatic treatment including treatment of pneumothorax and oxygen therapy. In progressive patients, lung transplantation is indicated in Europe and America, but this remains difficult in Japan. The main obstacle to lung transplantation in Japan, a lack of donors, can be attributed to three factors: (1) brain death is not accepted by the Japanese, (2) most Japanese prefer not to damage the corpses of their kin, and (3) in Japan there are few deaths from traffic accidents and, due to strict gun control, almost none from guns. Therefore, the patients diagnosed with LAM should be informed of the current state of management and therapeutic outcome, instructed not to smoke and to avoid catching colds and other stresses that might promote the progression of LAM, and then given symptomatic therapy.

References

1. Silverstein EF, Eilis K, Wolff M, Jaretzki A III. Pulmonary lymphangioleiomyomatosis. Am J Roentgenol 1974; 120:832–850.
2. Corrin B, Liebow AA, Friedman PJ. Pulmonary lymphangioleiomyomatosis: a review. Am J Pathol 1975; 79:347–382.
3. Taylor JR, Ryu J, Colby TV, Raffin TA. Lymphangioleiomyomatosis: clinical course in 32 patients. N Engl J Med 1990; 323:1254–1260.
4. Wahedha I, Cooper S, Williams J, Paterson IC, Britton IC, Tattersfield AE. Relation of pulmonary lymphangioleiomyomatosis to use of the oral contraceptive pill and fertility in the UK: a national case control study. Thorax 1994; 49:910–914.
5. Kitaichi M, Nishimura K, Itoh H, Izumi T. Pulmonary lymphangioleiomyomatosis: a report of 46 patients including a clinicopathologic study of prognostic factors. Am J Respir Crit Care Med 1995; 151:527–533.
6. Viskum K. Pulmonary lymphangioleiomyomatosis. Monaldi Arch Chest Dis 1993; 48:233–236.
7. Uzzo RG, Libby DM, Darracott LE, Vahghman ED, Levey SH.

Lymphangioleiomyomatosis and bilateral angiomyolipomas in a patient with tuberous sclerosis. J. Urol 1994; 151:1612–1615.
8. Scully RE, Mark EJ, McNeely WF, McNeely BU. Case records of the Massachusetts General Hospital. N Engl J Med 1994; 330:1300–1306.
9. Castro M, Shepherd CW, Gomez MR, Lie JT, Ryu JH. Pulmonary tuberous sclerosis. Chest 1995; 107:189–195.
10. Yamanaka A, Saiki A. Hamartoangiomyomatosis—for the differential diagnosis of chronic obstructive lung disease. Hai-to-Shin 1970; 17:171–181 (in Japanese).
11. Onodera H, Kobayashi Y, Akahagi T, Sako M, Hayashi H, Ozeki T, Taniike K, Takenaka A, Tokuda H, Kitaichi M, Izumi T. A case of diffuse pulmonary hamartoangiomyomatosis (HAM). Nippon-Kyobu-Rinsyo 1986; 45:243–248 (in Japanese).
12. Saiki A, Ibata H. Hamartoangiomyomatosis. Igaku-no-Ayumi 1991; (suppl):478–483 (in Japanese).

2

Perspectives on Lymphangioleiomyomatosis in France

JEAN-FRANÇOIS CORDIER and ROMAIN LAZOR,
and the Groupe d'Etudes et de Recherche sur les Maladies "Orphelines" Pulmonaires

Hôpital Louis Pradel-Université Claude Bernard
Lyon, France

I. Introduction

Lymphangioleiomyomatosis (LAM) is a rare disorder affecting exclusively women and characterized by a nonmalignant proliferation of smooth muscle cells throughout the interstitial lung structures and the lymphatic network, including that of the abdomen and thorax. It is often associated with angiomyolipoma of the kidney. The disease may manifest at different sites, but the most frequently (and often the only) involved organ is the lung. Pulmonary LAM has been individualized and characterized progressively in the last 50 years. It is now diagnosed with increasing frequency in France, although it is not clear whether the incidence of the disorder is really increasing or if it is more easily recognized by physicians.

II. Early Cases of Lymphangioleiomyomatosis in France

The first case of LAM was reported by von Stössel in Berlin, Germany, in 1937; he referred to it as "muscular cirrhosis of the lung" (1). The second case was described in 1937 as "chylous effusion due to leiomyosarcoma" by Burrell and

Ross in London (2). The third case was published by Rosendal in 1942 in Copenhagen and described as "diffuse myomatosis and cyst formation in the lung" (3). All three case reports clearly emphasized the muscular interstitial lung disease.

The next and first French case was reported in 1950 by Roujeau et al. (4), who described it as "diffuse pulmonary lymphangiectasis, chylous pneumonia and chylothorax, after puerperal thrombosis of the left subclavian vein." A 40-year-old woman experienced a phlebitis of the left arm shortly after delivery. A few months later, she developed a progressively increasing dyspnea. A left chylothorax was diagnosed, together with reticulonodular opacities on chest x-ray. The patient reported an expectoration like "white cheese." A chylous ascitis subsequently developed. The patient underwent a thoracoscopy, which disclosed multiple cysts on the surface of the lung. She died a few months later from respiratory failure. At autopsy, diffuse pulmonary lymphangiectasis was found together with multiple bullae; however, the most striking abnormality at histological examination of the lungs was the presence of abundant smooth muscle fibers in association with the lymphatic cysts; muscular proliferation was also present in the mediastinal lymph nodes, "transforming them into leiomyomas." The authors interpreted the pleuropulmonary disease of their patient as a result of the thrombosis of the subclavian vein, and while they discussed at large the causes of chylothorax and lymphangiectasis, they did not comment on muscular interstitial hyperplasia.

The second French case was reported by Justin-Besançon et al. (5) in 1963 as a case of "acquired diffuse pulmonary lymphangiectasis with respiratory insufficiency and chylothorax." A 41-year-old woman presented with dyspnea and hemoptysis. She had reticular opacities on chest x-ray. Thereafter, a left chylothorax developed. Lymphangiography found distended lymphatics in the abdomen with large cystic ectasias; furthermore, a fistula was present between a lymphatic vessel and a renal calix. The lung function tests found reduced vital capacity and FEV_1/FVC ratio. Because of the recurrence of chylothorax after thoracentesis, the patient underwent a pleurectomy with concomitant pulmonary biopsy. The lung looked emphysematous, but a closer analysis found that the bullae differed from the usual emphysematous pattern. The overall architecture of the lung was roughly preserved, but the cavities were associated with lymphangiectasis. Smooth muscle cell proliferation was present in the wall of the cavities and lymphatics. The authors commented on the pathophysiology of chylothorax and lymphangiectasis and briefly on the presence of smooth muscle cells, suggesting analogies with "muscular sclerosis of the lung or diffuse pulmonary leiomyomatosis."

The next French reports on lymphangiomyomatosis were those by Françoise Basset and Jean Marsac (6–9). These reports emphasized the smooth muscle cell proliferation, the destruction process with cyst formation, the presence of hemosiderosis, and the vascular abnormalities. They also mentioned muscular proliferation within the mediastinal lymph nodes and the presence of renal and uterine leiomyomas. A detailed ultrastructural description confirmed the smooth muscle cell nature of the pulmonary infiltrate and further showed the presence of cells with morphological features intermediate between smooth muscle cells and fibroblasts (myofibroblasts) (7). Basset et al. (7) proposed that the condition would be more fully termed pulmonary lymphangio*leio*myomatosis (LAM). In addition to reviewing the lymphatic consequences of the disease, these studies stressed the fact that, although it could be considered an interstitial lung process, LAM was often associated with an obstructive ventilatory defect at lung function tests. A distinction was also made between the pulmonary and extrapulmonary forms of the disease.

Subsequent reports of French cases focused on specific aspects of the disease: the characteristic abnormalities of the lymphatic network observed at lymphangiography (10), the relationship of LAM to Bourneville's tuberous sclerosis (11), extrapulmonary disease without pulmonary involvement (12), pulmonary imaging (13), pathologic characterization of the smooth muscle cells and associated connective matrix (14), and treatment (15).

III. The French Registry of "Orphan" Pulmonary Diseases

The Groupe d'Etudes et de Recherche sur les Maladies "Orphelines" Pulmonaires (GERM"O"P) (Group for Study and Research on "Orphan" Pulmonary Diseases) was founded in 1993 by J.-F. Cordier, with the creation of a coordination center based in Lyon. The objectives of the group are (1) to hold a registry of some rare and complex pulmonary disorders (Table 1) for which diagnostic or therapeutic information is currently insufficient ("orphan" pulmonary diseases), (2) to implement retrospective studies to better characterize the clinical and pathological fea-

Table 1 Groups of Disorders Recorded by the GERM"O"P's Registry of "Orphan" Pulmonary Diseases

Alveolar hemorrhage syndromes (especially microscopic polyangiitis and Goodpasture's syndrome)
Alveolar lipoproteinosis
Amyloidosis of the lung
Bronchiolitis
Eosinophilic lung diseases
Lymphangioleiomyomatosis
Lymphoproliferative disorders of the lung
Pulmonary vasculitides

tures of these disorders, (3) to promote prospective studies to improve diagnosis and treatment, (4) to provide pulmonary physicians with updated practical guidelines for the care of patients with "orphan" pulmonary diseases, and (5) to help patients affected by these disorders, especially by providing information on their disease.

Thirty-nine French pulmonary university centers agreed to participate in the group and to collaborate in the registry and studies. Regional hospitals and private practice pulmonary physicians were also invited, and many agreed to participate. Several papers in French medical journals and through the Société de Pneumologie de Langue Française disseminated the information to pulmonary physicians, so it may be assumed that almost all of them have heard of the group. Furthermore, a newsletter is regularly sent to all interested and participating physicians. By June 1997, more than 800 cases had been reported to the coordination center by more than 200 participating pulmonary groups or physicians. Once a significant number of cases is reached for a given disorder, the registry is used to implement retrospective studies if they are deemed useful. Two such studies have already been completed: one on chronic idiopathic eosinophilic pneumonia (61 cases) (16), and one on postradiation bronchiolitis obliterans organizing pneumonia (15 cases) (17). Two other studies are currently ending: the present one on LAM, and one on alveolar lipoproteinosis (38 cases). In addition, several prospective studies are being implemented.

IV. Selection of LAM Cases

Starting in 1993, participating physicians were asked to report to the GERM"O"P registry all cases of pulmonary LAM they had diagnosed. These consisted of either historical cases from their files, prevalent cases, or incident cases. Case records were nominative for patients who gave written consent, and anonymous otherwise. In December 1996, a questionnaire was sent to all physicians who had reported one or more cases of LAM to the registry in order to obtain detailed information on the patients.

Diagnostic criteria of pulmonary LAM for entering cases in the study were as follows:

1. Characteristic pathologic findings on pulmonary biopsy

or

2. Typical cystic appearance on chest computed tomography (CT) *and* one of the following:
   characteristic pathological findings on lymph node biopsy
   typical angiomyolipoma of the kidney on imaging (with histological confirmation when available)

chylous ascites with abdominal lymphadenopathy on imaging
abdominal lymphadenopathy with typical ectatic and cystic appearance on lymphangiograms.

Cases with signs of Bourneville's tuberous sclerosis were excluded from further analysis.

V. Data on Pulmonary Lymphangioleiomyomatosis in France

At the closing date of the study (June 16, 1997), 80 cases of LAM had been reported to the registry. Questionnaires had been returned for all patients. After review, 11 cases were excluded because they did not fit inclusion criteria: 3 had Bourneville's tuberous sclerosis and 2 others had cerebral calcifications suggestive of this condition, 3 had an equivocal aspect on lung biopsy, and 3 had no lung biopsy and lacked the other mandatory criteria. The remaining 69 cases met the diagnostic criteria and were included in the present study. Sixty-four of these were French patients, and 5 were from other countries. Some data of this series are presented in this chapter.

A. Diagnosis of LAM

Histopathological diagnosis of pulmonary LAM was obtained by open lung biopsy or videoassisted thoracoscopy in 50 patients, by transbronchial lung biopsy in 2, and by examination of explanted lung following transplantation in 5 cases. Thus, diagnosis of pulmonary LAM was made on histopathological grounds in 57 of 69 cases (83%).

LAM was diagnosed in the absence of lung biopsy in the 12 other patients (17%). All had a typical cystic appearance on chest CT. The required additional criteria was met by histopathological diagnosis of LAM on lymph node biopsy in 5 cases (abdominal 3, thoracic 1, inguinal 1), presence of typical angiomyolipoma of the kidney on imaging in 4 (with histological confirmation in 2), chylous ascites with abdominal lymphadenopathy on imaging in 2, and typical findings on abdominal lymphangiogram in one.

B. Incidence of LAM

The 69 reported cases of pulmonary LAM were diagnosed between 1975 and 1996. Figure 1 shows the distribution of incident cases during four consecutive 6-year periods from 1973 to 1996. Only 4 cases occurred in 1973–78 and 5 cases in 1979–84, whereas 15 cases occurred in 1985–90 and 45 in 1991–96. Because incident cases of the first periods are likely to have been underdiagnosed, incidence of LAM was only estimated for the last period, although some instability

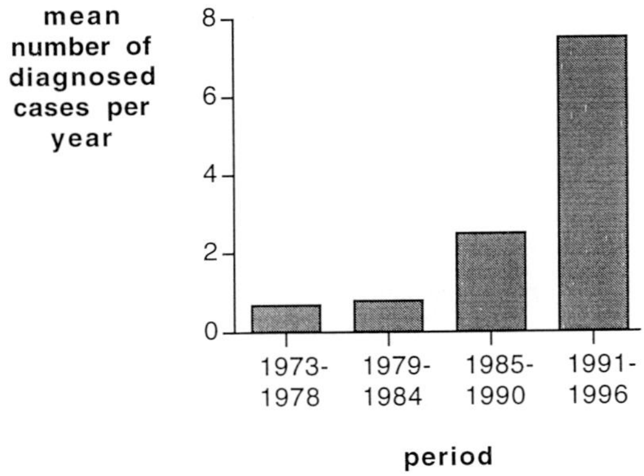

Figure 1 Distribution of 69 incident cases of LAM according to year of diagnosis during four consecutive 6-year periods between 1973 and 1996. Bars represent the average number of diagnosed cases per year.

of the incidence was still observed within this period (the number of cases recorded each year between 1991 and 1996 was, respectively, 6, 7, 5, 8, 14, and 5). Forty-one of these 45 cases occurred in French patients. Since the age at diagnosis ranged from 22 to 69 years, the annual incidence rate was estimated as the ratio of the average number of French cases per year during the 1991–96 period (6.8 cases) to the number of females aged 20–69 (18 189 638 individuals), as provided by the 1990 census (Institut National de la Statistique et des Etudes Economiques, Lyon, France). Thus, the crude annual incidence rate of LAM in France for the period 1991–96 was 0.4 per million per year in women aged 20–69.

C. Prevalence of LAM

At the reference date of the 1990 census (March 5), 17 French patients with *diagnosed* LAM were alive. Thus, the crude prevalence rate of *diagnosed* LAM in France on March 5, 1990, was 0.9 cases per million in women aged 20–69. At the same date, 14 other patients had respiratory symptoms attributable to the disease but diagnosed later (between 1991 and 1996). When including these *symptomatic* but yet undiagnosed cases, the overall number of patients alive with the disease at the reference date was 31. Thus, taking into account both *diagnosed* and *symptomatic* cases resulted in an overall prevalence rate of LAM in France on March 5, 1990, of 1.7 cases per million in women aged 20–69.

At the end of the 1991–96 period (i.e., on January 1, 1997), 49 French patients with *diagnosed* LAM were alive. Based on the 1990 census, the female population aged 20–69 at the same date was estimated to be 18 709 718 individuals (Institut National de la Statistique et des Etudes Economiques, Lyon, France). Thus, the crude prevalence rate of diagnosed LAM in France on January 1, 1997, was 2.6 cases per million in women aged 20–69.

D. Patient Characteristics

The 69 patients, all female, had a mean (±SD) age at onset of symptoms of 36.3 ± 9.6 years (range: 17.6–62.6). The mean age at diagnosis was 39.3 ± 9.6 years (range: 22.4–69.8). The age distribution at time of diagnosis is shown in Figure 2. No diagnosis was made before the age of 20. A marked increase in frequency occurred during the third and fourth decades of life, with a peak of occurrence between the ages of 30 and 34. The frequency progressively declined in older age groups, up to the age of 59 years. A few diagnoses were made between 65 and 69 years of age. The age distribution at time of first symptoms disclosed a very similar pattern and identical peak of frequency (data not shown).

The mean interval between onset of symptoms and diagnosis was 3.0 ± 4.5 years (range: 0–18.8) and the median interval was 1.0 year. Delays between onset of symptoms and diagnosis for all patients are summarized in Figure 3. In 53% of cases, the diagnosis of LAM was made within one year after the onset of symptoms. After the first year, the proportion of patients having their disease diagnosed increased more slowly over time: 20% remained undiagnosed after 5 years, and 10% after 10 years following onset of symptoms.

Sixteen of 67 (24%) patients were smokers at the time of their first symptoms. Use of oral contraceptives (before diagnosis) was recorded in 16 of 45

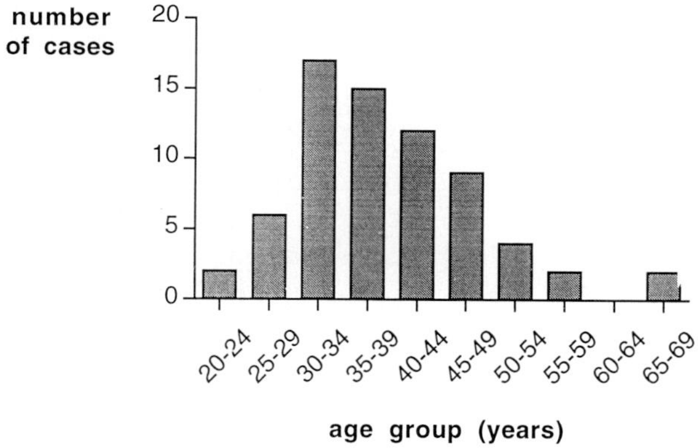

Figure 2 Distribution of 69 cases of LAM according to age at time of diagnosis. Bars represent the number of cases in each age group.

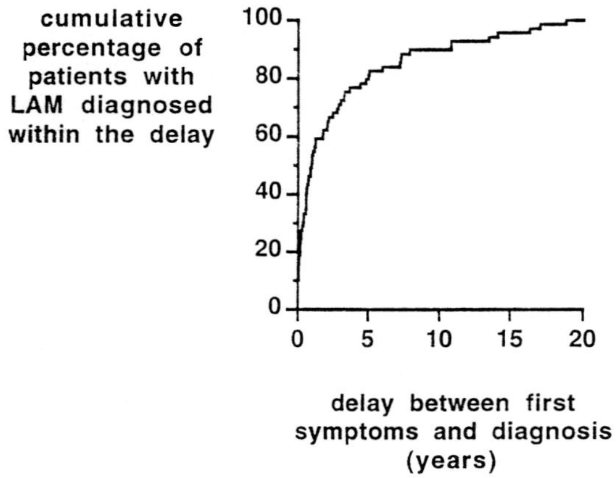

Figure 3 Delays between onset of symptoms and diagnosis in 69 patients with LAM.

(36%), and one or more pregnancies occurred before the first symptoms of LAM in 46 of 61 (75%). LAM was diagnosed after menopause in 7 of 54 patients (13%).

E. Clinical Manifestations

The initial symptoms were thoracic in 57 of the patients and extrathoracic in 5. Five other patients had both thoracic and extrathoracic symptoms, and 2 were asymptomatic.

The main respiratory manifestations at diagnosis consisted of dyspnea in 49 of 69 patients (71%), pneumothorax in 36 of 69 (52%), cough in 22 of 69 (32%), chylothorax in 14 of 69 (20%), and hemoptysis in 3 of 69 (4%).

Chest x-ray (apart from signs of pneumothorax or pleural effusion) was abnormal in 63 of 69 patients (91%), showing mainly interstitial opacities in 46 of 69 (67%) and cysts or bullae in 40 of 69 (58%). Chest CT was done in 66 patients and demonstrated pulmonary parenchymal abnormalities evocative of the cystic pattern of LAM in 66 of 66 (100%).

The most common abnormalities found at initial lung function tests are summarized in Table 2. Forty-two percent of patients had normal spirometry. Obstructive ventilatory defect was present in 35%. Restrictive (14%) or mixed (9%) patterns were less common. Lung hyperinflation was present in only 5%. Reduced carbon monoxide transfer factor (TL_{CO}) was found in 82% of cases, and hypoxemia was present in 60%.

The main extrarespiratory manifestations or associated tumors consisted of uterine leiomyomas in 23 of 65 patients (35%), renal angiomyolipomas in 20 of 65 (31%), abdominal lymph node enlargement or masses in 15 of 68 (22%), and chylous ascites in 6 of 69 (9%).

Table 2 Frequency of Abnormalities at Initial Lung Function Tests in 66 Patients with LAM

Abnormalities	Criteria	Number of patients	Percentage of patients
Normal spirometry		28/66	(42%)
Obstructive defect	$FEV_1/FVC < 70\%$	23/66	(35%)
Restrictive defect	TLC < 80% predicted, or VC < 80% predicted and $FEV_1/FVC > 70\%$	9/66	(14%)
Combined obstructive and restrictive defect	TLC < 80% predicted and $FEV_1/FVC < 70\%$	6/66	(9%)
Lung hyperinflation	TLC > 120% predicted	3/58	(5%)
Decreased TL_{CO}	$TL_{CO} < 80\%$ predicted	37/45	(82%)
Hypoxemia	$Pa_{O2} < 80$ mmHg	33/55	(60%)

FEV_1/FVC: Forced expiratory volume in one second/forced vital capacity; TLC: total lung capacity; VC: vital capacity; TL_{CO}: carbon monoxide transfer factor; Pa_{O_2}: arterial oxygen partial pressure.

F. Treatment

The management of patients after diagnosis was heterogeneous. Eleven of 68 (16%) patients had no hormonal treatment for 4.5 ± 4.3 years after diagnosis, 28 of 68 (41%) patients received one hormonal treatment, and 29 of 68 (43%) received two or more treatments (either simultaneously or consecutively). Forty-six patients received progestative hormones, 22 patients received tamoxifen, 14 patients received luteinizing hormone releasing–hormone (LHRH) agonists, 6 patients received somatostatin, and 5 patients underwent oophorectomy. Pleurodesis was performed in 40 of 69 patients (58%). Thirteen of 69 (19%) patients underwent lung transplantation.

G. Survival

Fifty-three patients were alive as of June 1997, with a mean follow-up from the time of their first symptoms of 8.6 ± 6.6 years. Eleven patients had died at the closing date of the study, after a mean interval of 6.2 ± 3.8 years after their first symptoms. Death could be attributed to LAM in 10 of 11 cases, either directly (respiratory failure in 3 cases, hemorrhage from renal angiomyolipoma in one case) or indirectly (postoperatively following pleurodesis in 3 cases, from complications of lung transplantation in 3 cases). One patient died from unrelated cause. Five patients were lost to follow-up, after a mean duration of 5.8 ± 8.2 years.

The probability of survival according to duration of the disease was evaluated by the Kaplan-Meier method. Results are shown in Figure 4. Onset of the disease was defined as the time of the first symptoms. The probability of being alive was 91% after 5 years, 79% after 10 years, and 71% after 15 years of dis-

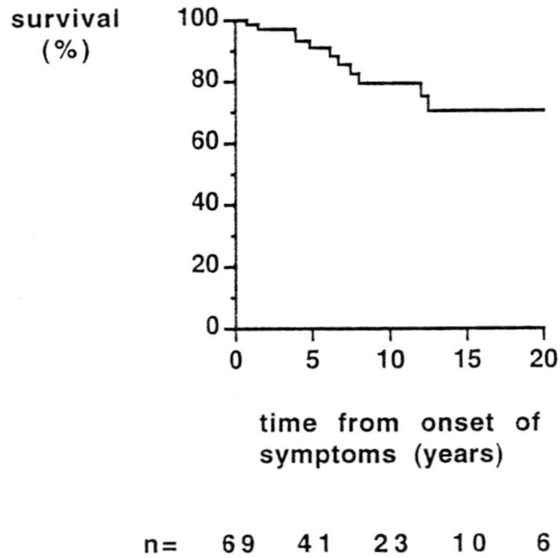

Figure 4 Kaplan-Meier plot of survival in 69 patients with LAM. *n* is the number of patients at risk at each time point.

ease duration. Survival at 8.5 years has been used as an endpoint in previous studies. In our series, the probability of survival at 8.5 years by the Kaplan-Meier method was 79%. The survival rate was slightly lower when considering the patients with effective 8.5-year follow-up or dying before this delay: 33 patients had a determined outcome at 8.5 years, of whom 24 were alive. Thirty-six other patients were followed for less than 8.5 years. The actual survival rate at 8.5 years was thus 24 of 33 (73%).

VI. Discussion

A. Incidence and Prevalence of LAM

This French series reports 69 cases of LAM, of which 60 cases were diagnosed after 1985. The number of cases diagnosed before 1985 in France, as reflected by our registry, was small: 9 cases. It was indeed probably greater, but some older cases were certainly unknown to the physicians participating in the GERM"O"P study, especially patients who died before 1985. However, from the cases published in the French literature or presented at national meetings, it is probable that this condition was rarely diagnosed in France before the 1980s.

It is worthwhile remarking further that 15 cases were diagnosed between 1985 and 1990, whereas 45 cases were diagnosed between 1991 and 1996. This increasing number of diagnoses of LAM in France may have several explanations. First, as already stated, it could be due to a memory bias, resulting in incomplete reporting of cases diagnosed in the 1970s and 1980s, especially if these patients were no longer alive at the time of the study. Alternatively, it may reflect the increasing awareness of chest physicians of the disease. The availability of CT all over the country could be a cause of improved diagnosis, since LAM imaging on high-resolution CT is extremely characteristic, with a differential diagnosis restricted to cystic histiocytosis X. In addition, our efforts through the GERM"O"P to promote the care of patients with "orphan" pulmonary diseases and to spread information on rare pulmonary disorders may have contributed to an increase in the index of suspicion of LAM since 1993. If CT and spread of information could conceivably have increased the number of diagnosed cases in recent years, it remains surprising that more reports (including autopsy reports) did not appear before 1985. If the increased number of diagnosed LAM only reflects improved diagnosis, one would expect a stabilization in the number of incident cases in the coming years. Finally, a true increase in disease incidence cannot be excluded.

The incidence and prevalence of LAM in other countries are not precisely known, as is the case for most "orphan" diseases, since there are currently a limited number of registries collecting the cases of such rare diseases from a definite population. From our data, the annual incidence rate of LAM in France between 1991 and 1996 was estimated as 0.4 cases per million per year in women aged 20–69 years, i.e., the population at risk. Not surprisingly, this incidence rate is low. The prevalence rate of diagnosed LAM on March 5, 1990, was 0.9 cases per million women aged 20–69. However, this figure did not reflect well the overall number of individuals with an active disease, since a significant proportion of them were undiagnosed at that time. Thus, while 17 patients with diagnosed LAM were alive on March 5, 1990, 14 others already had symptoms attributable to the disease but only subsequently diagnosed as LAM. Hence, using a broader definition of prevalence including both *diagnosed* and *symptomatic* cases resulted in a prevalence rate on March 5, 1990, of 1.7 cases per million women aged 20–69. Since most patients were diagnosed between 1991 and 1996, the highest prevalence was unsurprisingly found at the end of this period (January 1, 1997), reaching a prevalence rate of diagnosed LAM of 2.6 cases per million women aged 20–69. By analogy with data of 1990, the existence of symptomatic but undiagnosed cases of LAM at this later time point appears likely, but these were obviously missed by the present analysis.

In summary, the currently available data on LAM in France make it possible to estimate its incidence rate as 0.4 cases per million per year between 1991 and 1996 and its prevalence rate as 2.6 cases per million on January 1, 1997, in the population at risk (women aged 20–69). These figures obviously represent a minimal evaluation, since we cannot pretend that all French cases of LAM have been reported to our registry. However, since the registry is now widely known throughout the country and most chest physicians report to it their cases of rare disorders, it is likely that we have indeed collected most cases of LAM diagnosed in France during the last 6 years. It would be interesting to compare these figures with the epidemiologic trends of LAM in other countries, since comparing the data from different populations could help us to understand the genetic bases of the disease.

B. Patient Characteristics

The mean age at onset of symptoms in our series was 36.3 ± 9.6 years, and the mean age at diagnosis was 39.3 ± 9.6 years. The age characteristics of our patients did not markedly differ from those of previously published series (18–21). The distribution of our cases according to age at diagnosis showed a peak of frequency in the fourth decade of life. A significant number of patients were also diagnosed during their fifth decade.

The mean interval between the first symptoms and diagnosis in our series was 3.0 ± 4.5 years. A delayed diagnosis has generally been considered as the rule for this disorder. However, our data demonstrate that it is not always the case. As shown in Figure 3, more than half of our patients had their disease diagnosed within one year after their first symptoms. Diagnostic delays were longer for the other patients, with 20% remaining undiagnosed after 5 years, and 10% after 10 years following the onset of symptoms. However, a long delay does not necessarily reflect poor diagnostic skills or procedures, but could also be due to lesser severity or slower progression of the disease. The causes of diagnostic delays in our series remain to be analyzed in greater detail.

Most patients with LAM were nonsmokers in this series, in agreement with previous studies (18). At the present time, smoking has not been linked to the occurrence of LAM. The hypothesis that oral contraceptives are causally associated with the development of pulmonary LAM has been addressed in a case-control study (19), but no supportive evidence was found. The frequency of use of oral contraceptives was lower in our series (36%), as compared to the latter study (62%). In contrast, the percentage of patients who had one or more pregnancies before the onset of LAM was higher in our series (75% vs. 52%). The putative roles of oral contraceptives and pregnancy as risk factors for the development of LAM deserve further analysis. Cases of LAM diagnosed after menopause were reported to be uncommon (18,20,22). Accordingly, they accounted for 13% of cases in this series. It is likely that, in many cases diagnosed after menopause, disease started during childbearing age, but clearly progressed despite the occurrence of menopause. For example, one reported patient had a normal chest x-ray 3 years after menopause and 5 years before the onset of symptoms (22).

C. Thoracic Manifestations of LAM

The respiratory symptoms of LAM are nonspecific and consist mainly of dyspnea, cough, chest pain, and hemoptysis. Dyspnea was the most frequent initial symptom, occurring in 71% of our cases. Pneumothorax is a common presentation in patients with LAM (18,20,23–26), sometimes bilateral and severe (27–29), occurring in up to 81% of cases during the course of the disease (20). Pneumothorax was found at presentation in 52% of our patients, a frequency comparable to that of other series where it ranged from 39 to 53% (18,20,30). CT imaging done at the time of pneumothorax might contribute to earlier diagnosis of parenchymal abnormalities in those patients. In addition, the typical aspect of the lung surface at thoracoscopy or thoracotomy generally prompts pulmonary biopsy in patients undergoing these procedures for persisting or relapsing pneumothorax.

Manifestations resulting from involvement of the lymphatic system draining chyle are common in LAM. Chylothorax is a characteristic manifestation (18,20,23,25,31). It was present at diagnosis in 20% of our cases, and reached 39% in the series of Corrin et al. (21). Although the causes of chylothorax are numerous, spontaneous occurrence of chylothorax in a woman of childbearing age should raise the suspicion of LAM. Chylous expectoration occurring spontaneously (or after lung biopsy) is a rare but highly evocative manifestation of LAM (21,32,33). Chylous rhinorrhea is exceptional (34,35).

D. Chest Imaging

Chest x-ray is rarely normal at presentation in patients with LAM and usually shows a reticular, cystic, or honeycombing pattern, with possible Kerley B lines, and associated pleural effusion in some cases (13,18,20,21,23–26,31,36,37). In agreement with previous studies, lung parenchymal abnormalities were present in 91% of our patients at chest x-ray. High-resolution CT is superior to chest x-ray in the assessment of patients with LAM. It shows a characteristic pattern of bilateral and diffuse thin-walled cysts ranging from a few millimeters to several centimeters distributed throughout the central and peripheral parts of the lungs (13,36–40). In contrast to histiocytosis X, nodules are noticeably absent in patients with LAM. Chest CT was available in 66 patients of our series, and the typical abnormalities of LAM were present in all of them. In this study, we considered that CT findings were so characteristic of LAM that diagnosis could be confidently made in some cases without lung biopsy, if distinctive extrapulmonary features were present in addition to the typical chest CT findings. This occurred in 12 patients of the present series. Other CT abnormalities in patients with LAM include pleural effusions and mediastinal lymphadenopathy. Mediastinal lymph node involvement is common in LAM and is usually asymptomatic, although it may contribute to the development of chylothorax (23,25,26,31,39,41,42). An abdominal CT may be done during the same examination procedure as chest CT, and it may provide information on the subdiaphragmatic lesions associated with pulmonary LAM.

E. Lung Function Tests

Frequency of lung function test abnormalities disclosed some differences between our and other recent data (18,20). Forty-two percent of our patients had a normal initial spirometry, as compared to, respectively, 9% and 10% in the studies by Taylor et al. (20) and Kitaichi et al. (18). Obstructive ventilatory defect was the single most frequent abnormality at spirometry and was present in 35% of our cases, as compared to 78% and 29%, respectively, in the above-mentioned series. A restrictive defect was less common in our study (14%, vs. 31% and 26%). Similarly, our patients had less frequent $T_{L_{CO}}$ reduction (82%, vs. 96% and 97%) and hypoxemia (60%, vs. 77% and 81%). Taken together, these data suggest that our patients had less severe impairment at initial lung function tests and that testing was thus performed at an earlier stage of the disease. This, however, does not necessarily imply earlier diagnosis. Importantly, our results agree with other studies in that the most common abnormalities were respectively reduced $T_{L_{CO}}$, hypoxemia, and decreased FEV_1/FVC. Moreover, $T_{L_{CO}}$ reduction remained very frequent in our series (82%) despite a high rate of normal spirometry (42%), possibly reflecting an earlier disease stage. This suggests that reduced $T_{L_{CO}}$ may appear before any ventilatory defect in the natural history of LAM, and could in fact be the earliest functional abnormality. This hypothesis deserves further analysis.

F. Extrathoracic Manifestations of LAM

Extrathoracic involvement or associated tumors are common in LAM and may give rise to the first clinical manifestations of the disease.

Angiomyolipoma is a benign mesenchymal tumor consisting of fat, smooth muscle, and blood vessels. Angiomyolipomas of the kidney have characteristic CT features. They are present in up to 80% of patients with tuberous sclerosis and have also been reported with increasing frequency in patients with LAM (7,21,23,25,43–47). The frequency of diagnosed renal angiomyolipoma in the present study was 31% and was even lower in previous large series, probably because these had not been especially searched for. For example, in the series of Kitaichi et al. (18), renal angiomyolipoma was mentioned in only 4 of 46 cases. In contrast, in the series of Bernstein et al. (43) and Maziak et al. (46), where extrathoracic abnormalities were systematically examined by CT, the frequency of angiomyolipoma reached, respectively, 47% and 57% of cases.

Abdominal lymph node enlargement or lymphatic masses were detected in 22% of our patients and in up to 76% of patients of Chu et al. (44). Abdominal lymph node enlargement or lymphangiomyoma in LAM generally consists of spongy masses with smooth muscle cell proliferation and marked cystic dilatation of lymphatic channels containing chyle, which may be asymptomatic or manifest by associated complications such as chylous ascites (23,25,26,31,34,41,42,48–56). Abdominal lymph nodes are well demonstrated by CT scan (56). Lymphangiography, which is currently almost abandoned, has been used in patients with LAM to demonstrate characteristic dilatations of the abdominal lymphatic network with cystic and ectatic contrast-filled lymph nodes (7,10,23,25,57). Chylous ascites has been reported as a presenting feature in less than 10% of cases of LAM (18,20). In agreement with these data, the occurrence of chylous ascites was also uncommon in our patients (9%).

G. Treatment of LAM

Since LAM occurs almost exclusively in women of childbearing age, and because isolated but convincing reports have suggested disease exacerbation by pregnancy or estrogens, hormonal treatments have been widely used in LAM (15,18,20,55,58–67). These included mainly progestative drugs, antiestrogens, LHRH agonists, and oophorectomy. The interpretation of the effects of each treatment modality are difficult to assess in most reports, and no firm conclusion can be deduced from the literature at the present time. Kitaichi et al. (18) reviewed 40 evaluable treatments in 30 patients and observed objective improvement in only one case. Taylor et al. (20) observed two patients who improved with medroxyprogesterone, worsened when the dose was tapered, and improved again when it was increased. In their review of LAM treatment, Taylor et al. (20) concluded that medroxyprogesterone might be useful mainly in patients with chylous manifestations. Unfortunately, controlled therapeutic trials have not been conducted so far, and no convincing conclusions and treatment guidelines can be drawn from the small published series or isolated case reports.

Although definite proofs of efficacy are still lacking, hormonal treatment is presently considered to be indicated in patients with LAM (20). The treatment currently recommended by our group includes lynestrenol (a progestative drug derived from nortestosterone with a strong antigonadotropic and antiestrogen activity), often associated with tamoxifen. Additional measures may be useful for some manifestations of LAM. For instance, medium-chain triglyceride diet and diuresis may help to control chylous effusion (31).

Lung transplantation has emerged in recent years as a salvage procedure in patients with LAM and severe respiratory failure (68–70). A recent retrospective study reviewed 34 cases of lung transplantation for LAM (68). The actuarial survival rate calculated by the Kaplan-Meier method was 69% at one year and 58% at 2 years. LAM may recur after lung transplantation (68,71,72). In the present study, 13 patients underwent lung transplantation, of whom 9 are alive (3 died of complications related to transplantation, and one of massive abdominal hemorrhage). No recurrence of LAM has been observed so far in our cases.

H. Survival

The early reports of LAM up to the 1970s gave a pessimistic view of survival (21,25), with most patients dying within a few years after onset of the disease. However, in more recent series, survival appeared to be better (20). In the present study, Kaplan-Meier plot disclosed survival probabilities of 91% after 5 years, 79% after 10 years, and 71% after 15 years of disease duration. Survival at 8.5 years, used as an endpoint in previous series (18,20), was 79% by the Kaplan-Meier method, and 73% when considering the actual number of patients with a determined outcome at 8.5 years. These data are in very good agreement with those of Taylor et al. (20), who found that 78% of patients were still alive 8.5 years after onset of the disease. The probability of survival at 8.5 years was lower (38%) in the series by Kitaichi et al. (18). Since both the definition of disease onset and the characteristics of patients at diagnosis (especially the degree of respiratory impairment at lung function tests) are difficult to determine and compare in the published series, the reasons for differences in survival are not clear, and whether they result from different managements of the disease or from different study methods and analyzed populations remains to be determined. In any case, there is apparently a subgroup of patients who die rapidly within 5 years after onset of the disease (20), whereas a larger number of patients do not markedly deteriorate over years and survive longer. Kitaichi et al. (18) identified prognostic factors in LAM, with worse prognosis in patients with reduced FEV_1/FVC ratio, increased TLC, and a histologically predominantly cystic type (as opposed to a predominantly muscular type). Interestingly, LAM may present as abdominal lymphangiomyoma without apparent pulmonary involvement, the pulmonary parenchymal changes developing only subsequently and up to 14 years later (20).

VII. Goals for Clinical Research

Basic research in LAM is increasingly active and might lead to new and more efficient therapeutic strategies in the near future (73). In the meantime, both improving the management of patients with LAM worldwide and analyzing more accurately the clinical manifestations and complications of the disease may be reasonable goals to achieve.

Determining less aggressive and more sensitive and specific tools for clinical diagnosis of LAM is likely to directly benefit patients. High-resolution CT seems to be a very sensitive means of diagnosing early pulmonary LAM even in cases where chest x-ray is not conclusive, and it may be indicated in spontaneous pneumothorax occurring in women of childbearing age. In such cases, lung function tests with measurement of FEV_1/FVC ratio and TL_{CO} might also contribute to early detection of pulmonary LAM. Obtaining a pathologic diagnosis of pulmonary LAM may not require open-lung or videothoracoscopic lung biopsy. The recently available immunohistochemical characterization of smooth muscle cells in LAM (74–76) with anti–HMB-45 antibodies may help in diagnosing LAM in the small tissue specimens obtained by transbronchial biopsies (77–79).

Analyzing more meticulously the clinical, imaging, lung function tests, and pathologic features in both retrospective and prospective studies might provide clearer insights into prognostic factors and determine more precisely the respective consequences of smooth muscle cell proliferation, damage to lung structures, and chylous engorgement of the lymphatic network. Comparing subgroups of patients with rapidly progressive as opposed to smoldering disease course might also result in useful information.

Since LAM is associated with extrapulmonary lymphangioleiomyomatosis and angiomyolipoma, careful evaluation of patients with abdominal CT scan may help to assess these extrapulmonary manifestations and prompt diagnosis of their possible complications, thus improving the management of patients.

Tuberous sclerosis is associated in approximately 2.3% of cases with pulmonary lesions indistinguishable from those of LAM (80). Genetic studies in patients with LAM and tuberous sclerosis with and without pulmonary disease might help to characterize the possible common genetic basis of the pulmonary involvement. In this respect, cases of tuberous sclerosis with pulmonary LAM occurring in siblings (81,82) might be of special interest.

One of the most urgent goals in clinical research on LAM is to define and launch therapeutic trials in order to test the currently available hormonal treatments. As for all "orphan" pulmonary diseases, this can only be achieved through coordinated multicentric studies. The GERM"O"P has recruited a network of motivated French pulmonary physicians to do so. The formation of a European network is under study. A larger international collaboration of all North American, Asian, and European groups involved in the study of LAM should clearly not be missed.

Acknowledgments

This work was supported by a grant HCL-PNRC 93-005 from the Ministère de la Santé et de l'Action Humanitaire, and a grant FRC 97, France.

The following physicians participated in this study of the GERM"O"P by including one or more patients: H. Benzaquen (Paris), P. Blanc (Angoulème), F. Blanchon (Meaux), J. Capdeville (Foix), P. Carré (Tours), J.-M. Chavaillon (Antibes), M. Colas (Lyon), J.-F. Cordier (Lyon), J. Courdeau-Labourie (Tarbes), I. Court-Fortune (St Etienne), J.-C. Dalphin (Besançon), P. Fournel (St Etienne), C. Grange (Lyon), J.-P. Homasson (Chevilly Larue), G. Huchon (Paris), S. Labrune (Paris), J. Lacronique (Paris), D. Lauque (Toulouse), E. Lemarié (Tours), P. Léophonte (Toulouse), P. Leuenberger (Lausanne, Switzerland), J.-C. Meurice (Poitiers), B. Milleron (Paris), J.-F. Mornex (Lyon), J.-F. Muir (Rouen), M. Murris (Toulouse), L. Nicod (Genève, Switzerland), D. Pernet (Besançon), M. H. Pichot (Paris), M. Reynaud-Gaubert (Marseille), P. Romand (Thonon les Bains), P. Satre (Grenoble), A. B. Tonnel (Lille), T. Urban (Paris), D. Valeyre (Paris), J. Vergeret (Bordeaux), J.-F. Vodoz (Montreux, Switzerland), B. Wallaert (Lille).

The authors acknowledge Dr. Pascal Roy for his contribution to the analysis of the epidemiological data, and Ingrid Janin and Chantal Silarakis for data capture and secretarial work.

References

1. Von Stössel E. Über muskuläre Cirrhose der Lunge. Beitr Klin Tuberk 1937; 90:432–442.
2. Burrell LST, Ross JM. A case of chylous effusion due to leiomyosarcoma. Br J Tuberc 1937; 31:38–39.
3. Rosendal T. A case of diffuse myomatosis and cyst formation in the lung. Acta Radiol 1942; 23:138–146.
4. Roujeau J, Delarue J, Depierre R. Lymphangiectasie pulmonaire diffuse, pneumonie chyleuse et chylothorax, après thrombose puerpérale de la veine sous-clavière gauche. J Fr Med Chir Thor 1950; 5:488–503.
5. Justin-Besançon L, Péquignot H, Galey JJ, Renault P, Even P. Lymphangiectasies pulmonaires diffuses acquises avec insuffisance respiratoire et chylothorax. Sem Hop (Paris) 1963; 39:1179–1190.
6. Marsac J, Basset F, Broquie G, Rolland J, Soler P, de Saint-Florent G, Akoun G, Brocard H. Deux cas de lymphangiomyomatose pulmonaire diffuse avec étude ultrastructurale. Rev Fr Mal Resp 1975; 3:961–982.
7. Basset F, Soler P, Marsac J, Corrin B. Pulmonary lymphangiomyomatosis. Three new cases studies with electron microscopy. Cancer 1976; 38:2357–2366.
8. Marsac J, Blanchon F, Basset F, Bart-Emery MC, Brocard H. La lymphangiomyomatose. I. Etude clinique, radiologique et fonctionnelle respiratoire. Rev Fr Mal Resp 1978; 6:573–588.
9. Marsac J, Basset F, Soler P, Blanchon F, Chrétien J. La lymphangiomyomatose. II. Anatomo-pathologie, pathogénie, traitement. Rev Fr Mal Resp 1978; 6:589–602.

10. Léophonte P, Fabre J, Pris J, Eschapasse H, Delaude A. La lymphangiomyomatose pulmonaire. Aspects lymphographiques. A propos de 4 cas. Rev Fr Mal Resp 1978; 6:159–164.
11. Capron F, Ameille J, Leclerc P, Mornet P, Barbagellata M, Reynes M, Rochemaure J. Pulmonary lymphangioleiomyomatosis and Bourneville's tuberous sclerosis with pulmonary involvement: the same disease? Cancer 1983; 52:851–855.
12. Treilleux Salles I, Vitrey D, Berger F, Beurlet J, Patricot LM. Lymphangiomyomatose extrapulmonaire révélée par une entéropathie exudative d'évolution rapidement fatale. Ann Pathol 1989; 9:279–283.
13. Lenoir S, Grenier P, Brauner MW, Frija J, Remy-Jardin M, Revel D, Cordier JF. Pulmonary lymphangiomyomatosis and tuberous sclerosis: comparison of radiographic and thin-section CT findings. Radiology 1990; 175:329–334.
14. Peyrol S, Gindre D, Cordier JF, Loire R, Grimaud JA. Characterization of the smooth muscle cell infiltrate and associated connective matrix of lymphangiomyomatosis. Immunohistochemical and ultrastructural study of two cases. J Pathol 1992; 168:387–395.
15. Urban T, Kuttenn F, Gompel A, Marsac J, Lacronique J. Pulmonary lymphangiomyomatosis. Follow-up and long-term outcome with antiestrogen therapy; a report of eight cases. Chest 1992; 102:472–476.
16. Marchand E, Reynaud-Gaubert M, Lauque D, Wallaert B, Cordier JF, Tonnel AB. Chronic eosinophilic pneumonia (CEP). A clinical and follow-up study of 61 cases (abstr). Am J Respir Crit Care Med 1997; 155:A329.
17. Crestani B, Valeyre D, Bayle JY, Wallaert B, Cordier JF. Bronchiolitis obliterans organizing pneumonia primed by radiation therapy for breast carcinoma. A report of 15 patients (abstr). Am J Respir Crit Care Med 1997; 155:A332.
18. Kitaichi M, Nishimura K, Itoh H, Izumi T. Pulmonary lymphangioleiomyomatosis: a report of 46 patients including a clinicopathologic study of prognostic factors. Am J Respir Crit Care Med 1995; 151:527–533.
19. Wahedna I, Cooper S, Williams J, Paterson IC, Britton JR, Tattersfield AE. Relation of pulmonary lymphangioleiomyomatosis to use of the oral contraceptive pill and fertility in the UK: a national case control study. Thorax 1994; 49:910–914.
20. Taylor JR, Ryu J, Colby TV, Raffin TA. Lymphangioleiomyomatosis. Clinical course in 32 patients. N Engl J Med 1990; 323:1254–1260.
21. Corrin B, Liebow AA, Friedman PJ. Pulmonary lymphangiomyomatosis. A review. Am J Pathol 1975; 79:347–382.
22. Baldi S, Papotti M, Valente ML, Rapellino M, Scappaticci E, Corrin B. Pulmonary lymphangioleiomyomatosis in postmenopausal women: report of two cases and review of the literature. Eur Respir J 1994; 7:1013–1016.
23. Carrington CB, Cugell DW, Gaensler EA, Marks A, Redding RA, Schaaf JT, Tomasian A. Lymphangioleiomyomatosis. Physiologic-pathologic-radiologic correlations. Am Rev Respir Dis 1977; 116:977–995.
24. Sieker HO, McCarty KS Jr. Lymphangiomyomatosis. A respiratory illness with an endocrinologic therapy. Trans Am Clin Climatol Assoc 1987; 99:57–67.
25. Silverstein EF, Ellis K, Wolff M, Jaretzki AI. Pulmonary lymphangiomyomatosis. AJR 1974; 120:832–850.

26. Schiavina M, Fabiani A, Cornia B, DeBenedictis E, Poletti V, Pileri S, Zompatori M. Lymphangioleiomyomatosis: clinical course. Monaldi Arch Chest Dis 1994; 49:6–14.
27. Berkman N, Bloom A, Cohen P, Deviri E, Bar-Ziv Y, Shimon D, Kramer MR. Bilateral spontaneous pneumothorax as the presenting feature in lymphangioleiomyomatosis. Respir Med 1995; 89:381–383.
28. Graf-Deuel E, Knoblauch A. Simultaneous bilateral spontaneous pneumothorax. Chest 1994; 105:1142–1146.
29. Warren SE, Lee D, Martin V, Messink W. Pulmonary lymphangiomyomatosis causing bilateral pneumothorax during pregnancy. Ann Thorac Surg 1993; 55:998–1000.
30. Johnson SR, Tattersfield AE. Lymphangioleiomyomatosis: a UK survey (abstr). Thorax 1996; 51:A66.
31. Bradley SL, Dines DE, Soule EH, Muhm JR. Pulmonary lymphangiomyomatosis. Lung 1980; 158:69–80.
32. Khan SU, Mehta AC. Chyloptyses found in a patient with lymphangioleiomyomatosis. Chest 1995; 108:1775.
33. Puente Maestu L, Rodriguez Gonzalez-Moro JM, de Lucas Ramos P, Tarancon Llorente MC, Cubillo Marcos JM, Hernandez Fernandez J, Monturiol Rodriguez JM. A proposito de tres casos de linfangioleiomiomatosis pulmonar difusa. Rev Clin Esp 1990; 186:335–340.
34. Ardichvili D, Colard M, de Windt J. Syndrome de lymphangiomyomatose. Ann Anat Pathol (Paris) 1970; 15:307–320.
35. Molina C, Roche G, Baguet JC, Cheminat JC, Petit R, Chevalier A, Quintana M, Bourges M. Lymphangiomatose pulmonaire. A propos d'une observation avec étude clinique, histologique et ultrastructurale. Rev Fr Mal Resp 1976; 4:49–60.
36. Aberle DR, Hansell DM, Brown K, Tashkin DP. Lymphangiomyomatosis: CT, chest radiographic, and functional correlations. Radiology 1990; 176:381–387.
37. Muller NL, Chiles C, Kullnig P. Pulmonary lymphangiomyomatosis: correlation of CT with radiographic and functional findings. Radiology 1990; 175:335–339.
38. Rappaport DC, Weisbrod GL, Herman SJ, Chamberlain DW. Pulmonary lymphangioleiomyomatosis: high-resolution CT findings in four cases. AJR 1989; 152:961–964.
39. Sherrier RH, Chiles C, Roggli V. Pulmonary lymphangioleiomyomatosis: CT findings. AJR 1989; 153:937–940.
40. Templeton PA, McLoud TC, Muller NL, Shepard JA, Moore EH. Pulmonary lymphangioleiomyomatosis: CT and pathologic findings. J Comput Assist Tomogr 1989; 13:54–57.
41. Monteforte WJ, Kohnen PW. Angiomyolipomas in a case of lymphangiomyomatosis syndrome: relationships to tuberous sclerosis. Cancer 1974; 34:317–321.
42. Stovin PGI, Lum LC, Flower CDR, Darke CS, Beeley M. The lungs in lymphangiomyomatosis and in tuberous sclerosis. Thorax 1975; 30:497–509.
43. Bernstein SM, Newell JD Jr, Adamczyk D, Mortenson RL, King TE Jr, Lynch DA. How common are renal angiomyolipomas in patients with pulmonary lymphangiomyomatosis? Am J Respir Crit Care Med 1995; 152:2138–2143.
44. Chu SC, Horiba K, Usuki J, Avila NA, Chen CC, Travis WD, Ferrans VJ, Moss J.

Comprehensive evaluation of 25 patients with lymphangioleiomyomatosis (LAM) (abstr). Am J Respir Crit Care Med 1997; 155:A330.

45. Gawad KA, Knoefel WT, Izbicki JR, Schroder S, Broelsch CE. Generalised lymphangioleiomyomatosis presenting as a retroperitoneal tumour. Eur J Surg 1996; 162:583–585.
46. Maziak DE, Kesten S, Rappaport DC, Maurer J. Extrathoracic angiomyolipomas in lymphangioleiomyomatosis. Eur Respir J 1996; 9:402–405.
47. Tawfik O, Austenfeld M, Persons D. Multicentric renal angiomyolipoma associated with pulmonary lymphangioleiomyomatosis: case report, with histologic, immunohistochemical, and DNA content analyses. Urology 1996; 48:476–480.
48. Buhl L, Larsen KE, Bjorn-Hansen L. Lymphangioleiomyomatosis. Is fine needle aspiration cytodiagnosis possible? Acta Cytol 1988; 32:559–562.
49. Cornog JL, Enterline HT. Lymphangiomyoma, a benign lesion of chyliferous lymphatics synonymous with lymphangiopericytoma. Cancer 1966; 19:1909–1930.
50. Ernst JC, Sohaey R, Cary JM. Pelvic lymphangioleiomyomatosis. Atypical precursor to pulmonary disease. Chest 1994; 106:1267–1269.
51. Joliat G, Stalder H, Kapanci Y. Lymphangiomyomatosis: a clinico-anatomical entity. Cancer 1973; 31:455–461.
52. Merchant RN, Pearson MG, Rankin RN, Morgan WKC. Computerized tomography in the diagnosis of lymphangioleiomyomatosis. Am Rev Respir Dis 1985; 131:295–297.
53. Peh WCG, Law S, Fok M, Ngan H. Case report: lymphangiomyomatosis with spontaneous peritoneal rupture. Br J Radiol 1994; 67:605–608.
54. Shuman RL, Engelman R, Kittle CF. Pulmonary lymphangiomyomatosis. Ann Thorac Surg 1979; 27:70–75.
55. van Milligen de Wit AWM, Meilof-Planteydt MNM. Successful treatment of pulmonary lymphangioleiomyomatosis with oophorectomy and medroxyprogesteroneacetate: report of a case and brief review of the literature. Neth J Med 1990; 36:246–251.
56. Woodring JH, Howard RS II, Johnson MV. Massive low-attenuation mediastinal, retroperitoneal, and pelvic lymphadenopathy on CT from lymphangioleiomyomatosis. Case report. Clin Imaging 1994; 18:7–11.
57. Regnard JF, Levasseur P, Millat B, Gugenheim J, Oury M, Pouliquen E, Le Brigand H, Merlier M. La lymphangiomyomatose pulmonaire. A propos de six observations. Ann Chir 1987; 41:456–461.
58. Adamson D, Heinrichs WL, Raybin DM, Raffin TA. Successful treatment of pulmonary lymphangiomyomatosis with oophorectomy and progesterone. Am Rev Respir Dis 1985; 132:916–921.
59. Bevelaqua FA, Esptein H. Pulmonary lymphangiomyomatosis. Long-term survival in a patient with poor response to medroxyprogesterone. Chest 1985; 87:552–553.
60. Eisera NB, Venegoni E, Colombi R. Pulmonary lymphangiomyomatosis. J R Soc Med 1988; 81:607–609.
61. Eliasson AH, Phillips YY, Tenholder MF. Treatment of lymphangioleiomyomatosis. A meta-analysis. Chest 1989; 96:1352–1355.

62. McCarty KS Jr, Mossler JA, McLelland R, Sieker HO. Pulmonary lymphangiomyomatosis responsive to progesterone. N Engl J Med 1980; 303:1461–1465.
63. Radermecker MA, Broux R, Corhay JL, Limet R, Radermecker MF. Failure of buserelin-induced medical castration to control pulmonary lymphangiomyomatosis in two patients. Chest 1992; 101:1724–1726.
64. Rossi GA, Balbi B, Oddera S, Lantero S, Ravazzoni C. Response to treatment with an analog of the luteinizing-hormone-releasing hormone in a patient with pulmonary lymphangioleiomyomatosis. Am Rev Respir Dis 1991; 143:174–176.
65. Tomasian A, Greenberg MS, Rumerman H. Tamoxifen for lymphangioleiomyomatosis. N Engl J Med 1982; 306:745–746.
66. Zahner J, Borst MM, Worth H. Treatment of lymphangioleiomyomatosis. N Engl J Med 1991; 325:63–64.
67. Banner AS, Carrington CB, Emory WB, Kittle F, Leonard G, Ringus J, Taylor P, Addington WW. Efficacy of oophorectomy in lymphangioleiomyomatosis and benign metastasizing leiomyoma. N Engl J Med 1981; 305:204–209.
68. Boehler A, Speich R, Russi EW, Weder W. Lung transplantation for lymphangioleiomyomatosis. N Engl J Med 1996; 335:1275–1280.
69. Sleiman C, Mal H, Jebrak G, Darne C, Meeus E, Dubois F, Luisetti M, Fournier M, Pariente R, Andreassian B. Pulmonary lymphangiomyomatosis treated by single lung transplantation. Am Rev Respir Dis 1992; 145:964–966.
70. Wellens F, Estenne M, de Francquen P, Goldstein J, Leclerc JL, Primo G. Combined heart-lung transplantation for terminal pulmonary lymphangioleiomyomatosis. J Thorac Cardiovasc Surg 1985; 89:872–876.
71. Nine YS, Yousem SA, Paradis IL, Keenan R, Griffith BP. Lymphangioleiomyomatosis: recurrence after lung transplantation. J Heart Lung Transplant 1994; 13:714–719.
72. O'Brien JD, Lium JH, Parosa JF, DeYoung BR, Wick MR, Trulock EP. Lymphangiomyomatosis recurrence in the allograft after single-lung transplantation. Am J Respir Crit Care Med 1995; 151:2033–2036.
73. Kalassian KG, Doyle R, Kao P, Ruoss S, Raffin TA. Lymphangioleiomyomatosis: new insights. Am J Respir Crit Care Med 1997; 155:1183–1186.
74. Bacchi CE, Bonetti F, Pea M, Martignoni G, Gown AM. HMB–45. A review. Appl Immunohistochem 1996; 4:73–85.
75. Hoon V, Thung SN, Kaneko M, Unger PD. HMB-45 reactivity in renal angiomyolipoma and lymphangioleiomyomatosis. Arch Pathol Lab Med 1994; 118:732–734.
76. Tanaka H, Imada A, Morikawa T, Shibusa T, Satoh M, Sekine K, Abe S. Diagnosis of pulmonary lymphangioleiomyomatosis by HMB45 in surgically treated spontaneous pneumothorax. Eur Respir J 1995; 8:1879–1882.
77. Chan JKC, Tsang WYW, Pau MY, Tang MC, Pang SW, Fletcher CDM. Lymphangiomyomatosis and angiomyolipoma: closely related entities characterized by hamartomatous proliferation of HMB-45 positive smooth muscle. Histopathology 1993; 22:445–455.
78. Guinee DG Jr, Feuerstein I, Koss MN, Travis WD. Pulmonary lymphangio-

leiomyomatosis. Diagnosis based on results of transbronchial biopsy and immunohistochemical studies and correlation with high-resolution computed tomography findings. Arch Pathol Lab Med 1994; 118:846–849.

79. Bonetti F, Chiodera PL, Pea M, Martignoni G, Bosi F, Zamboni G, Mariuzzi GM. Transbronchial biopsy in lymphangiomyomatosis of the lung. HMB45 for diagnosis. Am J Surg Pathol 1993; 17:1092–1102.
80. Castro M, Shepherd CW, Gomez MR, Lie JT, Ryu JH. Pulmonary tuberous sclerosis. Chest 1995; 107:189–195.
81. Berg G, Zachrisson CG. Cystic-lungs of rare origin—tuberous sclerosis. Acta Radiol 1941; 22:425–436.
82. Rigault JY, Brun J, Rigault-Guillemot I, Galateau-Salle F, Boute V, Bertaux M. Les atteintes pulmonaires de la sclérose tubéreuse de Bourneville. Intérêts du dépistage précoce. A propos d'une forme familiale. Rev Mal Respir 1993; 10:366–370.

3

Clinical Experience with Lymphangioleiomyomatosis in the United Kingdom

MARC C. I. LIPMAN

Royal Free Hospital School of Medicine
London, England

ROLAND M. duBOIS

Royal Brompton Hospital
London, England

The Royal Brompton Hospital's position as a national cardiopulmonary referral center provides an unprecedented opportunity within the United Kingdom for the acquisition of extensive clinical experience and data collection on rare respiratory conditions. Lymphangioleiomyomatosis (LAM) is such a disease. Here we report the clinical findings of patients with LAM seen at this hospital over the last 20 years.

I. Methods

A retrospective case-note review was performed on all patients with LAM seen at the Royal Brompton for a clinical opinion over the 20 years from1976 to 1996. Subjects were located by searching clinical, pathological, radiological, and lung function databases.

The increasing advances in the diagnostic ability of high-resolution computed tomography (CT) scanning, as well as the appreciation that LAM has characteristic radiological appearances, were deemed sufficient justification to allow positive diagnoses of LAM to be made on the basis of either histological (lung tissue biopsy) or radiological (CT scan or chest radiograph) criteria. In practice, many cases had diagnostic confirmation performed by both methods.

Data extraction regarding time of onset of first and subsequent symptoms prediagnosis of LAM were performed in an accepted manner (1).

The sample size of the study population was large enough for means and 95% confidence intervals to accurately reflect the raw data. Two group comparisons were performed using two-tail student's *t*-test with paired or unpaired analyses as necessary.

II. Results

Twenty-two subjects were identified with LAM. In 14 cases the diagnosis was based initially on lung biopsy. Thirteen of these were thoracoscopic or open lung procedures, and one was via transbronchial biopsy. Ten of the 14 subjects had subsequent thoracic CT scans—in all cases these verified the tissue diagnosis. A primary radiological diagnosis was made in eight subjects. Seven of these had CT scans (two with subsequent tissue confirmation), and one had a diagnosis based on chest radiographic appearances. This case has been included in this analysis as it is felt that the patient's disease process in clinical and radiological terms was entirely consistent with LAM.

A. Clinical Presentation

All 22 subjects were premenopausal women. Twenty-one were of Caucasian origin, whereas one was of African descent. Their mean age at diagnosis was 35.5 years (Table 1). This was, on average, 4¾ years after the first onset of symptoms attributable to LAM. Fewer than half of the women had ever smoked cigarettes (9/22, or 41%), and only four were still smoking within one year of the first onset of symptoms. Two women were taking gynecological hormonal preparations prior to diagnosis. One was using a combined oral contraceptive pill, while the other was taking hormone-replacement therapy following oophorectomy for endometriosis. No family history of LAM was found in any of the 22 women.

Table 1 Age at Symptom Onset and Diagnosis Within the LAM Population

	Mean (95% confidence intervals)
Age at first symptoms (years)	30.7 (26.5–35.0)
Age at diagnosis (years)	35.5 (31.4–39.5)
Time from first symptoms—diagnosis (months)	56.6 (22.6–90.7)

n = 22.

Table 2 shows the range of symptoms both prior to diagnosis and also with disease progression in all 22 subjects. Although pneumothorax was the most common presenting symptom (seen in nine cases, four of which were right-sided, two left-sided, and three bilateral pneumothoraces), by the time of diagnosis persistent breathlessness was the most frequent subjective complaint (noted in 14 of 22, or 64% of patients). On further follow-up all 22 women developed progressive shortness of breath. Pneumothorax did not follow the same pattern in that recurrence post LAM diagnosis was relatively common (occurring in 5 of the 11 women with previous pneumothorax, and not limited to the previously affected side), although only one further woman developed pneumothoraces de novo during her illness. This finding was not explained either by the length of follow-up or by any differences in CT scan or histological lung tissue appearances in those who did or did not develop pneumothorax.

Other symptoms such as cough, hemoptysis, and presentation with pleural effusions were relatively rare (Table 2). One of the three subjects with chylous effusions also had chylous ascites and a retroperitoneal mass. Three other women had previous histories of renal angiomyolipoma prior to their final diagnosis. One woman subsequently shown to have LAM was noted to have an abnormal chest radiograph during a routine medical examination at another center several years prior to her clinical presentation. At that time she was symptom-free, although she subsequently developed hemoptysis and progressive breathlessness.

Clinical signs were often minimal or absent at the time of diagnosis, with almost half of the patients having no detectable physical abnormalities (Table 3). Crackles on auscultation were the only consistent clinical finding (9/22, or 41%). Pneumothorax was present at diagnosis in only two (9%) subjects, emphasizing the potential difficulty of diagnosis when LAM presents with pneumothorax.

Table 2 Frequency and Progression of Presenting Symptoms Within the LAM Population

	First symptom ($n = 22$)[a]	Subsequent symptoms prediagnosis	Subsequent symptoms postdiagnosis
Pneumothorax	9 (41%)	11 (50%)	12 (55%)
Progressive dyspnea	6 (27%)	14 (64%)	22 (100%)
Cough	3 (14%)	3 (14%)	3 (14%)
Pleural effusion	2 (9%)	3 (14%)	3 (14%)
Hemoptysis	1 (5%)	3 (14%)	4 (18%)

[a]One patient had an abnormal chest radiograph while asymptomatic.

Table 3 Clinical Signs Present at Diagnosis of LAM

Clinical signs at diagnosis	$n = 22$
None	10 (45%)
Crackles	9 (41%)
Pneumothorax	2 (9%)
Wheeze	1 (5%)
Pulmonary hypertension	1 (5%)
Clubbing	0 (0%)
Pleural effusion	0 (0%)
Ascites	0 (0%)

B. Physiological and Radiological Assessments at Diagnosis

Lung function results are summarized in Table 4. A marked obstructive defect was seen, with impaired spirometry, elevated residual volumes, and reduced transfer capacity after correction for lung volumes. Blood gases at rest on air revealed mild hypoxemia, although at the expense of hyperventilation (low-normal Pa_{CO_2}) (Table 4). These results provide a good physiological explanation of the subjects' complaint of exertional breathlessness.

Twenty-one subjects had chest radiograph reports documented at the time of diagnosis. All of these were abnormal, with the most common finding being reticulo-nodular shadowing (13/21, or 62% cases), followed by hyperinflation in seven cases and cysts and/or bullae in five (Table 5). Seventeen women had thoracic CT scans performed within 3 years of diagnosis. As expected, these were

Table 4 Lung Function at Diagnosis of LAM

Lung function at diagnosis	Mean (95% confidence intervals)
FEV1 [%], n = 20	45.8 (35.2 - 56.4)
FVC [%], n = 20	74.3 (62.5 - 86.1)
FEV1:FVC, n = 20	57.3 (46.8 - 67.8)
TLC [%], n = 18	105.7 (94.9 - 116.4)
RV [%], n = 16	168.9 (140.6 - 197.2)
DLCO [%], n = 20	41.3 (33.7 - 48.9)
KCO [%], n = 19	55.1 (40.6 - 69.6)
PaO_2 [kPa], n = 17	9.2 (8.3 - 10.1)
SaO_2 [%], n = 18	93.3 (91.7 - 94.9)
$PaCO_2$ [kPa], n = 17	4.5 (4.1 - 4.9)

Table 5 Chest Radiographic Features Present at Diagnosis of LAM

CXR appearance at diagnosis	*n* = 21
Reticulo-nodular shadowing	13 (62%)
Hyperinflation	7 (33%)
Cysts or bullae	5 (24%)
Pleural thickening	3 (14%)
Pneumothorax	2 (10%)
Pleural effusion	1 (5%)
Large pulmonary arteries	1 (5%)
Normal	0 (0%)

all abnormal, with cysts (15/17, or 88%) followed by reticular changes (7/14, or 41%) being the most common reported features (Table 6).

C. Specific Treatments for LAM

Apart from general supportive measures such as home oxygen therapy, which were prescribed as needed, 16 of the 22 (73%) women started either medical or surgical treatment to control their disease. Hormone receptor studies were performed in only four subjects. Here one woman was estrogen positive, one was both estrogen and progesterone positive, one was progesterone positive, and one was estrogen negative. The results of these studies did not influence future management decisions, and the different treatments used are detailed in Table 7. By far the most common drug prescribed was depot progestogen at a dosage of 300 mg per month (13/16, or 81%). In general this was well tolerated, being taken for a mean time of 45.6 months (95% CI = 19.6–71.7 months). Other drugs such as gonadotrophin hormone–releasing hormone (GnRH) analogs were used much less frequently (4/16, or 25% cases), and then only as a second-line therapy to

Table 6 CT Scan Appearances of LAM

CT thorax within 3 years of diagnosis	*n* = 17
Cysts	15 (88%)
Reticular shadowing	7 (41%)
Pneumothorax	4 (24%)
Pleural effusion	2 (12%)
Adenopathy	0 (0%)

Table 7 Therapies Used to Treat LAM

	Treatments	$n = 16$
Medical	Progestogens	13 (81%)
	GnRH analogues	4 (25%)
	Castration	1 (6%)
	Tamoxifen	1 (6%)
	Other	7 (44%)
Surgical	Transplant assessment	8 (50%)
	Transplant surgery	2 (13%)

[a]3 oral prednisolone (1 + cyclophosphamide); 3 inhaled steroids (1 concurrent asthma); 1 hormone replacement therapy.

progestogens. Inhaled or oral steroids were used in a total of six subjects, one of whom had a previous history of reversible airways disease.

Therapy with only one drug was used in 7 of 16 women (43%). However, a further 8 women were then switched to a second treatment when the first was deemed to have failed. Only one patient then moved to a third drug regime when the second was found to provide no benefit.

Lung transplant assessment was performed in eight subjects. All of these women had previously taken medical therapy. To date two patients have undergone successful single lung transplantation with a posttransplant survival and follow-up of 46 and 55 months, respectively. A further two patients are awaiting transplants, while two were excluded from transplantation on medical grounds and two women died within the time period of their assessments.

D. Survival and Outcome

At data censure (either death or last documented clinical review), 5 of the 22 women had died of LAM. Mean overall survival for the 22 subjects was 126.4 months (95% CI = 75.1–177.6 months). Follow-up, and therefore apparent survival, was longer in the five who died, although this did not reach statistical significance (mean and 95% CI for dead = 172 months, 27.9–316.1; mean and 95% CI for subjects alive at data censure = 112.9 months, 53.6–172.3 months).

Adequate follow-up data were available on 19 of the original 22 women. Of these, 12 (63%) were considered to have slowly progressive or stable disease on clinical grounds, while seven (37%) had a much more rapid decline. Serial lung function data recorded over an average of 5 years confirmed the great variability in outcome. For example, despite highly significant overall reductions in forced expiratory volume in one second (FEV_1, $p = 0.003$), forced vital capacity

Table 8 Change in Lung Function Over Time in LAM Population (mean and 95% confidence intervals shown)

	Diagnosis	Follow up	*p* value
FEV1 [%], $n = 15$	46.7 (34.8–58.6)	37.3 (24.6–49.9)	0.003
FVC [%], $n = 15$	77.2 (62.2–92.2)	65 (46.4–83.6)	0.02
FEV1:FVC, $n = 15$	55.8 (43.8–67.8)	51.3 (42.3–60.3)	0.15
TLC [%], $n = 12$	109.8 (93.1–126.5)	109.1 (93.6–124.6)	0.57
RV [%], $n = 12$	170 (126.6–213.4)	185.3 (150.8–219.9)	0.26
DLCO [%], $n = 13$	44.6 (35.3–54)	33.8 (23.7–43.8)	0.001
KCO [%], $n = 13$	59.8 (38.8–80.7)	49 (31–67)	0.004
PaO_2 [kPa], $n = 11$	9.4 (8.1–10.7)	8.7 (6.8–10.6)	0.32
SaO_2 [%], $n = 12$	92.8 (90.5–95)	89.3 (85–93.7)	0.03
$PaCO_2$ [kPa], $n = 11$	4.4 (3.9–4.9)	4.8 (4.2–5.3)	0.11

(FVC, $p = 0.02$), and transfer factor (DLCO, $p = 0.001$) (Table 8), a wide range of results were evident (Figs. 1 and 2). In general, lung obstruction and destruction progressed over time, though the ratio of FEV_1 to FVC did not change significantly during the follow-up period (Table 8 and Fig. 3). Despite a reduction in the oxygen saturations with time, no significant change was seen in either oxygen or carbon dioxide resting blood gas tensions during follow-up.

Baseline lung function did not appear to predict the rate of progressions or indeed clinical outcome. For example, Figure 2 shows that the patient with the lowest initial DLCO (diagnosis based on both histology and CT scans) had minimal further decline in lung function and had one of the longest overall survivals. The relatively short duration of progestogen drug therapy when compared to overall survival made it difficult to determine whether treatment had an effect in either reversing, stabilizing, or slowing up the disease process. Of the 12 women considered to have relatively benign disease, 7 used progestogens and 5 did not. Within the rapid progressors, 5 had been prescribed drug therapy and 2 had not.

III. Discussion

The findings from this study are largely consistent with the published literature. LAM was only seen in premenopausal women (1–3) with no apparent personal history of note (4). As found in previous studies, there was often a long delay between the first onset of symptoms and subsequent diagnosis (1,5). On the whole this could be explained by the nonspecific presentation of pneumothorax or slowly progressive breathlessness, which might have initially suggested less complex alternative diagnoses such as idiopathic pneumothorax, asthma, or emphy-

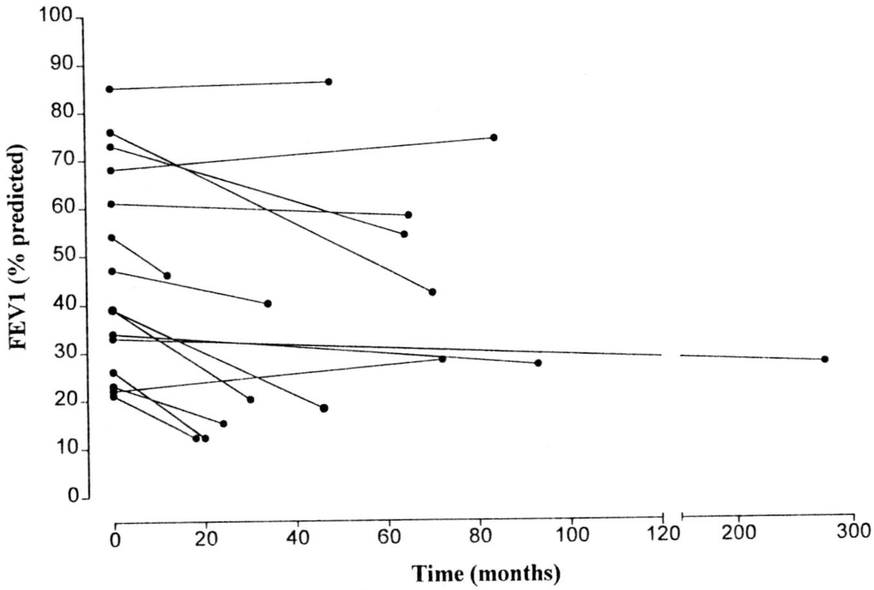

Figure 1 Changes in individual subjects' forced expiratory volume in 1 second (FEV_1) over time ($n = 15$).

sema (1). However, it is important to note that all chest radiographs were reported as abnormal at the time of diagnosis and that one subject had radiological abnormalities present while still asymptomatic. These data suggest that it should be possible to diagnose LAM at an earlier stage in its natural history than achieved in this and other studies (1,2).

Our study population had little evidence for extrapulmonary disease (three renal angiomyolipomas and one retroperitoneal mass). However, this may represent an underestimation as this is frequently asymptomatic (6).

Although lung tissue biopsy has long been regarded as the gold standard, and indeed may have some prognostic significance (2), thoracic CT scanning is now a widely accepted diagnostic modality. In our study over one third of women had a diagnosis of LAM based on initial CT scan findings, and all subjects scanned had abnormal radiology. CT, with its avoidance of tissue sampling error as well as its noninvasive nature, is increasingly used in the investigation of respiratory disease. This would be expected to lead to the earlier pickup of conditions such as LAM.

Lung function results were similar to those reported in previous studies (1–3). Subjects had marked obstructive features associated with significant paren-

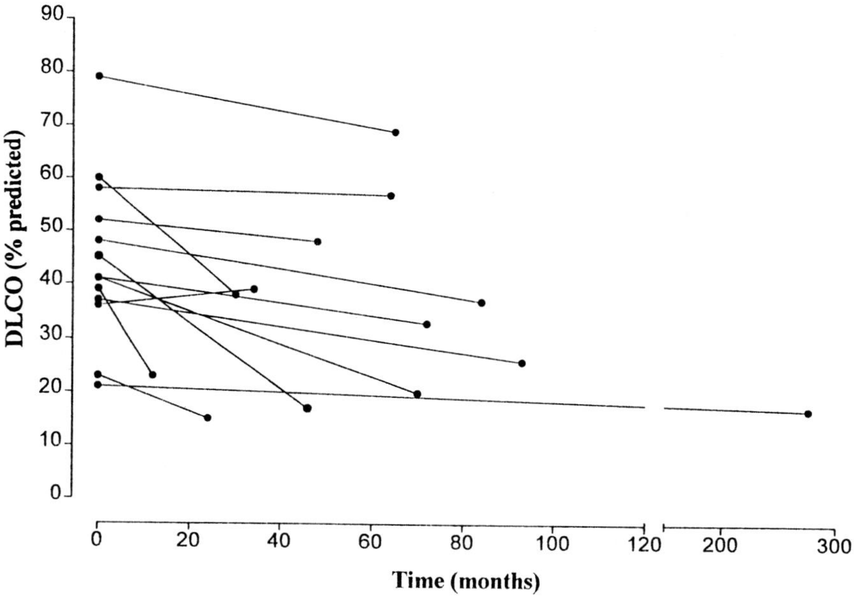

Figure 2 Changes in individual subjects' diffusing capacity (DLCO) over time ($n = 13$).

chymal lung damage. Again it is likely that these abnormalities were present for some time prior to diagnosis as serial lung function data revealed relatively gradual declines in lung physiology.

The majority of women started medical treatment for their condition. In most cases this was with depot progestogen preparations, which appeared to be well tolerated though of uncertain efficacy. Lung transplantation is a relatively new therapeutic option (5) which was considered in several of our patients. However, to date only 25% of those assessed have actually received a lung transplant, indicating the chronic shortage of organs available for donation.

Our patients had an overall survival time (from first symptoms to either death, in five cases, or last review) of approximately 10 years. This is in line with one large study (1), though longer than several others (2,3,7). There was, however, a relatively wide variation in survival times, with some subjects living for 20 years. No particular clinical or physiological measure appeared to predict a more rapid disease progression (2).

In conclusion this review of patients attending our center suggests that the clinical features and survival of our United Kingdom population is similar to that reported by other groups worldwide. An increased awareness of LAM together

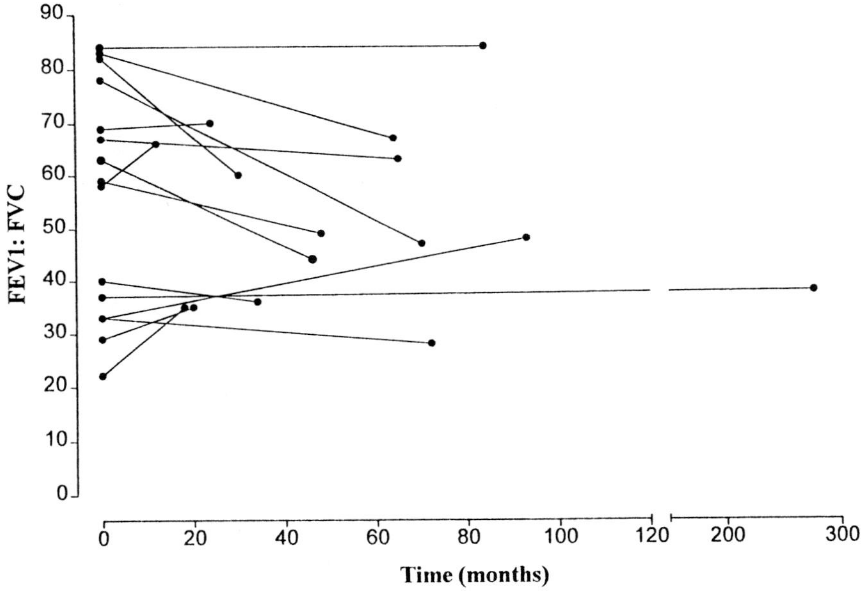

Figure 3 Changes in individual subjects' FEV_1:FVC ratio over time (n = 15).

with a greater use of noninvasive investigations may decrease the time from first symptoms to diagnosis, though whether this improves overall outcome remains unclear.

Acknowledgments

We would like to acknowledge the help of our colleagues at Royal Brompton Hospital in providing the clinical data used in this chapter.

References

1. Taylor JR, Ryu J, Colby TV, Raffin TA. Lymphangioleiomyomatosis: clinical course in 32 patients. N Engl J Med 1990; 323:1254–1260.
2. Kitaichi M, Nishimura K, Itoh H, Izumi T. Pulmonary lymphangioleiomyomatosis: a report of 46 patients including a clinicopathologic study of prognostic factors. Am J Respir Crit Care Med 1995; 151:527–533.
3. Corrin B, Liebow AA, Friedman PJ. Pulmonary lymphangioleiomyomatosis: a review. Am J Pathol 1975; 79:347–382.
4. Wahedna I, Cooper S, Williams J, Paterson IC, Britton JR, Tattersfield AE. Relation

to pulmonary lymphangioleiomyomatosis to use of the oral contraceptive pill and fertility in the UK: a national case control study. Thorax 1994; 49:910–914.
5. Boehler A, Speich R, Russi EW, Weder W. Lung transplantation for lymphangio leiomyomatosis. N Engl J Med 1996; 335:1275–1280.
6. Maziak DE, Kesten S, Rappaport DC, Maurer J. Extrathoracic angiomyolipoma in lymphangioleiomyomatosis. Eur Respir J 1996; 9:402–405.
7. Silverstein EF, Ellis K, Wolff M, Jaretzki A III. Pulmonary lymphangioleiomyomatosis. Am J Roentgenol 1974; 120:832–850.

4

Lymphangioleiomyomatosis
Clinical Aspects

KENNETH G. KALASSIAN, GERALD J. BERRY, and THOMAS A. RAFFIN

Stanford University Medical Center
Stanford, California

I. Introduction

More than 50 years ago, von Stössel (1) reported autopsy findings of diffuse cystic changes of the lung and dilated thoracic lymphatics in a premenopausal woman who died of respiratory failure of unknown etiology. He termed the process "muscular cirrhosis" of the lung. Shortly thereafter, Rosendal (2) reported a similar case in which he described his findings as "myomatosis" of the lung. These represent the first case reports of what is now known as lymphangioleiomyomatosis, a disease that has since both fascinated and frustrated the physicians who have had the uncommon opportunity to care for patients with this disease. Although much information has been accrued about the pathological and clinical manifestations of LAM, the molecular and cellular mechanisms responsible for the disease have remained a mystery and an effective treatment has yet to be defined. Advances in the techniques of molecular biology, however, have led to better characterization of the molecular features of the LAM cell and its kinship to cellular characteristics of another disease state, malignant melanoma. These advances have set the stage for elucidation of the molecular pathogenesis of LAM and for the future development of a definitive therapy.

II. Epidemiology

More than 300 cases of LAM are reported in the medical literature. The rarity of the disease makes estimates of incidence and prevalence difficult. It is suggested that there are no more than 3 cases per 100,000 population. The majority of those afflicted with the disease are premenopausal women. LAM has been reported, however, in a small number of postmenopausal women, the oldest reported being 72 years of age (3). The disease has also been reported in a man (4) and in a male bottlenose dolphin, *Turlops truncatus*, with a profoundly low testosterone level (5).

III. Pathology and Pathogenesis

The smooth muscle cells found in LAM are cytologically distinctive and phenotypically heterogeneous (6). Plump, spindle-shaped cells with round or ovoid nuclei and pale cytoplasm coexist with large polygonal cells with clear cytoplasm and epithelioid features (Fig. 1). The presence of alpha-smooth muscle–specific

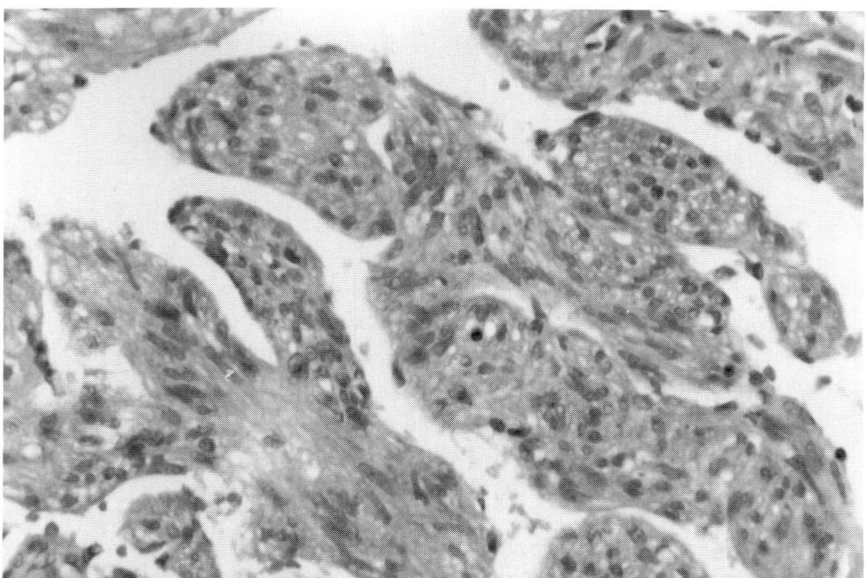

Figure 1 Light microscopy of an open lung biopsy specimen from a patient with LAM. Note the heterogeneous cellular morphology ranging from spindle-like cells to polygonal cells with epithelioid-like features.

actin in these cells confirms their myoid lineage (7). Electron microscopy demonstrates, nevertheless, that LAM cells have features unusual to smooth muscle cells such as multiply indented round to ovoid nuclei with prominent nucleoli, prominent microfilament bundles with dense bodies, and well-developed endoplasmic reticulum (8–10). Conspicuous are numerous electron-dense membrane-bound granules consisting of fine crystal-like lamellae (Fig. 2). Similar cells are found in angiomyolipomas of the kidney and liver as well as clear cell tumors of the lung (11,12). It has been proposed that the cellular heterogeneity represents various degrees of differentiation of a novel cell type related to tumors and tumor-like lesions associated with prominent vascular proliferation (13).

In addition to myoid markers, LAM cells stain with HMB-45, a monoclonal antibody derived from melanoma hybridomas which previously had been considered specific for melanocytic cell lines (Fig. 3). It is possible that HMB-45 staining of LAM cells represents cross-reactivity with an antigen similar, but distinct from, that of cells that display melanogenesis. That a characteristic staining pattern is identifiable in all HBM-45–reactive cells, including LAM cells, suggests that the reactive antigen in melanocytic cell lines and in LAM is the same. The HBM-45–reactive antigen in melanocytic cells has been localized to the cytoplasm and is associated with immature melanosomes (14). Expression cloning of the cDNA of the antigen, with subsequent cDNA sequence analysis and comparison with known sequences in genetic databases, has revealed total homology with the cDNA of Pmel 17, a gene important in the regulation of melanin biosynthesis (15).

The predilection of LAM for premenopausal women has led to the assumption that hormonal factors play an important role in the pathogenesis of the disease. The predilection of LAM for premenopausal women and reports of increased disease activity during pregnancy (16,17) and with exogenous estrogen administration (18) have stimulated investigation of the role of sex steroids in the abnormal smooth muscle proliferation of the disease. Analyses of estrogen and progesterone receptor expression in LAM cells have produced variable results (19–21). Interpretation is made more difficult by the use of varying techniques, either ligand binding assays or immunohistochemical methods, of receptor identification. It is unclear whether the variability represents methodological differences in receptor analysis or true heterogeneity in receptor expression (22).

The lesions of pulmonary LAM visible on light microscopy can be divided into two types: early, or active phase lesions, and late lesions (10). In the early lesions, abnormal accumulations of smooth muscle cells are found in the adventitia of the terminal bronchi, in the alveolar walls, and in the pleura. The alveolar/capillary interface is not involved. Involvement of the alveolar walls occurs in association with dilated emphysema-like alveolar spaces. Within the alveoli are found hyperplastic type II pneumocytes and hemosiderin-laden macrophages.

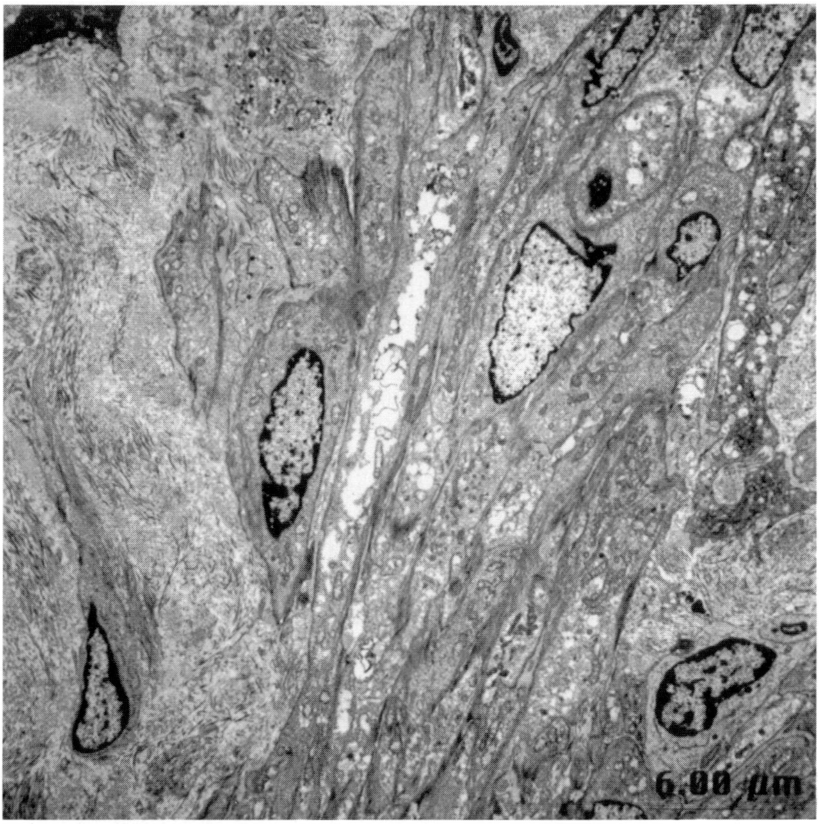

(A)

Figure 2 Features in LAM cells that are unusual in smooth muscle cells are seen in these electrons micrographs. These include (A) a multiply-indented nucleus (×2700) and prominent microfilaments with dense bodies, and (B) a well-developed endoplasmic reticulum (×25,000). Electron-dense membrane-bound granules are also found in melanoma cells and most likely represent the site of the antigen bound by the monoclonal antibody HMB-45.

The extracellular matrix of the smooth muscle cell infiltrate contains basement membrane components, fibrillar interstitial collagens, and fibronectin. At the periphery of the smooth muscle infiltrate, intense remodeling activity occurs with degradation of elastic fibers related to an imbalance in the elastase/α_1-proteinase system similar to the probable pathogenesis of emphysema (23). Fibronectin, the earliest matrix protein found in fibrogenesis, is present in abundance. Resi-

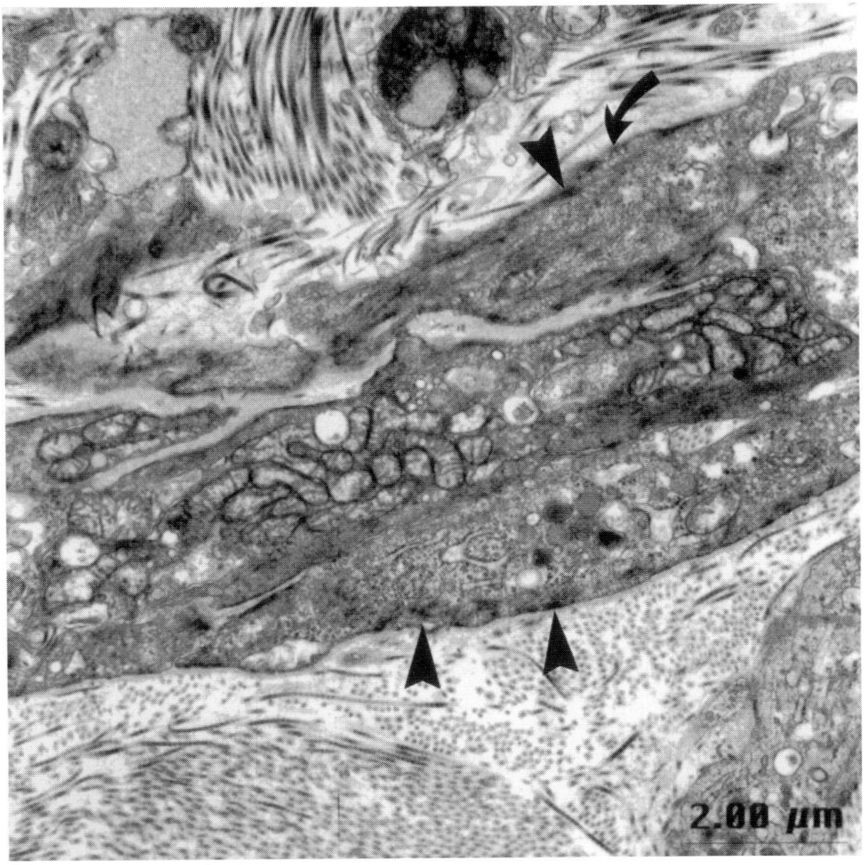

(B)

Figure 2 Continued.

dent lung interstitial cells, under the influence of the proliferating smooth muscle cells, increase their production of usual matrix proteins. In late lesions the smooth muscle accumulation, in association with increased collagen deposition, forms nodular aggregates. The markedly dilated alveolar spaces contain few hemosiderin-laden macrophages.

Macroscopically, the lungs of patients with LAM have multiple cystic spaces (Fig. 4), diffusely distributed without a peripheral or subpleural predilection, akin to emphysema (24). Dilated lymphatics form bleb-like lesions on the parietal and visceral pleural surfaces. On sectioning, focal areas of thickening in

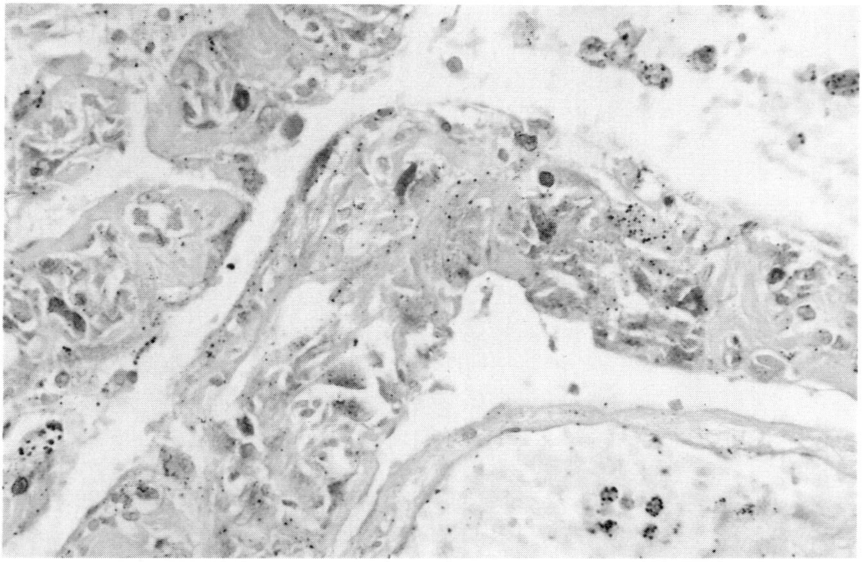

Figure 3 Light microscopy of lung LAM tissue stained with HMB-45, a monoclonal antibody derived from melanoma hybridomas. HMB-45 staining appears brown.

alveolar walls and septa are apparent and are surrounded by areas of normal lung parenchyma. Infiltration of pulmonary capillaries and venules results in obliteration of the pulmonary microvasculature producing hemorrhage and hemosiderosis. Abnormal smooth muscle proliferation occurs along lymphatics in peribronchovascular, lobular septal, and subpleural areas causing obstruction and marked dilatation. This proliferation is not confined to the lungs and occurs in extrapulmonary lymphatics, particularly those of the mediastinum and retroperitoneum. The other important extrapulmonary manifestation of the disease is its association with renal angiomyolipomas, hamartomatous lesions composed of smooth muscle, adipose tissue, and blood vessels that have been shown radiographically to be present in nearly 50% of patients with LAM (25).

IV. Clinical Characteristics

Patients with LAM most commonly present with exertional dyspnea and cough. Pneumothorax is often found on initial presentation. A minority of patients also have symptoms of chest pain, resting dyspnea, and hemoptysis. Physical exami-

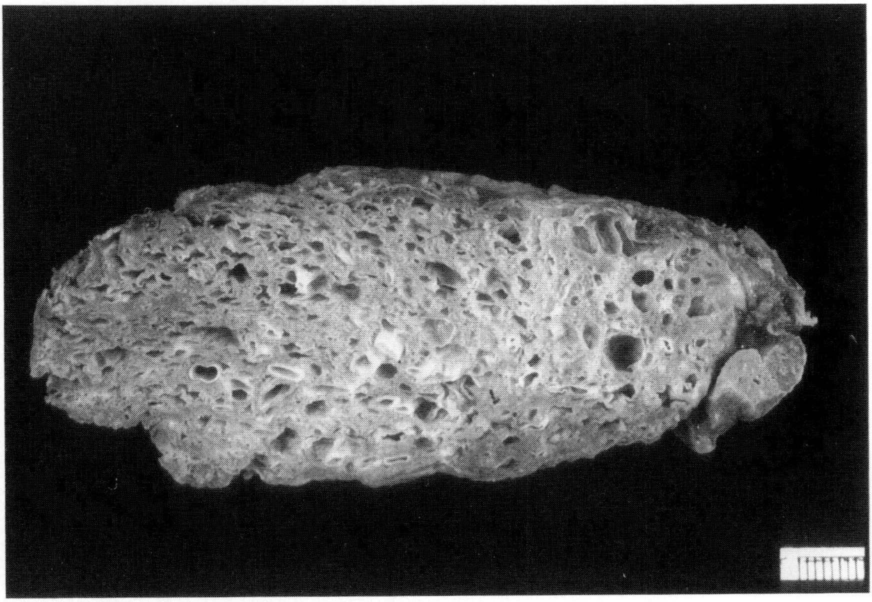

Figure 4 Macroscopic examination of the lungs of a patient with LAM. Multiple cystic spaces are diffusely distributed throughout the lungs. Markedly dilated lymphatics form bleb-like lesions on the pleural surface.

nation findings are nonspecific and include crackles, rhonchi, and, in a small number of patients, ascites (Table 1).

The predominant radiographic presentation is one of diffuse irregular linear opacities in a reticular pattern without a predominance for any one lung zone and with normal lung volumes (Fig. 5) (26). Sometimes radiographs reveal either a pneumothorax or a chylous pleural effusion. Cystic changes are uncommonly observed on chest radiograph and are usually recognized only when cyst size is greater than 1 cm. Over 50% of patients will have radiographic evidence of pneumothorax at the time of first presentation, and as many as 80% will develop a pneumothorax during the course of the disease (27,28). Pleural effusions, almost always chylous, are found in about 20% of patients (27). Hyperinflation may also be present. Computed tomography (CT) of the thorax (Fig. 6) most often reveals the presence of bilateral diffuse cystic airspace changes surrounded by areas of normal lung parenchyma (29–31). The majority of the cystic airspaces have walls of less than 2 mm. The size of the cysts correlates with disease extent and ranges from less than 0.5 cm to as great as 5 cm. Areas of airspace con-

Table 1 Clinical Findings at the Time of Presentation as Reported in the Two Largest Series of LAM Patients

	Taylor et al., 1990[a] (N = 32)	Kitaichi et al., 1995[b] (N = 46)
Symptoms		
Dyspnea		
Resting	0%	43%
Exertional	47	88
Cough	12	41
Chest Pain	12	14
Chyloptysis	0	0
Hemoptysis	9	39
Physical findings		
Crackles	NR	22
Wheezing	0	NR
Rhonchi	NR	14
Pleural effusion	0	11
Ascites	3	5
Chest radiography		
Normal	3	10
Reticular or reticulonodular changes	47	85
Cysts or bullae	12	45
Effusion	0	11
Pneumothorax	53	32
Hyperinflation	0	48

The differences in clinical findings suggest that the patients of Kitaichi et al. relative to the patients of Taylor et al., were diagnosed at a more advanced stage of disease.
NR = Not reported.
[a]From Ref. 27.
[b]From Ref. 28.

solidation presumably represent areas of hemorrhage. Semiquantitative scoring methods have been developed in an attempt to correlate the degree of radiologic abnormality with impairment in lung function (32). Although there is a better correlation with CT than with chest radiography, the correlation with pulmonary function in both cases is relatively low. The development of quantitative CT employing advanced image-processing techniques may result in a better correlation with physiologic measurements of disease severity (33).

In most patients with LAM, pulmonary function testing reveals the presence of obstruction with a reduced FEV_1 and FEV_1/FVC ratio (24,34,35). Lung

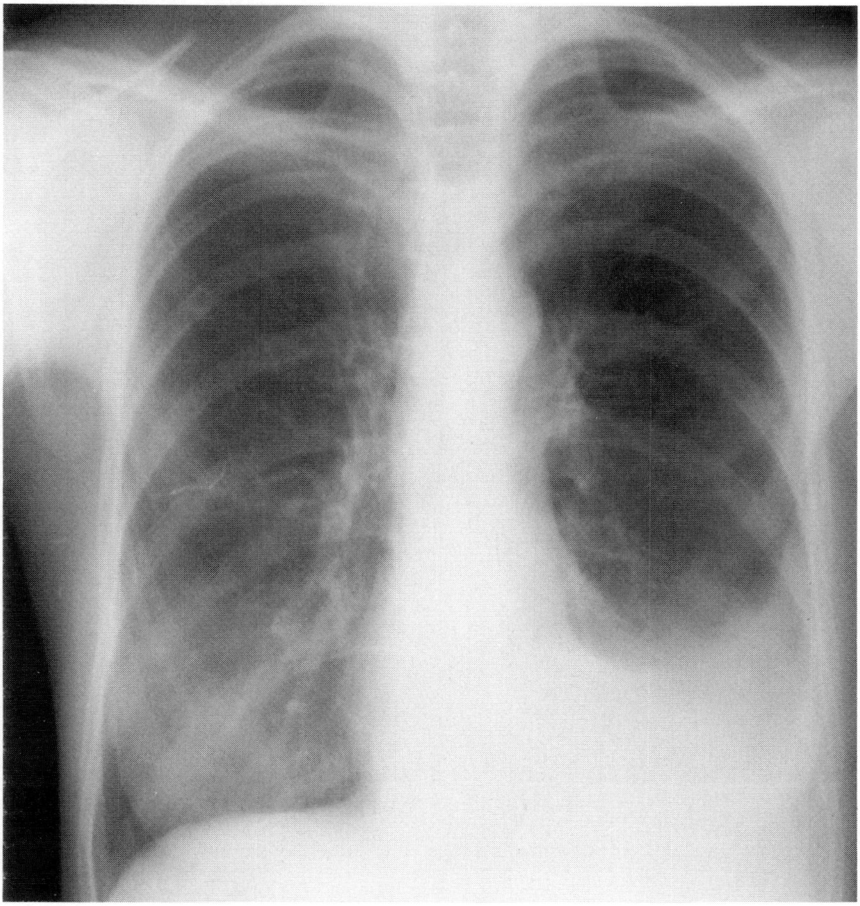

Figure 5 A posteroanterior chest radiograph from a patient with LAM. Reticular and reticulonodular opacities are present in the bases. There is a right chylous pleural effusion.

volumes are usually normal or increased and are reduced primarily in those patients who have large chylous effusions or who have undergone instrumentation of the thoracic cavity with or without pleurodesis. A reduction in elastic recoil forces, as evidenced by an increase in static compliance and a decrease in retractive force, contributes to airflow limitation. Maximal flow-static recoil curves suggest, however, that obstruction is primarily due to airway narrowing rather than the loss of elastic recoil (35). Diffusion of carbon monoxide is reduced due to both destruction of the alveolar-capillary interface as well as the presence

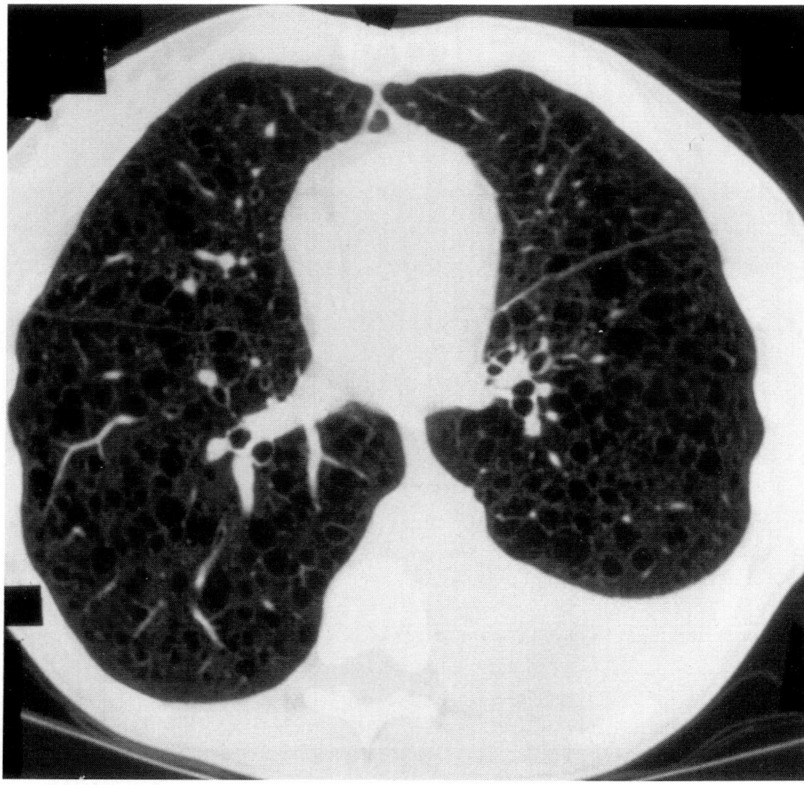

Figure 6 CT of the thorax from a patient with LAM. Bilateral cystic airspace changes 0.5–2 cm in diameter are surrounded by areas of normal lung parenchyma. A left chylous pleural effusion is also present.

of ventilation-perfusion abnormalities. Arterial blood gas analysis most often demonstrates hypoxemia without hypercapnia.

When cardiopulmonary exercise testing is performed in patients with LAM, impairment in exercise performance, as measured by percent of predicted maximum oxygen consumption and maximal work load, is significantly reduced (36). The reduction in exercise capacity is primarily due to ventilatory limitation. Airflow limitation results in a reduced ventilatory ceiling while ventilation-perfusion inequalities produce an excessive ventilatory response.

Misdiagnosis of LAM patients is common, often resulting in a significant delay between initial presentation and correct diagnosis (27) (Table 2). Any disease that manifests as cystic changes on chest radiograph or CT, such as emphysema or eosinophilic granuloma, may resemble LAM (29). Although correlation

Table 2 Differential Diagnosis in Patients with Suspected Lymphangioleiomyomatosis

Asthma
COPD
α_1-Proteinase deficiency
Eosinophilic granuloma
Benign metastasizing leiomyoma
Mesenchymal cystic hamartoma
Cystic pulmonary sarcoma
Metastatic stromal sarcoma
Tuberous sclerosis

of radiographic findings with clinical information is often suggestive, invariably pathologic examination of a lung tissue specimen is required for confirmation of the diagnosis of LAM. Lung tissue from LAM patients obtained by transbronchial biopsy, or even by open lung biopsy, may mimic numerous pathologic entities; most frequently benign metastasizing leiomyoma, mesenchymal cystic hamartoma, or the pulmonary sarcomas. The use of immunohistochemical staining with HMB-45, a monoclonal antibody derived from melanoma hybridomas which stains LAM cells as well as melanocytic lesions, has improved the usefulness of transbronchial biopsy in the diagnosis of LAM (37). HMB-45 staining in conjunction with transbronchial biopsy may obviate the need for violation of the integrity of the thoracic cavity by a more invasive biopsy procedure and thus eliminate a hindrance to future lung transplantation.

V. Prognosis and Survival

A reduction in FEV_1/FVC, an increase in TLC, and the presence of more mature and extensive lesions on pathological examination are poor prognostic factors (28). Quantitative CT, besides its potential to assess severity of disease, may also find a role as a prognostic tool (33). Kaplan-Meier plots of actuarial survival of patients with LAM (Fig. 7) in the two most recently reported series reveal a survival at 8.5 years of 78% and 38%, respectively (27,28).

VI. Treatment

No prospective, randomized clinical trials exist to evaluate the various therapeutic modalities that have been employed in the treatment of LAM. Current strategies for treatment are based on the results of empiric attempts with various therapies

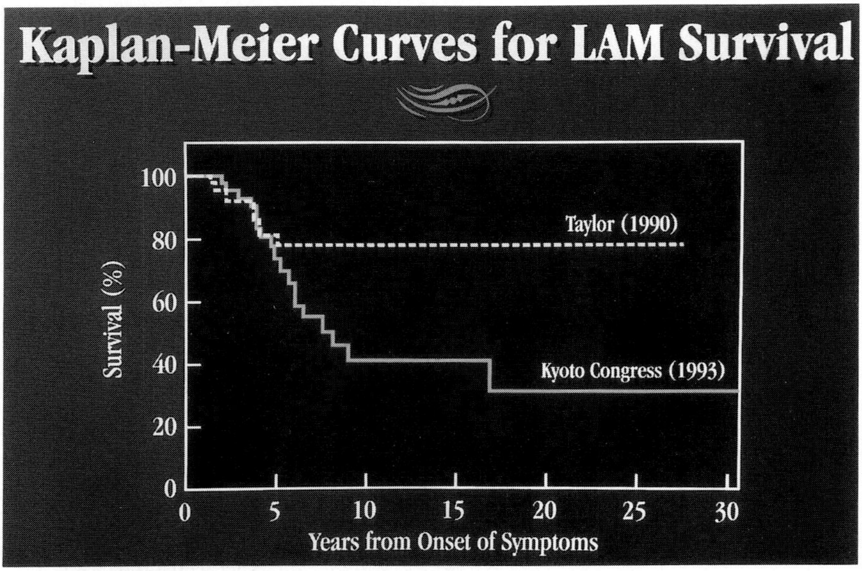

Figure 7 Kaplan-Meier plots of actuarial survival from the two largest and most recently reported series of LAM patients. The disparity in survival may be a function of sample sizes as well as the heterogeneity between the two populations as suggested by their different clinical characteristics (see Table 1).

as cited in isolated case reports or on assumptions based on evidence gleaned from the few existing small series of patients. The predilection of LAM for premenopausal women has led to the assumption that hormonal factors play an important role in the pathogenesis of the disease. Antiestrogen therapy has become the primary form of medical treatment. Ablation of ovarian function, by the administration of luteinizing-releasing hormone analogs (38,39), radiotherapy (40), and oophorectomy (41–45), has resulted in anecdotal reports of clinical benefit. The natural history of clinical deterioration has been significantly altered by these therapies in only rare instances. The use of alkylating chemotherapy agents and of interferon-α, with their significant toxicity and their lack of clearly demonstrated benefit, has been abandoned. Similarly, treatment with tamoxifen, because of its partial estrogen receptor agonist activity and the association of its use with exacerbation of disease, is uncommonly employed (27,46). There are no reports of the use of newer tamoxifen analogs, which lack partial agonist activity, in the treatment of LAM.

Progesterone has produced slowing of disease progression and, in a very small number of patients, clinical improvement (27,47–51). The purported mechanism of progesterone action involves downregulation of estrogen receptors but this remains unconfirmed. Response to progesterone therapy does not correlate with estrogen or progesterone receptor status but does correlate with the presence of chylous effusions or ascites (27). Commonly given in a dose of 400 mg as a monthly or bimonthly intramuscular injection, it may also be given in oral form as medroxyprogesterone acetate at a dose of 10–20 mg/day. Conversely, patients who are undergoing treatment with estrogen or estrogen receptor agonists (i.e., tamoxifen) should receive alternative therapy or have these medications discontinued. Pregnancy should be discouraged (16,17), and, as pregnancy may occur even while on progesterone therapy, barrier forms of contraception should be utilized.

The principles of care which apply to all patients with chronic lung disease also apply to patients with LAM. Adequate psychosocial support is crucial. As has been learned from the treatment of patients with breast cancer, lung cancer, and other serious diseases, participation in patient support groups and frequent contact with the treating physician so as to strengthen the patient-physician bond results in improvement in quality of life and may result in improved survival. The LAM Foundation (52), a national patient advocacy and support group, is an excellent resource.

LAM patients should routinely receive annual influenza vaccinations and polyvalent pneumococcal vaccine. The incidence of lower and upper respiratory tract infections in patients with LAM is most likely similar to that of patients with other chronic nonimmunologically mediated respiratory disease. Symptoms of infection should prompt a low threshold for treatment with antibiotics. Poor dentition, chronic sinusitis, and other abnormalities that predispose to lower respiratory tract infections should be aggressively addressed. It is the experience of the authors that the rare patient with LAM will, during course of the disease, develop airflow limitation that is responsive to bronchodilators. If deterioration in lung function occurs, a brief trial of bronchodilator therapy with inhaled β-agonists and anticholinergics may be warranted. Such airflow limitation is probably related to remodeling of the extracellular matrix by elastases and antielastases as described above and is likely not inflammatory in nature. Therefore, the benefit of inhaled corticosteroids would be expected to be minimal.

Cardiovascular fitness promotes physical as well as mental well-being, and an appropriate prescription for aerobic exercise should be provided to all patients capable of performing it. If the patient's impairment in lung function is severe, screening with exercise oximetry to observe for oxygen desaturation should be undertaken. If desaturation occurs, the initial phases of aerobic training may best be carried out through a supervised pulmonary rehabilitation program with supplemental oxygen provided as indicated. The utility of formal cardiopulmonary exercise testing is restricted to the realm of physiologic research and should not be routinely done.

The secondary complications of LAM are listed in Table 3. Most of those listed are found in most chronic lung diseases and are not complications specific to LAM. Acute and chronic respiratory failure are treated much as in any other noninflammatory obstructive lung disease including the use of noninvasive positive pressure ventilation and conventional mechanical ventilation as is clinically indicated. Guidelines for the treatment of lower respiratory tract infections in patients with chronic lung disease are also applicable to patients with LAM. Pneumothorax is often occult on posteroanterior chest radiograph. Any patient in which pneumothorax is suspected but difficult to confirm with standard chest radiography should promptly undergo CT imaging of the thorax. CT may also be useful for image-guided tube thoracostomy placement, particularly in patients with a complicated pleural space. Major hemoptysis is a rare complication, although death due to pulmonary hemorrhage has been reported.

In contrast, chylothorax, chylous ascites, and renal angiomyolipomas are rarely reported in association with any other primary pulmonary diseases. The effects of chyle loss may be classified as local, metabolic, or immunologic (53). Accumulation of chyle in the pleural space may lead to compression of the ipsilateral lung and atelectasis and, in the patient with limited respiratory reserve, acute respiratory failure. When chylous effusions become very large, mediastinal shift with hemodynamic compromise may occur. With prolonged chyle loss, protein, lipids, vitamins, and electrolytes are depleted. Hypoalbuminemia, hyponatremia, metabolic acidosis, and hypocalcemia develop in association with deficiencies of the fat-soluble vitamins A, D, E, and K. The main cellular component of chyle is T cells, and, with chyle loss, lymphopenia may develop resulting in an impairment in cell-mediated immunity (54).

Table 3 Secondary Complications of Lymphangioleiomyomatosis

Chronic respiratory failure
Acute respiratory failure
Lower respiratory tract infection
Pneumothorax
Major hemoptysis
Chylothorax
Chylous ascites
Renal angiomyolipomas

Treatment of chylous effusions begins with drainage via thoracentesis or tube thoracostomy. As for pneumothorax, tube thoracostomy placement is often best accomplished by under CT guidance. Losses of protein, electrolytes, and fat-soluble nutrients should be replaced. This may require the use of total parenteral nutrition. In order to reduce chyle flow, lipids are withheld with the exception of medium-chain triglycerides which are not transported by the intestinal lacteal system and thus are not a component of chyle. If these conservative measures fail to control chyle loss, a surgical approach may be indicated. Pleurodesis with tetracycline is often effective. Thoracoscopic ligation of chyle leaks, located preoperatively by lymphangiography and preoperatively by oral cream administration, has been successful in cases where pleurodesis has failed or has not been an option.

The major complications resulting from the presence of renal angiomyolipomas are retroperitoneal hemorrhage and hypertension resulting from invasion of the renal vein. Associated symptoms include flank or abdominal pain, a palpable mass, and hematuria. In the case of severe retroperitoneal hemorrhage, hypotension and marked anemia may also be present. In one recommended approach to management (55), symptomatic lesions greater than 4 cm in diameter, because of the high likelihood of the development of a major complication, should be treated with selective arterial embolization, enucleation, or partial nephrectomy. Total nephrectomy is rarely required and is reserved for instances in which other measures have failed. Patients with symptomatic lesions less than 4 cm in diameter should be monitored closely for prompt resolution of symptoms. If symptoms persist, angiography should be performed and embolization or surgical intervention should be considered. Asymptomatic lesions greater than 4 cm in diameter may be followed with semiannual imaging by CT or ultrasound. For asymptomatic lesions less than 4 cm imaging on an annual basis is sufficient.

The lack of an effective medical therapy for LAM has prompted treatment with lung transplantation. Patients who undergo transplantation often have severe airway obstruction with severe hyperinflation, have received instrumentation of the thoracic cavity or pleurodesis, and have had, and remain at high risk for, pneumothorax. These characteristics increase intraoperative and postoperative risk. Marked hemodynamic instability due to dynamic hyperinflation and intraoperative pneumothorax has been reported; in the latter case, institution of cardiopulmonary bypass was required (56,57). Most disturbing, however, are reports of recurrence of disease after transplantation (58,59). The technical challenges posed by LAM patients, combined with the medical and ethical dilemmas of transplantation for a systemic disease that may recur, make the issue of lung transplantation for LAM a complicated one. Medical and surgical advances in lung transplantation have resulted, however, in outcomes approaching that of transplantation for COPD, and transplantation will remain an important option for treatment for LAM patients who have progressed to respiratory failure.

VII. Future Directions

The absence of a cultured cell line or an animal model, combined with the rarity of LAM, have been obstacles to research regarding the biochemical and cellular processes responsible for the disease. Efforts at obtaining LAM cells in cell culture are underway. The discovery and characterization of the HMB-45–associated antigen in melanocytic cell lines may not only result in a better understanding of the molecular mechanisms at work in the disease but may also translate into the development of immunotherapeutic techniques for treatment of the disease (60). Elucidation of the role of hormonal control and the associated biochemical mechanisms will also be key to a better understanding of the disease process as well as to progress in creating an effective therapy. The National Institutes of Health has now committed to supporting research such as that described, thus providing hope that this fatal disease may in the future be overcome.

References

1. von Stössel E. Über muskulare Cirrhose der Lunge. Beitr Klin Tuberk 1937; 90:432–442.
2. Rosendal TR. A case of diffuse myomatosis and cyst formation in the lung. Acta Radiol 1942; 23:138–146.
3. Baldi S, Papotti M, Valente ML, Rapellino M, Scappaticci E, Corrin B. Pulmonary lymphangioleiomyomatosis in postmenopausal women: report of two cases and review of the literature. Eur Respir J 1994; 7(5):1013–1016.
4. Kang HW, Kim CJ, Kang SK, Lee KS, Lee CS, Kim YH. Pulmonary lymphangioleiomyomatosis in a male. J Korean Med Sci 1991; 6(1):83–85.
5. Rawson AJ, Patton GW, Brooks JS. Lymphangiomyomatosis in the Atlantic bottlenose dolphin (*Tursiops truncatus*). J Wildl Dis 1992; 28(2):323–325.
6. Bonetti F, Pea M, Martignoni G, Zamboni G, Iuzzolino P. Cellular heterogeneity in lymphangiomyomatosis of the lung [letter; comment]. Hum Pathol 1991; 22(7):727–728.
7. Matthews TJ, Hornall D, Sheppard MN. Comparison of the use of antibodies to alpha smooth muscle actin and desmin in pulmonary lymphangioleiomyomatosis. J Clin Pathol 1993; 46(5):479–480.
8. Basset F, Soler P, Marsac J, Corrin B. Pulmonary lymphangiomyomatosis: three new cases studied with electron microscopy. Cancer 1976; 39(6):2357–2366.
9. Kane PB, Lane BP, Cordice JW, Greenberg GM. Ultrastructure of the proliferating cells in pulmonary lymphangiomyomatosis. Arch Pathol Lab Med 1978; 102(12):618–622.

10. Peyrol S, Gindre D, Cordier JF, Loire R, Grimaud JA. Characterization of the smooth muscle cell infiltrate and associated connective matrix of lymphangiomyomatosis. Immunohistochemical and ultrastructural study of two cases. J Pathol 1992; 168(4):387–395.
11. Gaffey MJ, Mills SE, Askin FB, Ross GW, Sale GE, Kulander BG, Visscher DW, Yousem SA, Colby TV. Clear cell tumor of the lung. A clinicopathologic, immunohistochemical, and ultrastructural study of eight cases [see comments]. Am J Surg Pathol 1990; 14(3):248–259.
12. Pea M, Bonetti F, Zamboni G, Martignoni G, Fiore-Donati L, Doglioni C. Clear cell tumor and angiomyolipoma [letter; comment]. Am J Surg Pathol 1991; 15(2):199–202.
13. Bonetti F, Pea M, Martignoni G, Zamboni G. PEC and sugar [letter; comment]. Am J Surg Pathol 1992; 16(3):307–308.
14. Esclamado RM, Gown AM, Vogel AM. Unique proteins defined by monoclonal antibodies specific for human melanoma. Some potential clinical applications. Am J Surg 1986; 152(4):376–385.
15. Wagner SN, Wagner C, Hofler H, Atkinson MJ, Goos M. Expression cloning of the cDNA encoding a melanoma-associated Ag recognized by mAb HMB-45. Identification as melanocyte-specific Pmel 17 cDNA. Lab Invest 1995; 73(2):229–235.
16. Yockey CC, Riepe RE, Ryan K. Pulmonary lymphangioleiomyomatosis complicated by pregnancy. Kans Med 1986; 87(1):277–278, 293.
17. Hughes E, Hodder RV. Pulmonary lymphangiomyomatosis complicating pregnancy. A case report. J Reprod Med 1987; 32(7):553–557.
18. Shen A, Iseman MD, Waldron JA, King TE. Exacerbation of pulmonary lymphangioleiomyomatosis by exogenous estrogens. Chest 1987; 91(5):782–785.
19. Brentani MM, Carvalho CR, Saldiva PH, Pacheco MM, Oshima CT. Steroid receptors in pulmonary lymphangiomyomatosis. Chest 1984; 85(1):96–99.
20. Ohori NP, Yousem SA, Sonmez-Alpan E, Colby TV. Estrogen and progesterone receptors in lymphangioleiomyomatosis, epithelioid hemangioendothelioma, and sclerosing hemangioma of the lung. Am J Clin Pathol 1991; 96(4):529–535.
21. Berger U, Khaghani A, Pomerance A, Yacoub MH, Coombes RC. Pulmonary lymphangioleiomyomatosis and steroid receptors. An immunocytochemical study. Am J Clin Pathol 1990; 93(5):609–614.
22. Kinoshita M, Yokoyama T, Higuchi E, Yano H, Watanabe H, Rikimaru T, Ichikawa Y, Oizumi K. Hormone receptors in pulmonary lymphangiomyomatosis. Kurume Med J 1995; 42(3):141–144.
23. Fukuda Y, Kawamoto M, Yamamoto A, Ishizaki M, Basset F, Masugi Y. Role of elastic fiber degradation in emphysema-like lesions of pulmonary lymphangiomyomatosis [see comments]. Hum Pathol 1990; 21(12):1252–1261.
24. Corrin B, Liebow AA, Friedman PJ. Pulmonary lymphangiomyomatosis. A review. Am J Pathol 1975; 79(2):348–382.
25. Bernstein SM, Newell JD, Jr., Adamczyk D, Mortenson RL, King TE, Jr., Lynch DA. How common are renal angiomyolipomas in patients with pulmonary lymphangiomyomatosis? Am J Respir Crit Care Med 1995; 152(6 Pt 1):2138–2143.

26. Aberle DR, Hansell DM, Brown K, Tashkin DP. Lymphangiomyomatosis: CT, chest radiographic, and functional correlations. Radiology 1990; 176(2):381–387.
27. Taylor JR, Ryu J, Colby TV, Raffin TA. Lymphangioleiomyomatosis. Clinical course in 32 patients. N Engl J Med 1990; 323(18):1254–1260.
28. Kitaichi M, Nishimura K, Itoh H, Izumi T. Pulmonary lymphangioleiomyomatosis: a report of 46 patients including a clinicopathologic study of prognostic factors. Am J Respir Crit Care Med 1995; 151(2 Pt 1):527–533.
29. Rappaport DC, Weibrod GL, Herman SJ, Chamberlain DW. Pulmonary lymphangioleiomyomatosis: high-resolution CT findings in four cases. AJR Am J Roentgenol 1989; 152(5):961–964.
30. Templeton PA, McLoud TC, Muller NL, Shepard JA, Moore EH. Pulmonary lymphangioleiomyomatosis: CT and pathologic findings. J Comput Assist Tomogr 1989; 13(1):54–57.
31. Sherrier RH, Chiles C, Roggli V. Pulmonary lymphangioleiomyomatosis: CT findings [see comments]. AJR Am J Roentgenol 1989; 153(5):937–940.
32. Muller NL, Chiles C, Kullnig P. Pulmonary lymphangiomyomatosis: correlation of CT with radiographic and functional findings. Radiology 1990; 175(2):335–339.
33. Crausman RS, Lynch DA, Mortenson RL, King TE, Jr., Irvin CG, Hale VA, Newell JD, Jr. Quantitative CT predicts the severity of physiologic dysfunction in patients with lymphangioleiomyomatosis. Chest 1996; 109(1):131–137.
34. Carrington CB, Cugell DW, Gaensler EA, Marks A, Redding RA, Schaaf JT, Tomasian A. Lymphangioleiomyomatosis. Physiologic-pathologic-radiologic correlations. Am Rev Respir Dis 1977; 116(6):977–995.
35. Burger CD, Hyatt RE, Staats BA. Pulmonary mechanics in lymphangioleiomyomatosis. Am Rev Respir Dis 1991; 143(5 Pt 1):1030–1033.
36. Crausman RS J, CA, Mortenson RL, Ackerson LM, Irvin CG, King TE. Lymphangioleiomyomatosis: The pathophysiology of diminished exercise capacity. Am J Respir Crit Care Med 1996; 153:1368–1376.
37. Bonetti F, Chiodera PL, Pea M, Martignoni G, Bosi F, Zamboni G, Mariuzzi GM. Transbronchial biopsy in lymphangiomyomatosis of the lung. HMB45 for diagnosis [see comments]. Am J Surg Pathol 1993; 17(11):1092–1102.
38. Rossi GA, Balbi B, Oddera S, Lantero S, Ravazzoni C. Response to treatment with an analog of the luteinizing-hormone-releasing hormone in a patient with pulmonary lymphangioleiomyomatosis. Am Rev Respir Dis 1991; 143(1):174–176.
39. Radermecker M, Broux R, Corhay JL, Limet R, Radermecker M. Failure of buserelin-induced medical castration to control pulmonary lymphangiomyomatosis in two patients. Chest 1992; 101(6):1724–1726.
40. Flandes Aldeyturriaga J, Golpe Gomez A, Perez Rodriguez E. Lymphangioleiomyomatosis: the effectiveness of radiotherapy-induced ovarian function annulment. A case report. Respiration 1991; 58(3–4):214–218.
41. Adamson D, Heinrichs WL, Raybin DM, Raffin TA. Successful treatment of pulmonary lymphangiomyomatosis with oophorectomy and progesterone. Am Rev Respir Dis 1985; 132(4):916–921.

42. Banner AS, Carrington CB, Emory WB, Kittle F, Leonard G, Ringus J, Taylor P, Addington WW. Efficacy of oophorectomy in lymphangioleiomyomatosis and benign metastasizing leiomyoma. N Engl J Med 1981; 305(4):204–209.
43. Winter JA. Oophorectomy in lymphangioleiomyomatosis and benign metastasizing leiomyoma [letter]. N Engl J Med 1981; 305(23):1416–1417.
44. Logan RF, Fawcett IW. Oophorectomy for pulmonary lymphangioleiomyomatosis: a case report. Br J Dis Chest 1985; 79(1):98–100.
45. van Milligen de Wit AW, Meilof-Planteydt MN. Successful treatment of pulmonary lymphangioleiomyomatosis with oophorectomy and medroxyprogesterone-acetate: report of a case and brief review of the literature. Neth J Med 1990; 36(5-6):246–251.
46. Svendsen TL, Viskum K, Hansborg N, Thorpe SM, Nielsen NC. Pulmonary lymphangioleiomyomatosis: a case of progesterone receptor positive lymphangioleiomyomatosis treated with medroxyprogesterone, oophorectomy and tamoxifen. Br J Dis Chest 1984; 78(3):264–271.
47. Sawicka EH, Morris AJ. A report of two long-surviving cases of pulmonary lymphangioleiomyomatosis and the response to progesterone therapy. Br J Dis Chest 1985; 79(4):400–406.
48. McCarty KS, Jr., Mossler JA, McLelland R, Sieker HO. Pulmonary lymphangiomyomatosis responsive to progesterone. N Engl J Med 1980; 303(25):1461–1465.
49. Eliasson AH, Phillips YY, Tenholder MF. Treatment of lymphangioleiomyomatosis. A meta-analysis. Chest 1989; 96(6):1352–1355.
50. Burlew BP, Shames JM. Lymphangiomyomatosis: hormonal implications in etiology and therapy. South Med J 1991; 84(10):1247–1249.
51. Rajoub S, Blatt MW, Ritterspach J. Response to treatment with progesterone in a patient with pulmonary lymphangioleiomyomatosis. W V Med J 1995; 91(7):322–332.
52. LAM Foundation, Sue Byrnes, Executive Director. 10105 Beacon Hills Drive, Cincinnati, OH 45241.
53. Merrigan BA, Winter DC, and O'Sullivan GC. Chylothorax. Br J Surg 1997; 84:15–20.
54. Valentine VG, Raffin TA. The management of chylothorax. Chest 1992; 102(2):586–591.
55. Oesterling JE, Fishman EK, Goldman SM, Marshall FF. The management of renal angiomyolipoma. J Urol 1986; 135:1121–1124.
56. Popple C, Higgins TL, McCarthy P, Baldyga A, Mehta A. Unilateral auto-PEEP in the recipient of a single lung transplant. Chest 1993; 103(1):297–299.
57. Brusset A, Bonnette P, Hatahet Z, Loirat P, Bisson A, Fischler M. Single lung transplantation for pulmonary lymphangiomyomatosis. Unexpected need for extracorporeal circulation. Chest 1995; 107(1):278–282.
58. Nine JS, Yousem SA, Paradis IL, Keenan R, Griffith BP. Lymphangioleiomyomatosis: recurrence after lung transplantation. J Heart Lung Transplant 1994; 13(4):714–719.

59. O'Brien JD, Lium JH, Parosa JF, Deyoung BR, Wick MR, Trulock EP. Lymphangiomyomatosis recurrence in the allograft after single-lung transplantation. Am J Respir Crit Care Med 1995; 151(6):2033–2036.
60. Kalassian KG, Doyle R, Kao P, Ruoss SR, Raffin TA. New insights. Am J Respir Crit Care Med 1997; in press.

5

Lung Transplantation

Special Considerations and Outcome in LAM

ELBERT P. TRULOCK

Washington University School of Medicine
St. Louis, Missouri

I. Introduction

Pulmonary lymphangioleiomyomatosis (LAM) is a rare disease of uncertain pathogenesis that occurs almost exclusively in premenopausal women. The pathologic hallmark is the abnormal proliferation of smooth muscle around airways, blood vessels, and lymphatics in the lung. The common clinical manifestations include dyspnea, cough, and hemoptysis; progressive reticulonodular and/or cystic lung disease with obstructive, restrictive, or mixed pathophysiology; pneumothorax; and chylothorax (1,2). However, lesions can also be present in extrathoracic sites. Involvement of lymph nodes and lymphatics in the abdomen can cause chylous ascites, chyluria, and even chylous vaginal discharge, and renal angiomyolipomas have been detected in up to 47% of patients with LAM (3).

The natural history of pulmonary LAM is variable. Although the course is rather insidious in some patients, progressive lung disease ultimately leads to fatal respiratory complications in most cases. In several series, 22–50% of patients have died within 5 years of the onset of symptoms regardless of therapy (1,2,4,5).

Since 1983 lung transplantation has been performed for selected patients with a variety of end-stage diseases including LAM, and the results have been satisfactory (6–12). However, transplantation for LAM presents some unique problems and considerations. In this chapter, information on lung transplantation for LAM from the St. Louis International Lung Transplant Registry will be summarized, the experience at our center will be reviewed, and special issues in lung transplantation for LAM will be discussed.

II. Information from the Registry

In the January 1997 report, 6126 lung transplants had been recorded in the St. Louis International Lung Transplant Registry (13). The distribution of underlying diseases is shown in Table 1. LAM has been one of the less common indications for transplantation, accounting for only 1.5% of transplants in the registry.

The registry was queried on September 13, 1996, for additional information on recipients with a primary diagnosis of LAM (14); 82 cases were identified at that time and were analyzed further. Eighty recipients were female, but two were recorded as males (14). The mean age at the time of transplantation was 40 years (range, 23–55 years).

The registry does not contain information about complications, medical therapy, or lung function before transplantation, but these characteristics have been described in a multicenter survey of 34 recipients (12). In this study, approximately 75% of the patients had a pneumothorax, and all had medical treatment before transplantation. The majority had an obstructive pulmonary pathophysiologic pattern. The mean pretransplantation FEV_1 was 24 ± 12% of the predicted normal value, and the mean FEV_1/FVC ratio was 38 ± 12%.

Table 1 Indications for Lung Transplantation

Diagnosis	Number	% of transplants
Chronic obstructive pulmonary disease	1759	28.7
α_1-Antitrypsin deficiency emphysema	685	11.2
Idiopathic pulmonary fibrosis	960	15.7
Cystic fibrosis	932	15.2
Primary pulmonary hypertension	434	7.1
Eisenmenger's syndrome	131	2.1
Bronchiectasis	169	2.8
Sarcoidosis	91	1.5
Lymphangioleiomyomatosis	93	1.5
Retransplantation	169	2.8
Other	703	11.4
Total	6126	100.0

Source: St. Louis International Lung Transplant Registry, January 1997 Report.

The first lung transplant for LAM in the St. Louis Registry was performed in January 1988. The trend in annual activity is displayed in Figure 1. In recent years the number of procedures has reached a plateau of approximately 12–14 per year. No transplant center has reported a large experience with lung transplantation for LAM to the St. Louis Registry. Thirty-nine centers from the United States and abroad were represented among the 82 cases. One center reported 7 cases; two centers, 5 cases each; and five centers, 4 cases each.

The type of transplant operation and the actuarial survival after transplantation are depicted in Figure 2. For the group of 82 recipients, the survival rates were 76%, 56%, and 51% at 1, 3, and 5 years, respectively, after transplantation. These results are similar to the outcomes for all recipients in the St. Louis Registry (13), who had survival rates of 71%, 56%, and 45% at 1, 3, and 5 years, respectively, and to the results for all recipients in the Registry of International Society of Heart and Lung Transplantation (15) and the U.S. Scientific Registry (16). A formal statistical comparison of survival after single versus bilateral transplantation was not possible, but, considering the number of recipients in each group, a significant difference seems improbable.

On the date of the inquiry, 50 recipients were alive at their last follow-up, but 32 had died. The causes of death are tabulated in Table 2. As illustrated in Figure 2, mortality after lung transplantation for LAM is biphasic, and this pattern is typical of other diseases, too. The early, steep decline in survival is related to primary graft failure, infection, and other perioperative complications; the

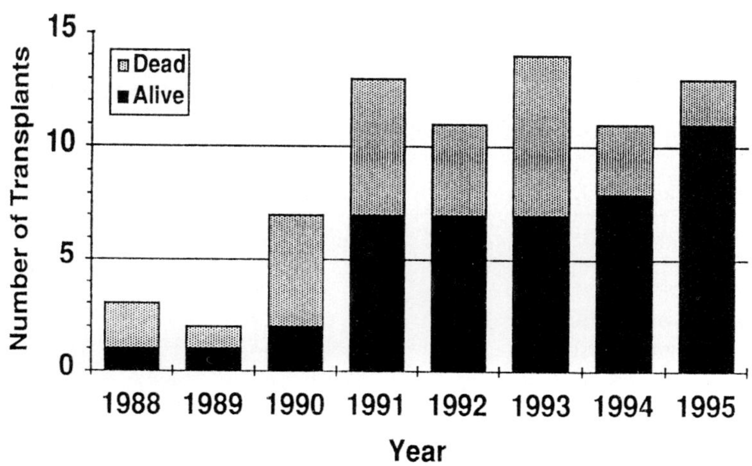

Figure 1 Lung transplant activity for LAM, by year, from the St. Louis International Lung Transplant Registry (September 13, 1996 query). The status of the recipients (dead or alive) as recorded in the Registry on the date of the query is shown.

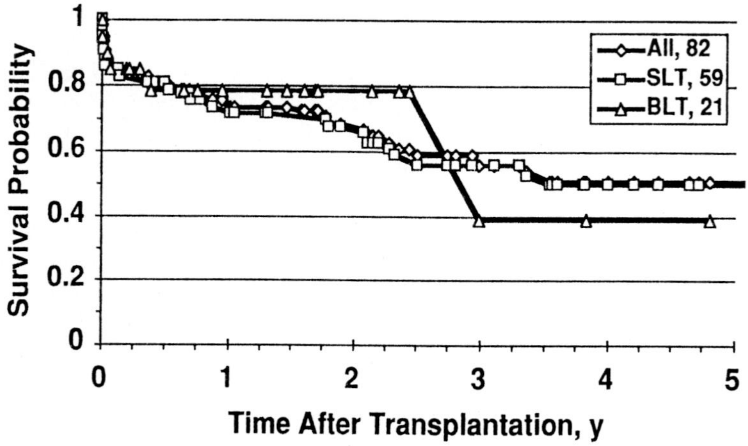

Figure 2 Actuarial survival of recipients with LAM after lung transplantation. Data from the St. Louis International Lung Transplant Registry; September 13, 1996. SLT, single lung transplantation; BLT, bilateral lung transplantation. Two recipients underwent an en bloc double lung transplant.

subsequent gradual attrition is caused mainly by infection and chronic allograft rejection.

III. Recipient Selection

Most lung transplant programs screen referrals and select candidates for lung transplantation according to standard protocols (17–20). In general, potential

Table 2 Causes of Death After Lung Transplantation for LAM

Cause of death	Number of deaths	% of deaths
Sepsis	9	28
Multisystem organ failure	5	16
Primary allograft failure	4	13
Rejection	4	13
Neoplasm	2	6
Cytomegalovirus infection	1	3
Other	6	19
Unknown	1	3
Total	32	

Source: St. Louis International Lung Transplant Registry; September 13, 1996.

recipients should be less than 60–65 years of age and in good health except for their lung disease. Since LAM afflicts relatively young women, the age criterion is not usually a factor, but some other aspects of LAM are pertinent. Although the lung is usually the only vital organ whose function is severely compromised, LAM is a systemic disease. Other common thoracic problems are pneumothorax and chylothorax (1,2), and extrathoracic involvement includes chylous ascites (1,2) and a frequent association with renal angiomyolipomas (3).

Pleurodesis, thoracotomy, and/or pleurectomy are frequently required for the management of complicated pneumothoraces or chylous pleural effusions before the disease reaches the stage for transplantation (12). These prior procedures increase the operative risk of hemorrhage, phrenic nerve injury, etc. A previous open lung biopsy or a simple pneumothorax that was treated by closed tube thoracostomy is not usually a deterrent to transplantation, but more complex cases must be decided individually. A previous thoracic procedure alone rarely precludes lung transplantation for LAM (12) or other diseases (21, 22), but if cardiopulmonary bypass is required for the operation, the morbidity and mortality may be increased (21).

Renal angiomyolipomas have been discovered in up to 48% of patients with LAM (3) and were present in 17% of the transplant recipients in a multicenter survey (12). These benign tumors are often asymptomatic, particularly if they are small. However, they can present as an abdominal mass if large enough, or hemorrhage into the tumor can cause flank pain and hematuria (3,23,24). Screening for angiomyolipomas with ultrasonography or computed tomography as part of the evaluation for transplantation is worthwhile because of the relatively high prevalence of the lesions and the potential for complications associated with them.

An expectant approach to management has been advised in patients without LAM (23,24), and these recommendations seem reasonable for patients with LAM. Asymptomatic or mildly symptomatic patients can be safely observed with radiographic follow-up at 6- to 12-month intervals regardless of tumor size, but if the size of the angiomyolipoma is greater than 4 cm, the patient should be apprised of possible complications. Patients with significant symptoms or complications should undergo angiography and be considered for embolization or for conservative surgery.

IV. Timing and Choice of Procedure

Transplantation is appropriate when other therapeutic options have been exhausted and when the patient's prognosis will be improved by the procedure. Quality of life is the prime motivation for transplantation for many patients, but prognosis should be the chief determinant of timing. Actuarial survival rates after transplantation for LAM (Fig. 2) can be compared with the prognosis of LAM without transplantation (1,2,4,5). However, each patient's clinical course must be synthesized into the final decision, too.

Prognostic factors have only recently been analyzed in patients with LAM. In a cohort of 46 patients from Japan, Korea, and Taiwan, a reduction in the FEV_1/FVC ratio and an increase in TLC at the first examination were associated with a poor outcome during the next 2–5 years (2). In the patients who died 2–5 years after their first examination, the mean FEV_1/FVC ratio was less than 50%, and the mean TLC was greater than 130% of the predicted normal value. Furthermore, patients with predominantly cystic lesions on their open lung biopsy had a poorer prognosis during the 2–5 years after their biopsy than those with muscular proliferation as the dominant histologic feature (2), and the extent of cystic changes, quantified by high-resolution computed tomography, has correlated closely with physiologic dysfunction (25).

Because the disease is relatively rare, the impact of the various therapeutic strategies—oophorectomy, tamoxifen, LH-RH, and progesterone—has not been resolved. Some reviews have suggested that improvement usually occurs in patients with chylous pleural effusions or ascites, whereas pulmonary parenchymal changes tend to stabilize or worsen (1,2). Nevertheless, survival rates in series reported in the era of antiestrogen treatments have been somewhat better than in earlier series (1,2,4,5), and medical treatment should precede transplantation unless the disease is already very advanced.

The median waiting time for lung transplantation in the United States was 553 days for patients who entered the waiting list in 1994 (16), and this inevitable delay must be incorporated into transplantation strategy. Some guidelines for planning the referral are proposed in Table 3, but prognostic implications have not been established for each of these. Transplantation may be premature for some patients who fulfill these criteria. However, postponement is simple, and urgent transplantation is impossible under the current donor lung allocation policy in the United States.

Heart-lung and lung transplantation have been performed for most end-stage lung diseases including LAM; however, heart-lung transplantation should

Table 3 Guidelines for Referring Patients with LAM for Transplantation

Progression of disease after adequate treatment
Extensive cystic disease on open lung biopsy or on high–resolution computed tomography
FEV_1/FVC ratio < 50% and/or TLC > 130% of the predicted normal value[a]
Hypercapnia
Pulmonary hypertension, in spite of adequate oxygenation

[a]For patients with predominant obstructive physiology.

be reserved for patients who cannot be treated by lung transplantation alone. Severe right ventricular dysfunction has been reversible after isolated lung transplantation for pulmonary hypertension (26–30), and cor pulmonale is not a contraindication to single or bilateral lung transplantation. Thus, unless there is some other cardiac problem, lung transplantation is the appropriate procedure for recipients with LAM.

Both single and bilateral lung transplantation have been performed for LAM, and the choice between these must be individualized. The most important consideration is the type and extent of any previous thoracic procedures. If one hemithorax has been spared, a single lung transplant on this side may be the most straightforward approach.

Single lung transplantation extends the limited supply of donor organs to more patients, but it provides less reserve lung function as a buffer for late complications, especially chronic allograft rejection. The remaining native lung can be an asset or a liability after SLT. If a severe complication develops in the allograft, even the diminished function of the native lung can be helpful during treatment and recovery, but the diseased native lung can also be a site for infection, pneumothorax, or other difficulties (12,31,32).

With the current donor shortage and long inherent waiting time, the best transplant procedure is the one that can be done when the patient needs it. If the patient is a candidate for either single or bilateral transplantation, these procedures are complementary because they broaden the range of donor sizes that can be used, e.g., bilateral transplantation with both lungs from a small donor or unilateral transplantation with one lung from a larger donor.

V. Institutional Experience and Commentary

Between July 1988 and October 1996, 332 lung transplant operations were performed in 327 patients at Barnes-Jewish Hospital. Eight recipients (2.4%) had LAM, including two (case 1 and case 5) with some features of tuberous sclerosis. A profile of the recipients and their outcome is presented in Tables 4, 5, and 6.

All patients were women whose disease began before menopause. The diagnosis of LAM had been made before the referral for lung transplantation in seven patients, and it was confirmed during the evaluation for transplantation in the other patient by review of excised tissue from a previous bullectomy. Although the patients had symptoms or signs of LAM for variable periods before diagnosis, the mean age was 36.8 years when the diagnosis was definitively established, and the average interval between diagnosis and transplantation was 5.3 years.

All recipients had been treated by surgical and/or medical hormonal manipulation before transplantation (Table 4). Four patients had received only medical therapy with medroxyprogesterone, and four had undergone an oophorectomy in addition to medical treatment. LAM recurred in the allograft in one recipient (case 3) from this series (11), and recurrence has been documented in a recipient at the university of Pittsburgh, too (10). The likelihood of recrudescence of LAM in the allograft is unknown, and the benefit of continuing medical treatment after transplantation is uncertain. However, medroxyprogesterone therapy after transplantation seems prudent.

Renal angiomyolipomas were detected in four patients before transplantation, but none required intervention preoperatively. Hemorrhage into a left renal angiomyolipoma occurred on two occasions, about 4 and 6 months after transplantation, in one recipient (case 6), and both episodes were successfully managed by embolization. A radiographically atypical (i.e., no visible fat by computed tomography) angiomyolipomas was incidentally discovered 5 years after transplantation in another recipient (case 2), who was participating in a screening study. A renal sparing resection was performed because the lesion could not be clinically or radiographically distinguished from a malignancy.

Two patients (case 3 and case 7) had a chylothorax before transplantation; one had been treated by ligation of the thoracic duct plus chemical pleurodesis, and the other by tube thoracostomy with chemical pleurodesis. Chylothorax complicated the early posttransplantation course of both recipients and required prolonged chest tube drainage, but posttransplantation chylothorax was not encountered in any other recipients.

Six patients had bilateral pneumothoraces before transplantation; two, who had chylothoraces, had not had a pneumothorax. Three of these had previous bilateral thoracotomies, two with chemical or surgical pleurodesis and one with bilateral pleurectomy; another had poor bilateral bullectomies and pleurectomies through a median sternotomy. A chemical or surgical pleurodesis had been performed in both hemithoraces in six patients and in one hemithorax in two patients (Table 4).

In spite of the extensive previous thoracic procedures, there were no intraoperative deaths or serious hemorrhagic complications. One patient (case 5) had transient bilateral diaphragmatic dysfunction and another (case 8) had a severe reperfusion lung injury that delayed their recovery, but both recipients ultimately achieved good lung function. As already described, two recipients (case 3 and case 7) required prolonged chest tube drainage for chylothorax, and small collections of chyle that did not compromise lung function remained after the tubes were removed.

The spirometric measurements before and after transplantation are tabulated in Table 5. Seven patients had predominately obstructive physiology, and one

Table 4 Profile of Recipients with LAM at Barnes-Jewish Hospital

Case	Age[a]	Treatment	Chylothorax	AML	Pneumothorax	Thoracic procedures
1	46	MP	No	Yes	Bilateral	Bilateral thoractomy and pleurectomy
2	44	MP	No	Yes	Bilateral	Left OLBx; bilateral tube thoracostomy and chemical pleurodesis
3	38	MP, TMX oophorectomy	Yes	Yes	None	Left thoracotomy, OLBx and thoracic duct ligation; right tube thoracostomy, chemical pleurodesis
4	31	MP	No	No	Bilateral	Right thoracotomy—OLBx, pleurodesis; left thoracotomy—bullectomy; pleurodesis
5	37	MP	No	Yes	Bilateral	Bilateral thoracotomy, bullectomy, and pleurodesis
6	32	MP oophorectomy	No	Yes	Bilateral	Median sternotomy, bilateral bullectomy, and pleurectomy
7	25	MP oophorectomy	Yes	No	None	Left OLBx; bilateral tube thoracostomy, and chemical pleurodesis
8	41	Leuprolide oophorectomy	No	No	Bilateral	Left thoracotomy, pleurodesis

[a]Age when diagnosis definitively established.
MP, Medroxyprogesterone; TMX, tamoxifen; AML, renal angiomyolipoma; OLBx, open lung biopsy.

Table 5 Outcome for Recipients with LAM at Barnes-Jewish Hospital

Case	Age[a]	Operation	Status[b]	Survival[b] (days)	Major posttransplant complication(s)
1	50	Left SLT	Dead	1226	BOS[c]
2	44	Left SLT	Alive	1993	BOS; resection of atypical renal AML
3	42	Right SLT	Dead	650	Chylothorax; disseminated aspergillosis[c]; recurrent LAM
4	38	Right SLT	Dead	781	BOS; pneumonia, PE, ARDS[c]
5	41	BLT	Alive	567	Diaphragmatic dysfunction
6	37	BLT	Alive	305	Hemorrhage from and embolization of renal AML
7	41	BLT	Alive	266	Chylothorax
8	42	Right SLT	Alive	50	Reperfusion lung injury

[a]Age at transplantation.
[b]Status and survival on October 1, 1996.
[c]Cause of death.
SLT, Single lung transplant; BLT, bilateral lung transplant; BOS, bronchiolitis obliterans syndrome; AML, angiomyolipoma; PE, pulmonary embolism; ARDS, adult respiratory distress syndrome.

Table 6 Spirometry of Recipients with LAM at Barnes-Jewish Hospital Before and After Lung Transplantation

	Pretransplantation		Posttransplantation, best		Posttransplantation, last	
Case	FVC, L(%)	FEV_1, L(%)	FVC, L(%)	FEV_1, L(%)	FVC, L(%)	FEV_1, L(%)
1	1.92 (53)	0.46 (16)	1.74 (48)	1.07 (36)	1.43 (40)	0.43 (15)
2	2.28 (66)	0.75 (28)	1.85 (57)	1.16 (43)	1.17 (36)	0.81 (30)
3	1.20 (38)	0.57 (21)	1.78 (54)	1.37 (50)	1.44 (44)	1.04 (38)
4	1.56 (41)	0.47 (18)	2.40 (63)	1.44 (45)	1.98 (52)	1.10 (35)
5	2.43 (66)	0.50 (16)	2.39 (65)	2.29 (75)	2.40 (65)	2.03 (67)
6	1.18 (32)	0.38 (12)	2.89 (77)	2.69 (86)	3.07 (82)	2.40 (76)
7	2.43 (78)	1.58 (60)	1.65 (53)	1.48 (56)	1.54 (50)	1.33 (51)
8	1.76 (45)	0.75 (29)	2.02 (63)	1.25 (47)	2.02 (63)	1.25 (47)
Mean, All[a]	1.76 (49)	0.55 (20)	2.09 (60)	1.59 (55)	1.88 (54)	1.30 (45)
Mean, SLT	1.74 (49)	0.60 (22)	1.96 (57)	1.26 (44)	1.61 (47)	0.93 (33)
Mean, BLT[a]	1.81 (49)	0.44 (14)	2.31 (65)	2.15 (72)	2.34 (66)	1.92 (65)

[a]Recipient 7, who had predominantly restrictive physiology, excluded from pretransplantation mean values to minimize distortion.

(case 7) a mild restrictive pattern coupled with severe diffusion impairment and hypoxemia. In the patients with an obstructive pattern, the mean FEV_1 was 0.55 ± 0.15 L (20 ± 6% of the predicted value), and the mean FVC/FEV_1 was 33 ± 10%. Spirometric parameters improved significantly after transplantation in the seven recipients with obstructive physiology. Not unexpectedly, lung function was substantially better after BLT than after SLT. Spirometry did not change significantly after transplantation in the recipient with the restrictive defect, but the diffusing capacity increased and oxygenation improved.

Lung function remained stable after transplantation unless a complication developed. Deterioration was associated with what ultimately proved to be recurrent LAM in one recipient (case 3) and with the evolution of bronchiolitis obliterans syndrome (BOS), a manifestation of chronic allograft rejection, in three recipients (cases 1, 2, and 4). Since both LAM and chronic allograft rejection are characterized by airflow limitation, the diagnosis of BOS (33) should not be made without considering this differential possibility. Unfortunately, transbronchial lung biopsy is relatively insensitive for detecting either obliterative bronchiolitis (34–36) or LAM, and a surgical biopsy may be the only way to make the distinction.

VI. Summary

Lung transplantation is an appropriate alternative for selected patients with end-stage lung disease associated with pulmonary LAM. While LAM presents some special problems, the results of transplantation for LAM have been comparable to other more common diseases.

References

1. Taylor JR, Colby TV, Raffin TA. Lymphangioleiomyomatosis: clinical course in 32 patients. N Engl J Med 1990; 323:1254–1260.
2. Kitaichi M, Nishimura K, Itoh H, Izumi T. Pulmonary lymphangioleiomyomatosis: a report of 46 patients including a clinicopathologic study of prognostic factors. Am J Respir Crit Care Med 1995; 151:527–533.
3. Bernstein SM, Newel Jr. JD, Adamczyk D, Mortenson RL, King Jr. TE, Lynch DA. How common are renal angiomyolipomas in patients with pulmonary lymphangiomyomatosis? Am J Respir Crit Care Med 1995; 152:2138–2143.
4. Silverstein E, Ellis K, Wolff M, Jaretzeki III A. Pulmonary lymphangioleiomyomatosis. Am J Roentgenol 1974; 120:12–50.
5. Corrin B, Liebow AA, Friedman PJ. Pulmonary lymphangioleiomyomatosis: a review. Am J Pathol 1975; 79:347–382.
6. Estenne M, de Francquen P, Wellens F, Leclerc J-L, Vanderhoeft P, Yernault J-C,

Primo G. Combined heart-and-lung transplantation for lymphangioleiomyomatosis [letter]. Lancet 1984; 1:275.
7. Wellens F, Estenne M, de Francquen P, Goldstein J, Leclerc JL, Primo G. Combined heart-lung transplantation for terminal pulmonary lymphangioleiomyomatosis. J Thorac Cardiovasc Surg 1985; 89:872–876.
8. Sleiman C, Mal H, Jebrak G, Darne C, Meeus E, Dubois F, Luisetti M, Fournier M, Pariente R, Andreassian B. Pulmonary lymphangiomyomatosis treated by single lung transplantation. Am Rev Respir Dis 1992; 145:964–966.
9. Lizotte PE, Whitlock WL, Prudhomme JC, Brown CR, Hershon JL. Lymphangiomyomatosis. Chest 1990; 98:1044–1045.
10. Nine JS, Yousem SA, Paradis IL, Keenan R, Griffith BP. Lymphangioleiomyomatosis: recurrence after lung transplantation. J Heart Lung Transplant 1994; 13:714–719.
11. O'Brien JD, Lium JH, Parosa JF, DeYoung BR, Wick MR, Trulock EP. Lymphangiomyomatosis recurrence in the allograft after single-lung transplantation. Am J Respir Crit Care Med 1995; 151:2033–2036.
12. Boehler A, Speich R, Russi EW, Weder W. Lung transplantation for lymphangioleiomyomatosis. N Engl J Med 1996; 335:1275–1280.
13. St. Louis International Lung Transplant Registry, January 1997 Report.
14. Pohl M, personal communication (from the St. Louis International Lung Transplant Registry).
15. Hosenpud JD, Novick, RJ, Bennett LE, Keck BM, Fiol B, Daily OP. The registry of the International Society for Heart and Lung Transplantation: thirteenth official report—1996. J Heart Lung Transplant 1996; 15:655–674.
16. Division of Transplantation, Bureau of Health Resources Development. 1995 Annual Report of the U.S. Scientific Registry for Transplant Recipients and the Organ Procurement and Transplantation Network—Transplant Data: 1988-1994. Rockville, MD: Health Resources and Services Administration, U.S. Department of Health and Human Services.
17. Marshall SE, Kramer MR, Lewiston NJ, Starnes VA, Theodore J. Selection and evaluation of recipients for heart-lung and lung transplantation. Chest 1990; 98:1488–1494.
18. Morrison DL, Maurer JR, Grossman RF. Preoperative assessment for lung transplantation. Clin Chest Med 1990; 11:207–215.
19. Trulock EP. Recipient selection. Chest Surg Clin NA 1993; 3:1–18.
20. Lynch JP, Trulock EP. Recipient selection. Semin Respir Crit Care Med 1996; 17:109–117.
21. Detterbeck FC, Egan TM, Mill MR. Lung transplantation after previous thoracic surgical procedures. Ann Thorac Surg 1995; 60:139–143.
22. Dusmet M, Winton TL, Kesten S, Maurer J. Previous intrapleural procedures do not adversely affect lung transplantation. J Heart Lung Transplant 1996; 15:249–254.
23. Steiner M, Goldman SM, Fishman EK, Marshall FF. The natural history of renal angiomyolipoma. J Urol 1993; 150:1782–1786.
24. Kennelly MJ, Grossman HB, Cho KJ. Outcome analysis of 42 cases of renal angiomyolipoma. J Urol 1994; 152:1988–1991.
25. Crausman RS, Lynch DA, Mortenson RL, King TE, Irvin CD, Hale VAE, Newell

JD. Quantitative CV predicts the severity of physiologic dysfunction in patients with lymphangioleiomyomatosis. Chest 1996; 109:131–137.
26. Pasque MK, Trulock EP, Kaiser LR, Cooper JD. Single-lung transplantation for pulmonary hypertension: three-month hemodynamic follow-up. Circulation 1991; 84:2275–2279.
27. Ritchie M, Waggoner AD, Dávila-Román VG, Barzilai B, Trulock EP, Eisenberg PR. Echocardiographic characterization of the improvement in right ventricular function in patients with severe pulmonary hypertension after single-lung transplantation. J Am Coll Cardiol 1993; 22:1170–1174.
28. Kramer MR, Valantine HA, Marshall SE, Starnes VA, Theodore J. Recovery of the right ventricle after single-lung transplantation in pulmonary hypertension. Am J Cardiol 1994; 73:494–500.
29. Bando K, Armitage JM, Paradis IL, Keenan RJ, Hardesty RL, Konishi H, Komatsu K, Stein KL, Shah AN, Bahnson HT, Griffith BP. Indications for and results of single, bilateral, and heart-lung transplantation for pulmonary hypertension. J Thorac Cardiovasc Surg 1994; 108:1056–1065.
30. Pasque MK, Trulock EP, Cooper JD, Triantafillou AN, Huddleston CB, Rosenbloom M, Sundaresan S, Cox JL, Patterson GA. Single lung transplantation for pulmonary hypertension: single institution experience in 34 patients. Circulation 1995; 92:2252–2258.
31. Horvath J, Dummer S, Loyd J, Walker B, Merrill WH, Frist WH. Infection in the transplanted and native lung after single lung transplantation. Chest 1993; 140:681–685.
32. Frost AE, Keller CA, Noon GP, Short HD, Cagle PT, Multiorgan Transplant Group. Outcome of the native lung after single lung transplant. Chest 1995; 107:981–984.
33. International Society for Heart and Lung Transplantation, Cooper JD, Billingham M, Egan T, Hertz MI, Higenbottam T, Lynch J, Maurer J, Paradis I, Patterson GA, Smith C, Trulock EP, Vreim C, Yousem S. A working formulation for the standardization of nomenclature and for clinical staging of chronic dysfunction in lung allografts. J Heart Lung Transplant 1993; 12:713–716.
34. Kramer MR, Stoehr C, Whang JL, Berry GJ, Sibley R, Marshall SE, Patterson GM, Starnes VA, Theodore J. The diagnosis of obliterative bronchiolitis after heart-lung and lung transplantation: low yield of transbronchial lung biopsy. J Heart Lung Transplant 1993; 12:675–681.
35. Yousem SA, Paradis I, Griffith BP. Can transbronchial biopsy aid in the diagnosis of bronchiolitis obliterans in lung transplant recipients? Transplantation 1994; 57:151–153.
36. Chamberlain D, Maurer J, Chaparro C, Idolor L. Evaluation of transbronchial lung biopsy specimens in the diagnosis of bronchiolitis obliterans after lung transplantation. J Heart Lung Transplant 1994; 13:963–971.

6

International Survey on Lung Transplantation in Lymphangioleiomyomatosis

ANNETTE BOEHLER, RUDOLF SPEICH, ERICH W. RUSSI, and WALTER WEDER

University Hospital Zurich
Zurich, Switzerland

I. Introduction

Over the last 10 years lung transplantation for lymphangioleiomyomatosis (LAM) has become a novel therapeutic option for patients with end-stage lung disease (1–7). Since most lung-transplantation centers deal with only a few LAM patients, we conducted an international survey between 1994 and 1995 to obtain information on transplantation for LAM (8). These data were updated in 1997 to further determine disease-associated factors and to elucidate intermediate term survival after lung transplantation for LAM.

II. Recruitment of Patients and Contributing Centers

To date 96 patients with LAM have received lung transplantation worldwide, which represents 1.5% of all lung transplant procedures performed (St. Louis International Lung Transplant Registry, January 1997).

We have been collecting information on patients undergoing lung transplantation for LAM since 1994 by questionnaire. Lung transplantation centers have been identified through the International Lung Transplant Registry, in St. Louis, or by personal contacts. A first analysis of the data was done in August 1995 (8). We reported on 34 patients, of which 18 were alive as of August 1995. Follow-up data of these patients were obtained in 1997 questionnaires. In addition, 12 new patients were included in the survey. A total of 16 transplantation centers contributed their data to this survey (see Table 1). Previous single case publications reported on five patients also included in this survey (1–3,5,6,9,10). Data on seven patients contained incomplete information and could not be used for all the calculations. In the following paragraphs data are expressed as means ± standard deviation. Overall survival was calculated with the use of Kaplan-Meier statistics (11).

III. Age, Sex, and Symptoms

LAM occurs exclusively in women, unless it is a feature of tuberous sclerosis where the male-to-female ratio is 1:5.

Table 1 Contributing Centers and Number of Patients

Center	Number of patients
Europe	
Hopital Universitaire Erasme, Bruxelles, Belgium	6
Universitätsspital, Zürich, Switzerland	4
Hospital Universitari Vall d'Hebron, Barcelona, Spain	3
Hopital Louis Pradel, Lyon, France	2
Universitätsklinik Wien, Wien, Austria	2
Medizinische Hochschule, Hannover, Germany	1
Hopital Beaujon, Clichy, France	1
North America	
Washington University, St. Louis, Missouri	10
Stanford University, Stanford, California	5 (one follow-up in Cedars Sinai)
University of Toronto, Ontario, Canada	4
University of Minnesota, Minneapolis, Minnesota	2
University Hospital London, Ontario, Canada	2
Cedars Sinai Medical Center, Los Angeles, California	1 (one additional patient underwent Tx in Standford)
McGill University, Montreal, Quebec, Canada	1
University of Alabama at Birmingham, Birmingham, Alabama	1
Virginia Commonwealth University, Richmond, Virginia	1

In this study all patients were women. The mean age at the onset of symptoms was 30 ± 8 years (range: 5–44). The age at the diagnosis of LAM was 34 ± 9 years (range 8–55). The interval between the first symptoms and diagnosis was 5 ± 6 years (range: 0–20). The age at transplantation was 41 ± 9 years (range: 23–55). The interval between the onset of symptoms and transplantation was 10 ± 6 years (range: 2–25).

A delay in the diagnosis of LAM is typical because the first symptoms are often uncharacteristic and tissue samples or high-resolution computed tomogram (CT) usually are needed to confirm the diagnosis. In this study the mean delay was 5 years, which is similar to the time observed by Taylor and colleagues (12). The mean interval of 10 years between the onset of symptoms and the time of lung transplantation can be compared to the natural history of LAM and matches the data reporting 10-year survival rates of 23 (13), 40 (14), and 78% (12). Kitaichi et al. (14) mention a potential benefit of hormonal therapy in their patients in comparison to an earlier series of untreated patients (13). All patients we studied had received some kind of hormonal treatment before developing end-stage disease.

IV. Clinical and Radiologic Characteristics at the Time of Diagnosis

Pulmonary complications due to a hamartomatous proliferation of smooth muscle cells along the bronchovascular structures lead to airway obliteration and consecutive development of cysts in the lungs (15,16).

Spontaneous pneumothorax is an early symptom of LAM at a time when the chest radiograph might still be normal. The diagnosis is often not made until the patient experiences repeated pneumothoraces or other symptoms, particularly shortness of breath. Typical concurrent or precedent features were a history of pneumothorax (33 patients), chylothorax (12), and chylous ascites (1). Chest radiographs showed hyperinflation (19 patients), cysts and bullae (19), and reticulonodular shadows (17) (Table 2).

High-resolution CT is a valuable tool for the early detection of parenchymal lung diseases (17). In our survey, all patients who were examined with CT showed the typical bilateral lung cysts.

V. Diagnosis of LAM

A histological diagnosis of LAM is still considered to be the gold standard. Because it is difficult to establish the diagnosis in small transbronchial biopsies, usually surgical biopsies are obtained. With the availability of video-assisted thoracoscopic biopsies, this procedure became less invasive. Additionally, HMB-

Table 2 Clinical and Radiological Characteristics in LAM Patients at the Time of Diagnosis

Clinical aspects:		
Shortness of breath	41/44	(93%)
History of pneumothorax	33/44	(75%)
Cough	15/44	(34%)
Chest pain	10/44	(23%)
History of chylothorax	12/44	(27%)
Hemoptysis	7/44	(16%)
Clubbing	5/44	(11%)
History of chylous ascites	1/44	(2%)
Chest radiography:		
Hyperinflation	19/41	(46%)
Cysts and bullae	19/41	(46%)
Reticulonodular shadows	17/41	(41%)
Pleural effusion	10/41	(24%)
Pneumothorax	4/41	(10%)
Normal	0/41	(0%)
Chest CT:		
Bilateral lung cysts	33/33	(100%)
Pleural effusion	8/33	(24%)
Hilar or mediastinal Lymphadenopathy	3/33	(9%)
Pneumothorax	2/33	(6%)
Extrapulmonary LAM (5 patients with tuberous sclerosis excluded)		
Lymph node involvement (8× retroperitoneal/4× mediastinal)	12/37	(32%)
Renal angiomyolipoma (4× unilateral/2× bilateral)	6/37	(16%)
Paraaortic abdominal angiomyolipoma	1/37	(3%)
Thoracic angiomyolipoma	1/37	(3%)
Pelvic myoma	1/37	(3%)
Ocular	1/37	(3%)

The ratio of positive findings over the total number of patients for whom data were available is shown.

Source: Ref. 8. Adapted with permission.

45, an immunohistochemical marker for melanogenesis, has been found to stain smooth muscle cells in LAM with high specificity. It is therefore conceivable that small specimens obtained by transbronchial biopsy may be sufficient to establish a firm diagnosis (18).

The diagnosis was established by surgical lung biopsy (34 patients), by high-resolution CT (9 patients), and in one patient by histologic examination of the explanted lung. Data were not available for two patients.

Apparently surgical lung biopsy was still considered in the majority of patients to be mandatory to establish the diagnosis of LAM. In about a quarter, however, the diagnosis was based on high-resolution CT alone and was confirmed histologically in the explanted lung after transplantation. Today, high-resolution CT is considered a reliable, noninvasive diagnostic method for LAM (19,20). However, patients with a history of smoking must be evaluated with painstaking care, since emphysema may mimic the radiologic pattern of LAM. Recently it has been shown that CT techniques able to quantitatively measures the cystic changes in LAM were able to assess disease severity and were correlated with physiologic measurements (21).

CT may reveal hilar or mediastinal lymph node enlargements, where the differential diagnosis should include LAM itself (22), and also other diseases such as tuberculosis and sarcoidosis (23).

VI. Functional Assessment at Time of Evaluation for Lung Transplantation

In order to define the appropriate timepoint to evaluate patients for lung transplantation, referral guidelines for most common lung diseases eventually treated by lung transplantation have been developed (24). These guidelines take into account that the current 2-year survival after lung transplantation ranges from 55 to 70% (St. Louis International Registry, January 1997) and that therefore the natural survival of the disease should be of lesser duration. Specific data for LAM, however, have not been available.

Generally, airflow limitation is the predominant functional feature in patients with LAM and is also the primary determinant of exercise limitation (25). Pulmonary function testing typically shows an obstructive ventilatory defect. A restrictive or combined obstructive-restrictive pattern typically occurs in patients who have received treatment for pneumothorax.

Thirty-six patients (84%) in our survey experienced severe obstructive ventilatory defects in the pretransplant period (Table 3). Four patients had restrictive patterns, and a combined obstructive and restrictive pattern was shown by three patients.

Although the mean FEV_1 value of all the obstructive patients was already low at 25 ± 12% (range: 10–66%), 92% of these patients showed values between 10 and 37% and only three patients were above this value. These measurements are lower than those reported in other series (15,26,27) and represent a selection of patients with end-stage pulmonary disease. Usually, an FEV_1 less than 25–30% of predicted is used as a threshold to consider lung transplantation. Carbon monoxide diffusing capacity was clearly decreased. Hypoxemia was present in 97%

Table 3 Pulmonary Function at Time of Evaluation for Lung Transplantation

Obstructive pattern	
(TLC $\geq$ 80%, FEV_1/FVC < 75%)	
Number of patients (%)	36/43 (84)
FEV_1 - % of predicted (range)	25 ± 12 (10–66)
FEV_1/FVC - % of predicted (range)	40 ± 13 (20-69)
Restrictive pattern	
(TLC < 80%, $FEV_1/FVC \geq$ 75%)	
Number of patients (%)	4/43 (9)
Combined obstructive and restrictive pattern	
Number of patients (%)	3/43 (7)
Decreased CO-diffusing capacity (DLCO < 80%)	
Number of patients (%)	35/35 (100)
% of predicted value (range)	24 ± 12 (10-59)
Hypoxemia	
(PO_2 > 80 mmHg)	
Number of patients (%)	34/35 (97)
Arterial P_{O_2} - mmHg (range)	54 ± 12 (40-79)
Hypercapnia	
(Pa_{CO_2} > 45 mmHg)	
Number of patients (%)	8/35 (23)

FEV_1: Forced expiratory volume in one second; FVC: forced vital capacity; TLC: total lung capacity; P_{O_2}: Partial pressure of oxygen.
Source: Ref. 8. Adapted with permission.

of the patients with a mean Pa_{O_2} of 54 ± 12 mmHg, whereas 23% of the patients showed hypercapnia.

VII. LAM in Tuberous Sclerosis

In recent years the border between pulmonary LAM and tuberous sclerosis has become less clear (28). However, there are still important clinical differences. LAM develops exclusively in females, whereas tuberous sclerosis affects both sexes. Furthermore, family history is common in tuberous sclerosis patients, while it has not been reported in patients with LAM.

Five patients diagnosed with tuberous sclerosis showed pulmonary LAM besides kidney, skin, and cerebral manifestations. One of them had cardiac, bone, and liver hamartomas, and another patient had uterus lipomas. The age of the onset of pulmonary symptoms was between 21 and 34 years, and the age at transplantation was between 23 and 46 years.

End-stage lung disease in tuberous sclerosis does not preclude lung transplantation. However, antiepileptic therapy may interfere with the immunosuppressive regimen in the posttransplant period. Severely reduced mental capacity might impede compliance with treatment after transplantation. In this survey we applied the classical diagnostic criteria for the diagnosis of tuberous sclerosis. In the revised classification of diagnostic criteria by Gomez (29), LAM in combination with, for example, renal angiomyolipoma would already be considered a feature of tuberous sclerosis. According to this classification at least six more patients in our survey would have fulfilled the diagnostic criteria of tuberous sclerosis. A relationship between LAM and angiomyolipomas is supported by recent immunohistochemical studies. It was shown that both pulmonary LAM and angiomyolipomas contain a distinctive phenotype of cells coexpressing muscle and a peculiar melanogenesis marker (HMB-45) (28,30–32).

VIII. Extrapulmonary Manifestations of LAM

Extrapulmonary manifestations of LAM (Table 2) consisted of lymph node involvement in 12 patients, renal angiomyolipomas in 6, para-aortic abdominal angiomyolipoma in one, and thoracic angiomyolipoma in one. As of August 1997, three patients showed severe bleeding of a renal angiomyolipoma in the posttransplant period, two of whom were treated with nephrectomy.

Extrapulmonary manifestations of LAM are common (22,33). Sixteen percent of the patients we studied (26% if patients with tuberous sclerosis are also included) had kidney involvement with unilateral or bilateral angiomyolipomas. This tumor is well known in patients with tuberous sclerosis and is less often reported in those with LAM (34), although depending on the criteria used to define tuberous sclerosis as mentioned above. Recently, the incidence of renal angiomyolipomas in patients with LAM was reported to be as high as 47% and 57% (35,36). Because these tumors are often asymptomatic, they might have been underestimated, unless extensive radiological examination is performed. So far, experience with the course of angiomyolipoma in patients who have received transplants is limited. Excessive retroperitoneal bleeding has been reported (37) in the nontransplant population. In our series, complications have been observed in three patients, but the follow-up time after lung transplantation is still short. An increased incidence of renal cell carcinoma in tuberous sclerosis patients with distinct clinical, pathological, and genetic features has been described (38) and must be considered in LAM patients as well.

In the posttransplant period, preexisting documentation of retroperitoneal and mediastinal lymphadenopathy and angiomyolipoma help to avoid diagnostic pitfalls.

IX. Hormonal Receptor Status and Treatment Before and After Lung Transplantation

The predominant occurrence of LAM in women during their reproductive years suggests the importance of hormonal status and smooth muscle cell proliferation secondary to estrogen stimulation. Treatment is therefore targeted against the production and effects of estrogens (13,39–43) but often remains ineffective. In vitro studies showed that cells cultured from LAM tissue exhibited a mitogenic response to estradiol (44). However, determination of tissue receptors for estrogen and progesterone has not bene proven to be of practical value (45).

In our survey the presence (+) or absence (–) of hormone receptors was reported in seven patients as follows (given as progesterone/estrogen): +/+ (1 patient), +/– (2 patients), –/+ (2 patients), and –/– (2 patients).

In the pretransplant period, 21 patients received steroids, 34 progesterone, and 11 antiestrogens as medical therapy. Eleven patients were treated by ovariectomy, and one had received a synthetic analog of luteinizing hormone–releasing hormone (LHRH). Twenty-three patients underwent multiple treatment modalities.

X. Lung Transplant Procedure

There were no treatment options for advanced pulmonary LAM until lung transplantation became available. The first successful transplantation for LAM—a combined heart-lung transplantation—was performed in 1983 (1,5) in a patient included in this survey.

The lung transplantation procedures included in this survey took place between 1983 and 1997. Single-lung transplant surgery was performed in 33 patients (16 right lungs and 17 left lungs), bilateral transplantation in 11, and 2 patients were treated with a heart-lung transplant. Cardiopulmonary bypass was used in 5 single and 6 bilateral procedures.

Lung transplantation surgery for LAM was mainly complicated by multiple pleural adhesions in over 50% (Table 4). Clinically described, they were moderate in 8 cases and severe in 13 cases. LAM as underlying cause was mentioned in 15 patients, prior pleurectomy after spontaneous pneumothorax together with LAM in 6 patients. LAM itself was suspected to be the main cause for the pleural adhesions as in most of the patients no prior surgery was performed. This is a specific feature of LAM, as other diseases (e.g., primary pulmonary hypertension or emphysema) do not cause adhesions by themselves. Marked hemorrhage occurred in 6 patients, 1 patient died intraoperatively, and repeated thoracotomy was necessary in 3 patients.

Table 4 Transplantation-Specific Surgical Problems in Patients with LAM

Previous surgery	
Pleurectomy: unilateral 7, bilateral 5	12/44 (27%)
Pleurodesis: unilateral 7, bilateral 9	16/44 (36%)
Surgical lung biopsy	34/44 (77%)
Intraoperative problems	
Moderate or severe adhesions:	21/39 (54%)
due to LAM	15
due to previous pleurectomy and LAM	6
Moderate-to-severe hemorrhage[a]	6/39 (15%)
Postoperative problems	
Reperfusion injury	2/39 (5%)
Bronchial stenosis/dehiscence	8/39 (21%)
Hematothorax	3/39 (8%)
Hemorrhage due to omentopexy	1/39 (3%)
Left phrenic nerve paralysis	2/39 (5%)
Cerebral embolism	1/39 (3%)

[a]One patient died during surgery, and three required a second thoracotomy.
Source: Ref. 8. Adapted with permission.

Enlargement of mediastinal lymph nodes did not cause an increase in the surgical complication rate.

XI. Survival After Lung Transplantation

Reported overall actuarial 1- and 2-year survival after lung transplantation are 71 and 63% (The St. Louis International Lung Transplant Registry, January 1997). Rates are 64 and 55% for patients with pulmonary fibrosis, and 77 and 69% for those with emphysema, respectively. In our survey, the actuarial 1- and 2-year survival (Fig. 1) of patients transplanted for LAM was 73 and 65%, respectively. The actuarial 3- and 5-year survival was 58 and 36%. Twenty-four patients (52%) were alive as of August 1997, which was 41 ± 31 months (range: 2–110 months) after transplantation. The 7 early deaths (within one month) were due to acute lung injury (4 patients), hemorrhage (1 patient), dehiscence of the bronchial anastomosis with sepsis (1 patients), and sepsis (1 patient). Fifteen patients died 2–58 months after transplantation due to infections (10 patients), bronchiolitis obliterans (3 patients), metastatic nephroblastoma transferred by the lung allograft (9) (1 patient), and one patient died after surgery for retransplantation. Five of the 10 patients who died of infection had previously received augmented immunosuppression for bronchiolitis obliterans (Table 5).

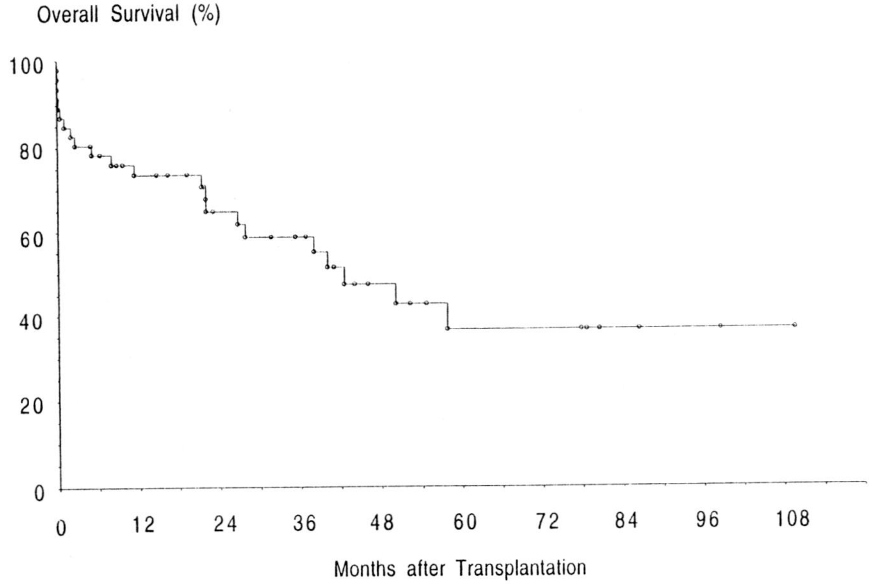

Figure 1 Overall survival (Kaplan-Meier curve) after lung transplantation for LAM in 46 patients. (From Ref. 8. Copyright © 1996 Massachusetts Medical Society. All rights reserved. Adapted with permission.)

So far, the longest survival after lung transplantation for LAM in our survey is 110 months.

XII. Functional Outcome After Transplantation

In general, impressive improvements in pulmonary function, gas exchange, and exercise tolerance after lung transplantation are achieved (46). Quality of life after single lung transplantation compared to bilateral lung transplantation remains an unsettled issue, since patients with a bilateral transplant seem to benefit from a greater functional reserve for eventually occurring subsequent complications. After single lung transplantation the forced expiratory volume in one second (FEV_1) usually reaches 50–60% of predicted, and even higher values are observed after bilateral transplantation.

In our survey the FEV_1 in single lung transplant recipients was 49 ± 16% of the predicted 6 months after surgery (range: 24–105%) and 48 ± 20% of the predicted one year after transplantation (range: 15–115%). The FEV_1 was 58 ± 5% of the predicted value after 6 months (range: 52–64%) after bilateral lung transplantation.

Table 5 Causes of Death in Patients after Lung Transplantation for LAM

Early death (<1 month)	
Acute lung injury	4x
Hemorrhage	1x
Dehiscence of bronchial anastomosis with sepsis	1x
Sepsis	1x
Late death (>1 month)	
Infection (5x during intensified immunosuppression in the presence of BO)	10x
BO	3x
Metastatic nephroblastoma transferred by the lung allograft	1x
After surgery for retransplantation	1x

XIII. Infection and Allograft Rejection After Transplantation

Whereas patients with LAM may experience posttransplant complications specific to their underlying disease, they also suffer from complications commonly observed in all lung transplant recipients, such as infection and acute and chronic allograft rejection.

Postoperative complications in our survey are listed in Table 6. Thirty-nine patients experienced 48 episodes of pneumonia. Forty-two acute rejection episodes had to be treated in 32 patients surviving more than one month.

Large cysts particularly in the remaining native lung were suspected to pose a major risk for infections in the posttransplant period after single lung procedure. The incidence of such infections was unexpectedly low as only two patients, both with invasive aspergillosis in the native lung, were reported. One of them died, and another patient successfully underwent pneumonectomy. All other infection episodes occurred in the transplanted lung, only occasionally affecting the native lung.

The most important obstacle to long-term survival after lung transplantation to date is bronchiolitis obliterans, regarded to be a form of chronic allograft rejection (47). Bronchiolitis obliterans was found in 17 of the 39 patients surviving longer than one month (40%). Bronchiolitis obliterans was the direct or indirect cause of death in 8 of the 22 patients who died (36%). Excluding the 7 patients who died <1 month after surgery, the percentage of patients who died with bronchiolitis obliterans rises to 53%. Thus, patients transplanted for LAM show a similar incidence of bronchiolitis obliterans as the general lung transplant population (48).

Table 6 Complications in Patients After Lung Transplantation for LAM

	No. of episodes	No. of patients
Pneumonia	48	39
Bacterial	21	15
CMV	13	10
Other viruses	4	4
Aspergillus sp[a]	5	5
Pneumocystis carinii	2	2
Nocardia sp.	1	1
Nontuberculous mycobacteria	3	3
Acute rejections (in patients with data available and surviving >1 month)	42 (1.3/patient)	32
Bronchiolitis obliterans in 39 patients surviving >1 month	17	17
LAM-specific complications	10	9
Pneumothorax after LTx (native lung)	12	5
Need for chest tube drainage	6	4
Chylothorax after LTx	3	3
Chylous ascites after LTx	1	1
Bleeding angiomyolipoma	3	3
Leading to nephrectomy	2	2
Recurrence of LAM in allograft	2	2
Other complications: bilateral cerebral cortical ischemia (1x), colitis due to clostridium difficile (2x), encephalitis of unknown origin (1x), urosepsis (2x), recurrent pneumatosis coli (1x), metastatic nephroblastoma (1x), posttransplant lymphoproliferative disease (2x), lung embolism (1x), cryptococcal cellulitis (1x), bilateral femoro popliteal arterial occlusion (1x).		

[a]Invasive aspergillosis occurred in the transplanted lung in three patients and in the native lung in two patients.

Source: Ref. 8. Adapted with permission.

XIV. Retransplantation for Bronchiolitis Obliterans

So far treatment of bronchiolitis obliterans is of limited effect, and to date the only effective therapy remains retransplantation. Four patients with bronchiolitis obliterans underwent retransplantation 19, 57, 58, and 79 months after the first transplantation. As first transplant all four patients had received a single graft. The following strategies have been chosen: Two bilateral transplants, one single transplant with the new graft replacing the old graft, and one single transplant with the new graft replacing the remaining native lung, leaving the old graft in place. In general, the outcome after retransplantation is less favorable compared to the first transplantation (49). In this study, one patient died after surgery, one patient died after 18 months because of sepsis, and two patients are alive 9 and 19 months after the retransplantation.

XV. LAM-Specific Complications After Transplantation

The most important posttransplantation complications of LAM consisted of 12 episodes of pneumothorax in the native lung after single-lung transplantation in five patients (Fig. 2). In four patients it caused mild-to-moderate chest pain. No severe functional impairment was reported since the function of the transplanted lung was sufficient for ventilation and perfusion. In one patient conservative therapy led to temporary success only, and the pneumothorax had to be treated surgically.

Three patients developed chylothorax posttransplant. In one patient, a right-sided chylothorax occurred 8 weeks after bilateral lung transplantation and resolved after thoracic duct ligation. Another patient had undergone thoracic duct ligation for chylothorax before transplantation. Nevertheless, a right-sided chylothorax developed in this same patient after single-lung transplantation was successfully treated with thoracotomy and diet containing medium-chain triglycerides. The third patient had a large right-sided chylothorax before receiving a heart-lung transplant; the chylothorax was evacuated intraoperatively. A left-sided chylothorax developed postoperatively in this patient and was managed successfully by needle aspiration. Chylothorax has to be seen as a leakage of chylous fluid from dilated and torn lymphatic vessels in the mediastinum after single-lung procedures as well as after bilateral and heart-lung transplantations.

As mentioned above, bleeding of angiomyolipoma remains an important complication in these patients also after transplantation.

Cyclosporine-induced nephropathy is a common complication in all solid organ transplant recipients due to long-term immunosuppressive therapy. In addition, in LAM patients LAM-specific renal manifestations can further impair

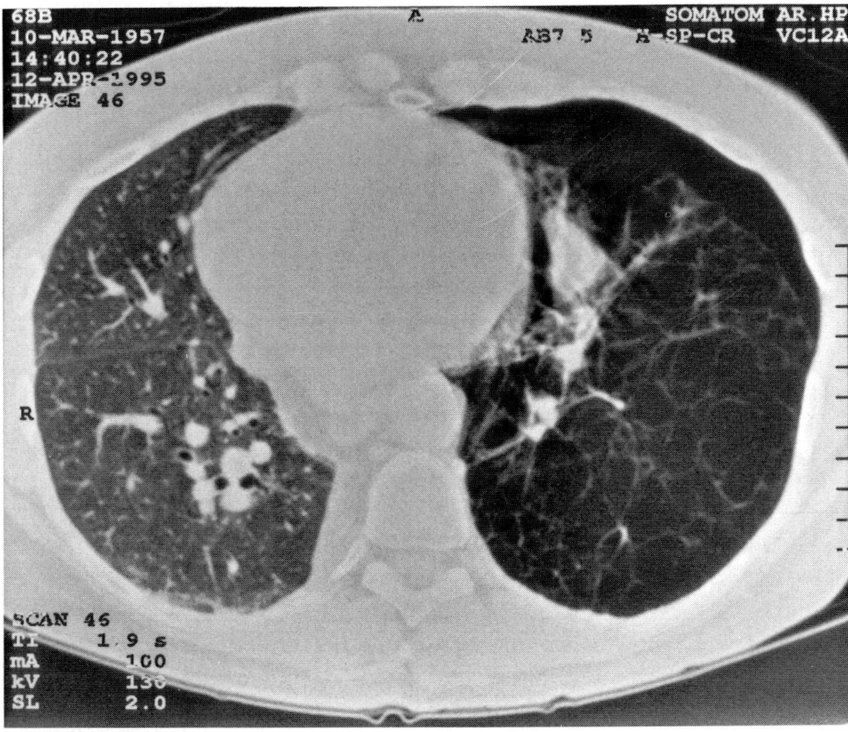

A

Figure 2 (A) Chest-CT of a 38-year-old patient 2 years after single right lung transplantation for LAM. The native left lung shows the typical findings of multiple and evenly distributed cystic spaces with coexisting pneumothorax. (B) Radiologic findings on plain chest film in the same patient.

kidney function directly (by large angiomyolipomas or cystic transformation) or indirectly (by bleeding angiomyolipomas with consecutive therapeutic arterial embolization or nephrectomy). In our series, seven patients showed a marked impairment of renal function occasionally requiring dialysis.

Osteoporosis after solid organ transplantation is a well-known side effect of cyclosporine and high-dose steroid therapy. As most LAM patients already have received ablative hormonal treatment for LAM before lung transplantation (e.g., antiestrogens, progesterone, ovarectomy), they carry an additional risk to develop severe osteoporosis due to long-term estrogen deficiency. In our survey four patients developed multiple vertebral osteoporotic fractures.

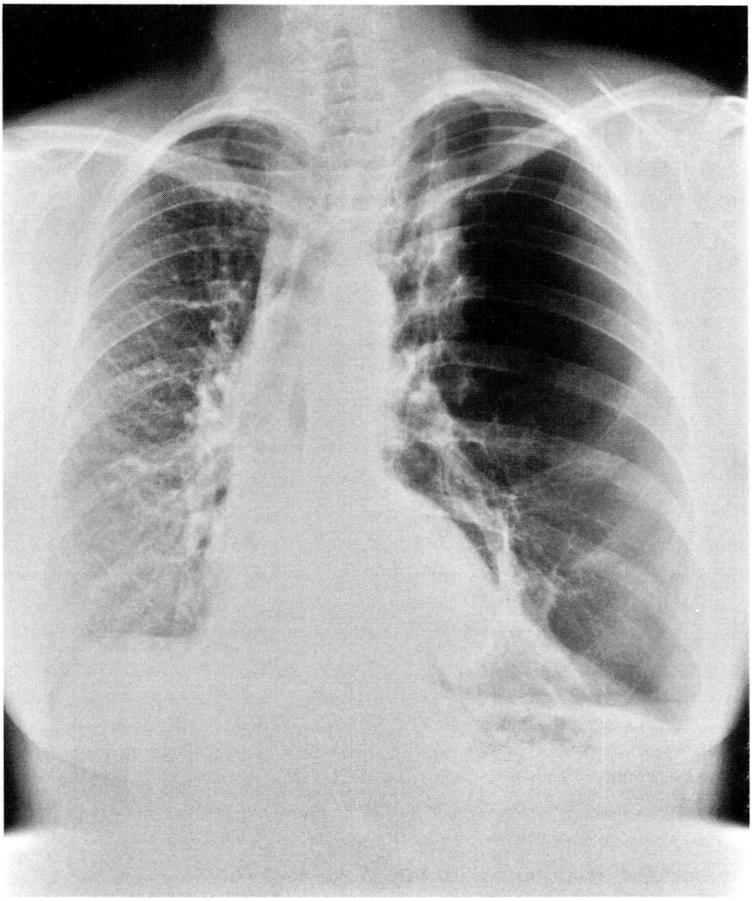

B

Figure 2 Continued.

XVI. Recurrence of LAM

Recurrent LAM in the lung allograft has been found at autopsy in one patient in our study, who died of disseminated *Aspergillus* infection (3). Another patient was diagnosed with recurrent LAM in the transplanted lung showing smooth muscle cells staining positively for HMB-45 in a transbronchial biopsy specimen. Two patients with recurrent LAM in the allograft after single-lung transplantation were published earlier (3,4). In each case, the graft came from a male donor. One of these patients is included in this series (3). Progressive airway obstruction was suggestive of obliterative bronchiolitis, but postmortem examinations revealed characteristic findings of LAM in the transplanted lungs. In contrast to the other patient described (4) the patient included in our study (3) had no evidence of obliterative bronchiolitis, suggesting that the obstructive ventilatory defect was due to the recurrence of LAM.

Disease recurrence should be considered in the differential diagnosis when pulmonary function deteriorates after lung transplantation for LAM. Recurrence of underlying disease in the lung allograft has been described in other diseases requiring lung transplantation: sarcoidosis (50,51), giant-cell pneumonia (52), and diffuse panbronchiolitis (53). A beneficial role of hormonal therapy after transplantation for LAM is not proven, and in the majority of patients in this survey, including the patients with recurrent disease, hormonal therapy was discontinued after transplantation.

XVII. Conclusion

This updated international survey includes data from different centers on patients transplanted for LAM. Aspects of this rare disease were identified that could potentially affect the outcome after lung transplantation. Lung transplantation offers a valuable therapeutic option for LAM patients with end-stage disease, and results are comparable to those in patients transplanted for other diseases. Survival data demonstrate the value of lung transplantation in this setting, taking into account some of the various problems associated with pulmonary and extrapulmonary LAM.

Acknowledgment

The authors are most grateful to the participating lung transplant centers for contributing their data. We are especially indebted to Joel D. Cooper, MD, and the St. Louis International Lung Transplant Registry.

References

1. Wellens F, Estenne M, de Francquen P, Goldstein J, Leclerc JL, Primo G. Combined heart-lung transplantation for terminal pulmonary lymphangioleiomyomatosis. J Thorac Cardiovasc Surg 1985; 89:872–876.
2. Sleiman C, Mal H, Jebrak G, Darne C, Meeus E, Dubois F, Luisetti M, Fournier M, Pariente R, Andreassian B. Pulmonary lymphangiomyomatosis treated by single lung transplantation. Am Rev Respir Dis 1992; 145:964–966.

3. O'Brien JD, Lium JH, Parosa JF, Deyoung BR, Wick MR, Trulock EP. Lymphangiomyomatosis recurrence in the allograft after single-lung transplantation. Am J Respir Crit Care Med 1995; 151:2033–2036.
4. Nine JS, Yousem SA, Paradis IL, Keenan R, Griffith BP. Lymphangioleiomyomatosis: recurrence after lung transplantation. J Heart Lung Transplant 1994; 13:714–719.
5. Estenne M, de Francquen P, Wellens F, et al. Combined heart and lung transplantation for lymphangioleiomyomatosis. Lancet 1984; 1:275.
6. Estenne M, Ketelbant P, Primo G, Yernault JC. Human heart-lung transplantation: physiologic aspects of the denervated lung and post-transplant obliterative bronchiolitis. Am Rev Respir Dis 1987; 135:976–978.
7. Kalassian KG, Doyle R, Kao, P, Ruoss S, Raffin TA. Lymphangioleiomyomatosis: new insights. Am J Respir Crit Care Med 1997; 155:1183–1186.
8. Boehler A, Speich R, Russi EW, Weder W. Lung transplantation for lymphangioleiomyomatosis. N Engl J Med 1996; 335:1275–1280.
9. Knoop C, Jacobovitz D, Antoine M, de Francquen P, Yernault JC, Estenne M. Donor-transmitted tumors in lung allograft recipients: report on two cases. Transplantation 1994; 57:1679–1680.
10. Boehler A, Speich R, Russi EW, Meyenberger C, Weder W. Pneumatosis intestinalis and active cytomegaloviral infection after lung transplantation. Chest 1995; 107:582–583.
11. Kaplan EL, Meier P. Nonparametric estimation from incomplete observations. J Am Stat Assoc 1958; 53:457–481.
12. Taylor JR, Ryu J, Colby TV, Raffin TA. Lymphangioleiomyomatosis: clinical course in 32 patients. N Engl J Med 1990; 323:1254–1260.
13. Silverstien E, Ellis K, Wolff M, Jaretzki A. Pulmonary lymphangioleiomyomatosis. Am J Roentgenol 1974; 120:12–50.
14. Kitaichi M, Nishimura K, Itoh H, Izumi T. Pulmonary lymphangioleiomyomatosis: a report of 46 patients including a clinicopathologic study of prognostic factors. Am J Respir Crit Care Med 1995; 151:527–533.
15. Corrin B, Liebow AA, Friedman PJ. Pulmonary lymphangioleiomyomatosis. Am J Pathol 1975; 79:347–382.
16. Bradley SL, Dines DE, Soule EH, Muhm JR. Pulmonary lymphangiomyomatosis. Lung 1980; 158:69–80.
17. Webb WR, Stein MG, Finkbeiner WE, Im JG, Lynch D, Gamso G. Normal and diseased isolated lungs: high-resolution CT. Radiology 1988; 166:81–87.
18. Guinee DJ, Feuerstein I, Koss M, Travis W. Pulmonary lymphangioleiomyomatosis. Diagnosis based on results of transbronchial biopsy and immunohistochemical studies and correlation with high-resolution computed tomography findings. Arch Pathol Lab Med 1994; 118:846–849.
19. Rappaport DC, Weisbrod GL, Herman SJ, Chamberlain DW. Pulmonary lymphangioleiomyomatosis: high-resolution CT findings in four cases. Am J Roentgenol 1989; 152:961–964.
20. Nishimura K, Izumi T, Kitaichi M, Nagai S, Itoh H. The diagnostic accuracy of high-

resolution computed tomography in diffuse infiltrative lung diseases. Chest 1993; 104:1149–1155.

21. Crausman R, Lynch D, Mortenson R, King TJ, Irvin C, Hale V, Newell JJ. Quantitative CT predicts the severity of physiologic dysfunction in patients with lymphangioleiomyomatosis. Chest 1996; 109:131–137.
22. Woodring JH, Howard 2nd RS, Johnson MV. Massive low-attenuation mediastinal, retroperitoneal, and pelvic lymphadenopathy on CT from lymphangioleiomyomatosis. Case report. Clin Imaging 1994; 18:7–11.
23. Sider L, Field LR, Courser JR JI, Yolandis AV, Martin GJ. Recurrent pneumothorax and adenopathy. Chest 1995; 107:860–862.
24. Andreassian B, Pariente R, Duchatelle JP, Mal H, Jebrak G. Selection criteria and preoperative management. Obstructive and restrictive lung disease. In: Patterson G, Couraud L, eds. Lung Transplantation. Vol. 3. New York: Elsevier, 1995:35–51.
25. Crausman R, Jennings C, Mortenson R, Ackerson L, Irvin C, King TJ. Lymphangioleiomyomatosis: the pathophysiology of diminished exercise capacity. Am J Respir Crit Care Med 1996; 153:1368–1376.
26. Carrington CB, Cugell DW, Gaensler EA, et al. Lymphangioleiomyomatosis: physiologic-pathologic-radiologic correlations. Am Rev Respir Dis 1977; 116:977–995.
27. Burger CD, Hyatt RE, Staats BA. Pulmonary mechanics in lymphangioleiomyomatosis. Am Rev Respir Dis 1991; 143:1030–1033.
28. Bonetti F, Chiodera P. Lymphangioleiomyomatosis and tuberous sclerosis: Where is the border? [editorial]. Eur Respir J 1996; 9:399–401.
29. Gomez MR. Phenotypes of the tuberous sclerosis complex with a revision of diagnostic criteria. In: Johnson WG, ed. Tuberous Sclerosis and Allied Disorders. New York: The New York Academy of Sciences, 1991:1–7.
30. Tanaka H, Imada A, Morikawa T, Shibusa T, Satoh M, Sekine K, Abe S. Diagnosis of pulmonary lymphangioleiomyomatosis by HMB45 in surgically treated spontaneous pneumothorax. Eur Respir J 1995; 8:1879–1882.
31. Chan J, Tsang W, Pau M, Tang M, Pang S, Fletcher C. Lymphangiomyomatosis and angiomyolipoma: closely related entities characterized by hamartomatous proliferation of HMB-45-positive smooth muscle [see comments]. Histopathology 1993; 22:445–455.
32. Pea M. Bonetti F, Zamboni G, Martignoni G, Riva M, Colombari R, Mombello A, Bonzanini M, Scarpa A, Ghimenton C, et al. Melanocyte-marker-HMB-45 is regularly expressed in angiomyolipoma of the kidney. Pathology 1991; 23:185–188.
33. Spencer JA, Smith MJ, Golding SJ. Lymphangioleiomyomatosis with unusual calcific retroperitoneal lymphangiomyoma: CT findings. Eur J Radiol 1992; 14:192–194.
34. Kerr LA, Blute ML, Ryu JH, Swensen SJ, Malek RS. Renal angiomyolipoma in association with pulmonary lymphangioleiomyomatosis: forme fruste of tuberous sclerosis. Urology 1993; 41:440–444.
35. Maziak D, Kesten S, Rappaport D, Maurer J. Extrathoracic angiomyolipomas in lymphangioleiomyomatosis. Eur Respir J 1996; 9:402–405.

36. Bernstein S, Newell JJ, Adamczyk D, Mortenson R, King TJ, Lynch D. How common are renal angiomyolipomas in patients with pulmonary lymphangiomyomatosis? Am J Respir Crit Care Med 1995; 152:2138–2143.
37. Blute ML, Malek RS, Segura JW. Angiomyolipoma: clinical metamorphosis and concepts for management. J Urol 1988; 139:20–24.
38. Bjornsson J, Short MP, Kwiatkowski DJ, Petri Henske E. Tuberous sclerosis-associated renal cell carcinoma. Am J Pathol 1996; 149:1201–1208.
39. Eliasson AH, Phillips YY, Tenholder MF. Treatment of lymphangioleiomyomatosis. A meta-analysis. Chest 1989; 196:1352–1355.
40. Clemm C, Jehn U, Wolf-Hornung B, Siemon G, Walter G. Lymphangiomyomatosis: a report of three cases treated with tamoxifen. Klin Wochenschr 1987; 65:391–393.
41. Rossi GA, Balbi B, Oddera S, Lantero S, Ravazzoni C. Response to treatment with an analog of the luteinizing-hormone-releasing hormone in a patient with pulmonary lymphangioleiomyomatosis. Am Rev Respir Dis 1991; 143:174–176.
42. Radermecker M, Bronx R, Corhay JL, Limet R, Radermecker M. Failure of buserelin-induced medical castration to control pulmonary lymphangiomyomatosis in two patients. Chest 1992; 101:1724–1726.
43. Klein M, Krieger O, Ruckser R, Rosen A, Waldner R, Preis P, Beck A. Treatment of lymphangioleiomyomatosis by ovariectomy, interferon alpha 2b and tamoxifen—a case report. Arch Gynecol Obstet 1992; 252:99–102.
44. Torres VE, Björnsson J, King BF, Kumar R, Zincke H, Edell ES, Wilson TO, Hattery RR, Gomez MR. Extrapulmonary lymphangioleiomyomatosis and lymphangiomatous cysts in tuberous sclerosis complex. Mayo Clin Proc 1995; 70:641–648.
45. Ohori N, Yousem S, Sonmez-Alpan E, Colby T. Estrogen and progesterone receptors in lymphangioleiomyomatosis, epithelioid hemangioendothelioma, and sclerosing hemangioma of the lung. Am J Clin Pathol 1991; 96:529–535.
46. Ettinger NA. Single-lung transplantation: results. In: Patterson G, Couraud L, eds. Lung Transplantation. Vol. 3. New York: Elsevier, 1995: 363–378.
47. Kelly K, Hertz MI. Obliterative bronchiolitis. In: Maurer JR, ed. Surgical Approaches to End-Stage Disease: Lung Transplantation and Volume Reduction. Vol. 18. Philadelphia: W. B. Saunders, 1997:319–338.
48. Sundaresan S, Trulock EP, Mohanakumar T, Cooper JD, Patterson GA. Prevalence and outcome of bronchiolitis obliterans syndrome after lung transplantation. Ann Thorac Surg 1995; 60:1341–1346.
49. Novick RJ, Stitt L, Schafers HJ, Andreassian B, Duchatelle JP, Klepetko W, Hardesty RL, Frost A, Patterson GA. Pulmonary retransplantation: Does the indication for operation influence postoperative lung function? J Thorac Cardiovasc Surg 1996; 112:1504–1513.
50. Johnson BA, Duncan SR, Ohori NP, Paradis IL, Yousem SA, Grgurich WF, Dauber JH, Griffith BP. Recurrence of sarcoidosis in pulmonary allograft recipients. Am Rev Respir Dis 1993; 148:1373–1377.
51. Yeatman M, McNeil K, Smith JA, Stewart S, Sharples LD, Higenbottam T, Wells FC, Wallwork J. Lung transplantation in patients with systemic diseases: an eleven-year experience at Papworth Hospital. J Heart Lung Transplant 1996; 15:144–149.

52. Frost AE, Keller CA, Brown RW, Noon GP, Short HD, Abraham JL, Pacinda S, Cagle PT. Giant cell interstitial pneumonitis: disease recurrence in the transplanted lung. Am Rev Respir Dis 1993; 148:1401–1404.
53. Baz MA, Kussin PS, Van Trigt P, Davis RD, Roggli VL, Tapson VF. Recurrence of diffuse panbronchiolitis after lung transplantation. Am J Respir Crit Care Med 1995; 151:895–898.

7

The Registry for Individuals with Lymphangioleiomyomatosis

EUGENE J. SULLIVAN, GERALD J. BECK, and JAMES K. STOLLER

The Cleveland Clinic Foundation
Cleveland, Ohio

I. Introduction

A Registry for Individuals with LAM has been proposed recently as a way of enhancing current understanding of the clinical features, natural history, and current therapy practices for individuals with lymphangioleiomyomatosis (LAM). The purpose of this chapter is to describe the objectives and design of this proposed Registry. Specifically, we first address the definition and rationale for registries in general, followed by a description of the rationale for a registry specifically to examine LAM. This section summarizes current knowledge regarding the natural history of LAM, highlighting the inadequacy of available information that requires larger coordinated, multicenter effort. Finally, we describe the objectives of the proposed Registry and the current concept of the Registry structure that is designed to meet these objectives.

II. Definition and Rationale for Registries

In the context of biomedical research, a registry may be defined as a mechanism to collect information about a single disease or clinical condition. While not a constant feature of registries, most registries are conducted at multiple different sites or centers because a registry is usually required when the condition under study is sufficiently uncommon that no one single center can assemble a large, representative cohort of affected individuals. By accruing individuals at many different sites, the number of individuals identified can be increased and the opportunity to describe the full spectrum of variation in the index condition is enhanced.

Depending on the objective, a registry may be cross-sectional (or a "single-state" registry) or the registry can assess longitudinal follow-up of participating subjects. Registries that collect only cross-sectional information identify and characterize participants once and may be likened to a mailing list or roster. Information from a cross-sectional registry is therefore limited to a single-state description of participants. In contrast, a longitudinal registry conducts serial evaluations of participants over time in order to describe temporal changes in the index condition or to observe the response to a changing circumstance, including therapy. Not surprisingly, registries that have the goal of describing the natural history of a condition are longitudinal registries. Indeed, because the need to better understand the natural history of a condition is frequently the impetus for forming a registry, most registries are longitudinal.

Besides the LAM Registry described in this chapter, there are several current examples of registries that have been conducted under the auspices of the National Heart, Lung, and Blood Institute. For example, the Primary Pulmonary Hypertension (PPH) Registry was initiated in 1981 with the goal of characterizing the natural history and describing treatment experience with primary pulmonary hypertension, a relatively uncommon and erstwhile poorly understood condition (1). The Primary Pulmonary Hypertension Registry included 32 clinical centers and recruited 194 subjects. With publications from the Registry first appearing in 1987, this registry has contributed important insights about primary pulmonary hypertension. For example, the PPH Registry allowed study of high-dose calcium channel blockers and of intravenous prostacyclin as therapy for primary pulmonary hypertension. Similarly, the PPH Registry demonstrated that demographic and pulmonary function test measurements were poor predictors of survival, but that hemodynamic variables (i.e., right atrial pressure, pulmonary artery pressure, and cardiac index) were independent survival predictors.

Another example of an NHLBI-sponsored registry is the Registry for Patients with Deficiency of α_1-Antitrypsin (2). Initiated in 1988, this registry included 37 clinical centers in the United States and Canada and recruited 1129 eligible subjects (adults with severe deficiency of α_1-antitrypsin) between March 1989 and October 1992 with follow-up extending through April 1996. Having assembled the largest cohort of individuals with severe deficiency of α_1-antitrypsin, the registry has already contributed important insights. For example, the fact that 30% of participants report being retired early for medical reasons despite a mean age of 46 years emphasizes the debilitating nature of α_1-antitrypsin deficiency. Other important observations from the registry regarding the baseline and longitudinal features of participants and the natural history of α_1-antitrypsin deficiency are both in press currently and forthcoming as analyses are finalized.

As the Registry for Individuals with Lymphangioleiomyomatosis is undertaken, it is hoped that similar important contributions about this sparsely studied and relatively poorly understood condition will also be possible. The rationale for forming an LAM Registry is reviewed below.

III. The Rationale for a Registry for Individuals with Lymphangioleiomyomatosis: Inadequacy of Available Information About LAM

The major rationale for a LAM Registry is that because LAM is an uncommon condition, available studies include small numbers of individuals with relatively short follow-up intervals and so available information about pathophysiology, natural history, and optimal therapy is incomplete. Specifically, the main shortcomings in the available information regarding this disease occur in three areas: (1) clinical characteristics and natural history of LAM, (2) cellular and molecular mechanisms of the proliferation of LAM cells and pulmonary parenchymal destruction, and (3) effectiveness of current and future therapies for the disease. By accruing a large cohort of individuals with LAM, the objective of the Registry is to garner data to address each of these areas.

With regard to deficiencies of current understanding about the clinical features and natural history of LAM, there have been several case series that characterized the disease manifestations (3–6), the largest of which included 46 subjects (3). While these studies provide useful descriptions regarding the common disease manifestations, they also serve to illustrate the diverse nature of these manifestations and current uncertainties about prognosis. For instance, the mean age of onset of symptoms attributable to LAM has frequently been reported to be early in the fourth decade of life (3,4,6), but the range of ages of onset is quite broad, from as early as 11 (7) and 17 (6) to as late as the seventh decade (3,4). Further, while LAM is felt to be slowly progressive in general, leading eventually to respiratory failure and death, the natural history of the disease seems to be quite variable. In Corrin's 1975 review of 28 cases (6), 11 patients were noted to have died 1–10 years after the onset of symptoms. However, other patients were noted to still be alive up to 17 years after the onset of symptoms. In fact, one patient was said to have remained "virtually asymptomatic" after 9 years, without radiographic progression of the disease (6). There have been reports of patients who remained alive 19 (8), 27 (9), and 28 (10) years after the development of the pneumothorax that was the presenting symptom of LAM. Conversely, Banner et al. (8) reported two patients who died less than 3 years after the development of their first symptom of LAM, a pneumothorax. In the report of Taylor et al., (4) 25 of 32 patients (78) were alive 8.5 years after the onset of the disease, but in a more recent series of 46 LAM patients from Japan, Korea, and Taiwan, only 10 of 26 (38%) were alive after 8.5 years (3). The features that were shown to portend a poorer prognosis in this study (i.e., reduced FEV_1/FVC, an elevated TLC percent predicted, and histology revealing predominantly cysts rather than extensive smooth muscle proliferation) seemed to be indicators of more severe disease (3). One factor that has been postulated to play a role in disease progression is the patient's hormonal status. Several cases have been reported in which the pulmonary symptoms developed or worsened during pregnancy (5,11–16) or with the administration of exogenous estrogens (17), although a case-control study performed in the United Kingdom failed to detect any association between LAM and the use of oral contraceptives (18). In summary, the current literature provides a fair description of common clinical manifestations of the disease, but it also reveals a broad spectrum of disease manifestations and a variable understanding of natural history while shedding little light on any potential factors that may predict or influence survival.

As discussed elsewhere in this text, the histopathologic hallmark of this disease is the proliferation of atypical smooth muscle cells (so-called LAM cells) throughout the lung. With regard to gaps in the current understanding of the cellular and molecular mechanisms of LAM, little is known regarding the nature of these cells, why they proliferate, or how their proliferation results in the dramatic destruction of the normal pulmonary parenchyma and cyst formation. Although inconsistent, the finding of estrogen and progesterone receptors in these cells (19–21) has raised the possibility of hormonal regulation in the process. Receptors for HMB-45, a monoclonal antibody that recognizes antigens on the surface of melanoma cell lines, have been found on LAM cells (22), although the significance of this finding is not clear. It has been suggested that the emphysema develops because of airflow obstruction related to narrowing of the lumina of bronchioles and small bronchi by the proliferating LAM cells (6,11). However, the emphysematous airspaces are not always seen in anatomic association with airway luminal compromise (11), leading some authors to postulate other mechanisms of parenchymal destruction (23).

Finally, there are significant gaps in the current understanding of the mechanisms of action and effectiveness of currently utilized treatments for the disease. No randomized trial of any treatment is available, and the paucity of individuals with the disease and the wide variability in the natural history of the disease have frustrated attempts to assess the efficacy of currently available therapy. Understanding treatment efficacy is further frustrated by the currently poor understanding of the cellular and molecular mechanisms that drive LAM cell proliferation. It seems apparent that corticosteroids and cytotoxic agents offer no benefit (5,11,24–27). Mediastinal, retroperitoneal, and whole lung irradiation have also been attempted without apparent success (5). Given the occurrence of the disease in women of childbearing years, reports of clinical worsening with exogenous estrogen administration, and the demonstration of estrogen and progesterone receptors in the proliferating LAM cells, many clinicians have attempted to use hormonal manipulation therapeutically. Treatment with oophorectomy (8,15,28), progesterone (12–16,29,30), luteinizing hormone–releasing hormone (LHRH) agonists (24,29,31), tamoxifen (12,15,16,32), or combinations of these (15,30,33,34) has been the subject of many case reports or small uncontrolled series. Responses to such treatments have been quite variable, and no definitive conclusion can be drawn from these reports. Based on an experience with 32 patients, Taylor et al. (4) observed no therapeutic benefit from oophorectomy or antiestrogen therapy with tamoxifen. There was some evidence that progesterone was beneficial in at least some patients with LAM, and the investigators recommended its use in all symptomatic patients with LAM. Interestingly, combining their patients with those in the literature, they found no correlation between tissue estrogen or progesterone receptor status and response to hormonal therapy (4). In 1989, Eliasson et al. performed a meta-analysis of 30 previously reported cases and concluded that oophorectomy, progesterone, or both were the most effective treatments (14). Finally, there is an emerging experience with lung transplantation in patients with end-stage LAM (35–38), but even the most recent and largest report from 16 different transplant centers described only 34 lung transplant recipients. The 18 surviving subjects have been followed for a mean duration of 33 months (range 3–74 months) (38).

In summary, it is these gaps in the current understanding of LAM, the desire to advance this understanding, and the realization that such advancement will require a multicenter, long-term study that has spurred interest in the current LAM Registry.

IV. Proposed Objectives and Structure of the Registry for Individuals with Lymphangioleiomyomatosis

In an effort to further our understanding of the clinical characteristics, natural history, molecular mechanisms, and efficacy of treatments of LAM, a large, multicenter registry has been proposed. The specific aims of this Registry are as follows:

1. To characterize the clinical features of subjects with LAM, including clinical signs and symptoms as well as demographic, radiographic and physiologic features
2. To assess the natural history of the disease and identify clinical features which may predict or influence disease progression
3. To examine the clinical features of individuals referred for lung transplantation and to assess the efficacy of this therapy
4. To collect biopsy specimens from participants to enable future scientific research into the molecular mechanisms of the disease
5. To assemble a cohort of patients and an organizational framework which may be utilized for future clinical treatment trials

Based upon data from the LAM Foundation (personal communication) as well as the opinion of a recent NIH-sponsored Working Group on LAM, it is estimated that there are currently approximately 200–400 identified LAM patients in the United States. Inclusion of these individuals in the Registry with recruitment of additional eligible participants from many centers would therefore represent the largest cohort of LAM patients ever reported and would allow a definitive description of the clinical features of the disease. The central collection of biopsy specimens as well as surgically explanted lungs would provide ample material with which to pursue future studies into the molecular characteristics of LAM. Analysis of the course of the disease in the context of the various nonrandomized treatment strategies may shed some light on the efficacy of currently utilized treatments, although it is recognized that a randomized trial would be necessary to reach definitive conclusions. While such a randomized treatment trial is not part of the Registry as it is currently proposed, the Registry would clearly provide the organizational framework as well as an established means of identifying potential subjects for the purpose of such a future trial.

In order to address these objectives, the LAM Registry will collect and follow a cohort of individuals who satisfy established criteria for the diagnosis of LAM (Table 1). The subjects will be followed over the duration of the study with periodic visits to collect information regarding symptoms, treatments, and physiologic function. For the purpose of the Registry, the diagnosis of LAM will

Table 1 LAM Registry: Eligibility Criteria

Diagnostic lung biopsy[a]
Characteristic features on high-resolution chest CT in the appropriate clinical setting[b]

[a]Reviewed by expert pathology panel.
[b]The clinical setting is considered appropriate in female subjects of any age who demonstrate any of the following features: dyspnea, cough, hemoptysis, chyloptysis, chylous ascites, pneumothorax, pleural effusion, extrapulmonary angiomyolipoma, or abnormal pulmonary function studies.

be considered "established" on the basis of a confirmatory lung biopsy and/or a characteristic high-resolution chest CT scan in the appropriate clinical setting. The clinical setting will be considered "appropriate" in female subjects of any age who demonstrate any of the following features: dyspnea, cough, hemoptysis, chyloptysis, chylous ascites, pneumothorax, pleural effusion, extrapulmonary angiomyolipoma, or abnormal pulmonary function studies. The CT scans will be reviewed by a panel of expert radiologists who will collectively make the determination if the scans are sufficiently characteristic of LAM to merit inclusion into the study. Because the histopathology of LAM is identical to that seen in the lungs of some patients with tuberous sclerosis (TS) and the stigmata of TS may be subtle, the clinical distinction between these two diseases may be difficult (5,39,40). Therefore, the LAM Registry will include all patients meeting the above criteria, regardless of whether stigmata of TS are present. Those patients with an established diagnosis of TS may be examined separately in the data analysis.

Potential Registry participants will be evaluated and entered into the Registry through six major clinical centers located across the country. The six currently participating clinical centers are: Stanford University, The Mayo Clinic Foundation, the National Jewish Medical and Research Center, The Cleveland Clinic Foundation, New England Medical Center, and the National Institutes of Health. In order to maximize recruitment, the Registry will not require that all participants be seen at the clinical centers. Individual practicing physicians who may be remote from a participating clinical center will be invited to contribute information about their patients. Each clinical center will be able to enter these subjects into the Registry on the basis of information submitted by the non-Registry physicians, provided they meet the established eligibility criteria.

At entry into the Registry, various data will be acquired (Table 2). Such data will include demographic features, symptoms, signs, medical and surgical history, medication history, current or past treatments for LAM, results of pulmonary function test and radiographic studies, and family history. Certain types of data, including symptoms, medications, and pulmonary functions, will be collected on an annual basis thereafter. In those patients who undergo lung transplantation, data will also be collected regarding the early and late complications of transplant as well as evidence of the recurrence of the disease in the transplanted lung. Patients will be followed for the duration of the study, which is currently expected to be 5 years.

Notably, the Registry is designed as an observational cohort study with no effort being made to randomize patients or to dictate therapies. To characterize the natural history of LAM in individuals receiving different types of treatment currently, the Registry will collect and analyze information regarding therapies

Table 2 LAM Registry: Initial Data Element Categories

Demographic features
(e.g., age, race, smoking status)
Functional status and quality of life
Signs and symptoms
(e.g., dyspnea, cough, hemoptysis, pain, weight gain/loss, edema, pneumothorax)
Past medical history and hospitalizations
(e.g., comorbid conditions, date of first diagnosis of LAM, pregnancy history)
Medication history
(e.g., prescription medications used with approximate dates or use with particular attention to hormonal medications)
Family history
Diagnosis and treatment of LAM sequelae
(e.g., thoracenteses, chest tubes, pleurodeses, etc.)
Pulmonary function testing
Radiographic studies
(descriptive features of chest x-rays and computed tomography)
Tissue specimens
(descriptive features of biopsy specimens)

utilized and patient outcomes. However, by virtue of the observational nature of the data, firm conclusions regarding therapeutic efficacy are not expected.

As presented in Figure 1, the organizational structure of the Registry will include several other components in addition to the 6 clinical centers. A steering committee consisting of representatives of each of the clinical centers, the data coordinating center, and the NIH will oversee the conduct of the Registry as a whole. The central office of the Registry, termed the data coordinating center, will be located at the Cleveland Clinic Foundation. The study design and data analysis group will be charged with the task of finalizing the protocol, data forms, and manual of operations, addressing issues of data quality control as well as subsequent analysis of the data generated. The data management group will oversee the day-to-day process of data entry and database management. A death review committee will review details of all deaths of Registry subjects and assign a cause of death for entry into the database. The data coordinating center will also oversee the activity of the three "Cores" included in the Registry design (Fig. 1). These Cores include an Imaging Core, a Tissue Core, and a Pulmonary Function Core. The Imaging Core will consist of three expert chest radiologists who will review all chest x-rays and chest CT scans with standardized criteria for the dual purposes of verifying the appropriateness of the diagnosis of LAM and scoring the extent, distribution, and characteristics of the radiographic abnormalities. The

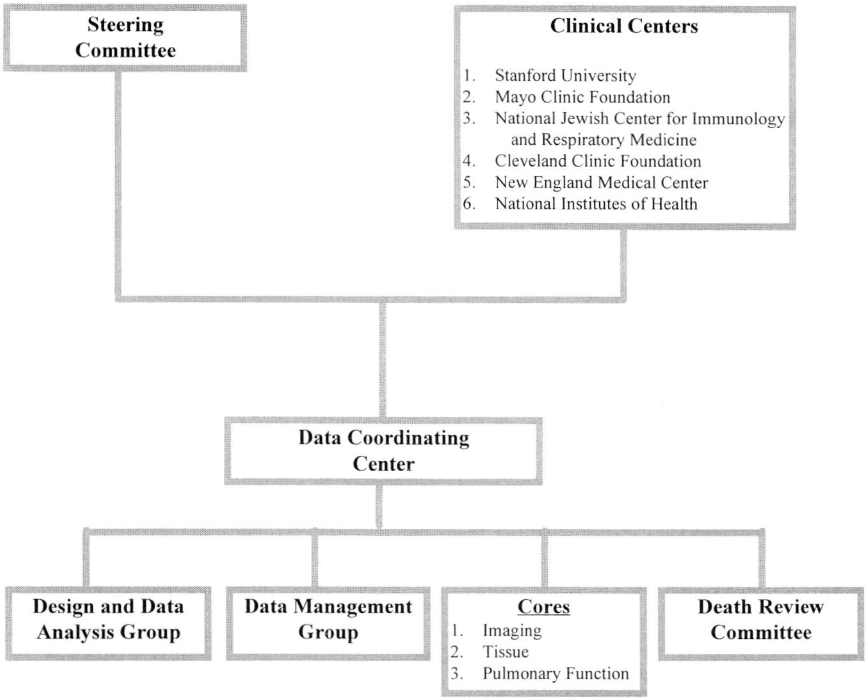

Figure 1 Organizational chart of the Registry for Individuals with Lymphangioleiomyomatosis.

scores generated by this team will be entered into the database for subsequent analysis and correlation with other data. As with other registries (e.g., Registry for Individuals with α_1-Antitrypsin Deficiency) the task of the Pulmonary Function Core will be to review the submitted pulmonary function data for the purposes of quality control. The Tissue Core, located at the National Institutes of Health, will serve two critical roles. First, it will review the pathology specimens of potential Registry participants in order to verify the diagnosis of LAM and to evaluate the extent, severity, and characteristics of the pathologic findings. As with the Imaging Core, the descriptive data generated by the Tissue Core will be entered into the database for subsequent analysis. Second, the Tissue Core will serve as the repository of all tissue specimens collected under the auspices of the Registry. This will include transbronchial, thoracoscopic, or open lung biopsy specimens, as well as explanted whole lungs from lung transplant recipients. This tissue will subsequently be made available upon request to qualified investigators after review of the proposed research project by the Steering Committee.

V. Summary

There is much to be learned regarding this rare and intriguing disorder, which strikes young women with devastating outcome. It is hoped that the development of a large multicenter Registry of Individuals with LAM will further our understanding of many aspects of the disease and provide a stimulus and material for further investigations.

References

1. Dantzker DR. Primary pulmonary hypertension: the American experience. Chest 1994; 150:26S–28S.
2. The Alpha 1-Antitrypsin Deficiency Registry Study Group. Prepared by: Schluchter MD, Barker AF, Crystal RG, Robbins RA, Stocks JM, Stoller JK, Wu MC. A registry of patients with severe deficiency of alpha 1-antitrypsin: design and methods. Chest 1994; 106:1223–1233.
3. Kitaichi M, Nishimura K, Itoh H, Izumi T. Pulmonary lymphangioleiomyomatosis: a report of 46 patients including a clinicopathologic study of prognostic factors. Am J Respir Crit Care Med 1995; 151:527–533.
4. Taylor JR, Ryu J, Colby TV, Raffin TA. Lymphangioleiomyomatosis: clinical course in 32 patients. N Engl J Med 1990; 323:1254–1260.
5. Silverstein EF, Ellis K, Wolff M, Jaretzki A. Pulmonary lymphangiomyomatosis. Am J Roentgenol 1974; 120:832–850.
6. Corrin B, Liebow AA, Friedman PJ. Pulmonary lymphangiomyomatosis: a review. Am J Pathol 1975; 79:347–382.
7. Awai K. Fujikawa K, Sato T, Nishioka Y, Azuma K, Sasaki Y, Ito K, Hiramoto T, Daido K, Sakano T, Nanbu S, Yonehara S. Pulmonary lymphangiomyomatosis. Rad Med 1990; 8:132–135.
8. Banner AS, Carrington CB, Emory WB, Kittle F, Leonard G, Ringus J, Taylor P, and Addington WW. Efficacy of oophorectomy in lymphangioleiomyomatosis and benign metastaaizing leiomyoma. N Engl J Med 1981; 305:204–209.
9. Bevelaqua FA, Epstein H. Pulmonary lymphangiomyomatosis. Long-term survival in a patient with poor response to medroxyprogesterone. Chest 1985; 87:552–553.
10. Sawicka EH, Morris JR. A report of two long-surviving cases of pulmonary lymphangioleiomyomatosis and the response to progesterone therapy. Br J Dis Chest 1985; 79:400–406.
11. Carrington CB, Cugell DW, Gaensler EA, Marks A, Redding RA, Schaaf, Tomasian A. Lymphangioleiomyomatosis: physiologic pathologic radiologic correlations. Am Rev Respir Dis 1977; 116:977–995.
12. Hughes E, Hodder RV. Pulmonary lymphangiomyomatosis complicating pregnancy, a case report. J Reprod Med 32:553–557.
13. McCarty KS, Mossler JA, McLelland R, Sieker HO. Pulmonary lymphangiomyomatosis responsive to progesterone. N Engl J Med 1980; 303:1461–1465.

14. Eliasson AH, Phillips YY, Tenholder MF. Treatment of lymphangioleiomyomatosis: a meta-analysis. Chest 1989; 196:1352–1355.
15. Urban T, Kuttenn F, Gompel A, Marsac J, Lacronique J. Pulmonary lymphangiomyomatosis. Follow-up and long-term outcome with antiestrogen therapy; a report of eight cases. Chest 1992; 102:472–476.
16. Yockey CC, Riepe RE, Ryan K. Pulmonary lymphangioleiomyomatosis complicated by pregnancy. Kansas Med 1986; 87:277–293.
17. Shen A, Iseman MD, Waldron JA, King TE. Exacerbation of pulmonary lymphangioleiomyomatosis by exogenous estrogens. Chest 1987; 91:782–785.
18. Wahedna I, Cooper S, Williams J, Paterson IC, Britton JR, Tattersfield AE. Relation of pulmonary lymphangioleiomyomatosis to use of the oral contraceptive pill and fertility in the UK: a national case control study. Thorax 1994; 49:910–914.
19. Brentani MM, Carvalho CRR, Saldiva PH, Pacheco MM, Oshima CTF. Steroid receptors in pulmonary lymphangiomyomatosis. Chest 1984; 85:96–99.
20. Graham ML, Spelsberg TC, Dines DE, Payne WS, Bjornsson J, Lie JT. Pulmonary lymphangiomyomatosis: with particular reference to steroid-receptor assay studies and pathologic correlation. Mayo Clin Proc 1984; 59:3–11.
21. Colley MH, Geppert E, Franklin WA. Immunohistochemical detection of steroid receptors in a case of pulmonary lymphangioleiomyomatosis. Am J Surg Pathol 1989; 13:803–807.
22. Bonetti F, Chiodera PL, Pea M, Martignoni G, Bosi F, Zamboni G, Mariuzzi GM. Transbronchial biopsy in lymphangiomyomatosis of the lung: HMB45 for diagnosis. Am J Surg Pathol 1993; 17:1092–1102.
23. Fukuda Y, Kawamoto M, Yamamoto A, Ishizaki M, Basset F, Masugi Y. Role of elastic fiber degradation in emphysema-like lesions of pulmonary lymphangiomyomatosis. Hum Pathol 1990; 21:1252–1261.
24. Rossi GA, Balbi B, Oddera S, Lantero S, Ravazzoni C. Response to treatment with an analog of the luteinizing-hormone-releasing hormone in a patient with pulmonary lymphangioleiomyomatosis. Am Rev Respir Dis 143:174–176.
25. Tomasian A, Greenberg MS, and Rumerman H. Tamoxifen for lymphangiomyomatosis. N Engl J Med 1982; 306:745–476.
26. Luna CM, Gene R, Jolly EC, Nahmod N, Defranchi, HA, Patino G, Elsner B. Pulmonary lymphangiomyomatosis associated with tuberous sclerosis: treatment with tamoxifen and tetracycline-pleurodesis. Chest 1985; 86:473–475.
27. Bush JK, McLean RL, Sieker HO. Diffuse disease due to lymphangiomyoma. Am J Med 1969; 46:645–654.
28. Kitzsteiner KA, Mallen RG. Pulmonary lymphangiomyomatosis: treatment with castration. Cancer 1980; 46:2248–2249.
29. Radermecker M, Broux R, Corhay J, Limet R, Radermecker M. Failure of Buserelin-induced medical castration to control pulmonary lymphangiomyomatosis in two patients. Chest 1992; 101:1724–1726.
30. Sieker HO, McCartty KS. Lymphangiomyomatosis: a respiratory illness with an endocrinologic therapy. Trans Am Clin Clim Assoc 1987; 99:57–67.
31. Maheux R, Parent J, Samson Y, Jean C, Farid NR. Utilization of luteinizing hor-

mone-releasing hormone agonist in pulmonary leiomyomatosis. Fertility and Sterility 1987; 48:315–317.
32. Clemm C, Jehn U, Wolf-Hornung B, Siemon G, Walter G. Lymphangiomyomatosis: a report of three cases treated with tamoxifen. Klin Wochenscher 1987; 65:391–393.
33. Adamson D, Heinrichs WL, Raybin DM, Raffin TA. Successful treatment of pulmonary lymphangiomyomatosis with oophorectomy and progesterone. Am Rev Respir Dis, 1985; 132:916–921.
34. Svendsen TL, Viskum K, Hansborg N, Thorpe SM, Nielsen NC. Pulmonary lymphangioleiomyomatosis: a case of progesterone receptor positive lymphangioleiomyomatosis treated with medroxyprogesterone, oophorectomy and tamoxifen. Br J Dis Chest 1984; 78:264–271.
35. Nine JS, Yousem SA, Paradis IL, Keenan R, Griffith BP. Lymphangioleiomatosis recurrence after lung transplantation. J Heart Lung Transplant 1994; 13:714–719.
36. Wellens F, Estenne M, de Francquen P, Goldstein J, Leclerc JL, and Primo G. Combined heart-lung transplantation for terminal pulmonary lymphangioleiomyomatosis. J Thorac Cardiovasc Surg 1985; 89:872–876.
37. Sleiman C, Mal H, Jebrak G, Darne C, Meeus E, Dubois F, Luisetti M, Fournier M, Pariente R, Andreassian B. Pulmonary lymphangiomyomatosis treated by single lung transplantation. Am Rev Respir Dis 1992; 145:964–966.
38. Boehler A, Speich R, Russi EW, and Weder W. Lung transplantation for lymphangioleiomyomatosis. N Engl J Med 1996; 335:1275–1280.
39. Capron F, Ameille J, Leclerc P, Mornet P, Barbagellata M, Reynes M, Rochemaure J. Pulmonary lymphangioleiomyomatosis and Bourneville's tuberous sclerosis with pulmonary involvement: the same disease? Cancer 1983; 52:851–855.
40. Valensi QJ. Pulmonary lymphangiomyoma, a probable forme frust of tuberous sclerosis. Am Rev Respir Dis 1973; 108:141–1415.

8

Lymphangioleiomyomatosis
Differential Diagnosis

ROBERT S. CRAUSMAN

Memorial Hospital of Rhode Island
and Brown University School of Medicine
Providence, Rhode Island

FRANCIS X. McCORMACK

University of Cincinnati Medical Center
Cincinnati, Ohio

TALMADGE E. KING, Jr.*

National Jewish Medical and Research Center
and University of Colorado Health Sciences Center
Denver, Colorado

I. Introduction

Pulmonary lymphangioleiomyomatosis (LAM) is an uncommon cause of progressive dyspnea in premenopausal women. The typical medical history of such a patient generally reveals a delayed or missed diagnosis despite years of respiratory symptoms. As a consequence, most women with confirmed LAM have advanced, irreversible disease. The late identification of LAM study subjects may be partially responsible for the dismal prognosis and poor response to treatment in reported series (1,2). Conceptually, the diagnosis and treatment of patients in an earlier phase of disease offers the best hope for a response.

The diagnosis of LAM is delayed because we do not think of it until characteristic signs develop, such as recurrent pneumothorax or chylous effusions. It does not occur to us earlier because: (1) it is rare, probably affecting less than 1000 people in the United States, (2) the chest roentgenographic findings can be very subtle, and (3) the most common symptoms, such as dyspnea on exertion, do not help to discriminate LAM from much more common diseases that present

**Current affiliation*: San Francisco General Hospital and University of California School of Medicine, San Francisco, California with obstructive physiology such as asthma and chronic obstructive pulmonary disease (COPD).

The primary responsibility for early recognition rests with the primary care physician. It is probably more reasonable to expect generalists to recognize when a lung disease is behaving in a fashion that is unlike asthma or COPD than to try to familiarize all physicians with the protean manifestations of LAM. Therefore, in this chapter we will contrast the presentation of common diseases such as asthma and emphysema with that of LAM. The objective is to promote early referral to a specialist when uncertainty about the cause of a patient's dyspnea exists. Once considered by a physician who is familiar with the disease, the diagnosis of LAM is rarely difficult. It is unlikely that we will be able to determine the efficacy of various treatments unless we can identify LAM patients before respiratory reserves are exhausted and lung architecture is irreversibly distorted.

In this chapter, we will (1) review the clinical, pathologic, physiologic, and radiographic manifestations of LAM and (2) discuss the features of LAM that distinguish it from the diseases with which it is most commonly confused.

II. Questionnaire

To better define the problems associated with delayed diagnosis in LAM, questionnaires were sent to 210 patients registered with the LAM Foundation (LF) as of March 1997. A similar questionnaire had been sent in March 1996. The number of respondents to the 1996 inquiry was 104, and at the time of this writing 101 patients (including 26 new patients) had responded to the 1997 questionnaire. Where possible, data were compiled from both questionnaires ($n = 130$). Of those who responded, 92% reported that they presently had symptoms due to LAM and 80% stated that their diagnosis was confirmed by biopsy of lung, kidney, or lymph node.

III. Clinical Presentation

Lymphangioleiomyomatosis is an idiopathic diffuse parenchymal lung disease that primarily affects young and middle-aged premenopausal women (1,3,4). It is rare and accounts for less then 1% of all patients referred to our tertiary care pulmonary disease center (NJMRC). The diagnosis of LAM is routinely delayed, and more than 50% of LF patients had symptoms for at least one year prior to diagnosis (Fig. 1). Caucasians represented more than 95% of the LF patients, and the mean age at diagnosis was approximately 35 years of age (Fig. 2) (1,4,5). Many patients were initially misdiagnosed as having asthma or allergies, emphysema, spontaneous pneumothorax, chronic bronchitis, or fibrosing pulmonary

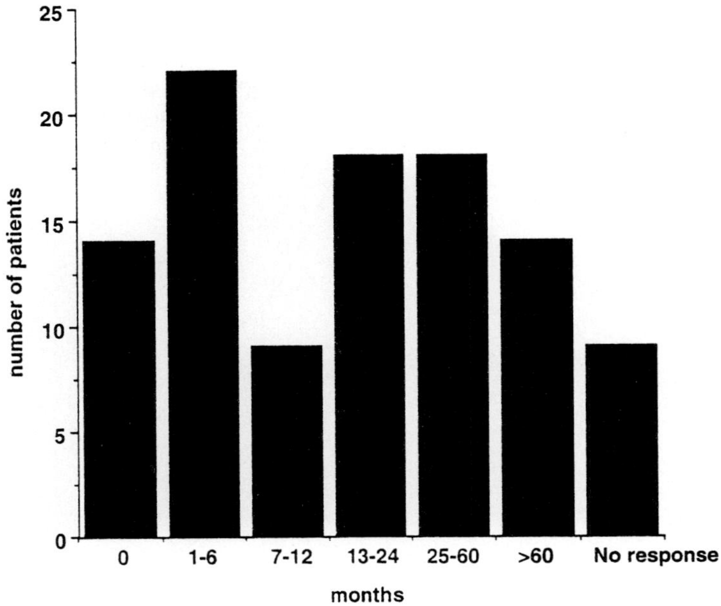

Figure 1 Duration of time elapsed from the onset of symptoms to the diagnosis of LAM for 104 LAM Foundation patients.

diseases such as idiopathic pulmonary fibrosis or pulmonary histiocytosis X (Fig. 3). Characteristic features of LAM including relentless decline in pulmonary function, lack of responsiveness to bronchodilators, pneumothorax, or cystic or chylous manifestations on chest x-ray (1,2) were the most common developments that prompted reevaluation that led to the correct diagnosis.

Dyspnea was the most common initial symptom (60%) and was present in most patients at diagnosis (1,4,5) (Table 1). Shortness of breath typically becomes quite limiting, and 74% of LF subjects reported dyspnea as their most troubling symptom. Dyspnea on exertion on ascending three flights of stairs was present in 77%, with one flight of stairs in 61%, with light housework in 40%, and with dressing in 21% ($n = 101$). Cough, phlegm production, and chest pain were infrequently reported as the symptoms prompting medical attention (<10%), but productive cough developed later in the course of disease in more than 30% of the subjects. Spontaneous pneumothorax was a common initial manifestation (48%) and eventually occurred in nearly all respondents (94%). The average age at first pneumothorax was 37 years (Fig. 2), and the average number of pneumothoraces per patient was 4.3 episodes. Recurrent pneumothorax or persistent

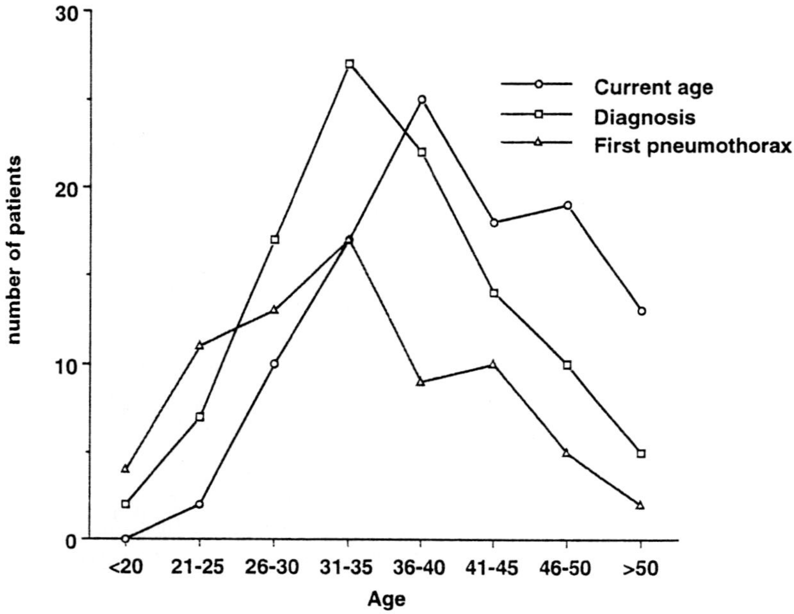

Figure 2 The current age (circle), age at the time of first pneumothorax (triangle), and age at the time of diagnosis (square) of LAM Foundation patients (n = 104).

bronchopleural fistula required pleurodesis, thoracotomy, or thoracoscopic surgery for more definitive therapy in 77% of patients (Table 2). Barotrauma and cyst rupture can still occur after pleural sclerosis and result in pneumomediastinum, pneumoretroperitoneum, pneumoretropharynx, or subcutaneous emphysema (6). Low-volume hemoptysis and/or chyloptysis, thought to be due to obstruction of small pulmonary vessels by proliferating smooth muscle cells (2), was reported by 44% of the LF subjects. Chylothorax, due to obstruction of the thoracic duct and other lymphatic vessels, was present in only a minority of patients at diagnosis (<10%) (7,8). Eventually, however, 50% of the patients developed this complication and 26% required drainage of the pleural space. Chylothorax can be difficult to treat, and repeated or continuous drainage is commonly associated with nutritional wasting and immunocompromise (9). Chyluria (10) (3%), chyloperitoneum (chylous ascites (13%) (11), and chylopericardium, due to abnormal connections between dilated lymphatics and the renal collecting system, peritoneal space, and pericardial sac, respectively, were also reported. Renal angiomyolipomata (AML) was very common (45%) in the LF population, and have been reported in more than 50% of patients referred for evaluation of pul-

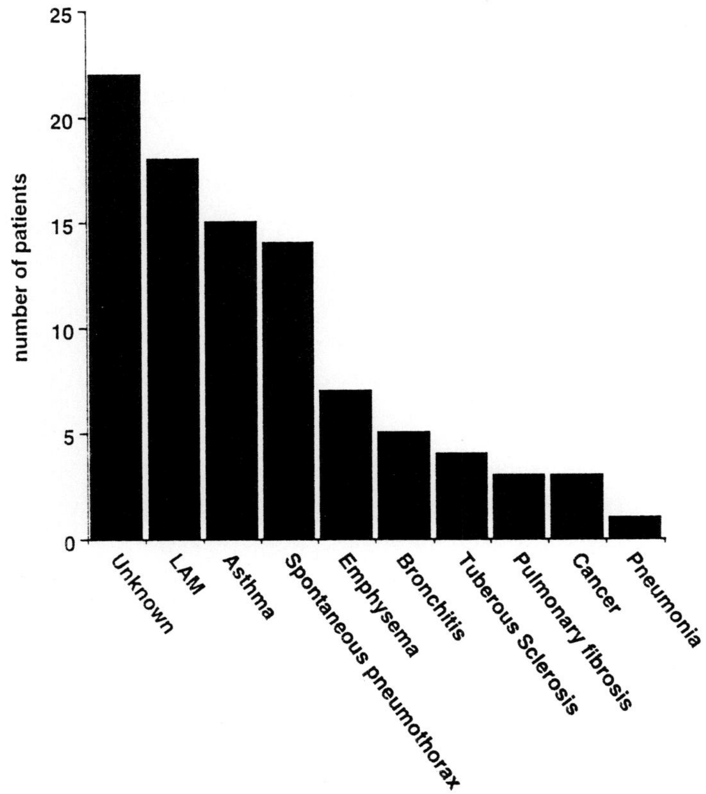

Figure 3 First diagnosis given to LAM Foundation patients who were ultimately diagnosed with LAM (n = 104).

monary LAM (12–14). These lesions are generally asymptomatic, unilateral, and benign, and do not commonly compromise renal function (15). Arterial embolization was used to control bleeding into AML in 3% of patients. Although 24% of the LF subjects had undergone nephrectomy for AML, this procedure is now infrequently recommended and may compromise candidacy for lung transplant.

Physical examination can be unrevealing, although end expiratory rales (22%), hyperinflation, decreased or absent breath sounds, ascites, intra-abdominal or adenexal masses, and clubbing (<5%) may be found. Pitted tooth enamel, hypopigmented macules, or angiofibromas in a patient with cystic lung disease suggest the diagnosis of pulmonary tuberous sclerosis rather than sporadic LAM (16).

Table 1 Symptoms and Manifestations of LAM in LAM Foundation Patients

	First symptom(s) or manifestation(s)[a]	Symptom(s) or manifestation(s) during course of disease[b]	Most troubling current symptoms or manifestation[b]
Dyspnea	60	79	74
Pneumothorax	48	94	4
Cough	7	41	1
Phlegm	0	32	0
Hemoptysis/Chyloptysis	3	44	0
Chest pain	3	—	3
Chylous effusion	2	50	2
Chyloperitoneum	—	13	—
Chyluria	—	3	—
Angiomyolipoma	—	45	—
Osteoporosis	—	23	—
Other	—	—	10
No response	3	0	6

The data are the number of subjects reporting each finding. Some patients reported more than one symptom in each category.
[a]$n = 130$.
[b]$n = 101$.

IV. Pulmonary Physiology

Unlike most other diffuse infiltrative processes of the lung, LAM patients are often hyperinflated with an increased total lung volume, increased thoracic gas volume and residual volume (RV). They are further reported to show evidence of airflow limitation with decreased FEV_1 and FEV_1/FVC and markedly reduced diffusion capacity for carbon monoxide (1,5,17,18). We have recently reported the pulmonary physiology and exercise performance of 16 subjects with LAM cared for at a tertiary care referral center (5). In a majority of subjects, increased gas trapping and significant airflow limitation was suggested by an increased RV, an increased RV/TLC ratio, and a decreased FEV_1. Only a minority of patients had improvement in airflow after bronchodilator administration.

Pulmonary mechanics studies have shown that mean elastic recoil is reduced and that upstream resistance (R_{US}) is increased in 70% of subjects. Burger and coworkers (18) reported that the loss of elastic recoil is the primary determinant of airflow limitation, although they found only minor changes in lung resistance. Our data would suggest that both a loss of elastic recoil and an increase

Table 2 Therapies Received for LAM by LAM Foundation Patients

Treatment or intervention	Percent
Oxygen[a]	43
Progestin therapy[a]	85
GnRH agonist[a]	14
Oophorectomy *for* LAM[a]	28
Drainage of chylous pleural effusion[b]	26
Pleurodesis, bleb resection, or pleurectomy[b]	77
Nephrectomy[b]	24
Renal arterial embolization[b]	4
Transplant	
Awaiting[a]	9
Received[a]	15
Denied[b]	7

[a] $n = 130$.
[b] $n = 101$.

in airway resistance contribute to the observed airflow limitation. The diffusing capacity of this group of patients is markedly reduced, and the alveolar-arterial oxygen difference is increased. Diminished exercise performance with a reduced oxygen consumption and low anaerobic threshold (5) is also seen. Thus, the primary determinants of exercise limitation in LAM are related to a combination of mechanical factors (i.e., decreased breathing reserve, work of breathing), gas exchange abnormalities, and destruction of the pulmonary vascular bed.

V. Chest Imaging Studies

Initial reports of roentgenographic changes in LAM described a pseudoreticular-nodular pattern of irregular shadows (Fig. 4). These opacities result from the compression of smooth muscle–rich interstitial tissue by more dilated cystic airspaces. Lymphatic obstruction with the development of Kerley B septal lines also contributes to the pattern. However, the chest radiograph findings in LAM are varied and can be normal early in the course of the disease and later demonstrate severe emphysematous-like changes. Cross-sectional studies show 33–62% of subjects to have hyperinflation with cystic dilatation of the airspaces producing relatively radiolucent lung fields (17,19–24). Pneumothorax can be an early feature, and chylous pleural effusion can develop at any time.

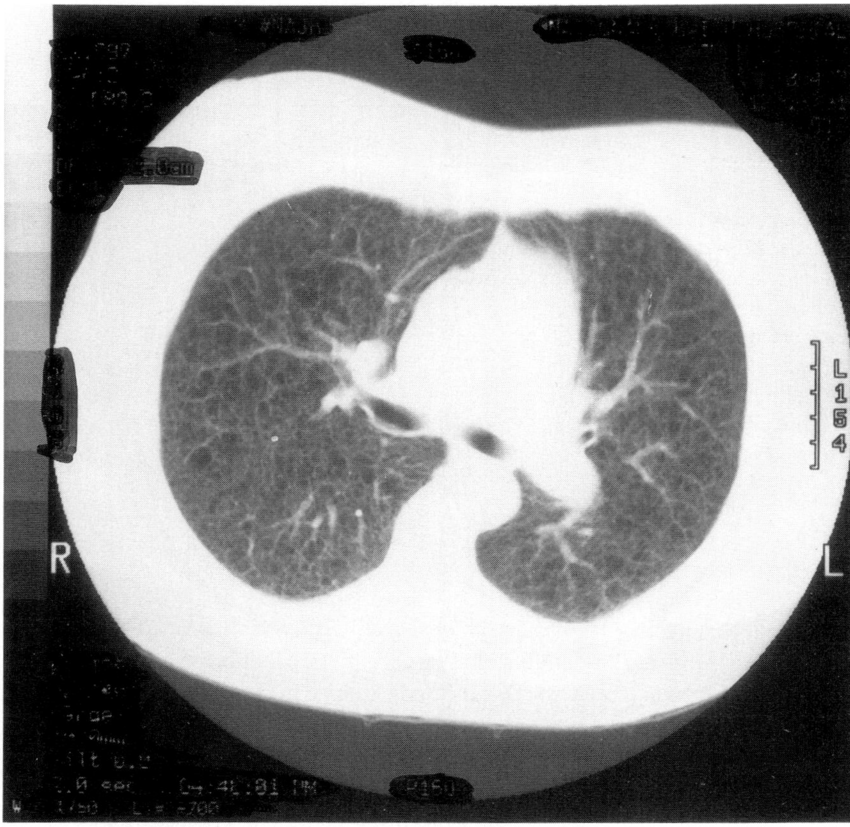

A

Figure 4 Pulmonary lymphangioleiomyomatosis. (A) Conventional CT scan shows bilateral small cysts. (B) The HRCT scan shows multiple thin-walled cystic airspaces of relatively uniform size. Characteristically, the cysts are distributed throughout the lungs and have thin but definable walls in the absence of reticular or nodular opacities.

The high-resolution (thin collimation) section is much more sensitive than routine chest radiography and the findings of diffuse, homogeneous, small (<1 cm diameter) thin–walled cysts can be pathognomonic in an appropriate clinical context. We have shown a close correlation between the degree of cystic parenchymal replacement in subjects with LAM as measured by quantitative chest high-resolution computed tomography (HRCT) and disease severity as determined by spirometry, diffusing capacity, lung volume, or exercise performance (20). Thus, chest HRCT may be both diagnostic and prognostic.

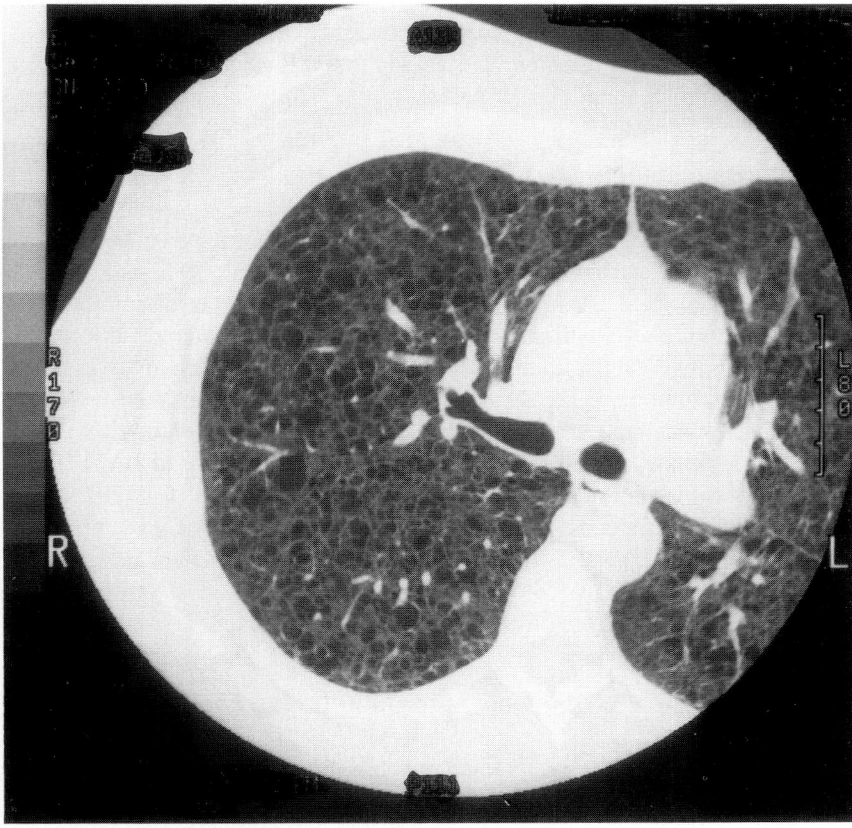

B

Figure 4 Continued.

VI. Lung Biopsy

LAM can be readily diagnosed by its characteristic histologic findings on examination of biopsy specimens obtained at thoracotomy. Video-assisted thoracoscopic lung biopsy has recently been shown to be an effective alternative surgical approach with lower morbidity (25). In a few reports, transbronchial lung biopsy has yielded an adequate sample for pathologic evaluation, especially when immunohistochemical stains with the monoclonal antibody HMB-45 or antibodies specific for smooth muscle components actin or desmin are used to improve diagnostic sensitivity and specificity (26,27). Tissue confirmation is usually recommended, although in some cases the diagnosis of LAM can be made based on a combination of characteristic clinical features, such as concomitant cystic lung disease, chylous pleural effusion, and an angiomyolipoma in a young woman without other known underlying diseases.

VII. Histopathology

LAM, pulmonary sarcoid, and pulmonary histiocytosis X each frequently demonstrate a "bronchovascular" pattern of histopathology (in all of these disorders, the primary pathology is organized in and around the bronchovascular structures). In LAM, the atypical smooth muscle proliferation that characterizes the condition also generally conforms to this distribution (2,17,28) but also involves other regions of the pulmonary interstitium. The infiltrating cells resemble vascular smooth muscle cells, but are often somewhat shortened and pleomorphic with an increased mitotic index. The second unique pathologic feature of LAM is the occurrence of diffuse, cystic dilatation of the terminal airspaces (5,17,20,29,30). Grossly and microscopically, the normal pulmonary architecture is distorted by multiple small cysts ranging from 0.1 cm to several centimeters in diameter (1,17,20,29). The mechanism by which interstitial smooth muscle proliferation causes cyst formation and emphysema-like disease is unknown.

VIII. Prognosis, Treatment, and Contributing Factors

Kitaichi et al. have shown that pulmonary function abnormalities are of prognostic value (2). An elevated total lung capacity (percent predicted TLC) and reduced FEV_1/FVC ratio are associated with poor survival 2–5 years after initial examination.

Treatment regimens have thus far been unsatisfactory, and many afflicted patients succumb to progressive respiratory failure within 10 years of the diagnosis. There have been few advances since the early recognition that female hormones likely play an important role in the pathogenesis. The treatments that 130 LF patients reported receiving are listed in Table 2. Oophorectomy (28%), progestins (85%), and more recently luteinizing hormone–releasing hormone analogs (14%) were the most common therapies (31,32). A recent metaanalysis summarized the results of 30 treated cases (33). Of these, 5 of 7 patients treated with oophorectomy stabilized or improved. Two patients who were treated with both oophorectomy and progesterone stabilized or improved by objective criteria. Only 4 patients out of 8 treated with progesterone alone demonstrated stabilization or improvement. Thus, combination therapy with oophorectomy and progesterone should be considered. Tamoxifen should probably be avoided given its partial agonist activity and anecdotal reports of disease exacerbation on this therapy (1,34). Chemical oophorectomy with LHRH analogs may ultimately replace surgical oophorectomy as the primary treatment of this disorder, especially if the cost of long-term medical therapy becomes practical (35). There is no role for either steroids or cytotoxic agents. Patients should avoid the use of estrogen-containing medications such as birth control pills or antiosteoporotic agents, which have been reported to exacerbate the disease (36) (Table 3). Over 80% of LF patients reported a history of birth control pill use, and 8% of those felt that their disease had become worse following this therapy. Fifty-four percent of the subjects had been pregnant at least once. Only 2% were diagnosed before their first pregnancy and 8% were diagnosed during pregnancy. Pregnancy in patients known to have LAM is generally discouraged since some patients report acceleration of symptomatology during or following pregnancy (16%), but this important issue has not been studied systematically. Over 40% of LAM patients re-

Table 3 Factors That May Complicate or Exacerbate LAM Reported by LAM Foundation Patients

Factor	Percent[a]
History of smoking	
Prior	43
Current	3
Birth control pill use	
Prior	83
Birth control pills made lungs worse	8
Pregnancy	
Prior history	54
Number of pregnancies	
0	18
1	20
2	6
3	6
>3	12
History of miscarriage	22
Diagnosis preceded first pregnancy	2
Diagnosis made during pregnancy	8
Had additional pregnancies after diagnosis	4
Pregnancy made lungs worse	16
Air travel	
History of lung problems with flying	13
Avoid air travel due to LAM	41

[a]$n = 101$.

ported a prior history of smoking, but few (3%) were current smokers. A few LAM patients have experienced pneumothoraces due to air travel, and although only 14% of LF subjects reported any flight-related lung problems, 41% avoid taking airplanes.

Lung transplantation should be considered as last resort therapy for patients with progressive, end-stage disease which has resulted in an unacceptable quality of life. In caring for patients with LAM, every effort should be made to maintain the integrity of the pleural space (by avoiding pleurodesis, if possible) and to maximize antiosteoporotic regimens to optimize candidacy for transplant. At the present time, 15% of living LF patients have received lung transplant, 9% are on waiting lists for transplant, and 7% have been denied transplant. The rate of perioperative complications, including chylothorax and bleeding due to adhesions, is slightly higher in patients with LAM who receive transplant, but the overall survival is similar to that of other disease groups (37). Two recent reports of recurrent disease in transplanted lungs have raised concerns regarding this therapy, but it should be emphasized that the graft was not threatened in either case (38,39). To date, there is no published experience with lung volume reduction surgery for patients with LAM, but progressive hyperinflation and graft compression led to the death of one single lung transplant patient despite surgical reduction of the native lung (M. Zamora, personal communication).

IX. Asthma

Patients with LAM are often misdiagnosed as having asthma early in their course. Asthma is a very common disorder with a prevalence of 4–5% in the United States and a broad range of clinical manifestations. It is a chronic illness that is characterized by episodic narrowing of the airways associated with a variable degree of inflammation and mucus production. Patients experience intermittent wheezing, cough, dyspnea, chest tightness, and/or nocturnal awakenings. Reversible airflow limitation and hyperinflation are its physiologic hallmarks. However, the presence of episodic expiratory wheezing is not sufficient to make the diagnosis of asthma, and LAM represents just one of the many pulmonary disorders that can present with wheezing.

The physical examination can be helpful in diagnosing asthma. Affected subjects can exhibit variable expiratory wheezing and rhonchi. Hyperresonance is present if there is also hyperinflation. Hyperinflation can also sometimes be recognized by a reduction in the distance between the thyroid cartilage and sternal notch. A pulsus paradoxus and the use of accessory muscles can also be present. However, these examination findings are nonspecific and can also be demonstrated in LAM.

Laboratory testing can be of assistance in making the diagnosis. Most subjects have elevated IgE levels and are also atopic on skin testing. Chest radiographic evidence of bronchial wall thickening is also a positive predictor. Neither cysts nor bullae are typical chest CT findings.

Untreated asthmatics most often demonstrate a limitation in airflow (reduced FEV_1 and FEV_1/FVC) that is improved (>15%) after the administration of an inhaled β_2-agonist. Lung function is most often normal between exacerbations.

The natural history of asthma is variable, although it is only rarely progressive in the absence of aggravating factors such as cigarette smoking. Typically, affected individuals suffer symptomatic flares punctuated by periods of normal lung function. The exacerbations themselves are only rarely fatal and most often respond well to routine management with bronchodilators or anti-inflammatory agents. In the more severely affected, the frequency, duration, and intensity of these exacerbations can be increased but are still followed by return to relatively normal function. Less commonly, the disease can be progressive and lead to chronic, persistent airflow limitation (40). Patients with LAM typically *do not* experience symptomatic exacerbations and remissions. This lack of variability, the absence of significant response to bronchodilators, and progressive decline in pulmonary function in a patient with a tentative diagnosis of asthma should prompt further evaluation.

Treatment with environmental control of aggravating factors, bronchodilators, and topical anti-inflammatory agents is most often sufficient to control this disorder. Less commonly, systemic steroids or cytotoxic therapies are required.

X. Emphysema

LAM is frequently misdiagnosed as emphysema, especially in patients with a history of cigarette smoking. However, symptomatic emphysema is unusual before age 40 even in the presence of heavy tobacco use. The diagnosis of α_1-antiprotease deficiency should be entertained and evaluated by obtaining serum levels of the inhibitor. In the absence of an inherited predisposition to emphysema, however, young to middle-aged women with this diagnosis should be screened for possible LAM. It is useful to review the clinical presentation of patients with emphysema, to contrast with that of LAM patients.

The diagnosis of emphysema in life is based on the clinical, radiologic, and functional presentation of the patient (41,42). The clinical manifestations are predominantly breathlessness, with or without cough, that progresses to severe disability. Early in the disease, the clinical examination may be of little value. As the severity increases, the physician is confronted by an anxious, thin, occasionally emaciated patient who demonstrates pursed-lip breathing. The patient may assume a forward leaning posture, and demonstrate prominent use of accessory muscles of respiration because of her need to further inflate an already overly inflated chest. Breath sounds are markedly diminished, and the heart sounds are faint. It is unusual to find a patient with "pure" emphysema. Although emphysema alone can result in a crippling and fatal disease, when hypoxemia and cor pulmonale supervene it is almost invariably associated with chronic bronchitis.

Obstruction to airflow is characteristically present in emphysema and predominantly results from a decrease in the elastic recoil of the lungs and collapsible airways (43). Pulmonary function studies typically also reveal increased total lung capacity, diminished elastic recoil, increased static compliance, and a decreased carbon monoxide diffusing capacity when clinically significant emphysema is present.

The chest radiograph is suggestive but not specific for the diagnosis of emphysema (Fig. 5). The presence of hyperinflation defined by a low, flat diaphragm and large retrosternal air space; cardiovascular changes with a narrow vertical heart, prominent pulmonary trunk, and large hilar vessels with rapid peripheral tapering; and signs of local vessel loss (bullae that are demarcated by a thick, white line or with no definite margins) increases the diagnostic accuracy of the plain chest film (44). Cases of mild emphysema are difficult to recognize by chest x-ray alone. High-resolution computerized tomography is a useful radiographic technique for detecting the morphologic changes of emphysema in life, which are rarely as homogeneous and diffuse as those seen in LAM (45) (Fig. 5). Parenchymal destruction in emphysema results in cystic spaces with margins that are characteristically much less distinct than those in LAM.

Lung biopsy is not necessary or recommended to make the diagnosis of emphysema. However, the study of lung specimens obtained at autopsy has revealed three anatomic subtypes of emphysema, which are based on the regions of the acinus that are primarily involved:

Panacinar emphysema is characterized by distention and destruction of all alveoli within the respiratory lobule. This type of emphysema is associated with α_1-antiprotease deficiency, which is a familial disease with clinical manifestations occurring by age 40 in subjects who have mutations of the Pi (protease inhibitor) gene.

Centriacinar emphysema is characterized by the destruction of the central part of the lobule. The proximal part of the acinus (respiratory bronchiole) is predominantly involved, with the peripheral alveolar ducts and the alveoli being relatively unaffected. There are two subdivisions of this form of lesion: (1) *Centrilobular* emphysema is classically associated with cigarette smoking. Most of the lung changes in centrilobular emphysema occur in the apices of the upper lobe, but spread downward as the disease progresses. This type is rare before the age of 40 and occurs without clinical manifestations in about one fourth of people who die with no history of lung disease and a normal chest radiograph. (2) *Focal* emphysema occurs in individuals exposed to the inhalation of coal dust (i.e., coal pneumoconiosis) and other mineral dust. This lesion is relatively uniform in distribution in the lungs and is characterized by the dilation of respiratory bronchioles, with the intense accumulation of dust-laden macrophages in and around the respiratory bronchioles.

Distal acinar emphysema involves the alveolar ducts and sacs, and vessels and airways, which abut the pleura. Mild airflow obstruction despite extensive bullous emphysema, and the spontaneous pneumothorax of young adults, are the clinical associations of this form of emphysema.

Most affected individuals stabilize their pulmonary function after smoking cessation. A number have an associated reactive airways abnormality, which can be treated with bronchodilator therapy, but the response is generally less than that seen in asthma. Recently, there has been considerable enthusiasm for lung volume reduction surgery as a treatment for this disorder, but the true benefit of this therapy must await the outcome of clinical trails.

XI. Primary Spontaneous Pneumothorax

Although the term primary spontaneous pneumothorax (PSP) is defined as a pneumothorax that occurs in the absence of underlying lung disease, in actuality most patients with PSP have abnormal lungs. This is based on studies that have shown that 80% of patients with PSP have apical subpleural blebs by chest CT (46) and nearly 100% who undergo thoracotomy for treatment of PSP have visible blebs on the surface of the lungs (47). Almost all patients with PSP are smokers, and the risk of PSP correlates closely with the level of cigarette consumption (48). Pneumothoraces are more common in tall thin persons and within several days after exposure to changes in atmospheric pressure (49). Before the diagnosis of PSP is established, the diseases most commonly associated with secondary pneumothoraces should be excluded, including chronic obstructive pulmonary disease, cystic fibrosis, and fibrosing interstitial lung disease. The symptoms of PSP are sudden onset dyspnea and unilateral chest pain and/or shoulder pain on the side of the lung collapse. The pathogenesis of PSP is thought to be related to airway inflammation and air trapping, and this is supported by histological evidence of inflammation at open lung biopsy and delayed washout on ventilation scanning. Drainage of air is generally recommended for pneumothoraces that involve more than 15% of the hemithorax, via simple aspiration or

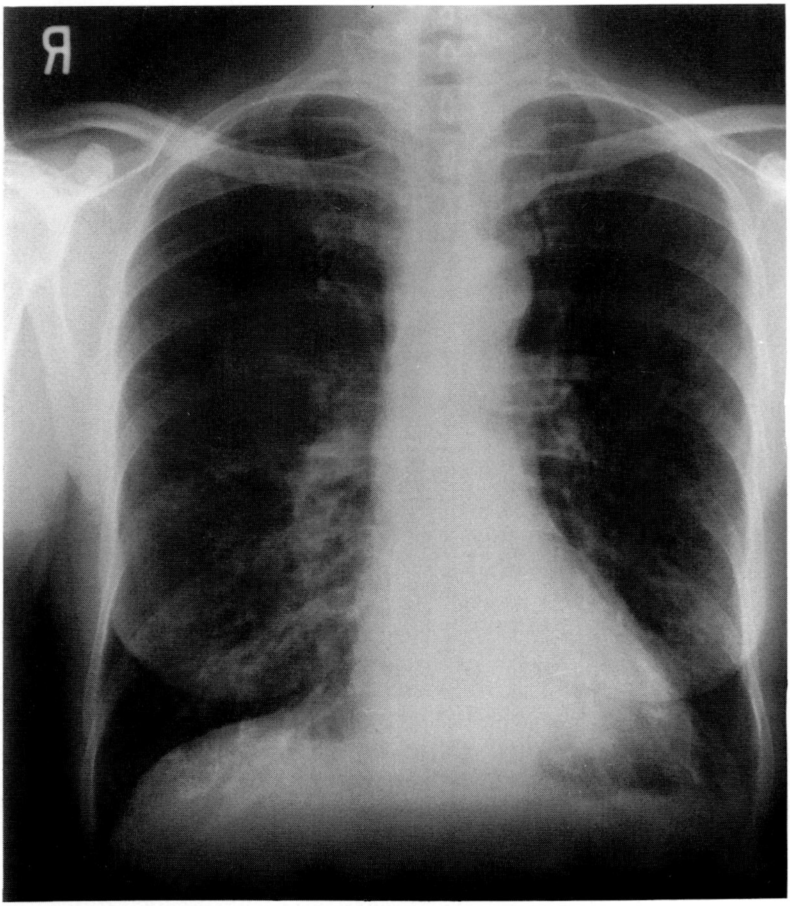

A

Figure 5 Advanced pulmonary emphysema. (A) Posteroanterior chest radiograph shows diminished vascularity in the central and peripheral zones. (B) High-resolution CT with thin section through the right upper lobe shows the characteristic pattern of emphysema definable as well-defined zones of diminished lung density, without definable walls. These air spaces are typically bounded peripherally by interlobular veins. Central or core lobular vessels can be identified. Despite their prominence, the interlobular septa are not actually thickened, and there is no evidence of prominent and irregular bronchovascular markings.

placement of a chest tube. Most air leaks seal within a few days (>90%), but pleural sclerosis or surgical treatment, including thoracoscopy or thoracotomy for sclerosis, ligation of bullae, laser ablation of blebs, pleurectomy, or wedge resection of lung, may become necessary for patients with persistent bronchopleural

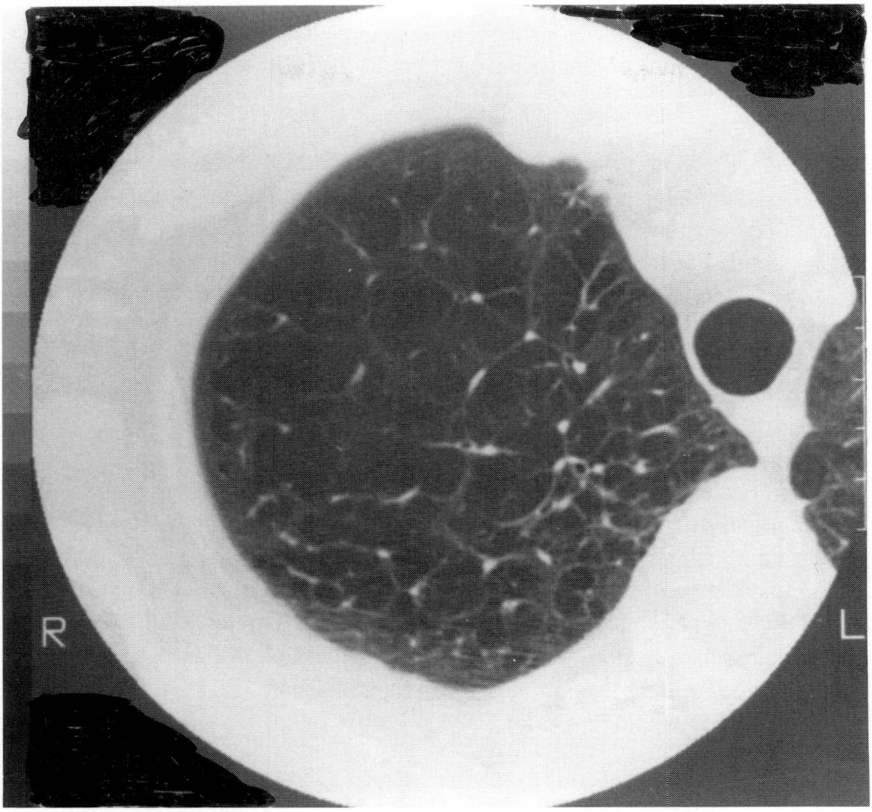

B

Figure 5 Continued.

fistulas. The diagnosis of LAM should be considered in all young women who present with pneumothorax, but especially in nonsmokers who do not have the typical body habitus or those with prolonged air leaks.

XII. Tuberous Sclerosis

Tuberous sclerosis (TS) is a rare (approximately 1 per 10,000 population) autosomal dominant disorder that affects men and women equally (16). Mental retardation, seizures, and adenoma sebaceum form the classic clinical triad. The features are highly variable, however, and some affected individuals have normal intelligence. In 1–3% of patients, TS is associated with pulmonary manifestations that are indistinguishable from those of LAM (50–53). When pulmonary involvement is present there is a marked female predominance (54), and the cases that have been reported in males have not been confirmed by biopsy (55,56). Like LAM, the onset of the lung disease occurs after puberty, generally discovered in the third decade of life. The lung histopathology is identical to that seen in sporadic LAM. Renal lesions, angiomyolipomata, also occur with high frequency and are frequently bilateral. Some have referred to LAM as a forme fruste of TS (51). Distinguishing sporadic LAM from pulmonary TS is usually not difficult, since most patients with pulmonary TS have skin and central nervous system manifestations of the disease (50). However, in equivocal cases, a CT of the brain is useful to identify calcified cortical tubers, which are characteristic of TS.

Given the compelling phenotypic similarities between TS and LAM, it is tempting to speculate that the two diseases may share common genetic roots. The fact that there have not been any reported cases of inherited LAM does not exclude a genetic basis for the disease. Indeed TS, which is clearly due to genetic mutation, occurs most frequently in a sporadic fashion affecting patients without a family history. The one third of TS cases that are familial have been mapped to two chromosomal loci, denoted TSC1 on 9q34 and TSC2 on 16p13.3 (57). Mutations of TSC2 have recently been discovered in two patients with pulmonary TS (A. Green, personal communication). This is an exciting finding that directly implicates the deficiency of the TSC2 gene product, tuberin (58), in the production of the lung lesion found in LAM. TSC1 and TSC2 are currently being evaluated as candidate loci in LAM.

XIII. Pulmonary Histiocytosis X

The clinical and radiographic manifestations of LAM can occasionally be mistaken for those of pulmonary histiocytosis X (PHX). PHX is an uncommon, smoking-related, interstitial lung disease that, like LAM, primarily affects young adults between 20 and 40 years of age (59,60). The true incidence and prevalence of PHX is unknown, and it is likely that some cases are misdiagnosed as idiopathic pulmonary fibrosis (IPF). Tobacco smoke is thought to be etiologic since nearly all affected individuals have a prior smoking history. Although PHX was once reported to be predominantly a male disease, this predilection probably reflected the demographics of smoking earlier in this century. More recent literature suggests an equal gender distribution. Like LAM, PHX is reported in Caucasians much more often than in persons of Asian or African descent.

Patients with PHX present to medical attention in a variety of ways. PHX is often an incidental diagnosis that is suggested by a screening chest roentgenogram. Like LAM, recurrent spontaneous pneumothorax can prompt the initial diagnostic evaluation. When symptomatic, most patients have cough, and, less frequently, dyspnea or generalized constitutional symptoms (60–62). PHX generally follows a more benign and protracted course than other fibrotic processes, such as idiopathic pulmonary fibrosis.

The Langerhans cell, a differentiated cell of the monocyte-macrophage line, is a prominent feature of the PHX lesion (61,63,64). Langerhans cells are distinguished by pale staining cytoplasm and large nuclei and nucleoli. Electron microscopy can demonstrate the classic pentalaminar cytoplasmic inclusion or Birbeck granule (X-body) within this cell. Early inflammatory lesions are centered around the smaller bronchioles and usually contain an admixture of eosinophils, lymphocytes, and neutrophils. These lesions often also involve pulmonary arterioles and venules (60,63). More advanced lesions extend widely into the parenchyma of the lung surrounding the bronchovascular structures and produce the so-called stellate lesions that are characteristic of this disorder (63–65). Although there are some remote histological similarities to pulmonary sarcoid, PHX is not a true granulomatous disorder. Interstitial fibrosis and small cyst formation with a mid to upper zone predominance occurs with advancing disease (66). The mechanism for cyst formation, as in LAM, is unknown.

Pulmonary function testing of subjects with PHX can demonstrate normal, obstructive, restrictive, or mixed patterns of abnormality (60,61,65, 67,68). In general, total lung capacity is well preserved with near normal airflow (60). The diffusing capacity is most often disproportionately reduced (60). This pattern of pulmonary function abnormality suggests pulmonary vascular involvement by the disease process. Airflow limitation occurs in a minority of patients and can sometimes be associated with reactive airways with significant improvement after bronchodilator administration (60).

We reviewed our experience with 23 patients with PHX (60) and found two major subgroups. The first group demonstrated normal total lung capacity with normal or near-normal airflow. This group had a normal elastic recoil with pulmonary mechanics testing. The second group demonstrated predominantly restrictive disease with reduced total lung volume and increased elastic recoil. Those in the restrictive group tended towards having more longstanding disease. Only a single subject demonstrated predominantly obstructive pulmonary dysfunction, although obstructive physiology with airflow limitation and hyperinflation is well described in the literature. Thus, while there is some overlap with patients with LAM who appear to develop progressive hyperinflation and airflow limitation (2,5,18), those with PHX tend to have either normal or a restrictive abnormality.

Clinically, we have observed that patients with established PHX demonstrate a level of activity limitation and exercise intolerance that is out of proportion to their pulmonary function abnormalities.

The radiographic appearance of PHX can be very characteristic (69,70), if not diagnostic (Fig. 6). Typically, there are reticular and nodular opacities with a middle to upper zone predominance and sparing of the costophrenic angles. On chest HRCT, the characteristic combination of multiple irregular-shaped cysts and nodules and interstitial thickening predominantly involving the middle to upper zone zones is considered diagnostic. Unlike the cysts seen in LAM, those seen in PHX are more often thick-walled and are less diffuse and less homogeneous in their distribution.

Unlike the predictable deterioration in lung function seen in LAM, the natural history of PHX is extraordinarily variable, with some patients experienc-

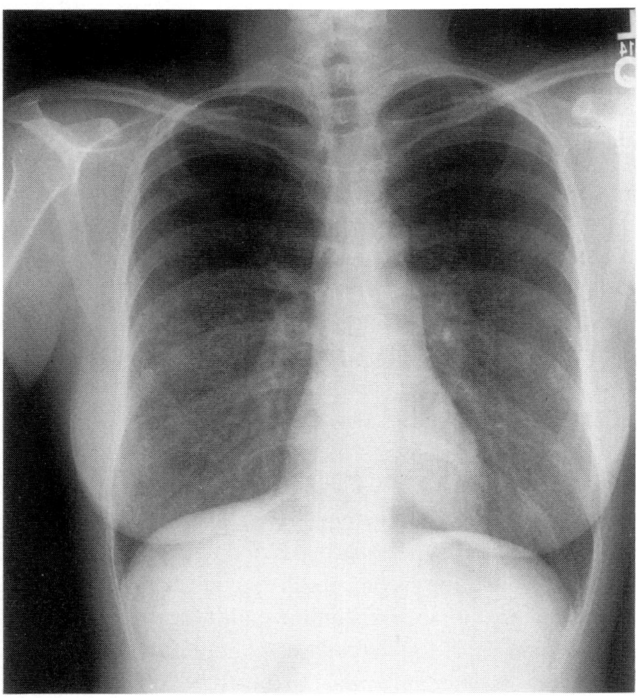

A

Figure 6 Pulmonary histiocytosis X. (A) Chest radiograph reveals reticulonodular opacities in mid-lung zones, cysts, costophrenic angle sparing, and preservation of lung volumes. (B) Conventional CT scan helps confirm the presence of bilateral reticulonodular opacities and cysts. (C) High-resolution CT with thin section shows more clearly that the reticular, nodular, or emphysematous changes on chest radiography are actually cysts. Few nodules are evident, and the cysts vary in size and may be larger than 10 mm. The cysts are bizzare in shape and may mimic bronchiectasis in some areas.

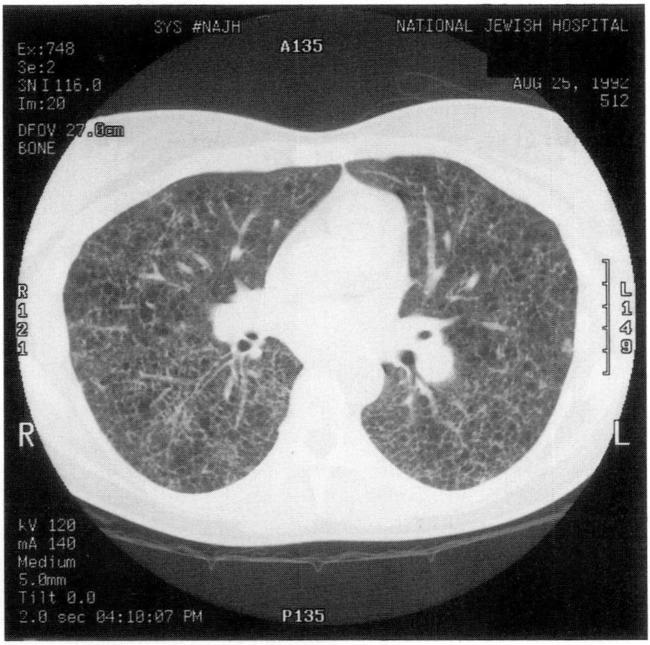

B

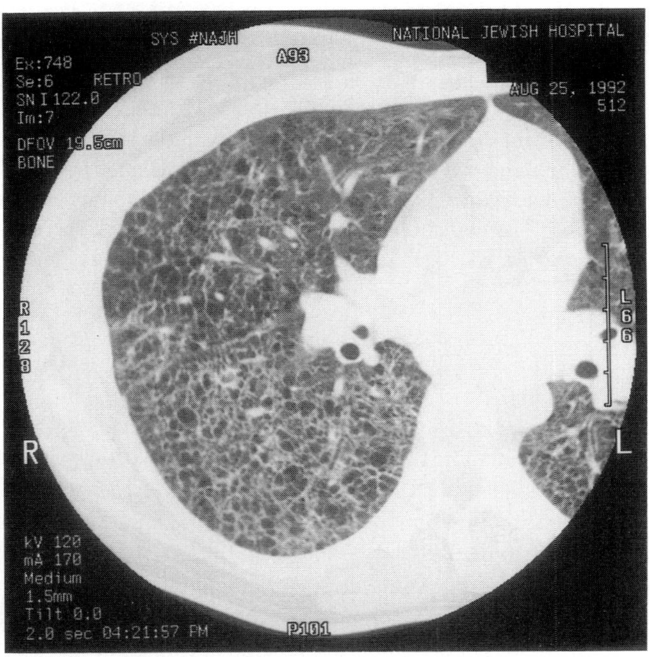

C

Figure 6 Continued.

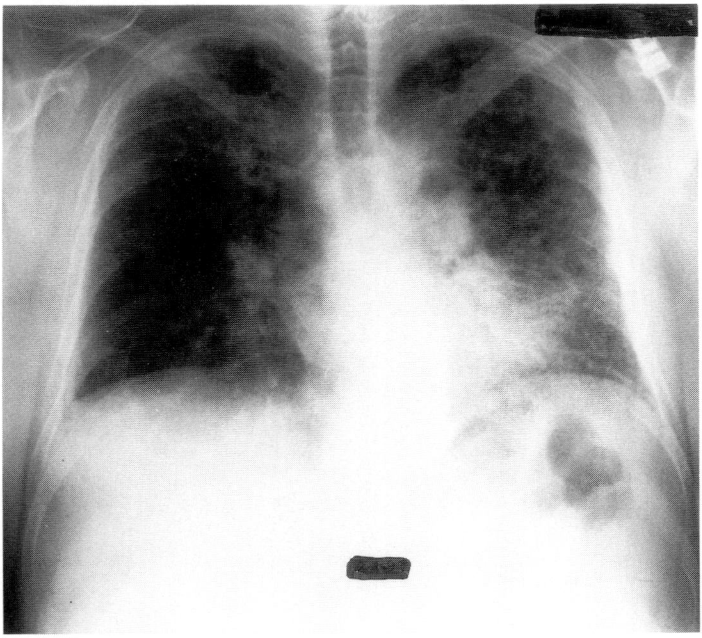

A

Figure 7 Idiopathic pulmonary fibrosis. (A) Posteroanterior chest radiograph in a patient with longstanding idiopathic pulmonary fibrosis shows diffuse reticular opacities and roentgenographic evidence of honeycombing especially in the left lung base. (B) High-resolution CT section through the right lung shows the characteristic pattern of subpleural parenchymal involvement with irregular reticular markings with tiny honeycomb cysts. (C) High-resolution CT section through the left lower lobe shows extensive parenchymal involvement with irregular reticular opacities containing numerous small honeycomb-like air spaces.

ing spontaneous remissions and others progressing to end-stage fibrotic lung disease. Most subjects demonstrate gradual progression with continued smoking, and most regressions have been in the setting of smoking cessation (71). Thus, it is incumbent upon treating physicians to counsel PHX patients regarding their unique susceptibility to cigarette smoke. Neither steroids nor cytotoxic therapy have been shown to be of any value in the treatment of PHX. Purine analogs (2-chlorodeoxyadenosine) have shown promise in the infantile form of histiocytosis X (72), but have not been studied in the adult form. Radiotherapy for symptomatic bone lesions can be used as a palliative measure.

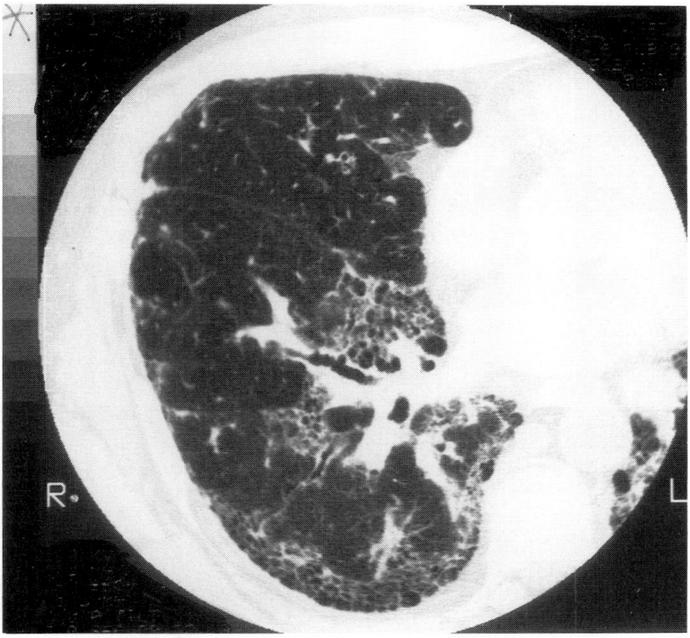

B

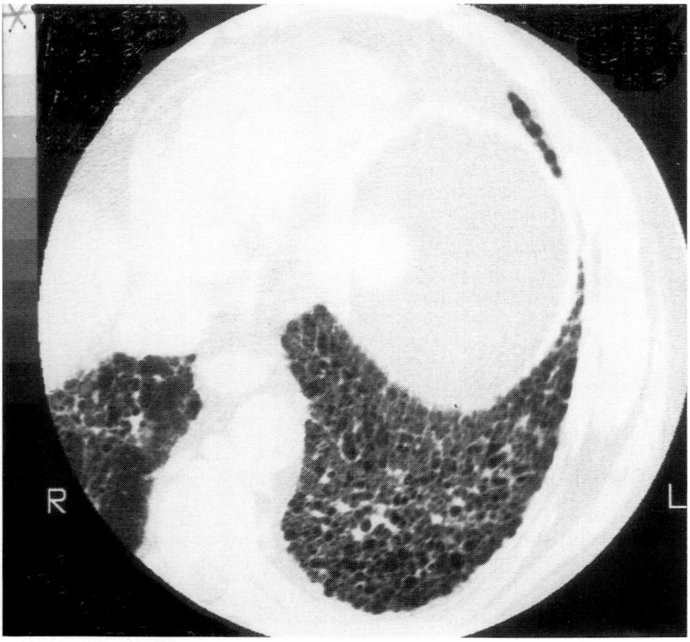

C

Figure 7 Continued.

XIV. Idiopathic Pulmonary Fibrosis

Idiopathic pulmonary fibrosis (IPF) is a chronic disease of middle-aged or elderly individuals that is characterized by the insidious onset of dyspnea, cough, digital clubbing, and interstitial opacities on chest x-ray (Fig. 7) (73). The diagnosis of IPF requires the exclusion of environmental exposures which are known to result in lung scarring, as well as underlying systemic diseases which can involve the lung, such as inflammatory arthritidies. Rarely IPF can be confused with LAM, especially in a smoker with concomitant emphysema (Fig. 8). In distin-

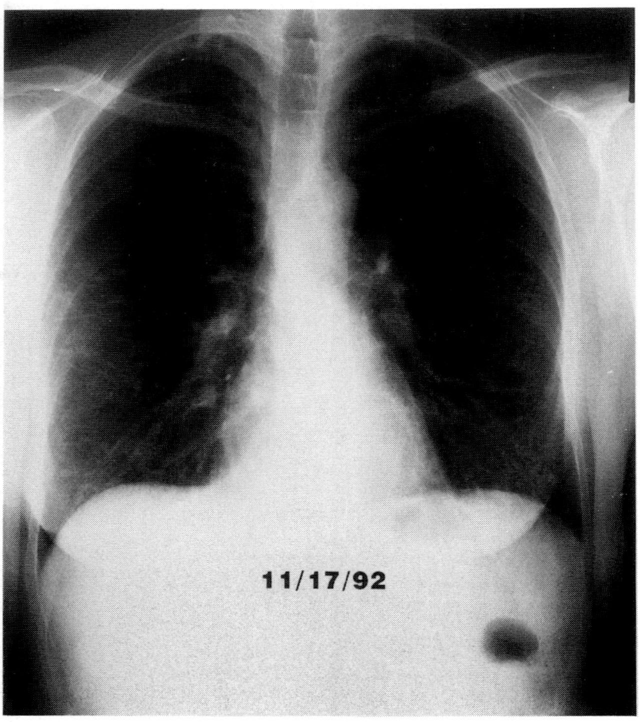

A

Figure 8 Idiopathic pulmonary fibrosis and pulmonary emphysema. (A) Posteroanterior chest radiograph in a 58-year-old woman with idiopathic pulmonary fibrosis and emphysema shows indistinct reticular opacities in the lower lung zones with diminished vascularity in the central and peripheral zones, especially in the upper lobes. (B) High-resolution CT section through the right upper lobe shows the characteristic pattern of emphysema with well-defined zones of diminished lung density without definable walls. (C) High-resolution CT section through the right lower lobe shows subpleural reticular opacities containing small honeycomb-like air spaces. The open lung biopsy show the pattern of usual interstitial pneumonitis.

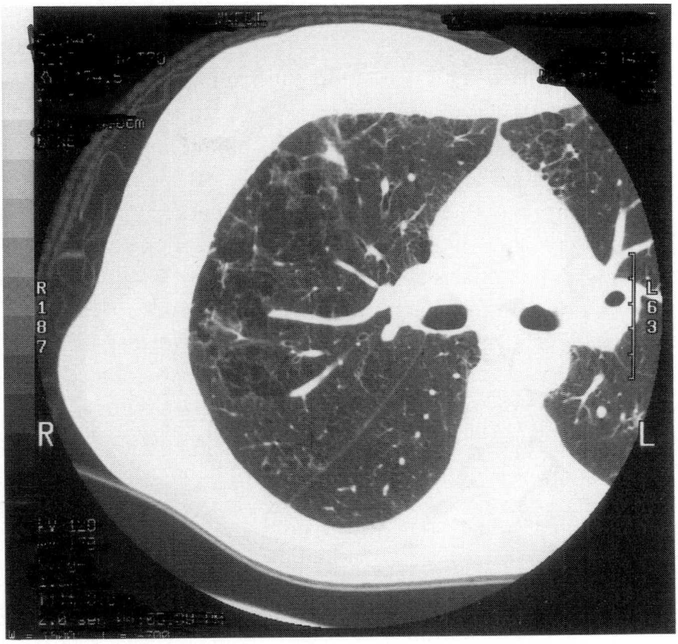

B

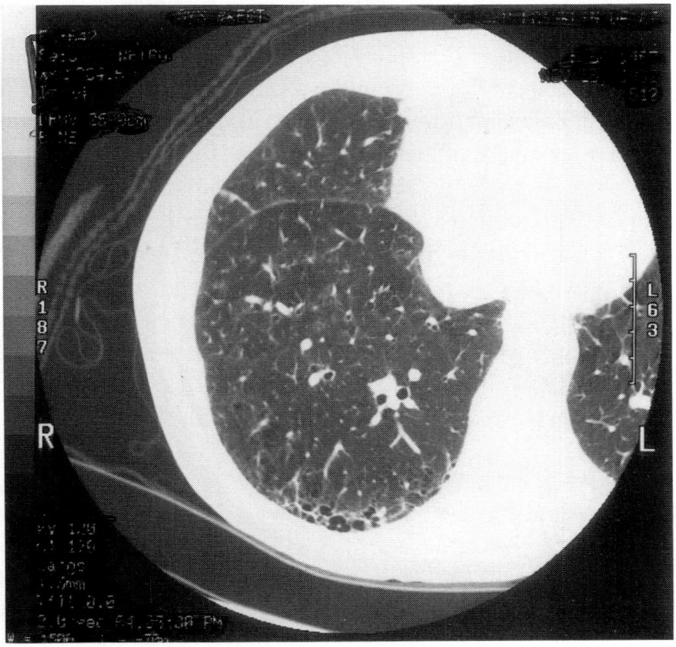

C

Figure 8 Continued.

guishing between the diseases, it is important to remember that IPF is uncommon before age 60. Pulmonary function tests reveal restrictive impairment (decreased static lung volumes) rather than the hyperinflation and airflow obstruction that is characteristic of LAM. The diffusing capacity for carbon monoxide is reduced, and arterial desaturation with exercise is one of the earliest manifestations of the disease. Lung biopsy with findings of usual interstitial pneumonia (UIP) is required to confirm the diagnosis of IPF. Smooth muscle proliferation and cystic change can be quite prominent histological features and can lead to confusion with the lesion in LAM. The intense fibrotic and inflammatory nature of the UIP lesion is not characteristic of LAM, however, and the experienced lung pathologist rarely has difficulty distinguishing the two diseases on biopsy specimens. The clinical course of IPF is relentlessly progressive, and the response to corticosteroid and cytotoxic therapy is routinely disappointing. The mean survival from diagnosis is 4–6 years after the onset of dyspnea. The pathogenesis of IPF is unknown.

XV. Conclusion

LAM is a degenerative lung disease of unknown etiology that affects only a small number of patients. Its impact upon these few individuals, however, is profound, with most of these young women dying within a decade of diagnosis due to progressive respiratory failure. It is likely that treatment strategies would have the greatest effect when instituted early in the course, before irreversible lung damage has developed. However, the disorder has an insidious presentation that is readily mistaken for other pulmonary diseases. It is therefore important for clinicians to become familiar with the typical manifestation of these more common conditions in order to more readily be able to distinguish them from LAM.

Further, LAM is prototypic for a number of diffuse pulmonary disease processes and provides a useful framework on which to consider (1) other diffuse parenchymal lung diseases characterized by cystic changes in the airspaces such as tuberous sclerosis (51–53), pulmonary histiocytosis X (60), and smoking-related pulmonary emphysema and (2) disorders such as asthma characterized by proliferation of smooth muscle cells around the airways.

Acknowledgments

The authors wish to thank Karlene Garinger, Joyce Beck, Don Scoralle, Betty Scoralle, Elizabeth Hillman, Alice Wheeler, and Sue Byrnes for their help with the questionnaire sent to LAM Foundation registrants; Martin Wallace and Dolly

Kervitsky National Jewish Medical and Research Center for their technical assistance; the referring physicians; and a special thanks to our patients for allowing up to participate in their care. This was supported in part by SCOR Grant No. NL-279353, National Heart Lung, and Blood Institute.

References

1. Taylor JR, Ryu J, Colby TV, Raffin TA. Lymphangioleiomyomatosis. Clinical course in 32 patients. N Engl J Med 1990; 323:1254–1260.
2. Kitaichi M, Nishmura K, Izumi T. Pulmonary lymphangioleiomyomatosis: a report of 46 patients including a clinicopathologic study of prognostic factors. Am J Respir Crit Care Med 1995; 151(2 Pt 1):527–533.
3. Berger JL, Shaff MI. Pulmonary lymphangioleiomyomatosis. J Comput Assist Tomogr 1981; 5:565–567.
4. Corrin B, Liebow A, Friedman P. Pulmonary lymphangioleiomyomatosis: a review. Am J Pathol 1975; 79:348–382.
5. Crausman RS, Jennings CA, Mortenson RL, Ackerson LM, Irvin CG, King TE, Jr. Lymphangioleiomyomatosis: the pathophysiology of diminished exercise capacity. Am J Respir Crit Care Med 1996; 153:1368–1376.
6. Crausman RS, Mellman D, Bloomfield EC, Jennings CA. Pulmonary barotrauma as the cause of pneumoretropharynx in pulmonary lymphangioleiomyomatosis. Am J Emerg Med 1996; 124:297–299.
7. Chuang ML, Tsai YH, Pang LC. Early chylopneumothorax in a patient with pulmonary lymphangioleiomyomatosis. J Formos Med Assoc 1993; 92:278–282.
8. Lieberman J, Agliozzo CM. Intrapleural nitrogen mustard for treating chylous effusion of pulmonary lymphangioleiomyomatosis. Cancer 1974; 33:1505–1511.
9. Nix JT, Albert M, Dugas JE, et al. Chylothorax and chylous ascites—a study of 302 selected cases. Am J Gastroenterol 1957; 28:40–55.
10. Gray RS, Carrington CB, Cornog JL. Lymphangiomyomatosis—report of a case with ureteral involvement and chyluria. Cancer 1975; 35:490–498.
11. Raymond AA, Isa MR, Abdullah T, Kudva MV. Lymphangioleiomyomatosis with chylous ascites. Singapore Med J 1993; 34:276–278.
12. Maziak DE, Kesten S, Rappaport DC, Maurer J. Extrathoracic angiomyolipomas in lymphangioleiomyomatosis. Eur Respir J 1996; 9:402–405.
13. Kerr LA, Blute ML, Ryu JH, Swensen SJ, Malek RS. Renal angiomyolipoma in association with pulmonary lymphangioleiomyomatosis: forme fruste of tuberous sclerosis? Urology 1993; 41:440–444.
14. Bernstein SM, Newell J, Jr., Adamczyk D, Mortenson RL, King T, Jr., Lynch DA. How common are renal angiomyolipomas in patients with pulmonary lymphangiomyomatosis? Am J Respir Crit Care Med 1995; 152:2138–2143.
15. Oesterling JE, Fishman EK, Goldman SM, Marshall FF. The management of renal angiomyolipoma. J Urol 1986; 135:1121–1124.

16. Gomez MR. Phenotypes of tuberous sclerosis complex with a revision of diagnostic criteria. Ann NY Acad Sci 1991; 614:1–7.
17. Carrington CB, Cugell DW, Gaensler EA, et al. Lymphangioleiomyomatosis. Physiologic-pathologic-radiologic correlations. Am Rev Respir Dis 1977; 116:977–995.
18. Burger CD, Hyatt RE, Staats BA. Pulmonary mechanics in lymphangioleiomyomatosis. Am Rev Respir Dis 1991; 143:1030–1033.
19. Brauner MW, Grenier P, Mouelhi M, Mompoint D, Lenoir S. Pulmonary histiocytosis X: evaluation with high resolution CT. Radiology 1989; 172.
20. Crausman RS, Lynch DA, Mortenson RL, et al. Quantitative CT predicts the severity of physiologic dysfunction in patients with lymphangioleiomyomatosis. Chest 1996; 109:131–137.
21. Hede J, Jurik AG. Lymphangioleiomyomatosis. Diagnostic imaging approach to a rare disease in women. Rofo Fortschr Geb Rontgenstr Neuen Bildgeb Verfahr 1991; 582–584.
22. Merchant RN, Pearson MG, Rankin RN, Morgan WK. Computerized tomography in the diagnosis of lymphangioleiomyomatosis. Am Rev Respir Dis 1985; 131:295–297.
23. Nishimura K, Kitaichi M, Izumi T, et al. Correlation of CT and pathologic findings of pulmonary lymphangioleiomyomatosis. Nippon Kyobu Shikkan Gakki Zasshi 1990; 28:691–697.
24. Sherrier RH, Chiles C, Roggli V. Pulmonary lymphangioleiomyomatosis: CT findings. Ajr Am J Roentgenol 1989; 153:937–940.
25. Bensard DD, McIntyre RCJ, Waring BJ, Simon JS. Comparison of video thoracoscopic lung biopsy to open lung biopsy in the diagnosis of interstitial lung diseases. Chest 1993; 103:765–770.
26. Matthews TJ, Hornall D, Sheppard MN. Comparison of the use of antibodies to alpha smooth muscle actin and desmin in pulmonary lymphangioleiomyomatosis. J Clin Pathol 1993; 46:479–80.
27. Hoon V, Thung SN, Kaneko M, Unger PD. HMB-45 reactivity in renal angiomyolipoma and lymphangioleiomyomatosis. Arch Pathol Lab Med 1994; 118:732–734.
28. Templeton PA. McLoud TC, Muller NL, Shepard JA, Moore EH. Pulmonary lymphangioleiomyomatosis: CT and pathologic findings. J Comput Assist Tomogr 1989; 13:54–57.
29. Sobonya R, Stuart Q, Fleishman J. Pulmonary lymphangioleiomyomatosis: quantitative analysis of lesions producing airflow limitation. Hum Pathol 1985; 16:1122–1128.
30. Bischoff HG, Mannle C, Wiedemann K, Vogt-Moykopf I. Bilateral giant distended cysts in lymphangioleiomyomatosis of the lung as a rare cause of inflow obstruction. Anasth Intensivther Notfallmed 1989; 24:341–344.
31. Brock ET, Votto JJ. Lymphangioleiomyomatosis: treatment with hormonal manipulation. NY State J Med 1986; 86:533–536.
32. Klein M, Krieger O, Ruckser R, et al. Treatment of lymphangioleiomyomatosis by ovariectomy, interferon alpha 2b and tamoxifen—a case report. Arch Gynecol Obstet 1992; 252:99–102.

33. Eliasson AH, Phillips YY, Tenholder MF. Treatment of lymphangioleiomyomatosis. A meta-analysis. Chest 1989; 96:1352–1355.
34. Svendsen TL, Viskum K, Hansborg N, Thorpe SM, Nielsen NC. Pulmonary lymphangioleiomyomatosis: a case of progesterone receptor positive lymphangioleiomyomatosis treated with medroxyprogesterone, oophorectomy and tamoxifen. Br J Dis Chest 1984; 78:264–271.
35. Rossi GA, Balbi B, Oddera S, Lantero S, Ravazzoni C. Response to treatment with an analog of the luteinizing-hormone-releasing hormone in a patient with pulmonary lymphangioleiomyomatosis. Am Rev Respir Dis 1991; 143:174–176.
36. Shen A, Iseman MD, Waldron JA, King TE. Exacerbation of pulmonary lymphangioleiomyomatosis by exogenous estrogens. Chest 1987; 91:782–785.
37. Boehler A, Speich R, Russi EW, Weder W. Lung transplantation for lymphangioleiomyomatosis. N Engl J Med 1996; 335:1275–1280.
38. O'Brien JD, Lium JH, Parosa JF, DeYound BR, Wick MR, Trulock EP. Lymphangiomyomatosis recurrence in the allograft after single-lung transplantation. Am J Respir Crit Care Med 1995; 151:2033-2036.
39. Nine JS YS, Paradis IL, Keenan R, Griffith BP. Lymphangioleiomyomatosis: recurrence after lung transplantation. J Heart Lung Transplant 1994; 13:714–719.
40. Dodge R, Cline MG, Burrows B. Comparisons of asthma, emphysema, and chronic bronchitis in a general population sample Am Rev Respir Dis 1986; 133:981–986.
41. National Heart Lung and Blood Institute, Division of Lung Diseases. The definition of emphysema. Am Rev Respir Dis 1985; 132:182–185.
42. Statement ATS. Standards for the diagnosis and care of patients with chronic obstructive pulmonary disease (COPD) and asthma. Am Rev Respir Dis 1987; 136:225–244.
43. Petty TL, Silvers GW, Stanford RE. Mild emphysema is associated with reduced elastic recoil and increased lung size but not with airflow limitation. Am Rev Respir Dis 1987; 136:867–871.
44. Thurlbeck WM, Simon G. Radiographic appearance of the chest in emphysema. Am J Roentgenol 1978; 130:429–440.
45. Hruban RH, Meziane MA, Zerhouni EA, et al. High resolution computed tomography of inflation-fixed lungs: pathologic–radiographic correlation of centrilobular emphysema. Am Rev Respir Dis 1987; 136:935–940.
46. Lesur O, Delorme N, Fromaget JM, Bernadac P, Polu JM. Computed tomography in the etiologic assessment of idiopathic spontaneous pneumothorax. Chest 1990; 98:341–347.
47. Gobbel WGJ, Rhea WGJ, Nelson IA, Daniel RAJ. Spontaneous pneumothorax. J Thoracic Cardiovasc Surg 1963; 46:331–345.
48. Bense L, Eklund G, Wiman LG. Smoking and the increased risk of contracting spontaneous pneumothorax. Chest 1987; 92:1009–1012.
49. Scott GC, Berger R, McKean HE. The role of atmospheric pressure variations in the development of spontaneous pneumothoraces. Am Rev Respir Dis 1989; 139:659–662.
50. Castro M, Shepherd CW, Gomez MR, Lie JT, Ryu JH. Pulmonary tuberous sclerosis. Chest 1995; 107:189–195.

51. Jozwiak S. Pulmonary lymphangioleiomyomatosis: a "forme fruste" of tuberous sclerosis? Am J Roentgenol 1990; 155:419.
52. Stovin P, Lum C, Flower D, Darke C, Beeley M. The lungs in lymphangiomyomatosis and in tuberous sclerosis. Thorax 1975; 30:497–509.
53. Capron F, Ameille J, Leclerc P, et al. Pulmonary lymphangioleiomyomatosis and Bourneville's tuberous sclerosis with pulmonary involvement: the same disease? Cancer 1983; 52:851–855.
54. Swyer J HJ, Garvan J. Pulmonary tuberous sclerosis. Q J Med 1971; 40:115.
55. Borberg A. Clinical and Genetic Investigations into Tuberous Sclerosis and Recklinhausen's Neurofibromatosis: Contribution to Euclidation of Interrelationship and Augenics of the Syndromes. Copenhagen: Ejnar Munksgaard, 1951.
56. Harris JO, Waltuck BL, Swenson EW. The pathophysiology of the lungs in tuberous sclerosis: a case report and literature overview. Am Rev Respir Dis 1969; 100:379–387.
57. Povey S, Burley MW, Attwood J, et al. Two loci for tuberous sclerosis: one on 9q34 and one on 16p13. Ann Hum Genet 1994; 58:107–127.
58. Consortium TECTS. Identification and characterization of the tuberous sclerosis gene on chromosome 16. Cell 1993; 75:1305–1315.
59. Hance AJ, Cadranel J, Soler P, et al. Pulmonary and extrapulmonary Langerhans' cell granulomatosis (histiocytosis X). Semin Respir Med 1988; 9:349–368.
60. Crausman RS, Jennings CA, Tuder RM, Ackerson LM, Irvin CG, King T, Jr. Pulmonary histiocytosis X: pulmonary function and exercise pathophysiology. Am J Respir Crit Care Med 1996; 153:426–435.
61. Basset F, Corrin B, Spencer H, et al. Pulmonary histiocytosis X. Am Rev Respir Dis 1978; 118:811–820.
62. Marcy TW, Reynolds HY. Pulmonary histiocytosis X. Lung 1985; 163:129–150.
63. Travis WD, Borok Z, Roum JH, et al. Pulmonary Langerhans cell granulomatosis (histiocytosis X). A clinicopathologic study of 48 cases. Am J Surg Pathol 1993; 17:971–986.
64. Auld D. Pathology of eosinophilic granuloma of the lung. Arch Pathol 1959; 63:113–131.
65. Friedman PJ, Leibow AA, Sokoloff J. Eosinophilic granuloma of lung. Medicine 1981; 60:385–396.
66. Aguayo SM, Schwarz M, Mortenson RL, et al. Differentiation of eosinophilic granuloma of the lung from other interstitial lung diseases using clinical, physiologic, and bronchoalveolar lavage criteria. Am Rev Respir Dis 1990; 141:A319.
67. Chusid EL. Pulmonary eosinophilic granuloma: aspects of pulmonary function. Mt Sinai J Med 1961; 33:116.
68. Hoffman L, Cohn JE, Guenster EA. Respiratory abnormalities in eosinophilic granuloma of the lung: long term study of 5 cases. N Engl J Med 1961; 267:377–389.
69. Aguayo SM, Schwarz MI, Mortenson RL. The role of the chest radiograph in the evaluation of disease severity and clinical course in eosinophilic granuloma. Am Rev Respir Dis 1990; 141:A61.
70. Lacronique J, Roth C, Battesti JP, Basset F, Chretien J. Chest radiological features

of pulmonary histiocytosis X: a report based on 50 adult cases. Thorax 1982; 37:104–109.
71. Von Essen S, West W, Sitorius M, Rennard S. Complete resolution of roentgenographic changes in a patient with pulmonary histiocytosis X. Chest 1990; 98:765–768.
72. Saven A, Foon KA, Piro LD. 2-Chlorodeoxyadenosine-induced complete remissions in Langerhans-cell histiocytosis. Ann Int Med 1994; 121:430–432.
73. King TE, Jr. Idiopathic pulmonary fibrosis. In: Schwarz MI, King TE, Jr., eds. Interstitial Lung Disease. Hamilton: B.C. Decker Inc., 1998: 597–644.

9

The Psychosocial Aspects of Chronic Pulmonary Disease and Lymphangioleiomyomatosis

PAULINE BARNES, KATERI GABRIELE, and MARY EHRMANTRAUT

National Heart, Lung and Blood Institute
National Institutes of Health
Bethesda, Maryland

Health is a state of complete physical, mental and social well-being and not merely the absence of disease or infirmity. (1)

I. Introduction

Chronic pulmonary disease results in irreversible loss of pulmonary function. The course varies greatly. It can be insidious and/or have remissions or recurrences. Variations within the same disease suggest that other factors, such as heredity and environment, may play a role in the clinical presentation. Like many chronic illnesses, chronic pulmonary disease requires adaptation by the individual and family.

Approximately 14 million persons in the United States suffer from chronic obstructive pulmonary disease (COPD) (2). Asthma, another chronic pulmonary disease, affects 12.4 million adults and children in the United States (3). Alpha$_1$-antitrypsin deficiency, a hereditary form of emphysema that can strike in early and middle adulthood, affects 70,000–100,000 individuals in the United States, although there are probably many more patients who have been misdiagnosed (4). Another disease that probably is underdiagnosed is lymphangioleiomyomatosis

(LAM). There are estimates that it affects approximately 2000 women in the United States, with about 100 new cases diagnosed each year worldwide (5).

LAM is a rare progressive lung disorder that affects primarily women of childbearing age. The symptoms usually appear between the ages of 17 and 47, with the average age being 33 (6). At the present time, as part of a National Institutes of Health clinical research protocol, 44 patients ranging in age from 23 to 54 are being followed. These patients have had a diagnosis of LAM for from 1 to 18 years.

The organs that are affected by LAM include the lung, kidney, and retroperitoneum. The chest x-ray may have fine reticular or linear and nodular densities, and the chest computerized tomography (CT) scan shows sharply demarcated cysts of various sizes in the lungs (7,8). Atypical smooth muscle proliferation can be found around and within the airways, blood vessels, and lymphatic channels (5,9).

The diagnosis of LAM can be made by biopsy in conjunction with the CT scan (6). The average time from presentation of symptoms to diagnosis is 44 months (6). Many patients are misdiagnosed with disorders such as COPD, asthma, bronchitis, interstitial lung disease (ILD) of unknown cause, idiopathic pulmonary hemosiderosis, and sarcoidosis (6). Since most physicians are unfamiliar with LAM, some patients may have a delay in diagnosis and treatment. Although for some patients more than 5 years transpired before diagnosis, the majority were diagnosed within the first year of the onset of symptoms.

The etiology of LAM is unknown, but because the disease occurs almost exclusively in premenopausal women and there is acceleration during pregnancy, hormonal influences are thought to play a role in its pathogenesis (10). During profound hormonal manipulation such as pregnancy, regression of symptoms and signs as well as progression have been reported (5). The prognosis for LAM is poor. Although most patients die within 10 years from the time of diagnosis, some have lived as long as 20 years (6). The treatment of LAM is limited to estrogen suppression through chemical and mechanical methods. Eventually all individuals with LAM will be faced with the decision to be evaluated for lung transplantation.

II. Quality of Life

Patients with chronic pulmonary disease must confront the impact of their illness on a daily basis. Quality of life becomes a very important outcome in determining the effect of disease on the individual's life. Quality of life is, however, subjective. The functional outcome and course of the illness and the therapy provided to the patient affect quality of life (11). Quality of life is multidimensional, consisting of four domains: physical status and occupational function, somatic sensation, psychological status, and social interactions (11).

A. Physical Status and Occupational Function

This first domain of quality of life, physical status and occupational function, refers to the person's perception of strength, energy, and the ability to carry out activities of daily living (ADLs) (11). Many physical changes occur that can affect daily life; the individual may notice a decreased exercise tolerance, no longer being able to walk, climb stairs, carry groceries, or do housework as effortlessly as in the past. In LAM, which affects a relatively young female population, these physical changes are unexpected and bewildering to the individual, the family, and/or the significant other. As the pulmonary disease progresses, the ability of the individual to perform ADLs declines. Oxygen therapy may be required to assist in maintaining ADLs that are perceived as important to the person. If employment has physical requirements, the individual may be unable to perform the work, with resulting effects on income, health insurance, and career goals.

B. Somatic Sensations

Somatic sensations refer to symptoms experienced by the individual. Somatic sensations associated with chronic pulmonary illness (e.g., shortness of breath, dyspnea on exertion, cough, wheeze, and fatigue) affect the individual's perceived quality of life (11). These signs may progress insidiously, delaying the patient's visit to a physician until symptoms become intolerable.

The most common symptoms reported in LAM patients is dyspnea, with all LAM patients having had some degree of shortness of breath. Spontaneous pneumothorax occurs frequently in this patient population with resulting risk to health and limitations to activity (e.g., airplane travel). Patients may also present with one or more of the following clinical findings: hemoptysis, chyloptysis, chylous ascites, chylous effusion, chest pain, and/or angiomyolipomas. The symptoms associated with these findings (e.g., pain, dyspnea, fatigue, cough) have an influence on quality of life. These symptoms may inhibit the performance of activities that are important to the patient.

C. Psychological Aspects

A patient diagnosed with a chronic lung disease may exhibit anxiety, depression, and fear. Rare pulmonary diseases such as LAM can evoke feelings of fear related to diagnosis, diagnostic testing, therapy, and possibly poor prognosis. Individuals with LAM may find it difficult to locate a knowledgeable health care provider or current literature about the disease. The person is concerned with the unfamiliar terms, procedures, drugs, and therapeutic interventions.

The grieving process can affect a person's quality of life. The individual or family may be in denial over the diagnosis (12). Anger occurs when the person realizes that future goals may have to change due to the chronicity of the illness (12). There may be feelings of bitterness and frustration over having the illness. The person may mourn or feel sadness toward what has been lost and what is no longer possible in the future (12). The final stage of grieving is acceptance (12). The individual accepts the changes in life, looks toward the future, and adapts positively (12).

The patient and family must deal with the physical and psychological stress of chronic illness. Many people consider chronic illness as a stigma. "Normal" individuals may avoid the chronically ill person, leaving the patient with a feeling of low self-esteem. The individual sees changes in physical appearance; a loss of freedom results from dependence upon bronchodilator devices, the use of oxygen, and the need for caregivers.

The young female with LAM and her family have a number of stresses with which to cope. Prior to this diagnosis, the individual was healthy and now faces a grave prognosis. The sense of loss surrounding the issue of childbearing can also increase stress. Patients have had multiple miscarriages or termination of their pregnancy for medical reasons related to the disease. Losing the option to have children can create feelings of guilt and powerlessness. The limitations imposed by this disease extend to other social aspects of quality of life. For instance, changes in atmospheric pressure, such as flying, mountain climbing, and scuba diving, can exacerbate dyspnea and increase the risk of developing a pneumothorax. Individuals with LAM may be advised to avoid participation in these activities. This may negatively impact recreation or employment. The patient's perception of the disease is important, as it will influence ability to cope, to carry on with daily life, and to interact with others.

D. Social Interactions

Social interactions are the ability of the patient to participate in activities necessary for community living (11). The social contacts that a person may have include family, friends, work associates, and the general community. With any chronic pulmonary disease, the family's view toward illness and the help they provide to the patient (financial, psychological support) are critical to the patient's ability to adapt to the chronic condition (13). Family members affect the ability of the person to cope and may begin to assume new roles and responsibilities as the illness progresses (14–16). Since LAM affects women, it often places the spouse in a nontraditional role of caregiver (17).

Difficulties in communication may arise with chronic illness. Denial on the part of the patient, family, or others can lead to isolation. This fear and isolation can create problems with social intimacy. In our experience, patients have expressed concern about the stress that illness has imposed on their marriage. The impact of chronic illness on intimacy must be addressed to enhance the relationships and improve the quality of life.

There are certain misconceptions regarding sexuality in individuals with chronic illness, including women with LAM. Although women with LAM may have symptoms of fatigue, shortness of breath, vaginal dryness, and decreased libido (related to medications), they still have a need for closeness and intimacy. Fear, apprehension, anger, or anxiety about one's sexual performance or physical attractiveness may result in a reduced ability to be sexually intimate (18). There are many deterrents to sexual intimacy, some of which include the use of oxygen by the patient, the perception that the patient is frail, lack of interest, or discord in the relationship (19).

Strong support from friends may influence how the person perceives the illness. The support from the individual's work community (supervisor and peers) is critical in determining whether or not the individual will be able to continue to work. If the employer supports the individual by restructuring the person's roles and responsibilities, the individual may continue to be a productive employee and maintain a sense of self-worth.

Since LAM is such a rare disease, it is not uncommon for a patient to feel isolated. Support groups within the community offer the patient a mechanism to adapt to illness in a positive way. Other individuals with chronic illness can best relate to the feelings that a patient with chronic pulmonary disease is experiencing.

E. Economic and Spiritual Aspects

Other domains affecting quality of life in chronic lung disease are economic, religious, and spiritual. The economic domain refers to financial aspects associated with lack of health insurance, loss of employment, and loss of income. LAM patients have expressed concerns regarding the financial burdens of medical costs, unemployment, and the loss of control over their lives. Culture and religion influence an individual's view of illness and death. Some individuals may find comfort in religion, while others may experience a partial or total loss of faith.

The average life expectancy for patients with LAM from time of diagnosis is 10 years (6,10). Because there is no single proven treatment and because of the shortened life expectancy, women with LAM may have a sense of uncertainty about the future. Women with LAM are in the prime of their lives and may not achieve their future goals related to career and family.

III. Psychological Impact of Therapy

A variety of treatments and supportive therapies are available for patients with chronic lung disease. These include medications, oxygen, pulmonary rehabilitation, lung transplantation, alternative therapies, and nutrition. The medications in the treatment of chronic pulmonary disease consist of, but are not limited to, bronchodilators and steroids. Most women with LAM are not treated with the usual pulmonary medications unless they have other pulmonary components to their disease, such as asthma. Different therapeutic interventions may be appropriate depending on the stage of the disease including surgical procedures such as bilateral oophorectomy, pleurodesis, and lung transplantation. None of the treatments for LAM have cured the disease, although there is some evidence that progesterone therapy, estrogen suppression, or oophorectomy may slow the progression (10,20). Therapies used to treat LAM may have a psychological impact because the end result is infertility.

The most commonly used medications in patients with LAM are listed in Table 1. Some individuals elect to discontinue the use of their prescribed medications due to the severity of side effects.

As the chronic lung disease progresses, the patient may require oxygen supplementation. Oxygen may help decrease dyspnea but may in fact have a negative psychological impact. The patient may feel a further loss of independence when she becomes tethered to the oxygen tank. Oxygen therapy is seen as progression of the disease, making it appear more visible. At first, compliance

Table 1 Medications Used to Treat LAM

Name	Purpose	Common side effects
Medroxyprogesterone acetate (Depoprovera, Provera)	Estrogen suppression	Weight gain, back pain, headache, mood changes, decreased libido, depression, osteoporosis
Leuprolide acetate (Lupron)	Ovarian estrogen and androgen suppression	Hot flashes
Tamoxifen citrate (Nolvadex)	Nonsteroidal antiestrogen	Hot flashes, visual disturbances
Megestrol acetate (Megace)	Estrogen suppression	Weight gain, hot flashes
Calcium/Vitamin D	Osteoporosis prevention	
Alendronate (Fosamax)	Osteoporosis treatment	Gastrointestinal irritation

Source: Physicians' Desk Reference. 51st ed. Montvale, NJ: Medical Economics Company, Inc., 1997.

with oxygen therapy may be an issue, but once the symptoms are allayed, the benefits of using oxygen are realized.

Pulmonary rehabilitation may be initiated as activity decreases and symptoms increase. The purpose of pulmonary rehabilitation is to decrease fatigue and increase endurance. It is a multidisciplinary approach that assists people with pulmonary disease and their families to gain and preserve the individual's maximum function within the community (22). Most of our LAM patients do not participate in a formal pulmonary rehabilitation program but try to maintain a physically active life within the constraints of their dyspnea. Formal pulmonary rehabilitation programs are recommended for those who will undergo evaluation for lung transplant.

Psychological symptoms of depression, anxiety, and fatigue are likely to improve through pulmonary rehabilitation. Being in a controlled environment under the supervision of the coordinator as well as the psychological support of other participants can be very comforting. The benefits gained by patients participating in pulmonary rehabilitation programs are improved stamina and increased independence. These benefits may lessen some of the burdens on the caregiver.

Lung transplantation is used when all other available treatments have proven ineffective and the patient's pulmonary disease has progressed to the point that life expectancy has been reduced to less than 2 years. Each lung transplantation center has specific criteria for patient selection. Considerations of lung transplantation that need to be taken into account by the recipient are scarcity of donor lungs (23), cost (24), quality of life (24), long-term survival rate (25), and potential new problems including rejection and infection. There have been two reported cases of LAM in transplanted lungs, and in both of these cases the donor lungs were from males (26,27). Transplantation is not a cure, but the exchange of one illness for another. It provides, however, the opportunity for prolonged life.

When patients with chronic lung disease such as LAM perceive that they are receiving little or no benefit from conventional therapy, they may be willing to experiment with other forms of treatment. The goal of alternative medical therapy ranges from managing symptoms to cure. The therapies range from home remedies to complex products (28). Alternative therapies may have no effect, be beneficial, or even have harmful effects on the patients. No matter which therapy is used, patients using alternative medicine need to be aware of the risks and/or benefits.

As with other lung diseases, patients with LAM expend additional energy with breathing, therefore, a well-balanced diet is essential. As the dyspnea increases, the caloric requirements may increase. However, it becomes more difficult for the patient to breathe and eat at the same time, which could result in inadequate caloric intake (32).

The goal of proper nutrition in chronic pulmonary disease is to maintain respiratory muscle mass, strength, and function to maximize the person's health status and quality of life. Poor nutrition can worsen symptoms and have a negative effect on the prognosis of disease (29).

Most research studies on nutrition and lung diseases have been limited to COPD or cystic fibrosis. There has been little research with LAM and its nutritional impact. A fat-free diet with medium-chain triglycerides has been used in LAM as supplementation for patients with chylous ascites and chylous effusions. Two case studies have reported improvement of chylous ascites after patients were placed on a fat-restricted diet with medium-chain triglyceride supplementation (30,31).

Several of our LAM patients have reported problems with chyluria, chylous ascites, chylous effusion, and/or chylous thorax. Some of these patients have been recommended for low-fat diet with medium-chain triglyceride supplements. Compliance is difficult because of the high cost of medium-chain triglyceride supplements and the limited selection of foods on the diet.

IV. Conclusion

Many burdens are imposed upon the individual with chronic pulmonary illness. The diagnosis of a chronic lung disease affects each person differently. Many people will acknowledge the physical aspects associated with chronic illness before they recognize and address the psychosocial aspects. Women with LAM are a unique subset because they are predominately in their childbearing years. The psychological impact of receiving a diagnosis with an average survival time of 10 years is devastating to the patient and family. With this disease come many physical, psychosocial, and financial barriers that need to be overcome.

The individual with LAM has symptoms of shortness of breath, which can affect activities of daily living. She is susceptible to spontaneous pneumothoraces resulting in frequent hospitalizations. Her travel by plane is limited, affecting her employment or recreation. She may no longer be able or advised to have children because of the effects of the current recommended treatment and impact that pregnancy may have on the progression of the disease. The medications have side effects including osteoporosis, weight gain, and decreased libido.

In addition to the hardship of having this disease, other psychosocial concerns are placed upon these women. Decreased libido may cause problems related to intimacy. The spouse or significant other may become the caregiver. The woman may feel isolated and begin to have concerns for the future of her children and family.

She may also have anxiety related to new financial problems. The frequent hospitalizations and the cost of therapy adds additional, unexpected expenses. Furthermore, these individuals must consider and ultimately plan for lung transplantation, the last option for treatment.

Despite this bleak outlook, women with LAM enrolled in the NIH study have remarkable resilience. They have demonstrated the ability to overcome barriers in part by being active participants in their health care and by seeking knowledge and understanding of their disease. These women have remained as active as their symptoms have allowed them to be. Many continue to be employed despite the fact that they may be on oxygen and/or awaiting lung transplantation.

References

1. World Health Organization (WHO). Constitutions of the World Health Organization. Basic documents. Geneva, Switzerland, 1948.
2. American Thoracic Society. Standards for the diagnosis and care of patients with chronic obstructive pulmonary disease. Am J Respir Crit Care Med 1995; 152:578–583.
3. National Center for Health Statistics. National Health Survey, 1982–1992.
4. Buist AS. Alpha 1-antitrypsin deficiency in lung and liver disease. Hosp Pract 1989; 24:51–59.
5. Viskum K. Pulmonary lymphangioleiomyomatosis. Monaldi Arch Chest Dis 1993; 48:233–236.
6. Taylor JR, Ryu J, Colby TV, Raffin TA. Lymphangioleiomyomatosis: clinical course in 32 patients. N Engl J Med 1990; 323:1254–1260.
7. Sherrier RH, Chiles C, Roggli V. Pulmonary lymphangioleiomyomatosis: CT findings. AJR 1989; 153:937–941.
8. Carrington CB, Cugell DW, Gaensle EA, Marks A, Redding RA, Schaaf JT, Tomasia A. Lymphangioleiomyomatosis: physiologic-pathologic-radiologic correlations. Am Rev Respir Dis 1977; 116:977–995.
9. Templeton PA, McLoud TC, Muller NL, Shepard JO, Moore EH. Pulmonary lymphangioleiomyomatosis: CT and pathologic findings. J Comput Assist Tomogr 1989; 13:54–57
10. Corrin B, Liebow AA, Friedman PJ. Pulmonary lymphangiomyomatosis. Am J Pathol 1975; 79:348–66.
11. Schipper H, Clinch JJ, Olweny CL. Quality of life studies: definitions and conceptual issues. In: Spilker B, ed. Quality of Life and Pharmoeconomics in Clinical Trials. 2d ed. Philadelphia: Lippincott-Raven, 1996:11–23.
12. Kahn AM. Coping with fear and grieving. In: Lubkin IM, ed. Chronic Illness: Impact and Interventions. 3d ed. Boston: Jones and Bartlett, 1995:241–259.
13. Woods N, Haberman M, Packard N. Demands of illness and individual, dyadic, and family adaptation in chronic illness. West J Nurs Res 1993; 15:10–30.

14. Friedman L, Nelson D, Smith F. Women with breast cancer: perception of family functioning and adjustment to illness. Psychosom Med 1988; 50:529–540.
15. Manne S, Zautra A. Spouse criticism and support: their association with coping and psychological adjustment among women with rheumatoid arthritis. J Personal Soc Psychol 1989; 56:608–617.
16. Sexton D, Munro B. Impact of a husband's chronic illness (COPD) on the spouse's life. Res Nurs Health 1985; 8:83–90.
17. Manne SL, Zautra AJ. Couples coping with chronic illness: women with rheumatoid arthritis and their healthy husbands. J Behav Med 1990; 13:327–342.
18. Sotile WM. Marital and family issues. In: Sotile WM. Psychosocial Interventions for Cardiopulmonary Patients: A Guide for Health Professionals. Illinois: Human Kinetics, 1996:137–159.
19. Birchfield ME. The chronic stage. In: Birchfield ME. Stages of Illness: Guidelines for Nursing Care. Bowie: Brady Communications Company, Inc., 1985:19–75.
20. Colby TV, Carrington CB. Interstitial lung disease. In: Thurlbeck WM, Churg AM, eds. Pathology of the Lung. New York: Thieme Medical Publishers, Inc., 1995:589–737.
21. Physicians' Desk Reference. 51st ed. Montvale, NJ: Medical Economics Company, Inc., 1997.
22. Fishman AP. Pulmonary rehabilitation research: NIH summary workshop. Am J Respir Crit Care Med 1994; 149:825–833.
23. Mentzer SJ, Reilly JJ, Caplan AL, Sugarbaker DJ. Ethical considerations in lung transplantation. Heart Lung Transplant 1994; 13:56–58.
24. Ramsey SD, Patrick DL, Albert RK, Larson EB, Wood DE. The cost-effectiveness of lung transplantation. Chest 1995; 108:1594–1601.
25. Kriett JM, Kaye MP. The registry of the international society for heart and lung transplantation: 8th official report. J Heart Lung Transplant 1991; 10:491–498.
26. O'Brien JD, Lium JH, Parosa JF, DeYoung BR, Wick MR, Trulock EP. Lymphangiomyomatosis recurrence in the allograft after single-lung transplantation. Am J Respir Crit Care Med 1995; 151:2033–2036.
27. Nine JS, Yousem SA, Paradis IL, Keenan R, Griffith BP. Lymphangioleiomyomatosis: recurrence after lung transplantation. J Heart Lung Transplant 1994; 13:714–719.
28. Cassileth BR, Chapman CC. Alternative and complementary treatments. In: Spilker B, ed. Quality of Life and Pharmacoeconomics in Clinical Trials. 2d ed. Philadelphia: Lippincott-Raven, 1996:421–425.
29. Mackay L. Nutritional status and chronic obstructive pulmonary disease. Nurs Standard 1996; 10:38–42.
30. Calvo E, Amarillas L, Mateos M, Orradre J, Gilsanz G, Alvarez-Sala J, Espinos D. Lymphangioleiomyomatosis, chylous ascites, and diet. Digest Dis Sci 1996; 41:591–593.
31. Calabrese PR, Frank HD, Taubin HL. Lymphangiomyomatosis with chylous ascites: treatment with dietary fat restriction and medium chain triglycerides. Cancer 1977; 40:895–897.

32. Chin R, Haponik EF. Nutrition, respiratory function, and disease. In: Shils ME, Olson JA, Shike M, eds. Modern Nutrition in Health and Disease. Philadelphia: Lea & Febiger, 1994:1374–1390.

10

Lymphangioleiomyomatosis

Imaging Features

NILO A. AVILA, CLARA C. CHEN, SHAN C. CHU, and JOEL MOSS

National Heart, Lung and Blood Institute
National Institutes of Health
Bethesda, Maryland

I. Introduction

LAM is characterized by hyperplasia of atypical smooth muscle along lymphatics in the thorax and abdomen. Typically, in the lung, the process starts as a micronodular proliferation along the lymphatic vessels in the bronchovascular bundles, interlobular septa, and pleura. Proliferation of atypical spindle cells along the bronchioles leads to air trapping and the development of cystic air spaces. Rupture of these spaces, and disruption of the pleural elastic laminae due to the growth of atypical spindle cells, result in pneumothoraces (1). Chronic lymphatic, airflow, and circulatory obstruction produces a remarkable spectrum of clinical and radiographic manifestations. These include focal hemorrhage and hemoptysis from venous obstruction, pneumothoraces, and airflow obstruction from impingement of the abnormal muscle on the lumina of bronchioles and small bronchi. The radiographic parenchymal changes are progressive, eventually leading to a diffuse honeycomb appearance (2).

II. Radiography and Computed Tomography of Pulmonary Disease

The chest radiography findings in LAM include reticular, reticulonodular, miliary, and honeycomb patterns (Fig. 1). These radiographic findings may precede, accompany, or postdate other chest findings such as pneumothoraces, pleural effusions, and hyperinflation (2). Radiographic findings may not be seen until late in the course of the disease. In some patients with recurrent pneumothoraces,

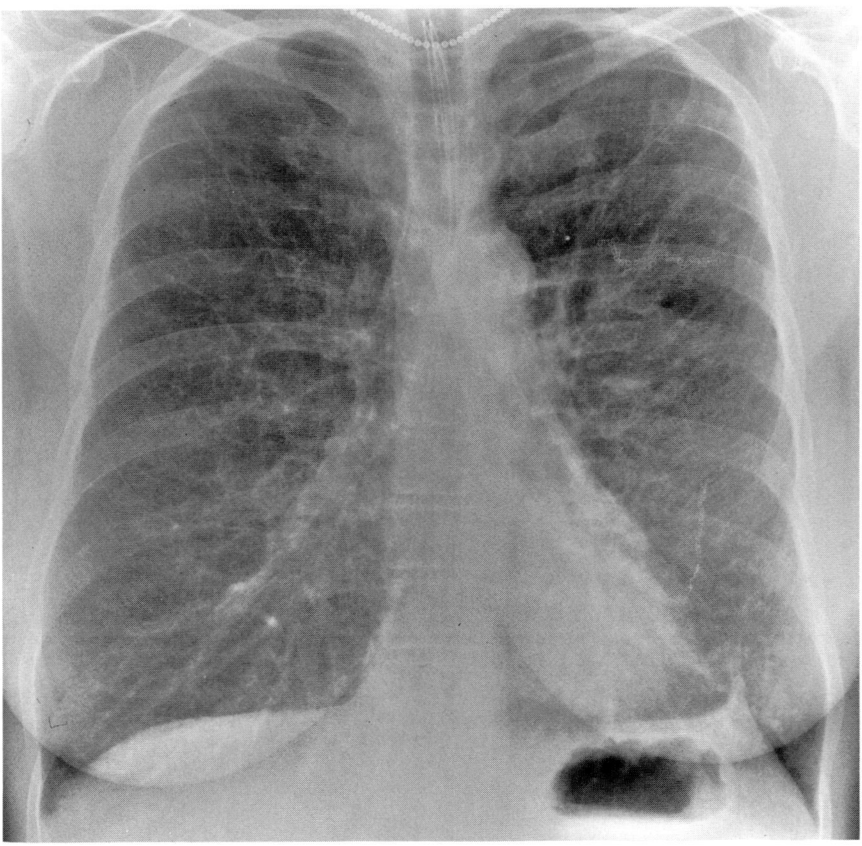

A

Figure 1 (A) Posterioranterior and (B) lateral chest radiographs demonstrate severe, diffuse interstitial lung changes in a patient with LAM.

extensive parenchymal abnormalities were seen at surgery that were not evident on radiographs (3).

The main finding on computed tomography (CT) consists of numerous thin-walled cystic air spaces of varying sizes surrounded by relatively normal lung parenchyma (3–9). CT is more accurate than chest radiography in defining the presence and extent of parenchymal cysts (8,9). The majority of cystic air spaces have walls ranging in size from faintly perceptible to approximately 2 mm thick and may be indistinguishable from emphysema on CT. The individual cyst walls are better displayed on high-resolution CT than on routine 10-mm-section CT (Fig. 2). No clear relationship has been demonstrated between the size of the pulmonary cysts and the severity of lung involvement. Some patients may have

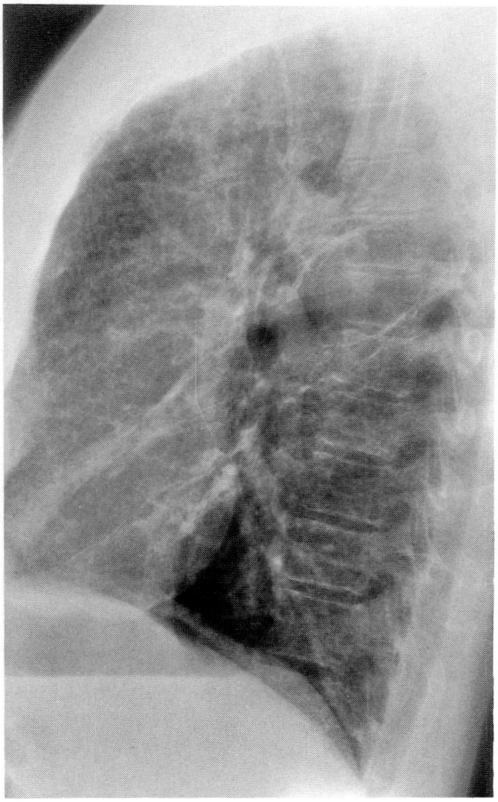

B

Figure 1 Continued.

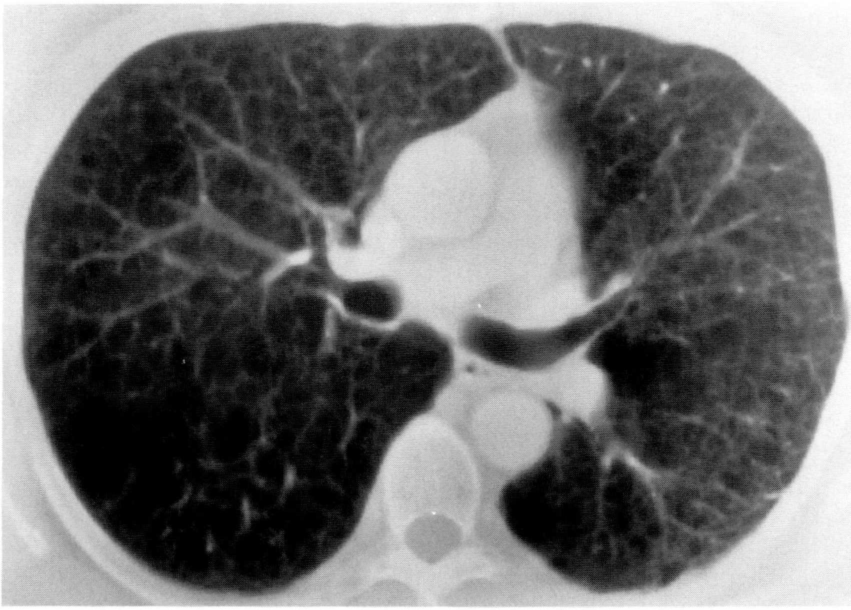

A

Figure 2 (A) Conventional, 10-mm axial computed tomography image of the chest in the same patient as Figure 1. Note diffuse, thin-walled parenchymal cysts and no evidence of interstitial lung disease. (B) High-resolution, 1-mm-thick axial CT image of the chest in the same patient. Note improved depiction of the parenchymal cysts compared to the conventional study (A).

tiny cysts diffusely involving the lung parenchyma, whereas others may have a few, scattered large cysts (Figs. 3 and 4).

Reticular patterns on chest radiographs of patients with LAM correspond to a cross-sectional appearance of innumerable, contiguous small cysts. Presumably, the reticulation observed on projectional images results from summation of numerous cyst walls (3,4,8–10). CT affords a more reliable depiction of the pulmonary interstitial pathology by virtue of superior contrast resolution and, with high-resolution techniques, reduced superimposition or volume-averaging effects (11,12). In most patients with cystic abnormalities on CT scans, only nonspecific, irregular, linear opacities are seen on chest radiographs. Only in advanced cases, when the cysts are greater than 1 cm in diameter, are they recognized readily on the radiographs (8,9).

The main advantage of CT is in demonstrating parenchymal abnormalities in symptomatic patients with normal or questionably abnormal findings on chest

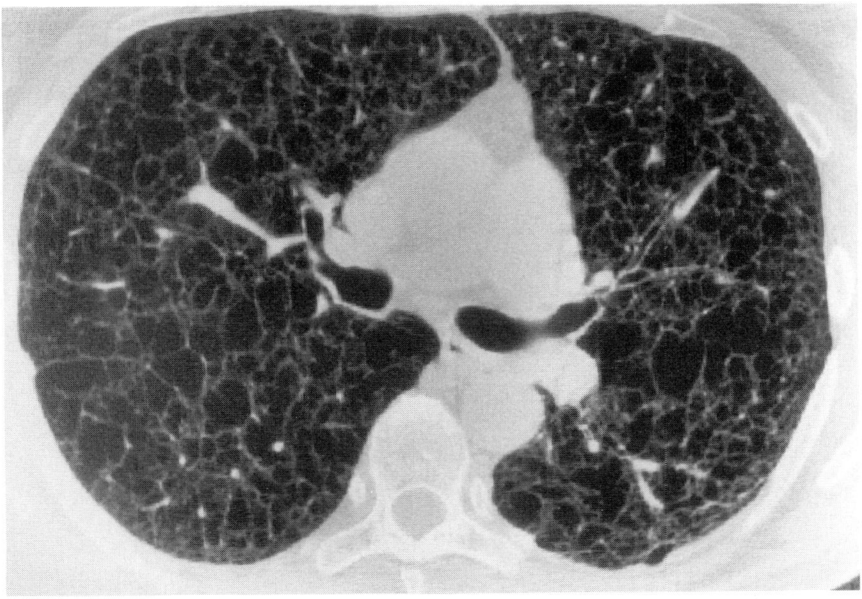

B

Figure 2 Continued.

radiographs, which may help to overcome the reluctance to proceed with lung biopsy (7). Normal findings on CT, however, do not exclude parenchymal disease. In one report, a patient with biopsy-proven LAM had no detectable abnormalities on thin-section CT scans obtained at 2-cm intervals (8).

LAM may also involve the hilar, mediastinal, and extrathoracic lymph nodes and may cause marked dilatation of the thoracic duct (Fig. 5). Rupture of dilated lymphatic vessels may result in chylous pleural effusion or ascites. Proliferation of cells in the walls of pulmonary veins may cause venous obstruction and lead to pulmonary hemorrhage, which may account for the small areas of air space consolidation seen in some patients (2,8,13).

III. Correlation of Radiography and CT with Pulmonary Function Tests

The chest radiographic assessment of disease includes both objective and subjective observations. Lung length measured in the posterior-anterior projection and the arc of the right hemidiaphragm measured from the left-lateral projection

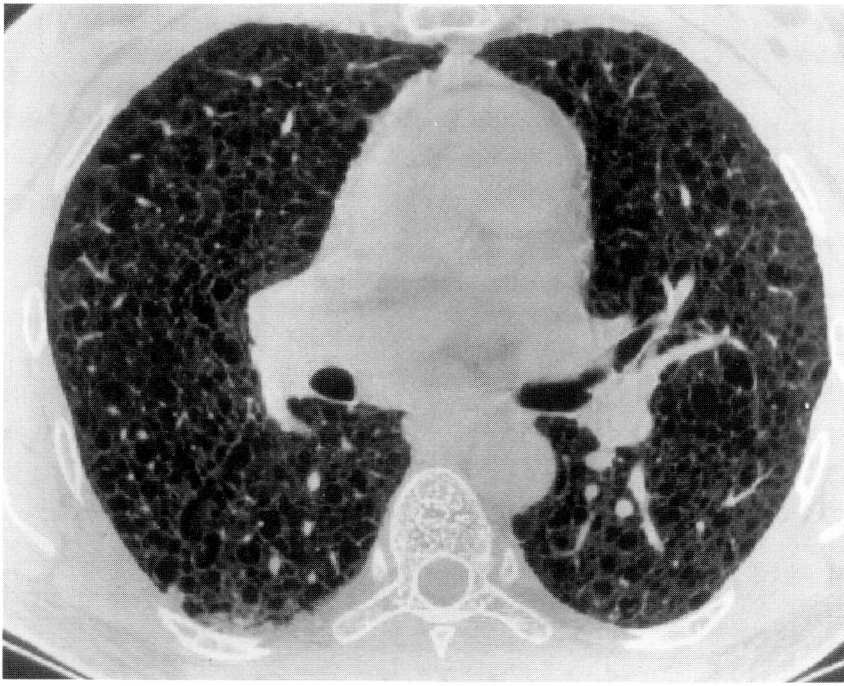

Figure 3 Axial CT image of the chest in a patient with LAM. Note diffuse involvement of the lung parenchyma, with numerous tiny thin-walled cysts.

have been used as measures of obstruction based on a previous report in patients with emphysema, in which these dimensions were significantly correlated with FEV_1/FVC, a functional measure of airflow obstruction (14). In patients with LAM, there is no significant relationship between lung length or the arc of the right hemidiaphragm and abnormalities in spirometry or gas diffusion; there is, however, a correlation between lung length and the percent predicted total lung capacity.

The pathophysiologic characteristics of LAM are clearly unique and would be expected to result in radiographic and functional abnormalities distinct from those seen in emphysema. In emphysema, TLC is generally in excess of 100% of predicted values (9). In LAM, there is no significant correlation between the extent of disease found at CT and the percent-predicted TLC (9). TLC is usually normal when calculated by means of helium equilibration (1,2). In contrast, a high correlation is observed between the extent of lung involvement found at CT and the percent predicted FEV_1/FVC ($r = -0.92$, $p < 0.002$) (9). The diffuse cystic

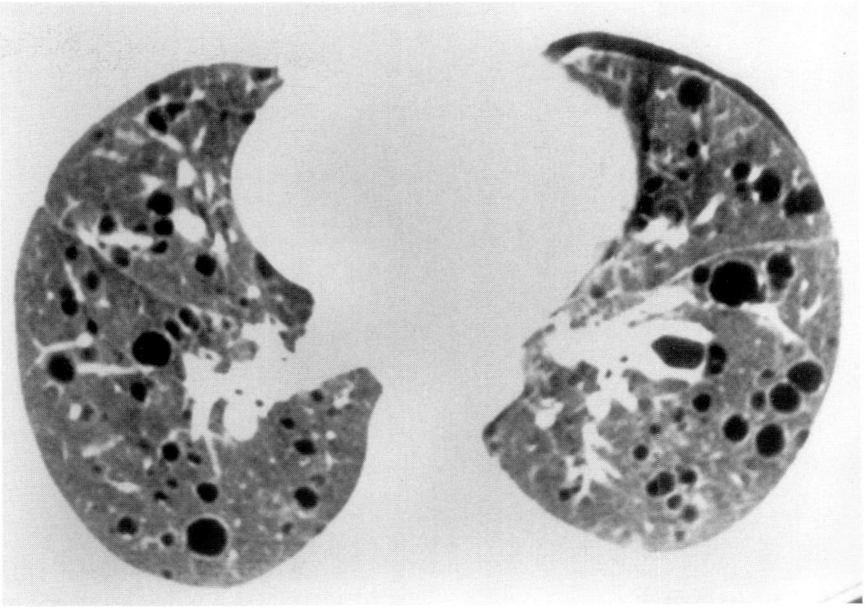

Figure 4 Axial CT image of the chest in a patient with LAM. Note large cysts scattered in the lung parenchyma. Note a small, left, anterior pneumothorax.

air spaces seen on CT may develop as a consequence of air trapping distal to small airways in which there has been smooth muscle proliferation and loss of alveoli, resulting in an obstructive ventilatory defect (1,2). In addition, extent of disease at CT correlates significantly with impairment in gas exchange as assessed by the carbon monoxide diffusing capacity (8).

IV. Ventilation/Perfusion Scintigraphy of Pulmonary Disease in LAM

Currently, ventilation and perfusion lung scanning of LAM patients is not performed routinely. The literature is limited to case reports. In 1992, Sleiman et al. (15) described bilateral heterogeneous perfusion defects in a LAM patient who was to undergo single lung transplantation. Similarly, Fanti et al. (16) reported diffuse heterogeneity in lung perfusion in a patient with LAM and severe dyspnea. A ventilation scan using Tc-99m Technegas demonstrated matching venti-

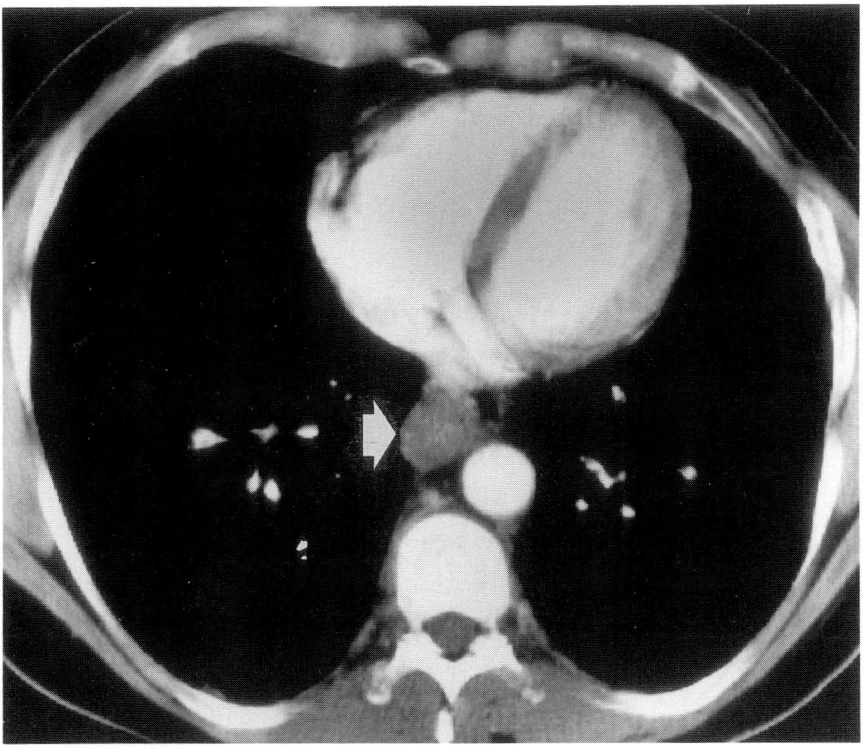

Figure 5 Axial CT image of the chest demonstrating dilatation of the thoracic duct (arrow).

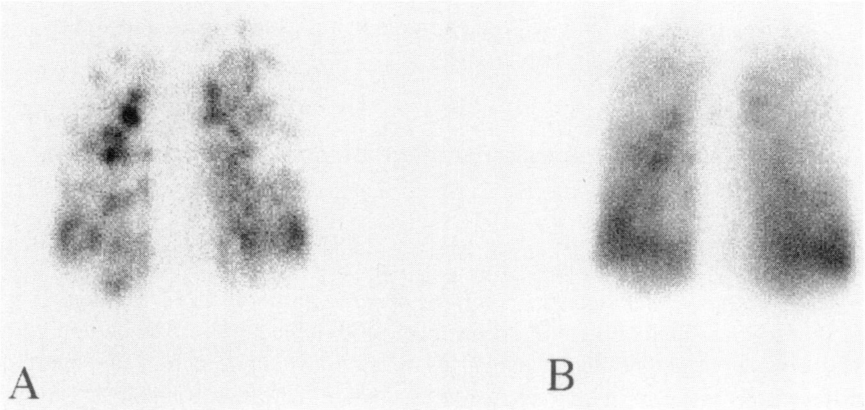

Figure 6 Posterior views of ventilation (A) and perfusion (B) scans in a patient with LAM show diffuse heterogeneity. Note the "speckling" pattern seen in the ventilation study.

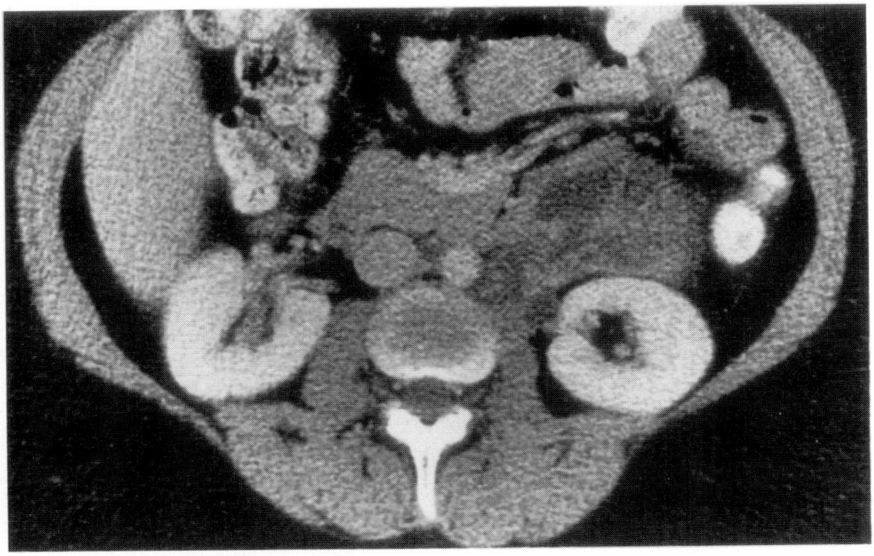

Figure 7 Axial CT image of the abdomen showing a large, left retroperitoneal mass separate from the kidney and containing areas of decreased attenuation.

lation/perfusion abnormalities. In addition, "well-defined hot spots" were described on the ventilation study, possibly correlating with uptake in cysts (16).

At NIH, aerosol ventilation/perfusion lung scanning in LAM patients has confirmed the frequent but nonspecific findings of diffuse, matched heterogeneity. Similar to the findings using Technegas, the frequent appearance of a "speckling"

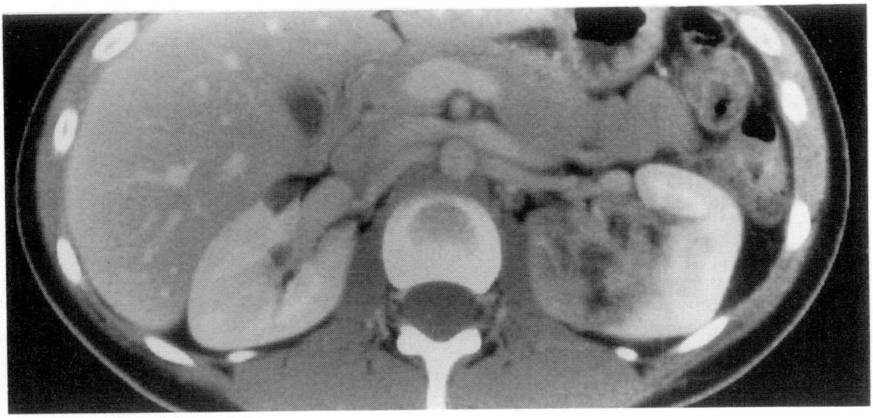

Figure 8 Axial CT image of the abdomen demonstrates a large angiomyolipoma arising from the medial aspect of the left kidney. The mass enhances heterogeneously and contains low attenuation material, consistent with fat.

pattern on our aerosol ventilation studies was noted. This pattern consists of multiple, small peripheral collections of activity and appears to be distinct from that seen in other pulmonary diseases (Fig. 6). It is quite striking at times, although the degree of speckling appears to vary from patient to patient. Further study is required to see if ventilation/perfusion scintigraphy has a role to play in the clinical management of patients with LAM.

V. MRI of Pulmonary Disease in LAM

Magnetic resonance imaging (MRI) of the lungs is technically difficult. Respiratory and cardiac motion causes blurring of pulmonary structures. MRI depends on many parameters, including proton density, tissue relaxation times, and blood flow. The density of lung parenchyma is less than any other tissue in the body, resulting in a low signal-to-noise ratio. The alveolar tissue/air interface induces local gradients, which affect magnetic field homogeneity leading to signal loss from intravoxel phase dispersion of spins. Despite these problems, several groups have explored the potential of MRI in lung imaging (17–19).

In a recent study, the lungs of patients with LAM showed a high signal intensity and a larger lung cross-sectional area on T_1-weighted images when compared to a control group. This abnormal signal is thought to be related to several factors, including abnormal proliferation of smooth muscle and dilated lymphatic vessels (20). This noninvasive technique, which does not involve the use of ionizing radiation, may be useful in the assessment of medical therapy and lung transplant procedures and for frequent follow-up of patients.

VI. Differential Considerations of Pulmonary Findings on Imaging Studies

Despite the very distinctive appearance of LAM at CT, the differential diagnosis must include tuberous sclerosis, histiocytosis X, idiopathic pulmonary fibrosis, and emphysema (6,8,21,22). Identical clinical, radiologic, and pathologic pulmonary changes may be seen in 1% of patients with tuberous sclerosis. Although tuberous sclerosis affects both sexes equally, the pulmonary changes have been described almost exclusively in women (8).

Parenchymal cysts are also a primary morphologic features of histiocytosis X. Frequently, the cyst wall in histiocytosis X is more variable in thickness than in LAM (23). In addition, micronodules, macronodules, or cavitary nodules are common in histiocytosis X and not described in LAM (22). Furthermore, histiocytosis X characteristically involves the upper two thirds of the lungs and spares the costophrenic angles, whereas LAM involves the lungs diffusely

(21,22). To differentiate between histiocytosis X and LAM, it may be necessary to perform high-resolution CT (HRCT), which displays the cyst walls much better than does conventional 10-mm-section CT.

Although parenchymal cysts are common in many interstitial lung diseases, they are particularly common in idiopathic pulmonary fibrosis (IPF). IPF is characterized by the presence of a reticular pattern and honeycomb spaces with a predominant distribution in the basilar and subpleural regions; in LAM, the distribution is more diffuse. In IPF, the honeycomb cysts are surrounded by abnormal parenchyma, whereas most of the cysts in LAM are surrounded by normal lung (5).

Pulmonary emphysema may be the most difficult disease to differentiate from LAM on HRCT. The cystic air spaces in LAM, compared to those in emphysema, tend to be more uniform, better defined, and less variable in size. These differences, however, may or may not be present, and the HRCT appearance of emphysema may mimic LAM (11). Correlation of the HRCT appearance with the patient's age, sex, and clinical presentation will aid in the differential diagnosis.

VII. Abdominal Findings in LAM

Abdominal involvement results from the proliferation of smooth muscle within the thoracic duct and lymphatic channels, with replacement of lymph nodes by smooth muscle (Fig. 7). The normal lymphatic routes are disrupted, resulting in diverted collaterals and large lymph cysts. Overdistention of these structures and collaterals may cause rupture and development of chylous ascites (24). Other forms of abdominal involvement include lymphaticoureteric and lymphaticovenous communications and intraadrenal adenopathy (2,17,25–27).

The incidence of renal angiomyolipomas in patients with LAM has been reported to be as high as 47% (28). Angiomyolipomas are uncommon benign neoplasms or hamartomas of mesenchymal origin. They consist of fat, smooth muscle, and blood vessels. Renal angiomyolipomas are usually found incidentally, but can present as abdominal masses or with flank or abdominal pain or hematuria (23,29). The CT diagnosis is made when a well-defined mass containing fat density is found within the renal parenchyma (Fig. 8). The smooth muscle found in pulmonary lymphangioleiomyomatosis is similar histologically and immunohistochemically to that found in angiomyolipomas (30,31).

The diagnosis of renal angiomyolipomas in some patients may precede the diagnosis of pulmonary LAM (28). Since CT may detect pulmonary LAM prior to the onset of symptoms, and since early diagnosis of the disease may lead to changes in management (e.g., avoidance of pregnancy, hormonal manipulation), it may be important to use high-resolution CT to screen young female patients with renal angiomyolipoma for the presence of LAM (28).

VIII. Management of Renal Angiomyolipomas

The recommended management of renal angiomyolipomas is based on tumor size and the presence of symptoms. Tumor size correlates well with the presence or absence of symptoms: 90% of all symptomatic lesions are 4 cm or larger, while 64% of all asymptomatic tumors are smaller than 4 cm (32). Angiomyolipomas that are 4 cm or larger and that cause significant symptoms are at risk for spontaneous rupture and massive hemorrhage (33).

Asymptomatic patients with lesions smaller than 4 cm in their greatest dimension may be followed with yearly ultrasonography or CT, whereas lesions measuring 4 cm or greater in diameter should be followed by semiannual ultrasonography or CT. Symptomatic patients with lesions smaller than 4 cm should be observed to determine whether their symptoms resolve promptly. Patients with a lesion smaller than 4 cm and in whom symptoms resolve can be followed with semiannual ultrasound or CT. Patients with persistent symptoms can undergo angiography and be considered for selective arterial embolization or conservative surgical intervention (enucleation or partial nephrectomy) (32).

A slightly modified approach to the management of isolated renal angiomyolipoma has been suggested for lesions greater than 4 cm in diameter. These patients may be divided into asymptomatic, mildly symptomatic, and severely symptomatic groups. Asymptomatic and mildly symptomatic patients may be followed conservatively with semiannual ultrasonography, but they should be warned of possible future complications. If any significant growth is seen, even without symptoms, embolization or conservative surgery should be considered to prevent further parenchymal damage. Patients with severe symptoms (e.g., uncontrollable pain, hemorrhage) should undergo embolization or conservative surgery (32). If surgery is contemplated for patients with LAM, one should consider operating before a worsening of the patient's pulmonary disease increases the risk of the procedure.

IX. Conclusion

LAM has a characteristic appearance on CT scans, consisting of cystic air spaces surrounded by normal lung. The size of the cystic spaces varies and does not correlate with severity of disease. CT may show parenchymal abnormalities, even in patients with normal chest radiographs and normal pulmonary function. The impairment in gas exchange seen in LAM correlates better with CT than with chest radiographic findings. In addition, CT is the imaging modality of choice in the diagnosis and follow-up of other coincidental chest and intraabdominal disease including lymph nodes and renal angiomyolipomas.

References

1. Braman SS, Mark EJ. Case records of the Massachusetts General Hospital: a 32-year-old woman with recurrent pneumothorax. N Engl J Med 1988; 318:1601–1610.
2. Carrington CB, Cugell DW, Gaensler EA, Marks A, Redding RA, Schaaf JT, Tomasian A. Lymphangiomyomatosis: physiologic-pathologic-radiologic correlations. Am Rev Respir Dis 1977; 116:977–995.
3. Berger JL, Shaff MI. Pulmonary lymphangioleiomyomatosis. J Comput Assist Tomogr 1981; 5:565–567.
4. Merchant RN, Pearson MG, Rankin RN, Morgan WKC. Computerized tomography in the diagnosis of lymphangioleiomyomatosis. Am Rev Respir Dis 1985; 131:295–297.
5. Templeton PA, McLoud TC, Muller NL, Shepard JO, Moore EH. Pulmonary lymphangioleiomyomatosis: CT and pathologic findings. J Comput Assist Tomogr 1989; 13:54–57.
6. Rappaport DC, Weibrod GL, Herman SJ, Chamberlain DW. Pulmonary lymphangioleiomyomatosis: high-resolution CT findings in four cases. AJR 1989; 152:961–964.
7. Sherrier RH, Chiles C, Roggli V. Pulmonary lymphangioleiomyomatosis: CT findings. Am J Roentgenol 1989; 153:937–940.
8. Muller NL, Chiles C, Kullnig P. Pulmonary lymphangiomyomatosis: correlation of CT with radiographic and functional findings. Radiology 1990; 175:335–339.
9. Aberle DR, Hansell DM, Brown K, Tashkin DP. Lymphangiomyomatosis: CT, chest radiographic, and functional correlations. Radiology 1990; 176:381–387.
10. Lenoir S, Grenier P, Brauner MW, Frija J, Remy-Jardin M, Revel D, Cordier J-F. Pulmonary lymphangiomyomatosis and tuberous sclerosis: comparison of radiographic and thin-section CT findings. Radiology 1990; 175:329–334.
11. Hruban RH, Meziane MA, Zerhouni EA, Khouri NF, Fishman EK, Wheeler PS, Dumler JS, Hutchins GM. High resolution computed tomography of inflation-fixed lungs: pathologic-radiologic correlation of centrilobular emphysema. Am Rev Respir Dis 1987; 136:935–940.
12. Murata K, Itoh H, Todo G, Kanaoka M, Noma S, Itoh T, Furuta M, Asamoto H, Torizuka K. Centrilobular lesions of the lung: demonstration by high resolution CT and pathologic correlation. Radiology 1986; 161:641–645.
13. Corrin B, Liebow AA, Friedman PJ. Pulmonary lymphangiomyomatosis: a review. Am J Pathol 1975; 79:348–367.
14. Reich SB, Weishelbaum A, Yee J. Correlation of radiographic measurements and

pulmonary function tests in chronic obstructive pulmonary disease. Am J Roentgenol 1985; 144:695–699.
15. Sleiman C, Mal H, Jebrak G, Darne C, Meeus E, Dubois F, Luisetti M, Fournier M, Pariente R, Andreassian B. Pulmonary lymphangiomyomatosis treated by single lung transplantation. Am Rev Respir Dis 1992; 145:964–966.
16. Fanti S, Monetti N, Schiavina M, Rimondi MR. Scintigraphic findings in a case of lymphangioleiomyomatosis. Clin Nucl Med 1995; 20:1034–1035.
17. Bergin CJ, Pauly JM, Macovaski A. Lung parenchyma: projection reconstruction MR imaging. Radiology 1991; 179:777–781.
18. Bergin CJ, Noll DC, Pauly JM, Glover GH, Macovaski A. MR imaging of lung parenchyma: a solution to susceptibility. Radiology 1992; 183:673–676.
19. Mayo JR, Mackay A, Muller NL. MR imaging of the lungs: value of short TE spin-echo pulse sequences. Am J Roentgenol 1992; 159:951–956.
20. Mohiaddin RH, Notohamiprodjio G, Schoser K. Magnetic resonance imaging of lung single intensity and dimensions in patients with advanced lung disease before and after single lung transplantation. Eur J Radiol 1995; 20:16–22.
21. Moore ADA, Godwin JD, Muller NL, Naidich DP, Hammar SP, Buschman DL, Takasugi JE, de Carvalho CRR. Pulmonary histiocytosis X: comparison of radiographic and CT findings. Radiology 1989; 172:249–254.
22. Bruaner MW, Grenier P, Mouelhi MM, Mompoint D, Lenoir S. Pulmonary histiocytosis X: evaluation with high-resolution CT. Radiology 1989; 172:255–258.
23. Malone MJ, Johnson PR, Jumper BM, Howard PJ, Hopkins TB, Libertino JA. Renal angiomyolipoma: 6 case reports and literature review. J Urol 1986; 135:349–353.
24. Naegeli, CD, Cordasco EM, Meden G, et al. Lymphangiomyomatosis—new concepts in pathogenesis and management—case reports. Angiology 1990; 41:957–963.
25. Collard M, Fievez M, Godart S, Toussaint JP. The contribution of lymphangiography in the study of diffuse lymphangiomyomatosis. Am J Roentgenol 1968; 102:466–470.
26. Frack MD, Simon L, Dawson BH. The lymphangiomyomatosis syndrome. Cancer 1968; 22:428–437.
27. Gray SR, Carrington CB, Cornog JL. Lymphangiomyomatosis: report of a case with ureteral involvement and chyluria. Cancer 1975; 35:490–498.
28. Bernstein SM, Newell JD, Jr., Adamczyk D, Mortenson RL, Talmadge EK, Jr., Lynch DA. How common are renal angiomyolipomas in patients with pulmonary lymphangiomyomatosis? Am J Respir Crit Care Med 1995; 152:2138–2143.
29. Walker DE, Barry JM, Hodges CV. Angiomyolipoma: diagnosis and treatment. J Urol 1976; 116:712–714.
30. Chan JKC, Tsang WYW, Pau MY, Tang MC, Pang SW, Fletcher CDM. Lymphangiomyomatosis and angiomyolipma: closely related entities characterized by hamartomatous proliferation of HMB-45 positive smooth muscle. Histopathology 1993; 22:445–455.
31. Bonetti F. Chiodera PL, Pea M, Martignoni G, Bosi F, Zamboni G, Mariuzzi GM. Transbronchial biopsy in lymphangiomyomatosis of the lung: HMB45 for diagnosis. Am J Surg Pathol 1993; 17:1092–1102.

32. Oesterling JE, Fishman EK, Goldman SM, Marshall FF. The management of renal angiomyolipoma. J Urol 1986; 135:1121–1124.
33. Steiner MS, Goldman SM, Fishman EK, Marshall FF. The natural history of renal angiomyolipoma. J Urol 1993; 150:1782–1786.

11

Histopathologic Studies on Lymphangioleiomyomatosis

WILLIAM D. TRAVIS

Armed Forces Institute of Pathology
Washington, D.C.

JIRO USUKI, KOJI HORIBA, and VICTOR J. FERRANS

National Heart, Lung and Blood Institute
National Institutes of Health
Bethesda, Maryland

Lymphangioleiomyomatosis (LAM) is a rare disorder that affects women primarily of reproductive age. It is characterized by an abnormal proliferation of smooth muscle cells (LAM cells) in the lungs as well as in the lymphatics and lymph nodes in the thorax and retroperitoneum (1–4). The disease is frequently associated with single or multiple angiomyolipomas (AMLs), which occur most frequently in the kidney (5–8). Pulmonary LAM is found in only 0.1–1% of patients with tuberous sclerosis (TS) (9–17). All patients with TS developing this complication are women (9–17).

I. Gross Pathology

The gross pathology in the lungs is distinctive, with diffuse, bilateral cystic changes throughout (Fig. 1). The lungs are enlarged, as in severe emphysema. Most cysts are 0.5–2 cm in size, but in some cases they can measure over 10 cm (4,18).

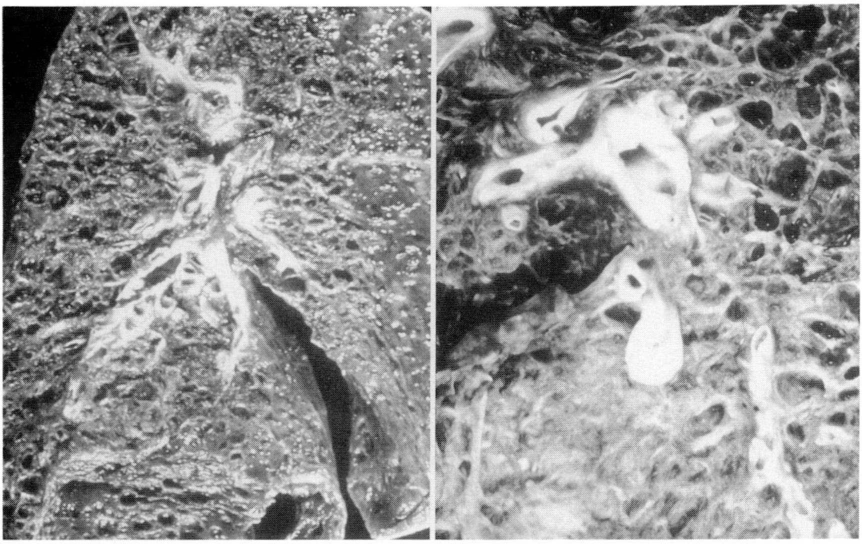

Figure 1 These gross photographs show diffuse cystic changes throughout the lung parenchyma. Details of these changes are shown at higher magnification in the panel at right.

II. Histology

At low magnification, the lungs show the same cystic pattern seen on gross examination (Figs. 2–4). This is one of the key histologic hallmarks of pulmonary LAM (4,18). In the early stages of the disease, LAM cells may be inconspicuous (Fig. 3). In these stages, the LAM cell infiltrates are often overlooked and the biopsy is misinterpreted as showing either emphysema or normal lung. The LAM cells are typically found in small clusters or nests at the edges of the cysts and along pulmonary lymphatics (Figs. 3,5–7). In advanced cases, the LAM cells can become so prominent that it is difficult to identify any normal lung structures. LAM cells infiltrate the walls of vessels and distal airways, leading to vascular destruction and microscopic foci of hemosiderosis (Fig. 4). Bronchiolar obliteration may occasionally be seen (18).

The proliferating LAM cells are round, oval, or spindle-shaped (Figs. 6 and 7). They grow in a haphazard arrangement, unlike the orderly, concentric, or parallel pattern of the smooth muscle cells normally present in the airways and blood vessels (4,18–20). The LAM cells have a moderate amount of eosinophilic cytoplasm, and their nuclei have a fine or vesicular chromatin. They are morphologically heterogeneous, with a spectrum ranging from small and round to

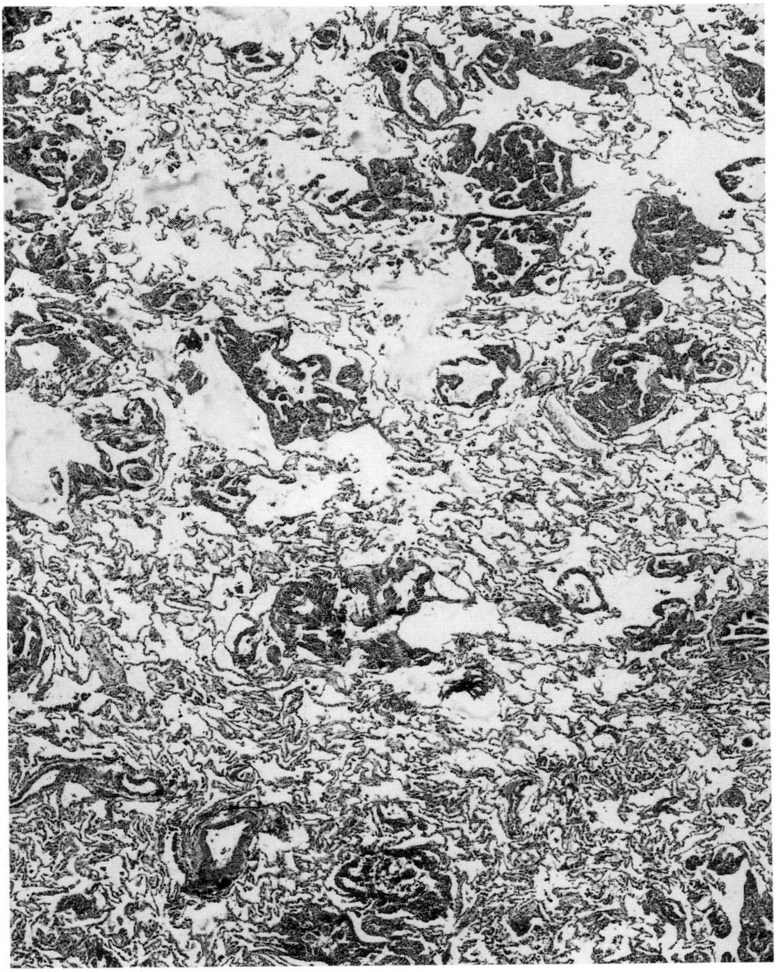

Figure 2 At low power, the lung shows multiple nodules of proliferating LAM cells, many of which surround cystic spaces similar to those found in emphysema. These spaces are generally empty, without cellular or fluid contents. (×16)

spindle-shaped, oval, and large epithelioid cells (Figs. 7 and 8) (4,18,21). Rare mitotic figures and cytologically atypical cells (Fig. 9) may be seen. When LAM cell infiltrates are present in transbronchial biopsy specimens, the diagnosis can be established definitively (Fig. 10) (20,22).

LAM cells also may infiltrate the thoracic duct and lymph nodes of the thorax or retroperitoneum (Fig. 11) (4,18,23). In such cases, the cellular proliferation tends to form masses of LAM cells. The term lymphangiomyoma is some-

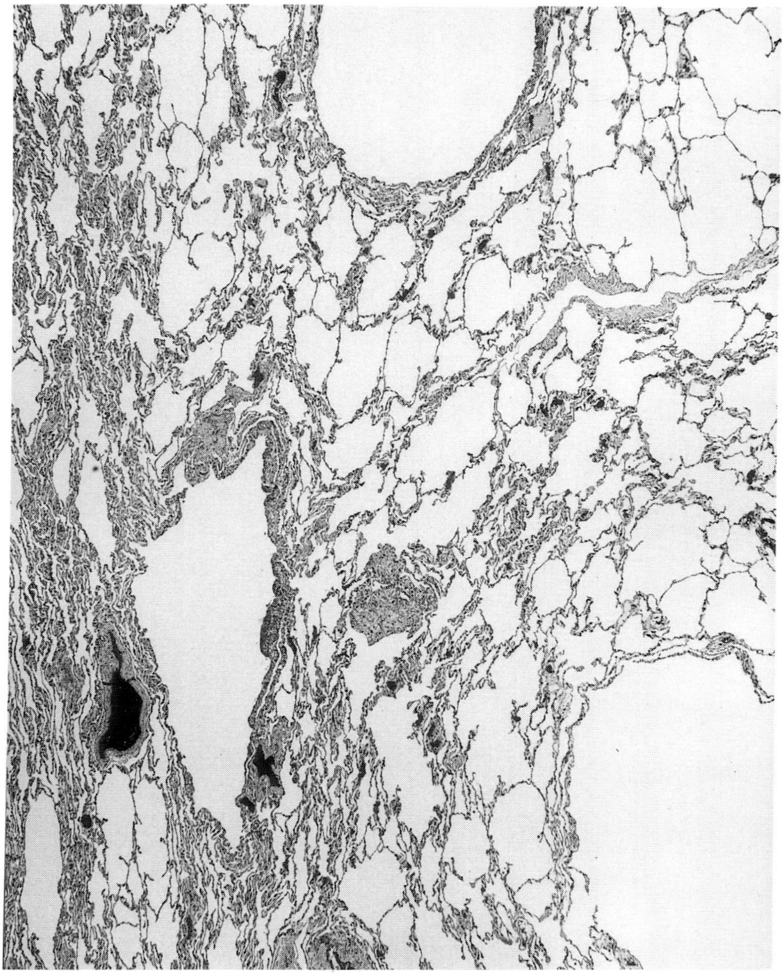

Figure 3 In this case the dominant findings is that of large cystic spaces surrounded by thin connective tissue and alveolar walls. LAM cells are inconspicuous, and only a tiny focus of these cells can be seen in this entire specimen (arrow). (×21)

times used to refer to a tumefactive growth of LAM cells in these lesions (24). In these masses, the cells tend to be more round to oval, rather than spindle-shaped, and often grow in papillary clusters (Fig. 11) (25). In one case, a lymphangiomyoma involving the thoracic duct contained tubules with cells resembling bronchial epithelium (26).

In the setting of pneumothorax, reactive eosinophilic pleuritis may be seen in the pleura (27–29). This is a nonspecific lesion, which can be found in pleu-

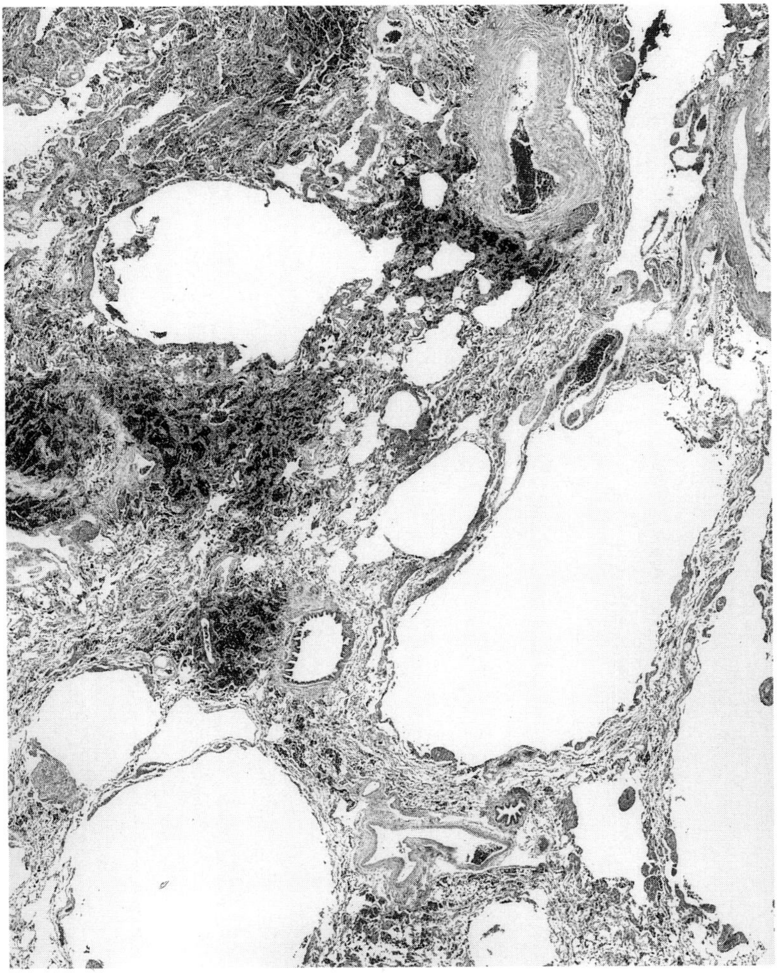

Figure 4 This specimen shows large cystic spaces with focal nodules of LAM cells. The dark areas of the interstitium represent extensive hemosiderin deposits due to hemorrhage. (×11.5)

ral biopsy specimens from patients who have had pneumothorax of any cause and is characterized by infiltration of lymphocytes, plasma cells, histiocytes, and eosinophils (Figs. 12 and 13). Strips of the inflamed pleura sometimes become partly detached from the underlying lung (Fig. 12). This is probably related to the rupture of the pleural surface that occurred with the pneumothorax. The number of eosinophils varies from scant to very large. Due to the many histiocytes

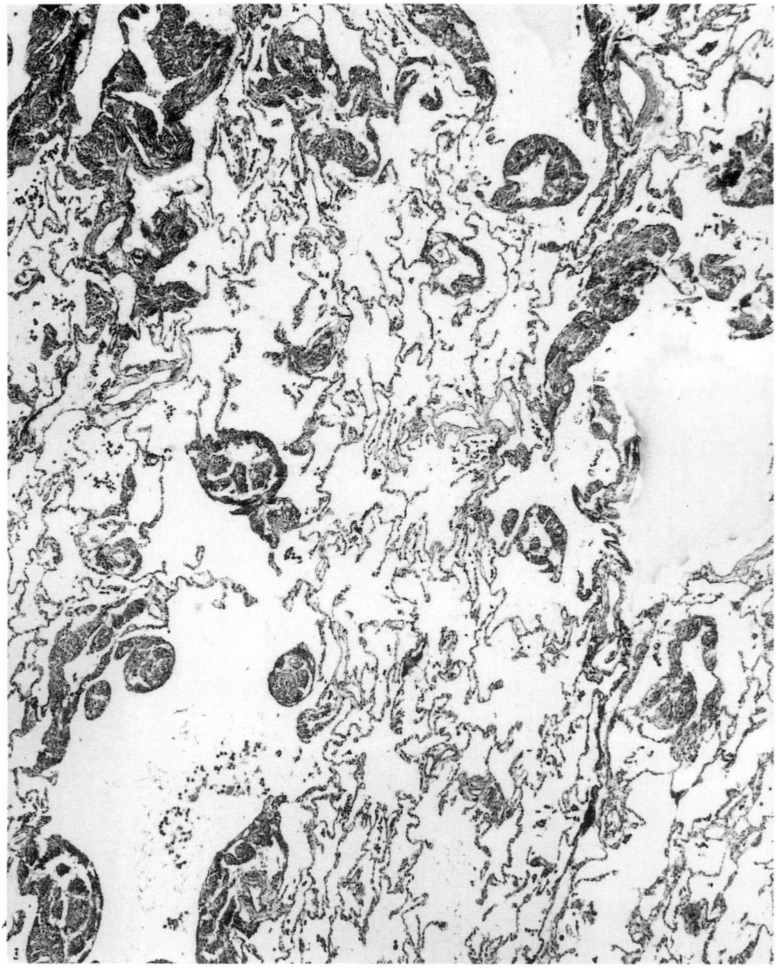

Figure 5 The walls of the cysts in this case are lined either by fragments of residual alveolar walls or by bundles of LAM cells, which in some instances form polypoid clusters protruding into the lumina of the cysts. (×31)

and their occasional convoluted nuclei, as well as the eosinophils, this lesion is occasionally mistaken for Langerhans cell histiocytosis (LCH or histiocytosis X). However, it is restricted to the pleura and does not cause diffuse interstitial nodular infiltrates with the characteristic stellate morphology of LCH. Occasional histiocytes in this lesion may stain immunohistochemically for S-100 protein; however, dense infiltrates of Langerhans cells are not seen.

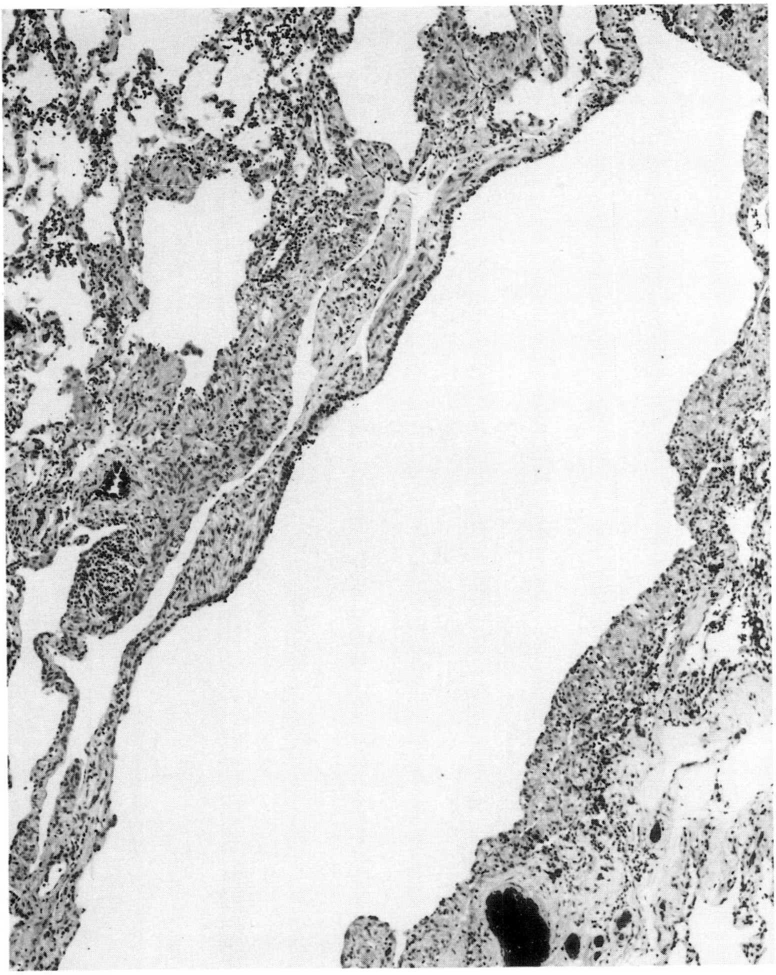

Figure 6 This cyst is lined by inconspicuous LAM cell infiltrates. (×60)

III. Immunohistochemistry and Electron Microscopy

LAM cells are immunohistochemically similar to normal smooth muscle cells in that they stain for α-smooth muscle actin (Fig. 14), desmin, and vimentin. However, they also show reactivity for HMB-45 antibody (Fig. 15). This reactivity is absent in other smooth muscle lesions of the lung (20,22,30). HMB-45 is a mouse monoclonal antibody that was originally developed against a melanoma extract (31). This antibody also reacts with normal fetal, neonatal, and adult

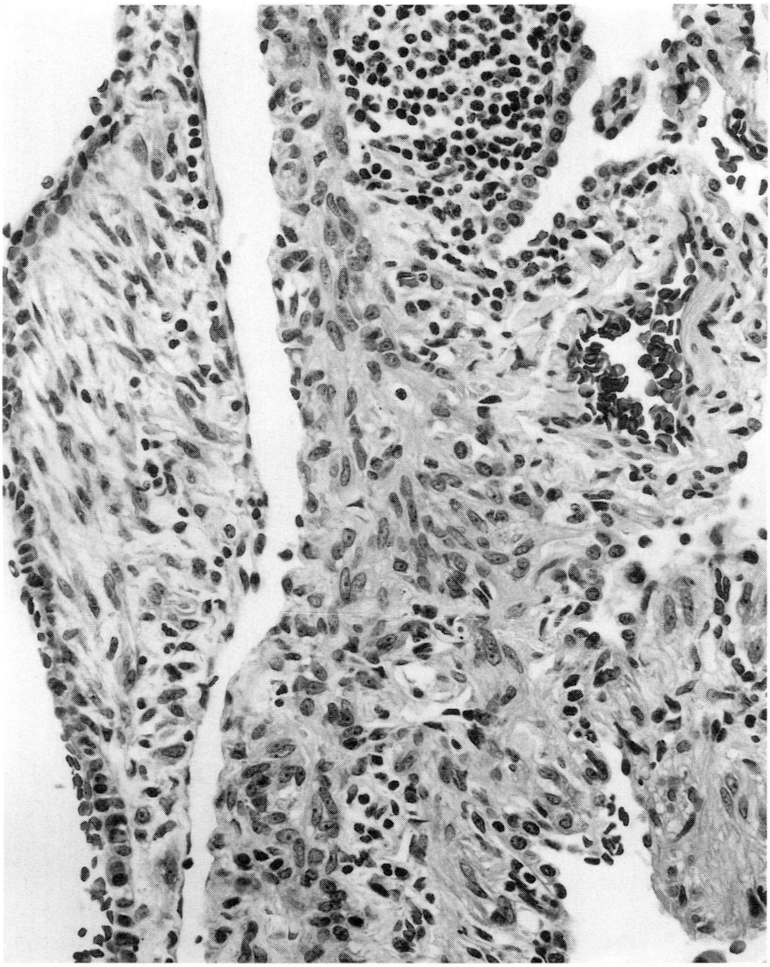

Figure 7 At higher power, the LAM cells appear round, oval, or spindle-shaped. Although they resemble smooth muscle cells, they are more haphazardly arranged than the muscle cells of vascular and alveolar walls. (×250)

melanocytes; neoplastic melanocytes in malignant melanomas; junctional nevi; prenatal and infantile human retinal pigmented epithelial cells; the smooth muscle cells in AML; and the cells in clear cell tumors of the lungs (22,31–33). A single renal cell carcinoma from a patient with tuberous sclerosis has also been demonstrated to stain positively with HMB-45 (34). It should be emphasized that not all of the LAM cells react with HMB-45. The percentage of reactive LAM cells varies from 20 to 70% in different patients (35). At the light microscopic level,

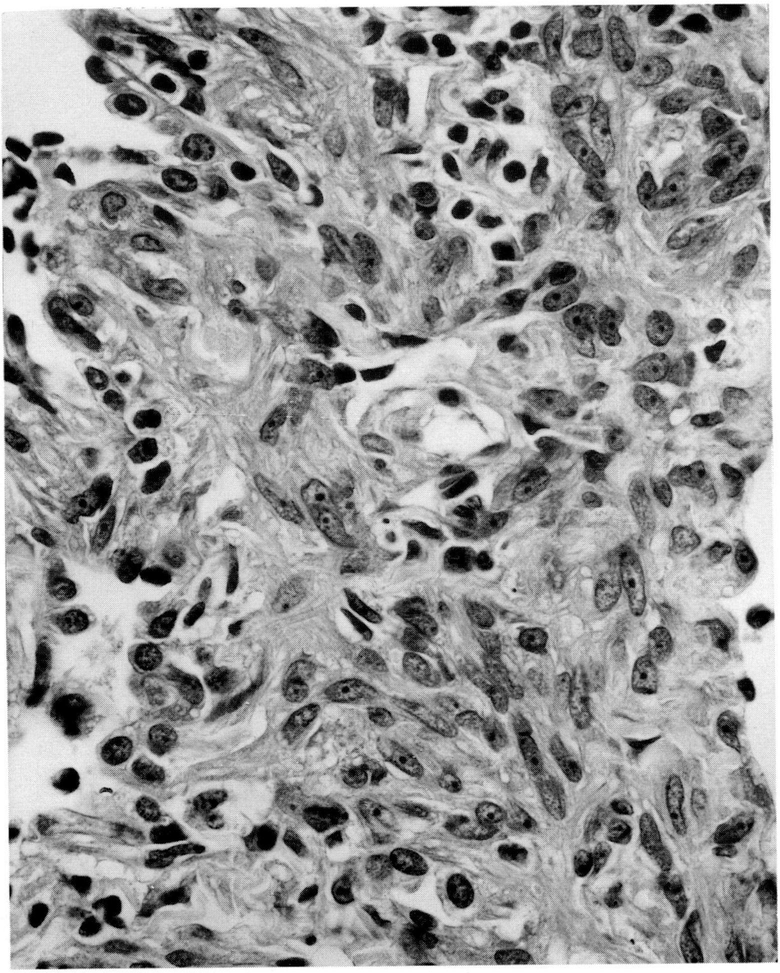

Figure 8 A moderate amount of cytoplasm is present in most of the LAM cells, and small nucleoli are seen in many of the nuclei. (×400)

the reactivity of LAM cells for HMB-45 is localized mainly in small cytoplasmic granules (Fig. 15).

Electron microscopic studies have shown that the immunoreactivity for HMB-45 in melanocytes is localized in stage 1 and 2 melanosomes (premalenosomes) and in the nonmelanized portion of stage 3 melanosomes (36). As described by Fukuda et al. (37), LAM cells share many ultrastructural features with normal smooth muscle cells (Fig. 16) (19,22). Electron microscopic reports have documented the occurrence of inclusions structurally similar to stage 1 and

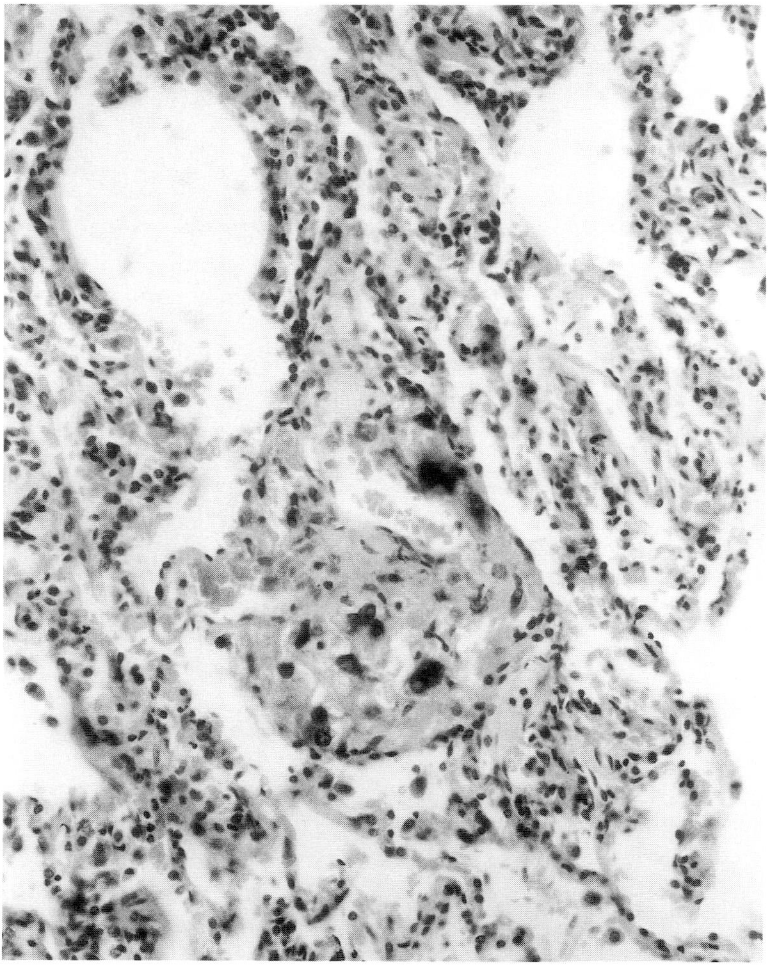

Figure 9 These LAM cells show marked cytologic atypia with nuclear enlargement and hyperchromasia. (×300)

2 melanosomes in LAM cells (Fig. 17) (22), and we have recently demonstrated, by means of ultrastructural labeling with HMB-45 conjugated with gold particles, the specific immunoreactivity of such inclusions with this antibody in LAM cells (Fig. 18). Other immunoelectron microscopic studies have shown that similar premelanosome-like structures are the sites of reactivity for HMB-45 in the smooth muscle cells in AMLs (32) and in the tumor cells of malignant melanomas and clear cell tumors of the lung (33,38). The significance of the presence of these structures in cells of nonmelanocytic lineage is not understood.

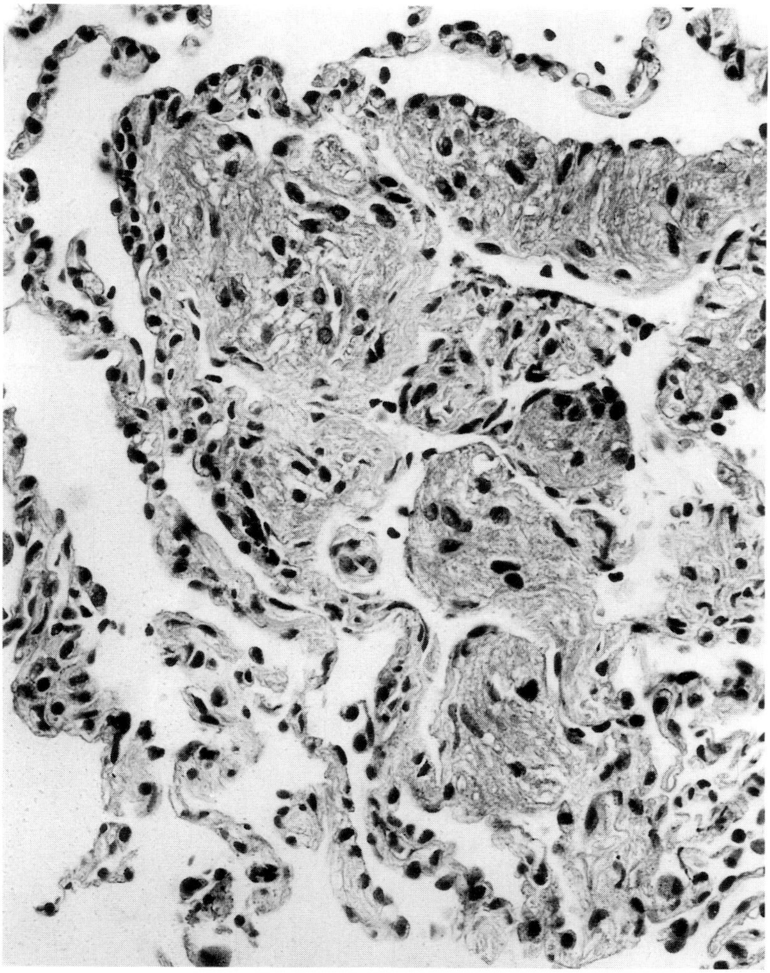

Figure 10 Cellular infiltrates diagnostic of LAM were present in this transbronchial biopsy. (×300)

IV. Lung Pathology in Tuberous Sclerosis

While TS patients are not exempt from other types of lung disease, LAM is regarded as the primary form of pulmonary involvement in women with TS (9,14,39,40). This issue has been debated in the literature, with some authors arguing that there are differences in the distribution of the lesions and the histological location of the smooth muscle, suggesting that LAM and pulmonary in-

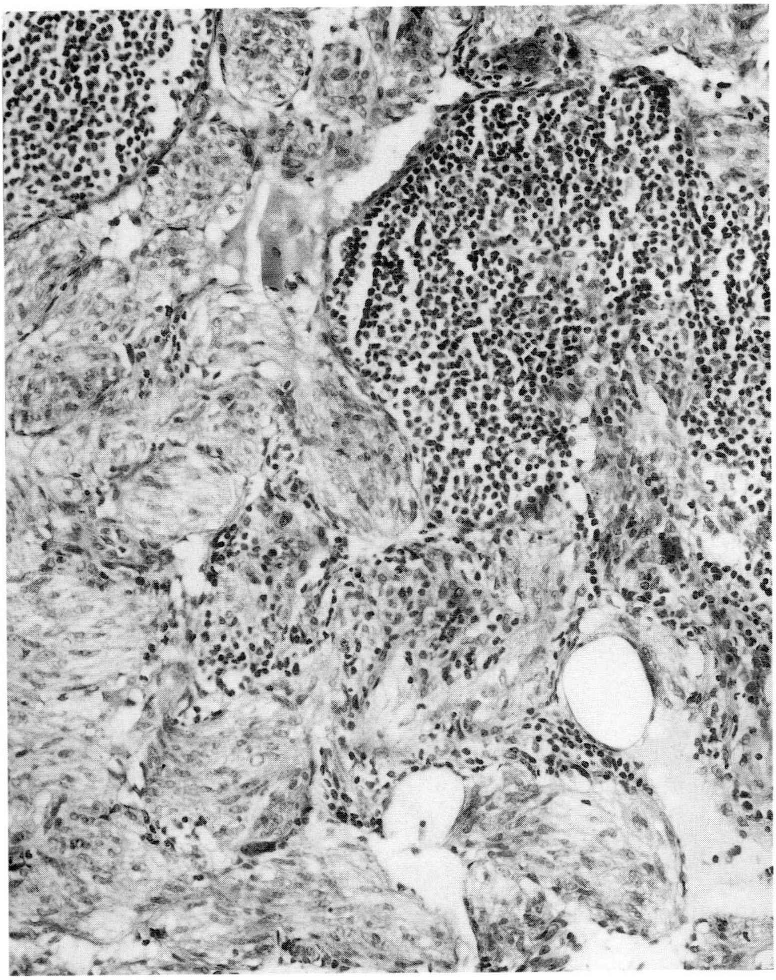

Figure 11 Retroperitoneal biopsy: LAM cell infiltrates surround lymphoid follicles that probably represent residual lymph node tissue. The LAM cells are growing in papillary arrangements interspersed with lymphatic spaces lined by endothelial cells. (×75)

volvement by TS are two separate processes (15). While pulmonary abnormalities occur in men with TS (16,41), details of the pathology in these cases are lacking or they suggest lesions other than LAM. Dwyer et al. reported two men with TS and pulmonary disease and reviewed the literature, including four additional cases (16). However, most of these reports provided either few or no details about the pathologic findings in the lung. One man reported by Dwyer et al. showed "diffuse infiltration by vascular plain muscle with widespread destruction of al-

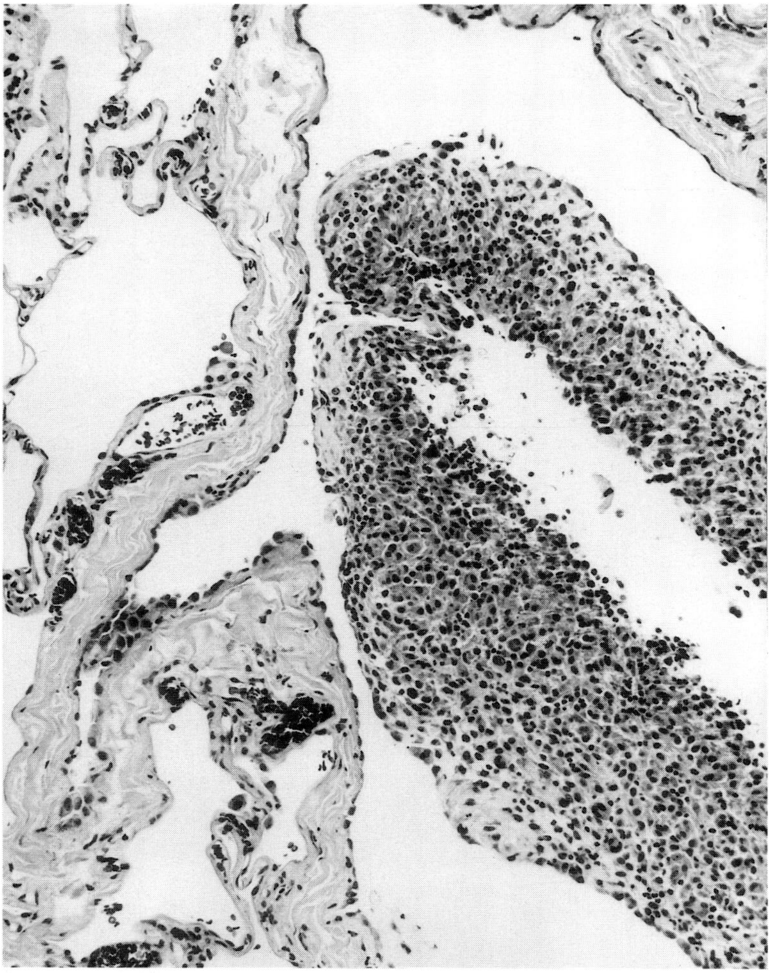

Figure 12 Reactive eosinophilic pleuritis, a secondary lesion associated with pneumothorax, is characterized by a pleural inflammatory infiltrate. (×125)

veoli and terminal bronchioles and hypertensive changes in the pulmonary arterial system." At autopsy, this case showed cystic changes and interstitial fibrosis typical of honeycomb lung (16). It is difficult to be sure what this lung disease represented, since no illustrations of the pathologic findings were provided, but the statement that there was "profound overgrowth of plain muscle and fibrous tissue" raises doubts that this was LAM, since fibrous tissue is usually not abundant in lesions of this disorder. The second male patient reported by Dwyer

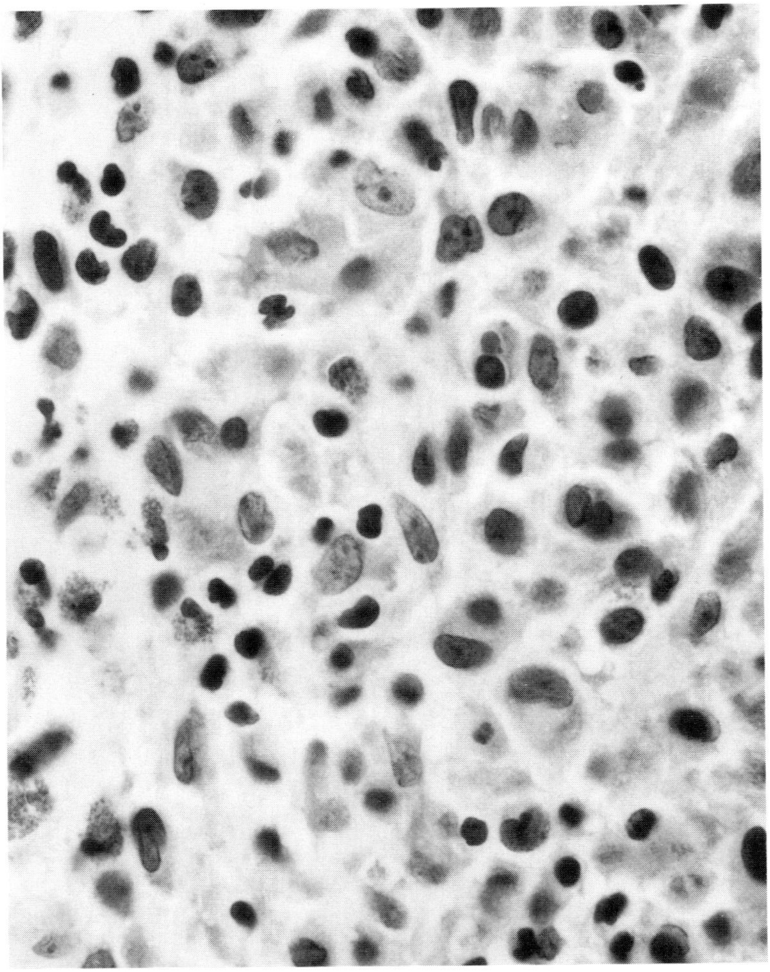

Figure 13 The infiltrate in reactive eosinophilic pleuritis consists of histiocytes, mesothelial cells, chronic inflammatory cells, and eosinophils. (×800)

et al. had no pathology description, but the chest radiographic findings of "an ill-defined opacity in the lower half of both lungs and a moderately large air cyst in the right lower lobe suggest a process other than LAM (16). One 12-year-old boy with TS, reported by Baar et al. in 1964, was described as having "pulmonary glomangiomata" (9,14,39,40,42). The illustrations in this paper do not represent LAM, but may be meningothelial-like nodules or so-called minute pulmonary chemodectomas, which are incidental findings of no known clinical significance (43).

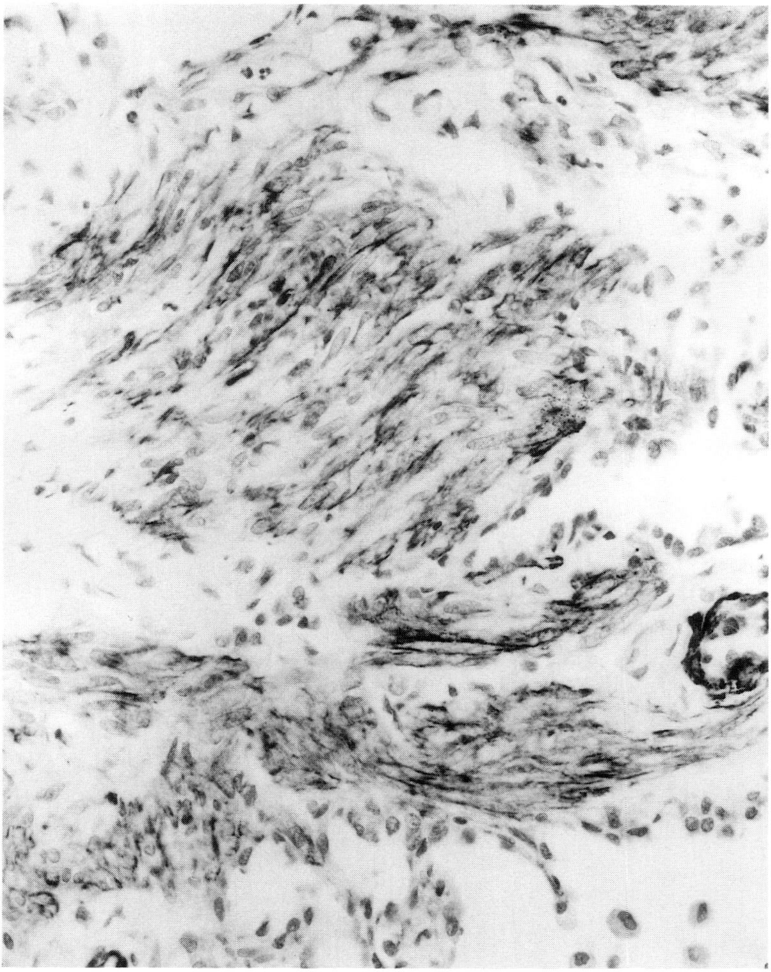

Figure 14 Immunostaining for α-smooth muscle actin shows a positive reaction in the cytoplasm of LAM cells and vascular smooth muscle cells. (Immunoperoxidase-hematoxylin, ×400)

Although there are few pathologic studies comparing the morphology of LAM in patients with and without TS, our impression is that the findings in the two disorders are identical (14,15,39,44,45).

The only distinguishing feature that may be seen in lung biopsies from TS patients is the lesion of multifocal micronodular pneumocyte hyperplasia (MMNPH) (46). These lesions have been reported previously under a variety of

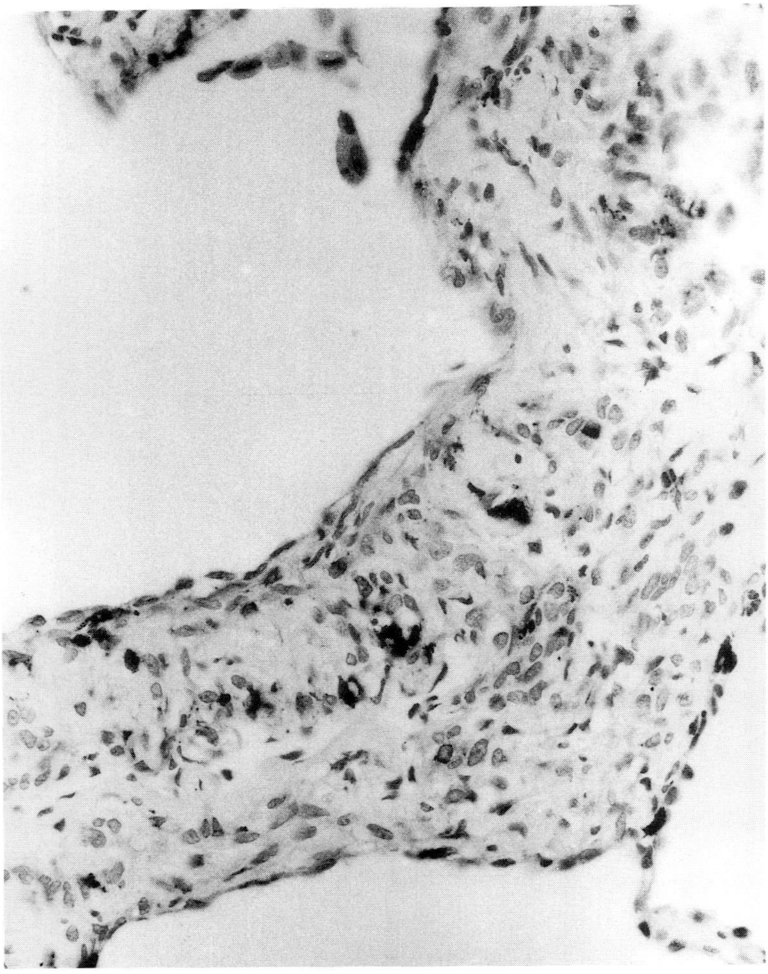

Figure 15 Immunohistochemical staining for HMB-45 shows a strongly positive reaction in many of the LAM cells. Note that some of the LAM cells are negative. (×300)

terms, including adenomatoid proliferations and atypical adenomatoid proliferations (14,18). More recently, the term MMNPH has been used (46). A case reported by Popper et al. in 1991 as a new entity (47) probably represents the same type of lesion described by Corrin et al. (18) and Lie et al. (14) as "adenomatoid proliferations" and illustrated by Spencer in his textbook on pulmonary pathology (48). These lesions are so distinctive that they are virtually pathognomonic of TS when identified in patients with LAM (46). At low magnification they appear as multiple, ill-defined, nodular areas of interstitial thickening measuring

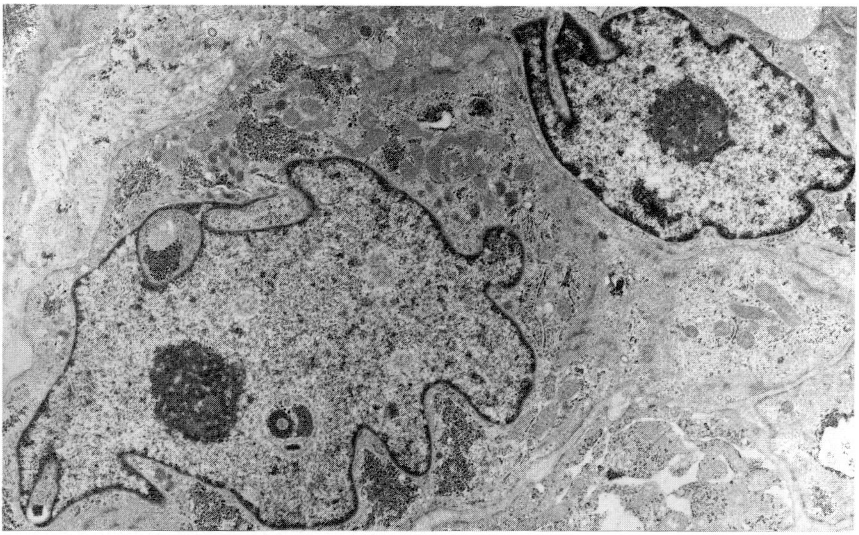

Figure 16 Transmission electron micrograph of LAM cell. Note the convoluted nucleus, the relatively large nucleolus, the bundles of actin microfilaments, glycogen particles and clusters of electron-dense, membrane-bound cytoplasmic granules. (×4000)

several millimeters in size (Figs. 19 and 20). The alveolar walls are slightly thickened by fibrous connective tissue and are lined by hyperplastic, cuboidal epithelial cells (46). These cells have the ultrastructural features of type II pneumocytes and stain for surfactant apoprotein, but not for Clara cell protein (46,47). Popper et al. speculated that these lesions cause "obstruction of the alveolar lymphatic vessels and alveolar ducts, resulting in an emphysema-like picture" (47). While lesions of MMNPH are occasionally situated adjacent to emphysema-like cysts, we suspect that these cysts are probably a manifestation of LAM, since they are frequently associated with LAM cells.

V. Angiomyolipoma

AMLs occur in association with LAM, both in patients with and without TS. While some have argued that the association of renal AMLs and LAM represents a form fruste of TS, this association is not uniformly accepted as sufficient for a diagnosis of TS. In patients with LAM and/or TS, AMLs also occur in extrarenal sites, such as the liver and retroperitoneum (49–52). We have seen a single case of pulmonary AML that occurred in a patient without TS, LAM, or AMLs elsewhere (Figs 21 and 22) (53). Interestingly, this tumor did not stain for HMB-45.

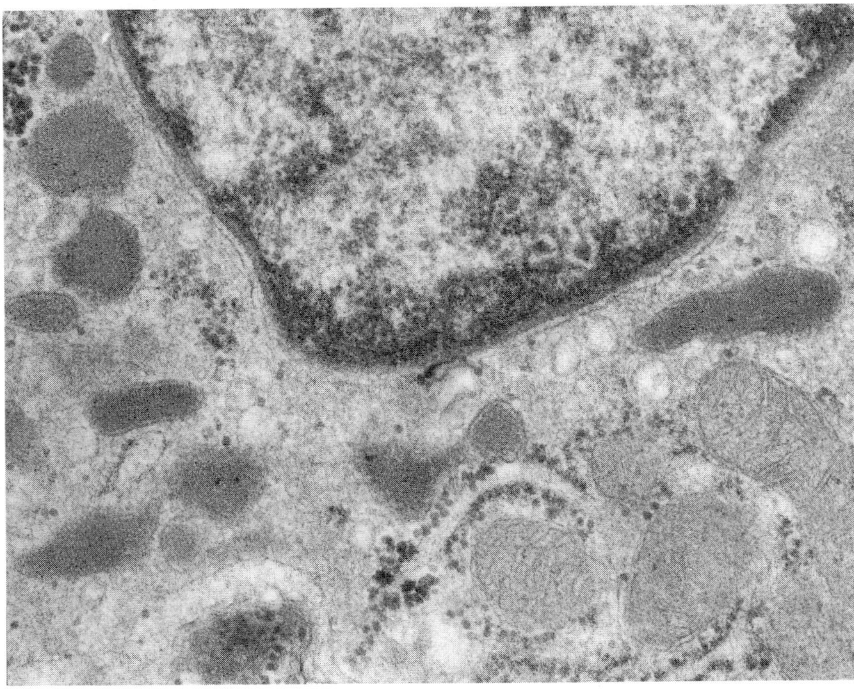

Figure 17 The electron-dense, membrane-bound cytoplasmic granules often exhibit an elliptical shape and their structure resembles that of stage one and stage two melanosomes (premelanosomes), being characterized by a striated, fine crystal-like lamellae. (×22,000)

The incidence of renal AML in LAM without associated TS was reported to be 15% (8), but recent radiologic studies have shown renal AMLs in up to 57% of patients (5,7,38,54–57). In a recent study using computerized tomography and ultrasonography, Chu et al. found evidence of renal AMLs in 60% of 35 patients with LAM (35). This incidence is similar to the 47 and 57% frequency found in radiologic studies by Maziak et al. and Bernstein et al., respectively (5,6). Twenty-two of these patients (63%) had solitary renal masses, nine (26%) had multiple masses, and six (17%) had bilateral involvement (35).

AMLs vary considerably in size, ranging from less than 1 cm up to 45 cm in diameter (58). Large tumors of this type may extend into the retroperitoneum. Histologically, AMLs consist of a mixture of smooth muscle, fat, and blood vessels (Fig. 23). The percentage of each of these components varies considerably. The blood vessels lack the normal inner and outer layer of elastic tissue seen in normal arterioles (5,8,38,54–57). The tumors are not encapsulated and may have

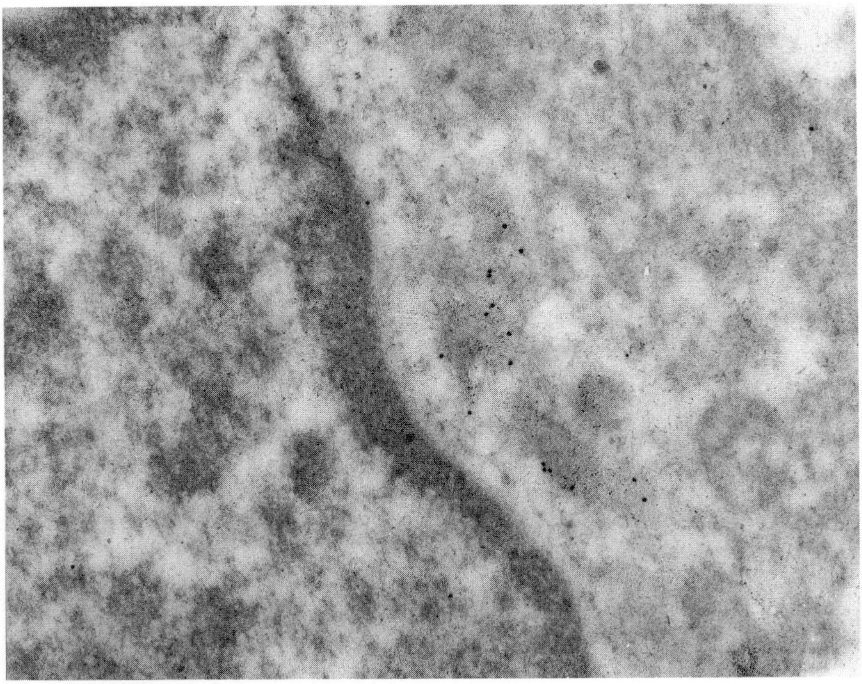

Figure 18 These premelanosome-like structures show a positive reaction with HMB-45 antibody labeled with gold particles (10 nm in diameter). (×22,000)

infiltrative borders. In some cases scattered microscopic nodules of smooth muscle cells may be seen in the surrounding kidney (59). The smooth muscle often appears to merge with the walls of medium-sized blood vessels. There is morphologic heterogeneity in the smooth muscle cells of AMLs, similar to that seen in LAM, with a spectrum ranging from spindle-shaped cells with moderate cytoplasm to epithelioid cells with abundant eosinophilic cytoplasm. Occasionally, the cytoplasm may be optically clear. Atypical nuclear features, such as enlargement and hypercromasia, may be present. Rare cases may have prominent epithelioid cells that may cause problems in distinction from renal cell carcinoma (60). Hemorrhage is a potential complication that may cause extensive hemosiderin deposition (61).

The immunohistochemical profile of the smooth muscle cells in AMLs is similar to that of LAM cells, with positive staining for smooth muscle actin, desmin, and HMB-45 (38,54,59,62). Electron-dense granules have also been demonstrated by electron microscopy in AML (32,59,63). Similar to those in LAM, these granules may represent melanosome-like structures. In the kidney,

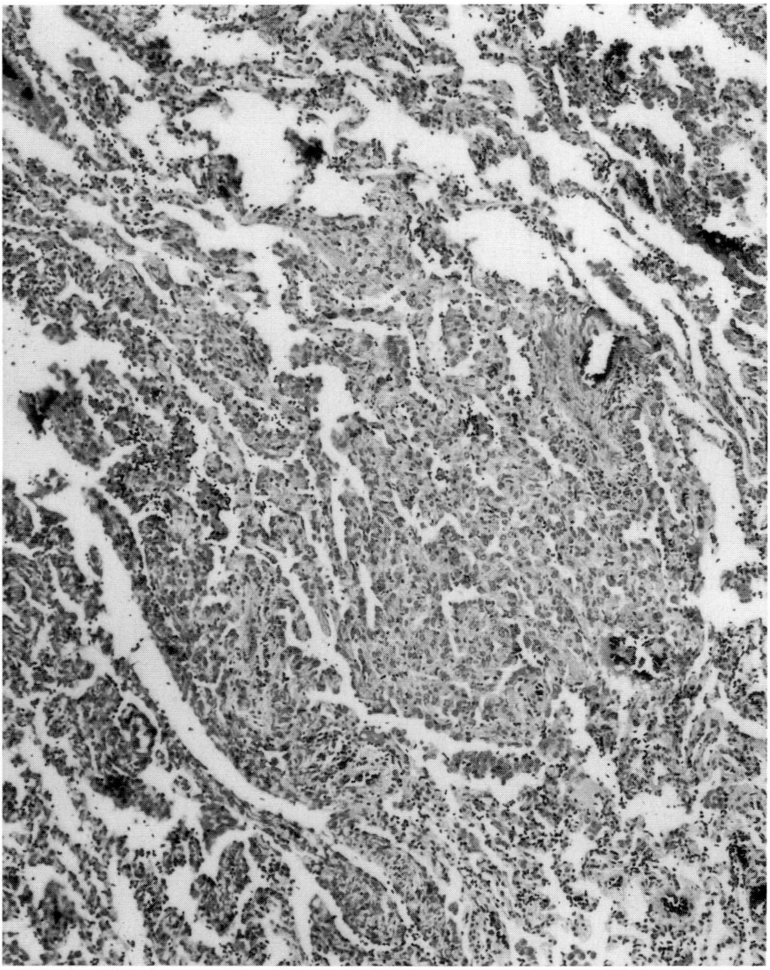

Figure 19 Multifocal micronodular pneumocyte hyperplasia (MMNPH) consists of ill-defined nodules associated with mild thickening of the interstitium. (×150)

AML is not the only lesion shown to be HMB-45 positive. According to one recent study, subcapsular leiomyomas may also stain positively for HMB-45 (64). The relationship of these subcapsular leiomyomas to AML is not clear, but the lesions reported in this study did not contain fat or abnormal blood vessels suggestive of AML. One renal cell carcinoma from a TS patient also was found to stain with HMB-45 (34), raising the question whether these tumors in TS patients differ from sporadic cases.

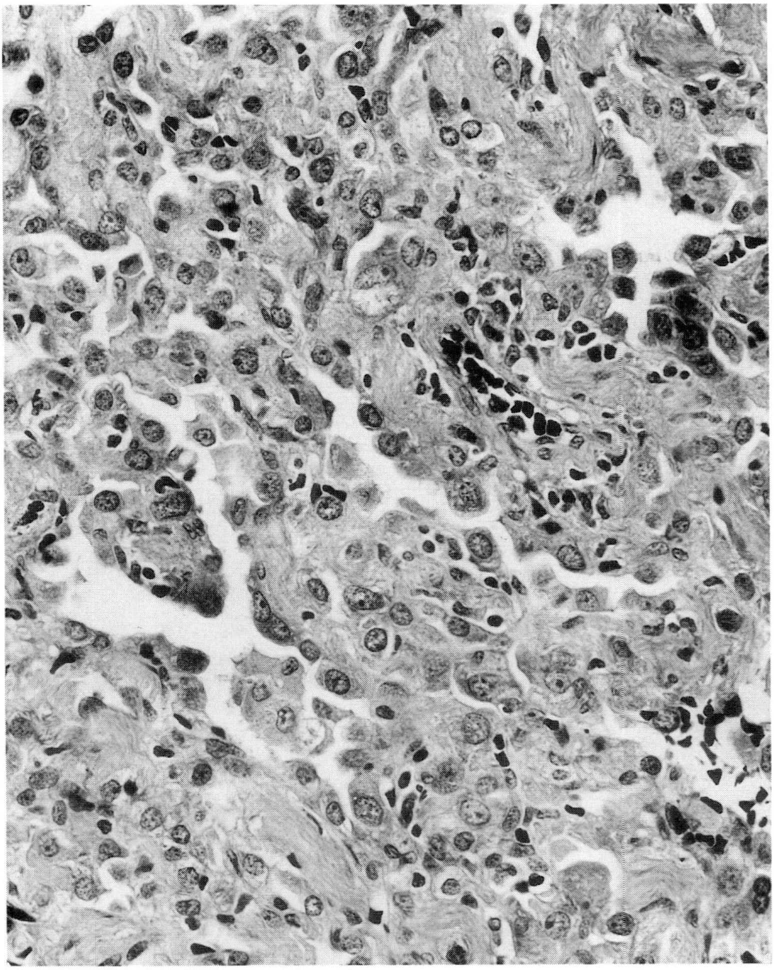

Figure 20 The alveolar walls in the nodules of MMNPH are lined by hyperplastic cuboidal-shaped type II pneumocytes, some of which protrude into the alveolar space in a hobnailed fashion. (×300)

VI. Clear Cell Tumors of the Lung

Clear cell tumors of the lung are extremely rare and are virtually always benign (33,38,65–68). Virtually all clear cell tumors have presented in the lung, but rare examples have occurred in other sites such as the rectum (69), pancreas (70), heart (71), and liver (71). They present as solitary coin lesions, several centimeters in

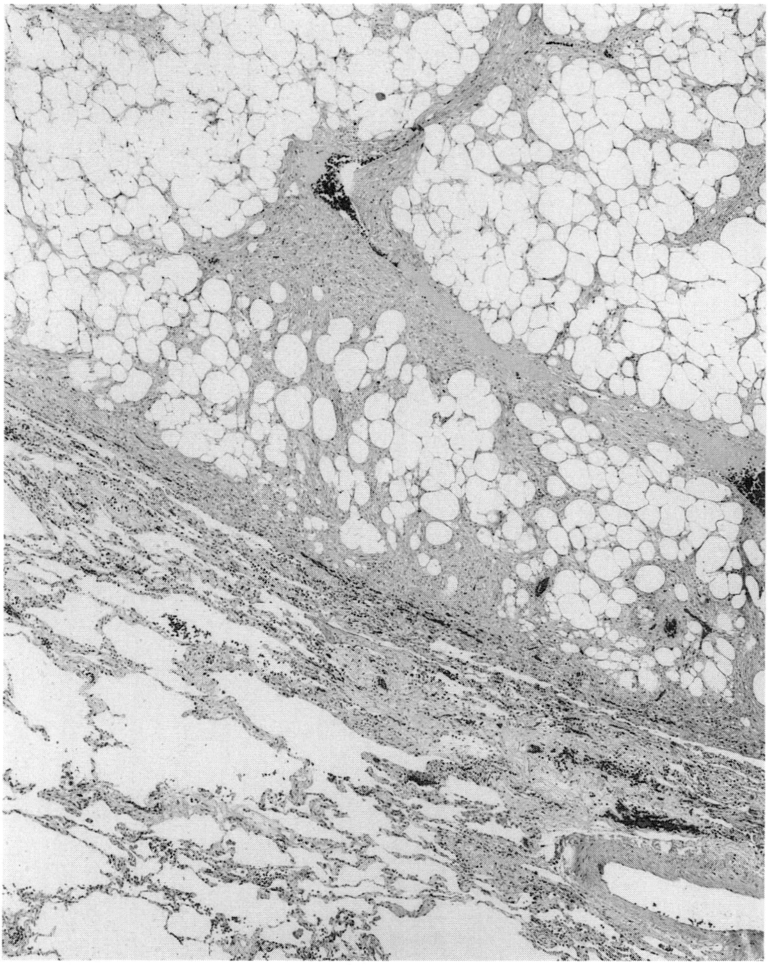

Figure 21 Pulmonary angiomyolipoma in a patient without tuberous sclerosis and LAM. The tumor is sharply circumscribed and surrounded by normal lung. (×30)

size. They form circumscribed masses consisting of tumor cells with abundant, clear cytoplasm (Fig. 24) that contains large amounts of glycogen (Fig. 25). The tumors may be vascular with thin-walled vessels sometimes with a hemangiopericytomatous pattern (Fig. 24). The abundant glycogen is well demonstrated by strong positive staining of the tumor cell cytoplasm (Fig. 25) with the periodic acid-Schiff stain. This reactivity is removed by digestion with diastase (Fig. 26). As mentioned previously, the tumor cells stain for HMB-45 (Fig. 27)

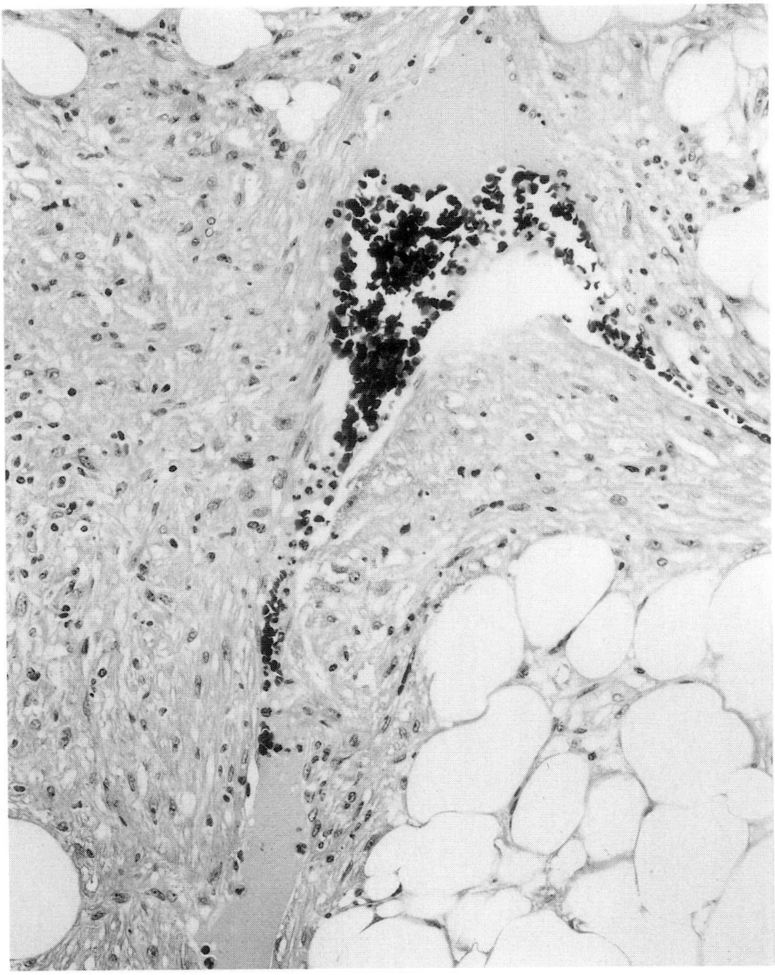

Figure 22 The angiomyolipoma in Figure 21 consists of smooth muscle cells, fat, and blood vessels. (×150)

and have melanosome-like cytoplasmic inclusions (33,66–68). These structures had been previously believed to represent neurosecretory granules, for which reason the tumors were thought to be derived from Kulchitzy cells. Their cellular origin remains to be determined (33,66–68). We have recently studied the first patient in whom the coexistence of TS, AML, clear cell tumor of the lung, and LAM was observed (Fig. 28) (65). This suggests that clear cell tumor of the lung may rarely represent the part of the tuberous sclerosis complex.

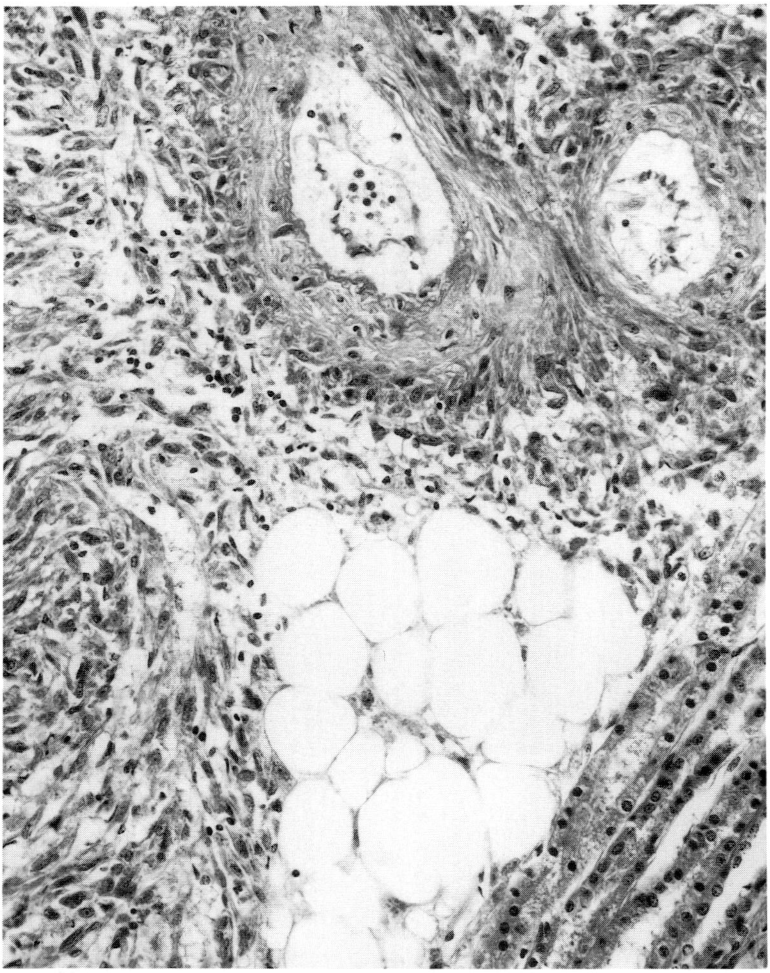

Figure 23 Renal angiomyolipoma. Renal tissue is infiltrated by a mass consisting of a mixture of spindle-shaped smooth muscle cells, blood vessels, and fat. (×75)

VII. Pathogenesis of LAM

Although the cause of LAM is unknown, three aspects of the pathogenesis of this disorder are worthy of special consideration: (1) the origin of the LAM cells; (2) the proliferation of these cells, and (3) the destruction of the lung parenchyma. The histologic, histochemical, and ultrastructural characteristics of LAM cells clearly correspond to those of smooth muscle cells. However, as indicated pre-

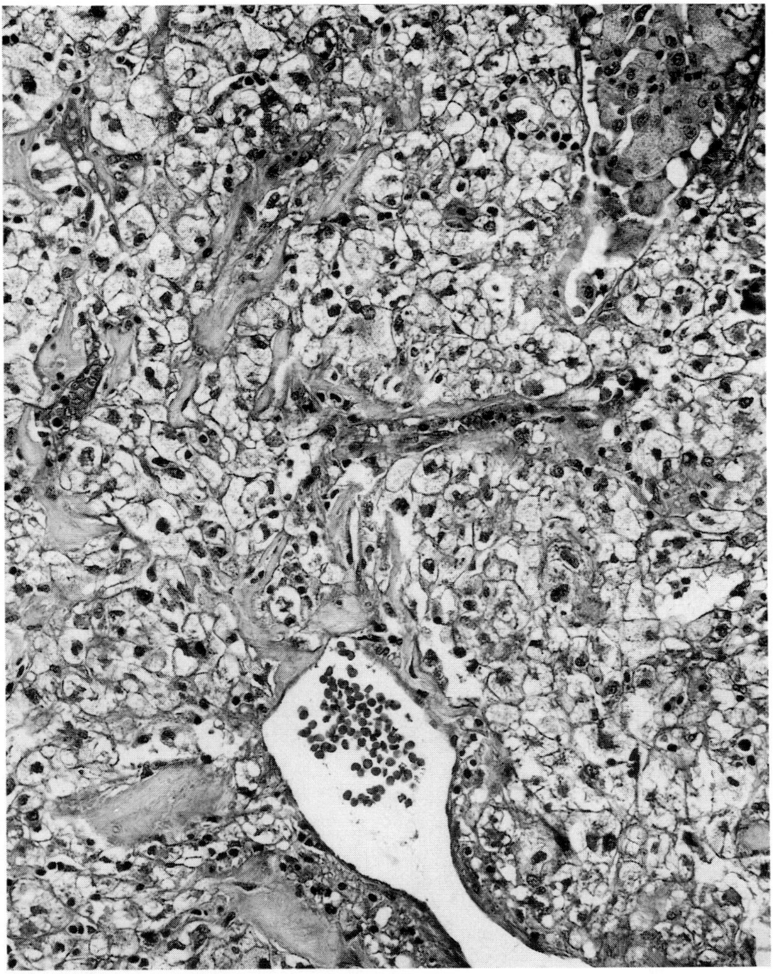

Figure 24 Clear cell tumor of the lung consists of a mass of cells with abundant clear cytoplasm. The slit-like vascular space (right) is thin-walled. (H&E ×150)

viously, LAM cells differ from other smooth muscle cells in their reactivity with HMB-45 (33,66–68). It has been suggested that LAM cells are derived from smooth muscle cells in pulmonary lymphatic vessels. Bonetti et al. have postulated the existence of a so-called perivascular epithelioid cell that could give rise to the cells in LAM, AMLs, and clear cell tumors of the lung (38). However, HMB-45 positive perivascular epithelioid cells are not seen in normal tissues or other pathologic settings (38). Our recent observation of a clear cell tumor of the lung in association with pulmonary LAM in a woman with tuberous sclerosis and

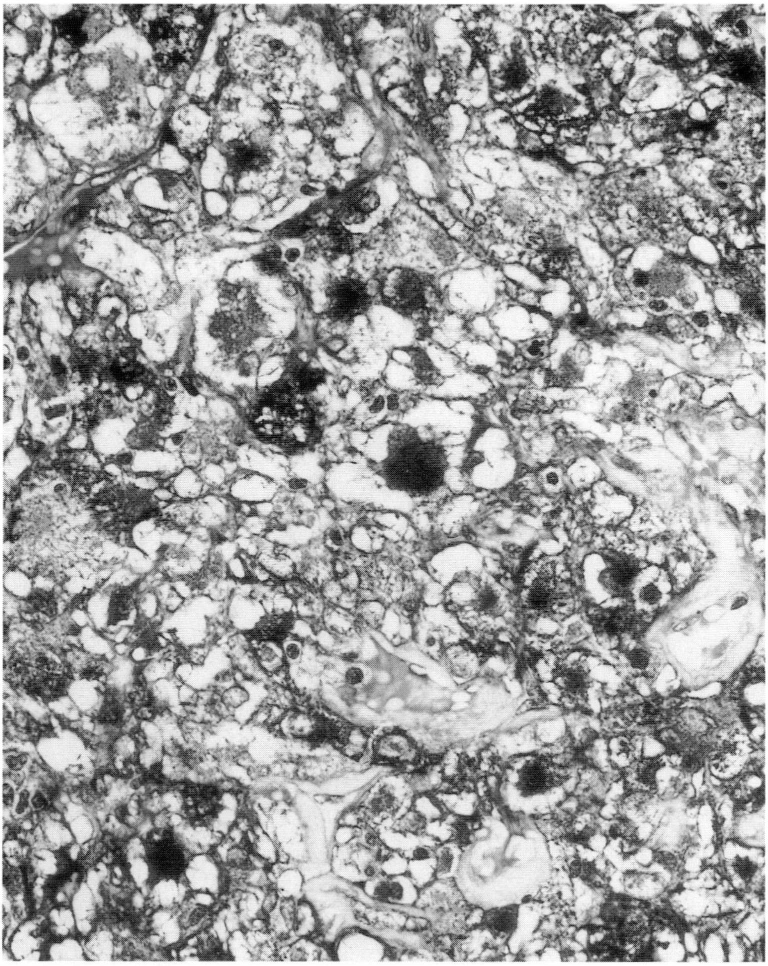

Figure 25 The cells in the clear cell tumor contain abundant glycogen. (Periodic acid Schiff ×300)

radiographic evidence of renal AML raises the possibility of a common histogenesis for all these lesions (Fig. 28) (65).

Little is known of the factors influencing the proliferation of LAM cells. The occurrence of LAM in women primarily of reproductive age has led to speculation that the LAM cell proliferation is hormonally driven. Estrogen receptors (ER) and/or progesterone receptors (PR) have been demonstrated by a variety of techniques in some LAM specimens (Fig. 29) (3,72–78). Immunhistochemical

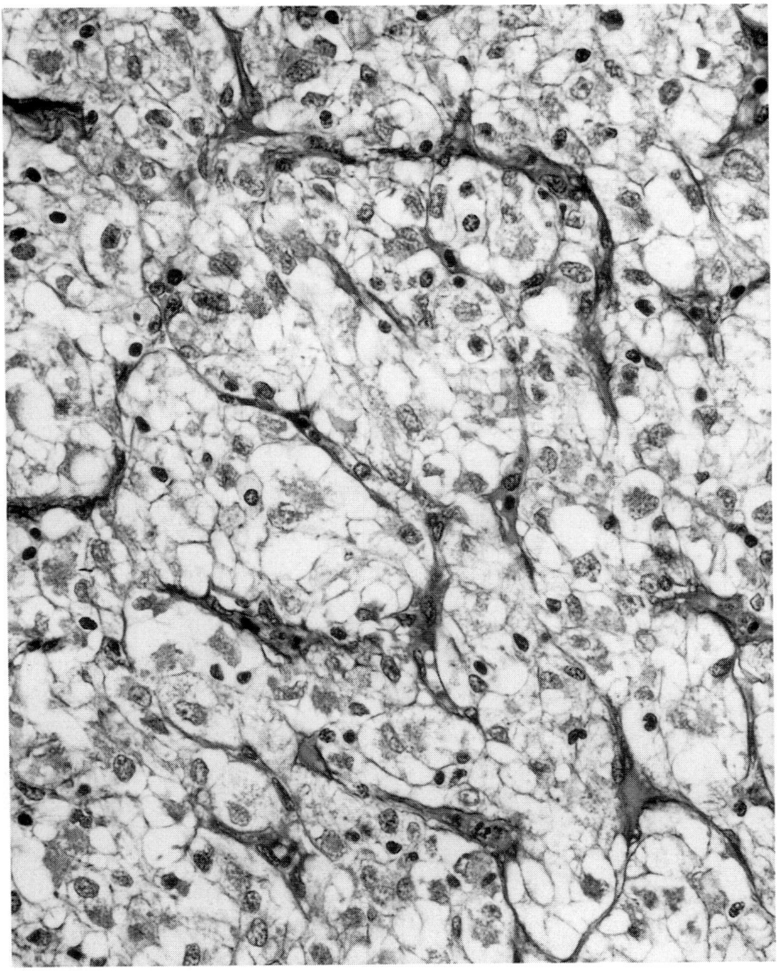

Figure 26 The glycogen in the clear cells is digested with diastase. (Periodic acid Schiff with diastase ×300)

studies have shown that both of these types of receptors are localized in the nuclei of the LAM cells. Smooth muscle proliferative activity is regulated by a variety of growth factors, including transforming growth factor beta (TGF-β) and platelet-derived growth factor (79–83). However, there has been little investigation concerning the potential role of such factors on the proliferation of LAM cells. A single immunohistochemical study of TGF-β in a spectrum of interstitial lung disorders showed strong staining in one case of LAM (84).

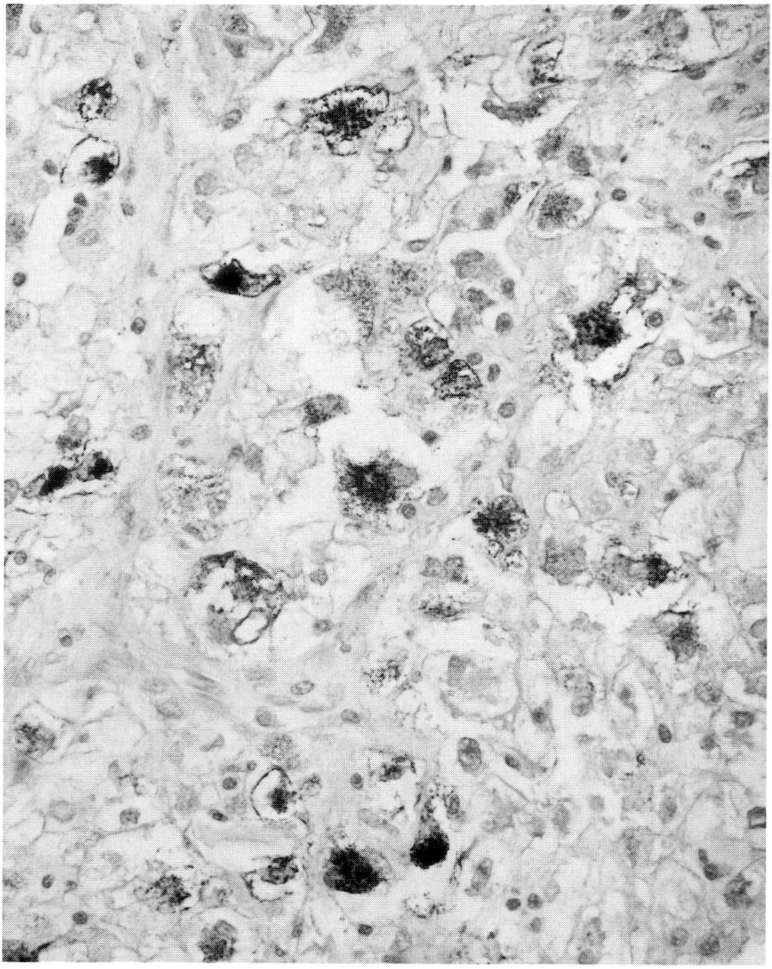

Figure 27 Many cells in the clear cell tumor stain positively for HMB-45. (Immunoperoxidase ×300)

The oncoprotein Bcl-2 is a suppressor of apoptosis. Bax, a promoter of apoptosis, forms heterodimers with Bcl-2. The ratio of Bcl-2 to Bax is thought to determine the survival or death of cells. The presence of Bcl-2 in hormone-responsive normal and malignant cells is associated with hormonal regulation. To investigate the expression of Bcl-2 in LAM and the relationship of this expression to estrogen receptor, the distribution of Bcl-2, Bax, and ER was studied immunohistochemically in paraffin sections of lungs from six patients with LAM (85). In normal lungs, no cells were positive for ER, but Bcl-2 was expressed in

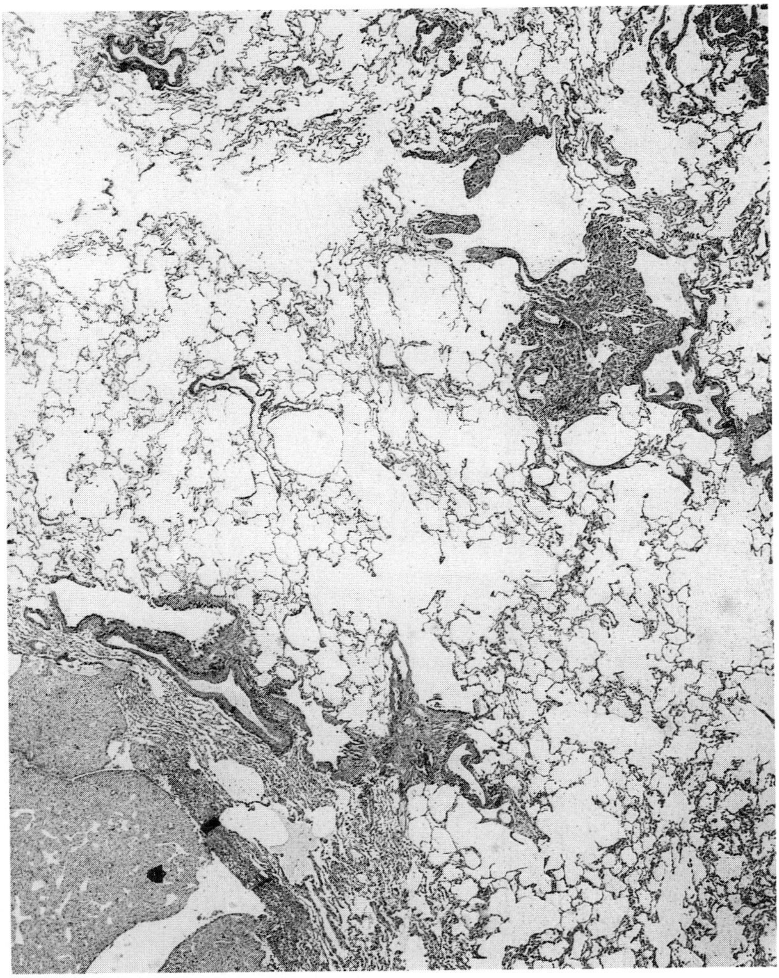

Figure 28 Clear cell tumor of lung adjacent to LAM infiltrates (arrow) and multifocal micronodular pneumocyte hyperplasia (arrowheads). (×7.5)

basal cells of the mucosa and in lymphocytes, and Bax was detected intensely in alveolar macrophages and weakly to moderately in epithelial cells of airways, vascular, bronchial, and bronchiolar smooth muscle cells and lymphocytes (85). Three of the six LAM samples were ER positive, with marked staining in LAM cells; these three samples also gave a positive reaction for Bcl-2 in the cytoplasm of the LAM cells (Fig. 30). The three ER-negative samples were Bcl-2 negative. In all 6 samples, most LAM cells gave a positive cytoplasmic reaction for Bax.

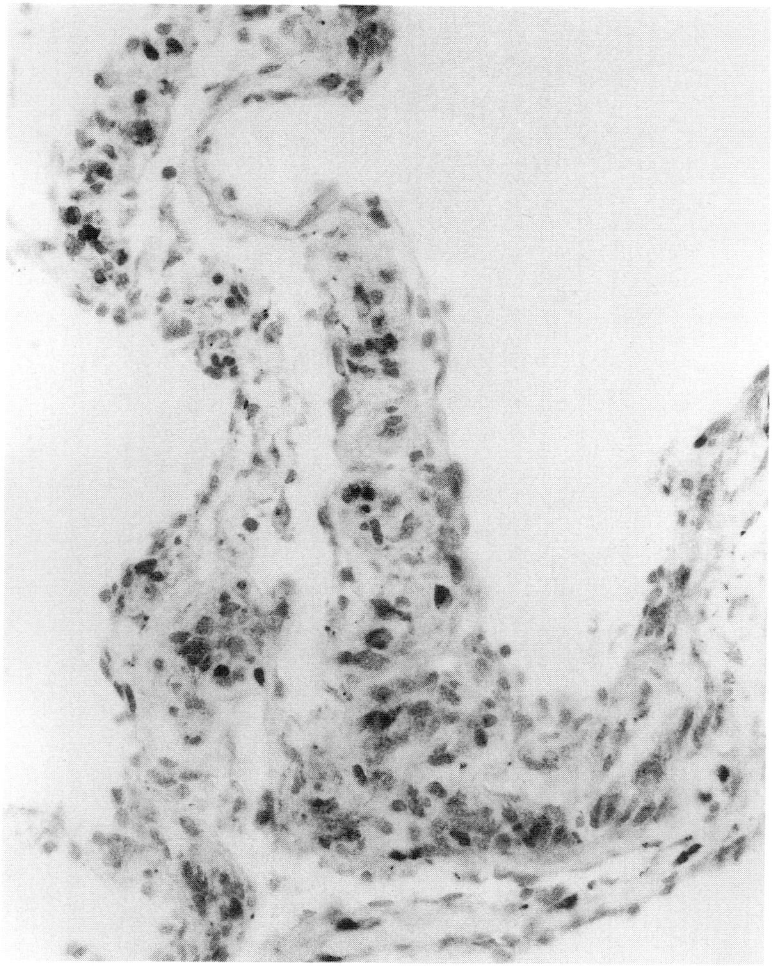

Figure 29 The reaction for estrogen receptors results in distinct nuclear staining of the majority of the LAM cells. (Immunoperoxidase ×400)

This reaction was more intense than that observed in normal smooth muscle cells. Double staining (peroxidase/alkaline phosphatase method) showed that >50% of Bcl-2–positive LAM cells were also positive for estrogen receptor. Immunofluorescence staining for confocal microscopy disclosed colocalization of Bcl-2 and Bax in the cytoplasm of LAM cells. The results of this study suggest that Bcl-2 expression in LAM cells may be related to hormonal regulation and contribute to the sustained life of these cells by changing the balance between Bcl-2 and Bax (85). The proliferative activity of LAM cells has been demonstrated in a recent

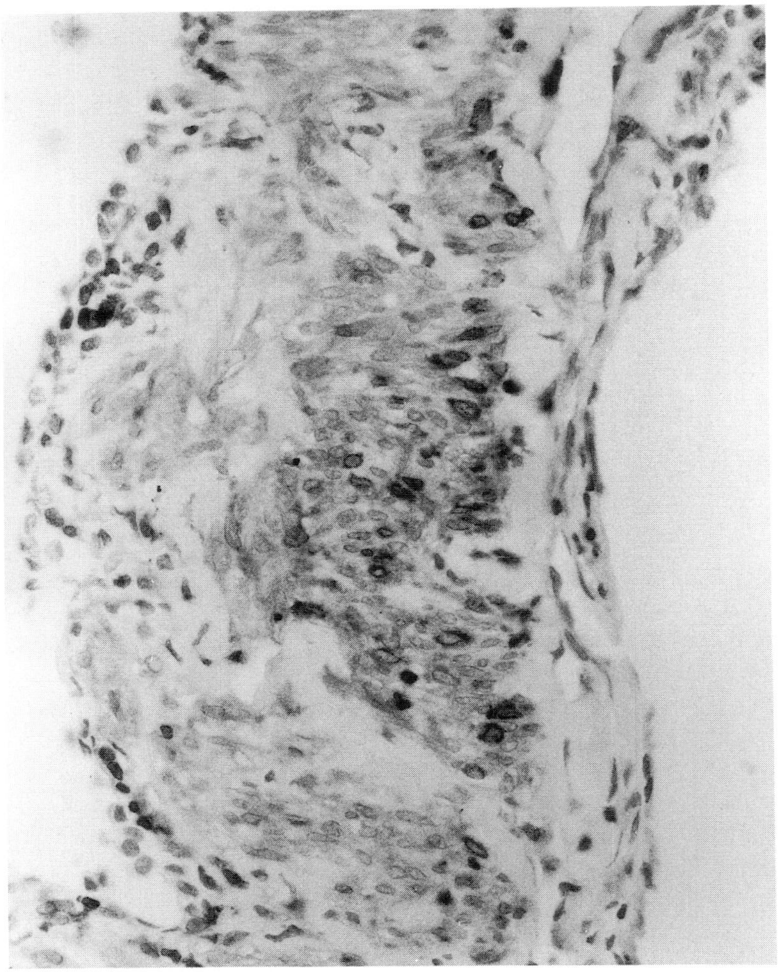

Figure 30 The reaction for Bcl-2 is weak to moderate in the cytoplasm of LAM cells. Intense perinuclear staining is seen in some cells. (Immunoperoxidase-hematoxylin ×400)

study from our laboratory (unpublished data) showing that 30–60% of the nuclei of these cells are immunohistochemically reactive for proliferating cell nuclear antigen (PCNA) (Fig. 31). We have also demonstrated, by dual immunolabeling, that there is an inverse relationship between the reactivity for PCNA and that for HMB-45 (86). The reason for this remains unknown.

The pathogenesis of the destruction of pulmonary tissue in LAM remains incompletely understood. It was initially speculated that the infiltration of bron-

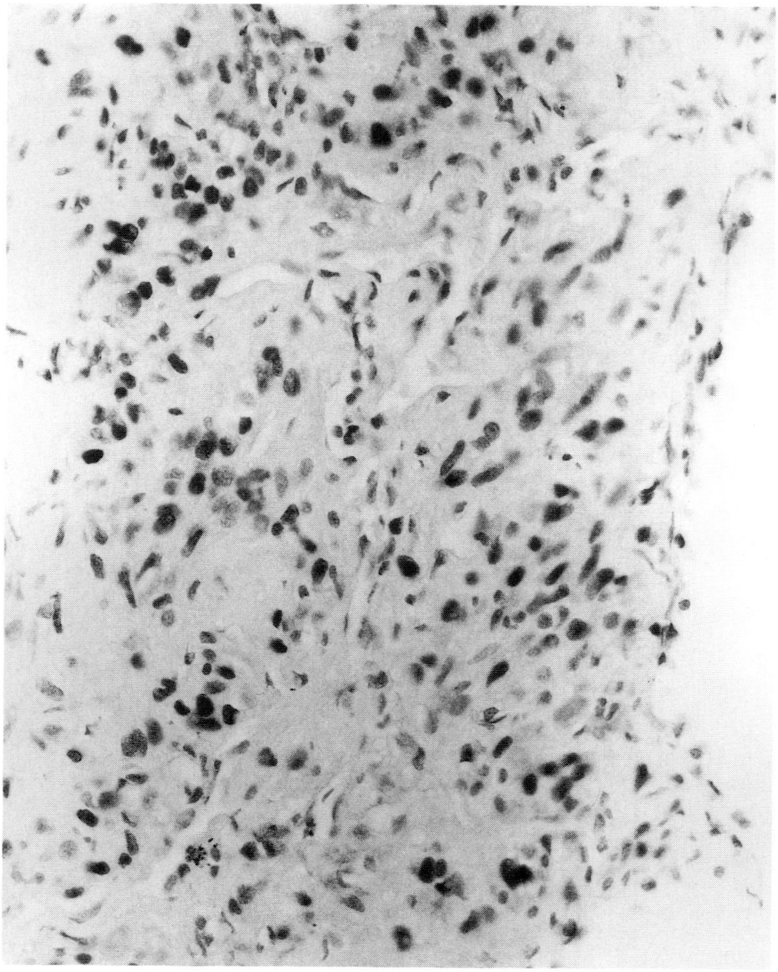

Figure 31 Immunostaining for PCNA (used as an indicator of mitotic activity) shows a nuclear reaction in approximately 70% of the LAM cells, thus demonstrating their proliferative activity. (Immunoperoxidase ×400)

chioles by LAM cells leads to mechanical obstruction of the airway, with air trapping and postobstructive dilatation of the airspaces (18). However, Sobonya et al. showed that there was little involvement of bronchioles by LAM cell infiltrates (87). Fukuda et al. demonstrated elastic fiber destruction in LAM and showed that this destruction is ultrastructurally similar to that seen in emphysema (37). These authors found immunohistochemically detectable α_1-antitrypsin reactivity in the

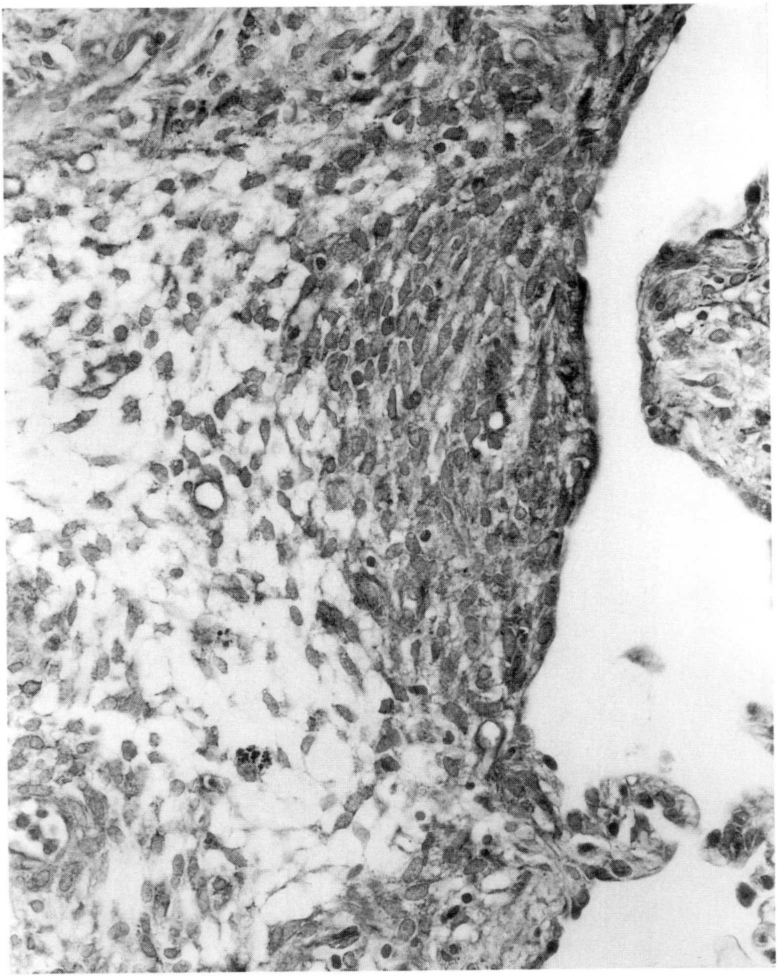

Figure 32 Benign metastasizing leiomyoma consists of a nodular pulmonary infiltrate of spindle-shaped cells. (×15)

damaged elastic fibers in LAM tissue. They suggested that this α_1-antitrypsin was actually complexed with elastase and that the cystic destruction in LAM is due to an imbalance in the elastase/α_1-antitrypsin system (a situation similar to that involved in the pathogenesis of emphysema). However, they did not identify the source of this elastolytic activity, as they were unable to detect neutrophil elastase or pancreatic elastase-1 in the LAM lesions (37). Thus, the binding of α_1-antitrypsin to damaged elastic fibers in LAM remains unexplained.

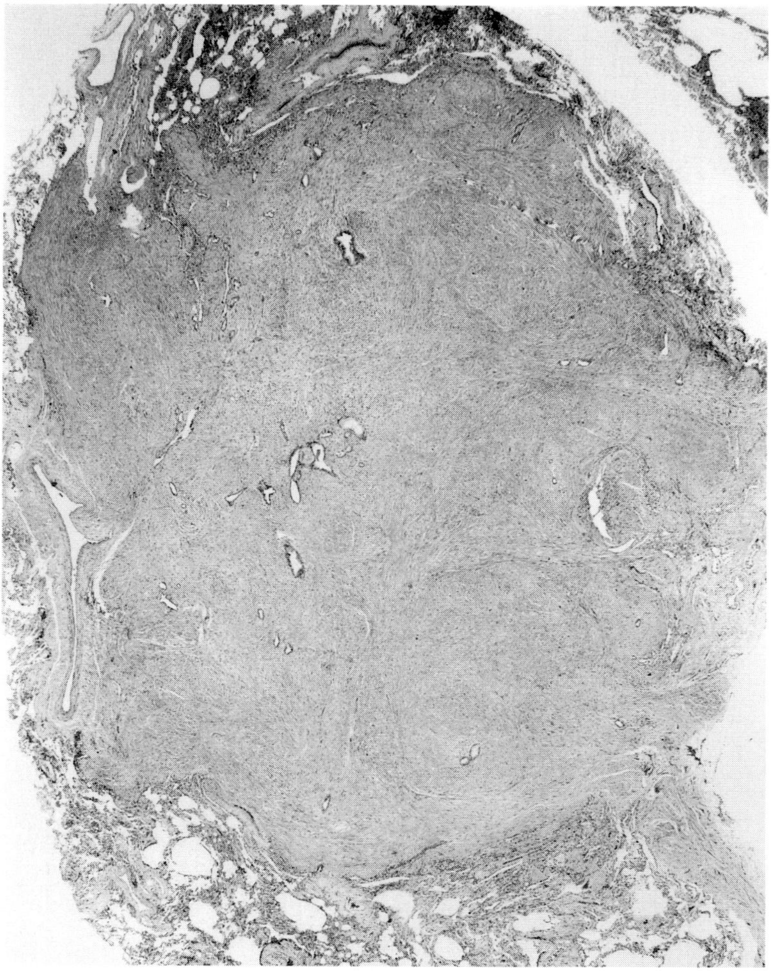

Figure 33 Benign metastasizing leiomyoma consists of a nodular pulmonary infiltrate of spindle-shaped cells. (×15)

Recent studies have demonstrated the importance of matrix metalloproteinases (MMPs) and their specific tissue inhibitors (TIMPs) in the mediation of a number of processes involving the destruction of components of the extracellular matrix, including collagenous and elastic fibers (88,89). To evaluate the role of MMPs and TIMPs in the pathogenesis of the structural damage and cystic lesions found in LAM, Hayashi et al. performed immunohistochemical studies of the localization of MMP-1, MMP-2, MMP-3, MMP-9, TIMP-1, TIMP-2, and

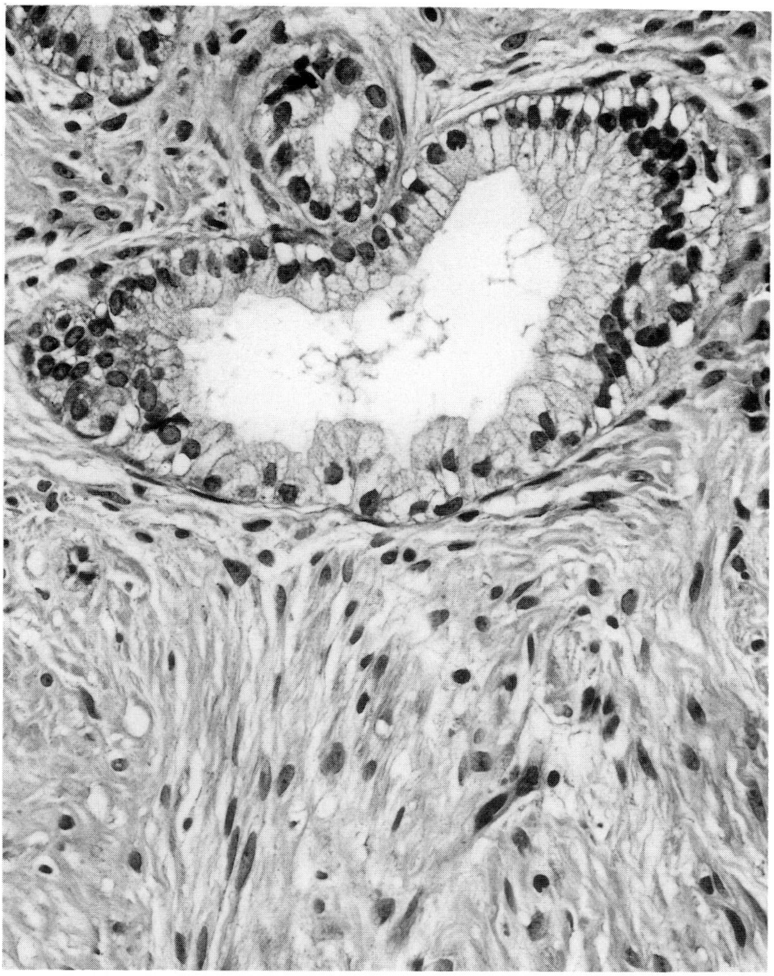

Figure 34 The cells in benign metastasizing leiomyoma have the morphology of smooth muscle without atypia, mitotic figures or necrosis, indicating a benign proliferation. Entrapped glandular epithelium is hyperplastic. (×300)

type IV collagen in sections of lung biopsy specimens from four patients with this disorder (90). These studies demonstrated increased immunoreactivity (compared to that in normal bronchiolar and vascular smooth muscle cells) of MMP-2 and, to a lesser extent, MMP-9 and MMP-1 in the LAM cells (Fig. 32). MMP-2 was also localized in some elastic fibers as well as in the basement membranes of LAM cells and overlying epithelial cells. The basement membranes in both of these sites often showed colocalization of MMP-2 and type IV collagen. Some

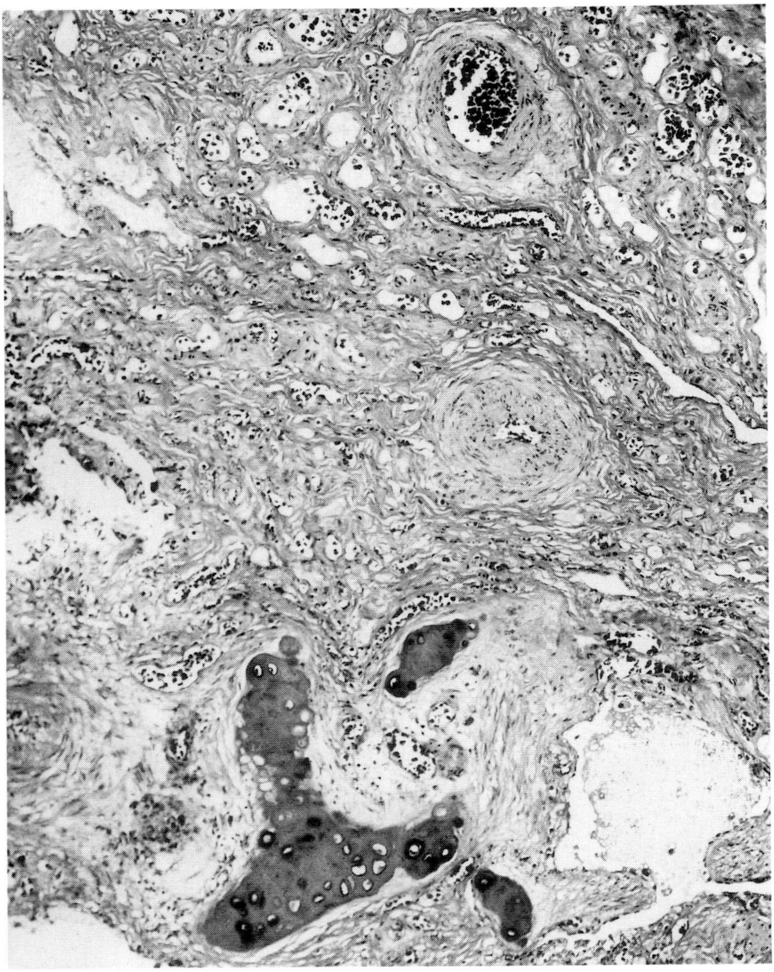

Figure 35 Angiomatosis in bottle-nosed dolphin. Adjacent to the bronchial cartilage within the pulmonary interstitium there is a proliferation of small blood vessels and capillaries. (×75)

epithelial basement membranes showing this colocalization were disrupted. These changes were not accompanied by increased immunoreactivity for TIMPs. Taken together with previous observations showing structural damage to elastic fibers and collagen fibrils, and with the absence of demonstrable neutrophil or pancreatic types of elastase, these findings suggest that MMP-2 and MMP-9 (both of which can degrade elastin as well as collagens) are responsible for the connective tissue destruction and cyst formation in LAM.

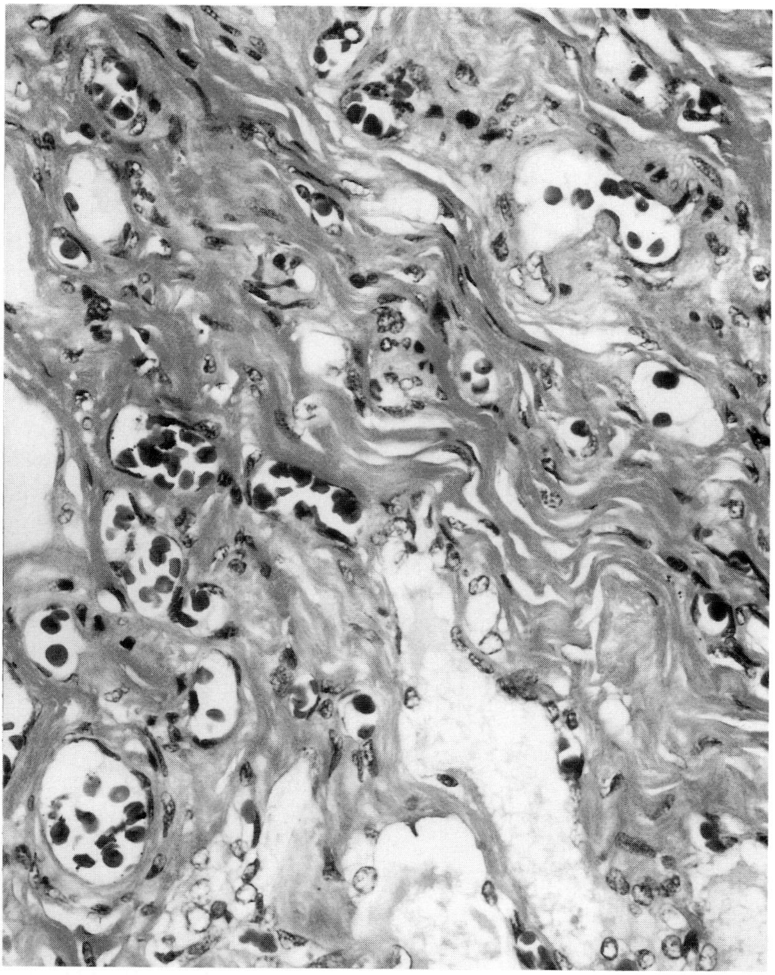

Figure 36 Higher magnification view of lesion of angiomatosis in bottle-nosed dolphin. These small blood vessels and capillaries are surrounded by a fibrous stroma. (×300)

VIII. Differential Diagnosis

Pulmonary LAM must be distinguished from other disorders characterized by abnormal proliferation of smooth muscle cells in the lung. These include the hyperplasia of interstitial smooth muscle cells that occurs in honeycomb fibrosis of various causes (particularly in idiopathic pulmonary fibrosis) (91), pulmonary hypertension (92), and emphysema, as well as smooth muscle cell neoplasms, such as benign metastasizing leiomyomas (BML) (93–96), leiomyosarcomas (96–100), and various cystic sarcomas.

BML has been confused with LAM; however, there is little similarity between these conditions, except that both are multicentric and affect smooth muscle cells (Figs. 33 and 34) (93–96). Reactive, hyperplastic epithelial elements admixed with the bundles of smooth muscle cells can sometimes be very prominent in BML and lead to confusion with hamartomas (Fig. 34) (99). BML typically causes multiple, bilateral, discrete nodules, in contrast to the diffuse parenchymal cystic changes and ill-defined smooth muscle infiltrates of LAM. BML is usually encountered in women with a prior history of uterine leiomyomas (94,96,97,101–104). The history often is so remote that it may be impossible to retrieve the original histologic slides. However, review of the slides from the hysterectomy specimen often shows features of a benign leiomyoma. Distinction of BML from metastatic low-grade leiomyosarcoma occasionally may be difficult if the histologic specimens from the lung and/or uterine lesions show atypical features, such as mitotic figures or cytologic atypia. Cystic changes may occur in BML and metastatic leiomyosarcoma (105) and can even present with pneumothorax (98). Estrogen and progesterone receptors may be positive in BML (106). Therefore, such markers cannot be relied upon for a distinction from LAM (106). Rarely, the differential diagnosis between LAM, BML, or metastatic leiomyosarcoma may be difficult in a small bronchoscopic biopsy containing a few strands of smooth muscle. Immunohistochemical staining for HMB-45 and correlation with the clinical history or high-resolution CT scan findings can be very helpful in making this distinction.

Muscular hyperplasia and cystic changes may occur in advanced interstitial fibrosis, but they are found in the presence of extensive and dense collagen deposits and remodeling of the lung architecture. Interstitial fibrosis is absent or inconspicuous in LAM. In emphysema, there is cystic destruction of the lung; however, LAM cell infiltrates are absent. Subtle infiltrates of LAM cells are sometimes overlooked histologically, and for this reason the diagnosis of LAM should be kept in mind when interpreting lung biopsy specimens from women of reproductive age (particularly if they have a history of pneumothorax).

LAM should not be confused with other entities bearing similar names, such as lymphangiomatosis, lymphangioma, and lymphangiectasis. Lymphangiomatosis is characterized by proliferation of endothelial-lined spaces along lymphatic routes, including those in the pleura, interlobular septa, and bronchovascular bundles (107). It often occurs in infants or young children of either sex. True lymphangiomas of the lung are extremely rare and are manifested by solitary coin lesions rather than be diffuse cystic lung disease (108). Lymphangiectasis simply represents dilation of lymphatics and is seen most often in children, especially after mechanical ventilation.

IX. Occurrence of LAM in Men

LAM has been reported in at least two male patients (109,110), and another male patient was reported in a series with 26 women studied by the urology group at the Mayo Clinic (111). However, none of these cases was well documented pathologically, and it is likely that the lesions in these cases represent disorders other than LAM. Although we were unable to obtain the histologic slides from these cases, we were able to obtain personal communications from Joanne S. Yi (University of California, San Diego, CA) and Jay H. Ryu (Mayo Clinic, Rochester, MN) indicating that the patients reported from Korea and Mayo Clinic did not have LAM. One case of mediastinal lymphangiomyoma (or LAM) was erroneously reported in a male patient (112). Wolff, confirming that the patient was female, subsequently corrected this error (113). Unfortunately, some of these reports have been cited in important articles published in major journals (114), perpetuating the misconception that LAM occurs in men.

X. LAM in Bottle-Nosed Dolphins

LAM has also been reported in a bottle-nosed dolphin (115). The slides from this case were referred to the Veterinary Pathology Department of the Armed Forces Institute of Pathology, where they were reviewed by Dr. Thomas Lipscomb and one of us (WT). The pathological findings did not resemble those in LAM and actually represent a lesion called angiomatosis, which is encountered in up to 20% of both male and female adult bottle-nosed dolphins. Histologically this consists of an interstitial and pleural proliferation of capillaries and small blood vessels within a fibrous stroma (Figs. 35 and 36).

XI. Summary

In summary, LAM is characterized histologically by two features: (1) proliferation of abnormal smooth muscle cells (LAM cells), which are distinguished from other types of smooth muscle cells by their reactivity with HMB-45 antibody (which reacts with premelanosome-like structures in LAM cells and in cells of melanocytic lineage), and (2) progressive destruction of pulmonary connective tissue and formation of multiple cysts. LAM can occur sporadically or in association with tuberous sclerosis. In either instance, it is associated with a high incidence of AMLs, which occur most frequently in the kidneys. In patients with tuberous sclerosis, LAM is frequently associated with multifocal micronodular pneumocyte hyperplasia. Diseases to be considered in the differential diagnosis of LAM include emphysema, pulmonary Langerhans cell histiocytosis (pulmonary histiocytosis X), reactive eosinophilic pleuritis, lymphangiomas, and other disorders characterized by proliferation of smooth muscle cells, such as idiopathic pulmonary fibrosis and other interstitial lung disorders associated with honeycombing and fibrosis, as well as tumors of smooth muscle cells, such as benign metastasizing uterine leiomyomas and leiomyosarcomas.

References

1. Kalassian KG, Doyle R, Kao P, Ruoss S, Raffin TA. Lymphangioleiomyomatosis: new insights. Am J Respir Crit Care Med 1997; 155:1183–1186.
2. Kitaichi M, Nishimura K, Itoh H, Izumi T. Pulmonary lymphangioleiomyomatosis: a report of 46 patients including a clinicopathologic study of prognostic factors. Am J Respir Crit Care Med 1995; 151:527–533.
3. Taylor JR, Ryu J, Colby TV, Raffin TA. Lymphangioleiomyomatosis. Clinical course in 32 patients. N Engl J Med 1990; 323:1254–1260.
4. Carrington CB, Cugell DW, Gaensler EA, Marks A, Redding RA, Schaaf JT, Tomasian A. Lymphangioleiomyomatosis. Physiologic-pathologic correlations. Am Rev Respir Dis 1977; 116:977–995.
5. Maziak DE, Kesten S, Rappaport DC, Maurer J. Extrathoracic angiomyolipomas in lymphangioleiomyomatosis. Eur Respir J 1996; 9:402–405.
6. Bernstein SM, Newell JDJ, Adamczyk D, Mortenson RL, King TEJ, Lynch DA. How common are renal angiomyolipomas in patients with pulmonary lymphangiomyomatosis? Am J Respir Crit Care Med 1995; 152:2138–2143.
7. Callol L, Villegas Fernandez FR, Calderon Alvarez J, Chillon MD, Gomez-Terreros FJ. Pulmonary lymphangiomyomatosis and kidney angiomyolipomas [letter]. Respiration 1993; 60:311.
8. Lack EE, Dolan MF, Finisio J, Grover G, Singh M, Triche TJ. Pulmonary and extrapulmonary lymphangioleiomyomatosis. Report of a case with bilateral renal angiomyolipomas, multifocal lymphangioleiomyomatosis, and a glial polyp of the endocervix. Am J Surg Pathol 1986; 10:650–657.
9. Lenior S, Grenier P, Brauner MW, Frija J, Remy-Jardin M, Revel D, Cordier JF. Pulmonary lymphangiomyomatosis and tuberous sclerosis: comparison of radiographic and thin-section CT findings. Radiology 1990; 175:329–334.
10. Luna CM, Genë R, Jolly EC, Nahmod N, Defranchi HA, Patino G, Elsner B. Pulmonary lymphangiomyomatosis associated with tuberous sclerosis. Treatment with tamoxifen and tetracycline-pleurodesis. Chest 1985; 88:473–475.
11. Liberman BA, Chamberlain DW, Goldstein RS. Tuberous sclerosis with pulmonary involvement. Can Med Assoc J 1984; 130:287–289.
12. Capron F, Ameille J, Leclerc P, Mornet P, Barbagellata M, Reynes M, Rouchemaure J. Pulmonary lymphangioleiomyomatosis and Bourneville's tuberous sclerosis with pulmonary involvement: the same disease? Cancer 1983; 52:851–855.
13. Rosenberg DM. Inherited forms of interstitial lung disease. Clin Chest Med 1982; 3:635–641.

14. Lie JT, Miller RD, Williams DE. Cystic disease of the lungs in tuberous sclerosis: clinicopathologic correlation, including body plethysmographic lung function tests. Mayo Clin Proc 1980; 55:547–553.
15. Stovin PG, Lum LC, Flower CD, Darke CS, Beeley M. The lungs in lymphangiomyomatosis and in tuberous sclerosis. Thorax 1975; 30:497–509.
16. Dwyer JM, Hickie JB, Garvan J. Pulmonary tuberous sclerosis. Report of three patients and a review of the literature. Q J Med 1971; 40:115–125.
17. Malik SK, Pardee N, Martin CJ. Involvement of the lungs in tuberous sclerosis. Chest 1970; 58:538–540.
18. Corrin B, Liebow AA, Friedman PJ. Pulmonary lymphangiomyomatosis. A review. Am J Pathol 1975; 79:348–382.
19. Basset F, Soler P, Marsac J, Corrin B. Pulmonary lymphangiomyomatosis: three new cases studied with electron microscopy. Cancer 1976; 38:2357–2366.
20. Guinee DG, Jr., Feuerstein I, Koss MN, Travis WD. Pulmonary lymphangioleiomyomatosis. Diagnosis based on results of transbronchial biopsy and immunohistochemical studies and correlation with high-resolution computed tomography findings. Arch Pathol Lab Med 1994; 118:846–849.
21. Bonetti F, Pea M, Martignoni G, Zamboni G, Iuzzolino P. Cellular heterogeneity in lymphangiomyomatosis of the lung [letter]. Hum Pathol 1991; 22:727–728.
22. Bonetti F, Chiodera PL, Pea M, Martignoni G, Bosi F, Zamboni G, Mariuzzi GM. Transbronchial biopsy in lymphangiomyomatosis of the lung. HMB45 for diagnosis. Am J Surg Pathol 1993; 17:1092–1102.
23. Gawad KA, Knoefel WT, Izbicki JR, Schroder S, Broelsch CE. Generalised lymphangioleiomyomatosis presenting as a retroperitoneal tumour. Eur J Surg 1996; 162:583–585.
24. Tsang WY, Chan JK. Primary leiomyomatosis of lymph node or nodal lymphangiomyoma? [letter]. Histopathology 1993; 23:393–394.
25. Bhattacharyya AK, Balogh K. Retroperitoneal lymphangioleiomyomatosis. A 36-year benign course in a postmenopausal woman. Cancer 1985; 56:1144–1146.
26. Stubbe Teglbjaerg P, Svendsen V. Lymphangiomyoma of the thoracic duct with previously undescribed epithelial tubules. Tumori. 178; 64:63–70.
27. Askin FB, McCann BG, Kuhn C. Reactive eosinophilic pleuritis: a lesion to be distinguished from pulmonary eosinophilic granuloma. Arch Pathol Lab Med 1977; 101:187–191.
28. McDonnell TJ, Crough EC, Gonzalez JG. Reactive eosinophilic pleuritis. A sequela of pneumothorax in pulmonary eosinophilic granuloma. Am J Clin Pathol 1989; 91:107–111.
29. Michal M. Havlicek F. Immunohistochemical phenotypes of histioeosinophilic granulomas of thymus and reactive eosinophilic pleuritis. Acta Histochem 1993; 94:97–101.
30. Chiodera F, Pea M, Martignoni G, Zamboni G, Maran M, Montresor C, Mombello A, Bonetti F. Transbronchial biopsies in lymphangioleiomyomatosis of the lung: MOAB HMB-45 is helpful for the diagnosis (abstr). Mod Pathol 1993; 6:129A.
31. Kapur RP, Bigler SA, Skelly M, Gown AM. Anti-melanoma monoclonal antibody

HMB45 identifies an oncofetal glycoconjugate associated with immature melanosomes. J Histochem Cytochem 1992; 40:207–212.
32. Kaiserling E, Krober S, Xiao JC, Schaumburg-Lever G. Angiomyolipoma of the kidney. Immunoreactivity with HMB-45. Light- and electron-microscopic findings. Histopathology 1994; 25:41–48.
33. Gaffey MJ, Mills SE, Zarbo RJ, Weiss LM, Gown AM. Clear cell tumor of the lung. Immunohistochemical and ultrastructural evidence of melanogenesis. Am J Surg Pathol 1991; 15:644–653.
34. Bjornsson J, Nascimento AG, Gujino SP. The expression of neural crest-associated markers in normal kidney and renal angiomyolipomas and carcinomas in patients with and without tuberous sclerosis (abstr). Mod Pathol 1995; 8:73A.
35. Chu SC, Horiba K, Usuki J, Avila NA, Chen CC, Travis WD, et al. Comprehensive evaluation of 35 patients with lymphangioleimyomatosis (LAM).
36. Schaumburg-Lever G, Metzler G, Kaiserling E. Ultrastructural localization of HMB-45 binding sites. J Cutan Pathol 1991; 18:432–435.
37. Fukuda Y, Kawamoto M, Yamamoto A, Ishizaki M, Basset F, Masugi Y. Role of elastic fiber degradation in emphysema-like lesions of pulmonary lymphangiomyomatosis. Hum Pathol 1990; 21:1252–1261.
38. Bonetti F, Pea M, Martignoni G, Doglioni C, Zamboni G, Capelli P, Rimondi P, Andrion A. Clear cell (sugar) tumor of the lung is a lesion strictly related to angiomyolipoma—the concept of a family of lesions characterized by the presence of the perivascular epithelioid cells (PEC). Pathology 1994; 26:230–236.
39. Castro M, Shepherd CW, Gomez MR, Lie JT, Ryu JH. Pulmonary tuberous sclerosis. Chest 1995; 107:189–195.
40. Hauck RW, König G, Permanetter W, Weiss M, Wöckel W, Fruhmann G. Tuberous sclerosis with pulmonary involvement. Respiration 1990; 57:289–292.
41. Harris JO, Waltuck BL, Swenson EW. The pathophysiology of the lungs in tuberous sclerosis. A case report and literature review. Am Rev Respir Dis 1969; 100:379–387.
42. Baar HS, Galindo J. Pulmonary glomangiomata and hamartoma in tuberous sclerosis. Arch Pathol 1964; 78:287–291.
43. Gaffey MJ, Mills SE, Askin FB. Minute pulmonary meningothelial-like nodules. A clinicopathologic study of so-called minute pulmonary chemodectoma. Am J Surg Pathol 1988; 12:167–175.
44. Lie JT. Cardiac, pulmonary, and vascular involvements in tuberous sclerosis. Ann NY Acad Sci 1991; 615:58–70.
45. Slingerland JM, Grossman RF, Chamberlain D, Tremblay CE. Pulmonary manifestations of tuberous sclerosis in first degree relatives. Thorax 1989; 44:212–214.
46. Guinee D, Singh R, Azumi N, Singh G, Przygodzki RM, Travis WD, Koss MN. Multifocal micronodular pneumocyte hyperplasia: a distinctive pulmonary manifestation of tuberous sclerosis. Mod Pathol 1995; 8:902–906.
47. Popper HH, Juettner-Smolle FM, Pongratz MG. Micronodular hyperplasia of type II pneumocytes—a new lung lesion associated with tuberous sclerosis. Histopathology 1991; 18:347–354.
48. Spencer H. Pathology of the Lung. 4th ed. New York: Raven Press, 1985:1043.

49. Fegan JE, Shah HR, Mukunyadzi P, Schutz MJ. Extrarenal retroperitoneal angiomyolipoma. South Med J 1997; 90:59–62.
50. Sola JE, Pierre-Jerome F, Sitzmann JV, Wheeler J, Bizzi A, Terotola SO. Multifocal angiomyolipoma in a patient with tuberous sclerosis. Clin Imaging 1996; 20:99–102.
51. Ben-Izhak O, Groissman G, Lichtig C. Hepatic angiomyolipoma in childhood: association with tuberous sclerosis [letter]. Pediatr Pathol Lab Med 1995; 15:213–217.
52. Maffezzini M, Vlassopoulos G, Simonato A, Bussani R, Silvestri F, Carmignani G. Renal angiomyolipoma with extrarenal involvement—in vascular, lymph-node and perirenal tissue. Reports of four cases. Scand J Urol Nephrol 1995; 29:327–329.
53. Guinee DG, Jr., Thornberry DS, Azumi N, Przygodzki RM, Koss MN, Travis WD, Unique pulmonary presentation of an angiomyolipoma. Analysis of clinical, radiographic, and histopathologic features. Am J Surg Pathol 1995; 19:476–480.
54. Hoon V, Thung SN, Kaneko M, Unger PD. HMB-45 reactivity in renal angiomyolipoma and lymphangioleiomyomatosis. Arch Pathol Lab Med 1994; 118:732–734.
55. McIntosh GS, Dutoit SH, Chronos NV, Kaisary AV. Multiple unilateral renal angiomyolipomas with regional lymphangioleiomyomatosis. J Urol 1989; 142:1305–1307.
56. Monteforte WJ, Jr., Kohnen PW. Angiomyolipomas in a case of lymphangiomyomatosis syndrome: relationships to tuberous sclerosis. Cancer 1974; 34:317–321.
57. Tawfik O, Austenfeld M, Persons D. Multicentric renal angiomyolipoma associated with pulmonary lymphangioleiomyomatosis: case report, with histologic, immunohistochemical, and DNA content analyses. Urology 1996; 48:476–480.
58. Katz DS, Poster RB. Massive renal angiomyolipoma in tuberous sclerosis. Clin Imaging 1997; 21:200–202.
59. Chan JK, Tsang WY, Pau MY, Tang MC, Pang SW, Fletcher CD. Lymphangiomyomatosis and angiomyolipoma: closely related entities characterized by hamartomatous proliferation of HBM-45-positive smooth muscle. Histopathology 1993; 22:445–455.
60. Eble JN, Amin MB, Young RH. Epithelioid angiomyolipoma of the kidney. A report of five cases with a prominent and diagnostically confusing epithelioid smooth muscle component. Am J Surg Pathol 1997; 21:1123–1130.
61. Chatterjee T, Heindel W, Vorreuther R, Englemann U, Lackner K. Recurrent bleeding of angiomyolipomas in tuberous sclerosis. Urol Int 1996; 56:44–47.
62. Chowdhury PR, Tsuda N, Anami M, Hayashi T, Iseki M, Kishikawa M, Matsuya F, Kanetake H, Saito Y. A histopathologic and immunohistochemical study of small nodules of renal angiomyolipoma: a comparison of small nodules with angiomyolipoma. Mod Pathol 1996; 9:1081–1088.
63. Liwnicz BH, Weeks DA, Zuppan CW. Extrarenal angiomyolipoma with melanocytic and hibernoma-like features. Ultrastruct Pathol 1994; 18:443–448.

64. Bonsib SM. HMB-45 reactivity in renal leiomyomas and leiomyosarcomas. Mod Pathol 1996; 9:664–669.
65. Flieder DB, Travis WD. Clear cell "sugar" tumor of the lung: Association with lymphangioleiomyomatosis and multifocal micronodular pneumocyte hyperplasia in a patient with tuberous sclerosis. Am J Surg Pathol 1997; 21:1242–1247.
66. Liebow AA, Castleman B. Benign clear cell ("sugar") tumors of the lung. Yale J Biol Med 1971; 43:213–222.
67. Gaffey MJ, Mills SE, Askin FB, Ross GW, Sale GE, Kulander BG, Visscher DW, Yousem SA, Colby TV. Clear cell tumor of the lung. A clinicopathologic, immunohistochemical, and ultrastructural study of eight cases. Am J Surg Pathol 1990; 14:248–259.
68. Gal AA, Koss MN, Hochholzer L, Chejfec G. An immunohistochemical study of benign clear cell ('sugar') tumor of the lung. Arch Pathol Lab Med 1991; 115:1034–1038.
69. Fetsch PA, Fetsch JF, Marincola FM, Travis WD, Batts KP, Abati A. Comparison of melanoma-associated membrane antigen (MART-1) to HMB-45: further evidence to support a common lineage for angiomyolipoma, lymphangioleiomyomatosis, and clear cell "sugar" tumor. Mod Pathol 1998; In press.
70. Zamboni G, Pea M, Martignoni G, Zancanaro C, Faccioli G, Gilioli E, Pederzoli P, Bonetti F. Clear cell sugar tumor of the pancreas. A novel member of the family of lesions characterized by the presence of perivascular epithelioid cells. Am J Surg Pathol 1996; 20:722–730.
71. Batts KP, Taxelaar HD. Extrapulmonary clear cell tumor ("sugar") tumor: a study of 3 cases (abstr). Mod Pathol 1996; 9:5.
72. Banner AS. Hormone receptors in lymphangioleiomyomatosis. Chest 1984; 85:3–4.
73. Berger U, Khaghani A, Pomerance A, Yacoub MH, Coombes RC. Pulmonary lymphangioleiomyomatosis and steroid receptors. An immunocytochemical study. Am J Clin Pathol 1990; 93:609–614.
74. Brentani MM, Carvalho CR, Saldiva PH, Pacheco MM, Oshima T. Steroid receptors in pulmonary lymphangiomyomatosis. Chest 1984; 85:96–99.
75. Colley MH, Geppert E, Franklin WA. Immunohistochemical detection of steroid receptors in a case of pulmonary lymphangioleiomyomatosis. Am J Surg Pathol 1989; 13:803–807.
76. Graham ML, Spelsberg TC, Dines DE, Payne WS, Bjornsson J, Lie JT. Pulmonary lymphangiomyomatosis: with particular reference to steroid-receptor assay studies and pathologic correlation. Mayo Clin Proc 1984; 59:3–11.
77. Kinoshita M, Yokoyama T, Higuchi E, Yano H, Watanabe H, Rikimaru T, Ichikawa Y, Oizumi K. Hormone receptors in pulmonary lymphangiomyomatosis. Kurume Med J 1995; 42:141–144.
78. Svendsen TL, Viskum K, Hansborg N, Thorpe SM, Nielsen NC. Pulmonary lymphangioleiomyomatosis: a case of progesterone receptor positive lymphangioleiomyomatosis treated with medroxyprogesterone, oophorectomy and tamoxifen. Br J Dis Chest 1984; 78:264–271.

79. Davis MG, Zhou M, Ali S, Coffin JD, Doetschman T, Dorn GW. Intracrine and autocrine effects of basic fibroblast growth factor in vascular smooth muscle cells. J Mol Cell Cardiol 1997; 29:1061–1072.
80. Engel L, Ryan U. TGF-beta 1 reverses PDGF-stimulated migration of human aortic smooth muscle cells in vitro. In Vitro Cell Dev Biol Anim 1997; 33:443–451.
81. Saltis J, Bobik A. Developmental regulation of transforming growth factor-beta 1 responses and vascular smooth muscle growth in spontaneously hypertensive rats. J Hypertens 1995; 13:1441–1448.
82. Thieszen SL, Dalton M, Gadson PF, Patterson E, Rosenquist TH. Embryonic lineage of vascular smooth muscle cells determines responses to collagen matrices and integrin receptor expression. Exp Cell Res 1996; 227:135–145.
83. Black PN, Young PG, Skinner SJ. Response of airway smooth muscle cells to TGF-beta 1: effects on growth and synthesis of glycosaminoglycans. Am J Physiol 1996; 271:L910–L917.
84. Corrin B, Butcher D, McAnulty BJ, Dubois RM, Black CM, Laurent GJ, Harrison NK. Immunohistochemical localization of transforming growth factor beta-1 in the lungs of patients with systemic sclerosis, cryptogenic fibrosing alveolitis and other lung disorders. Histopathology 1994; 24:145–150.
85. Usuki J, Horiba K, Chu SC, Matsumoto Y, Moss J, Ferans VJ; Immunoreactivity in pulmonary lymphangioleiomyomatosis and its association with estrogen receptor positivity. (submitted)
86. Matsumoto Y, Horiba K, Usuki J, Chu SC, Ferrans VJ, Moss J; Characterization of the melanosome-containing smooth muscle cells in lymphangioleiomyomatosis (LAM): inverse correlation between markers of cell proliferation and expression of melanosomal antigens in LAM and melanoma cells. (submitted)
87. Sobonya RE, Quan SF, Fleishman JS. Pulmonary lymphangioleiomyomatosis: quantitative analysis of lesions producing airflow limitation. Hum Pathol 1985; 16:1122–1128.
88. Stetler-Stevenson WG, Hewitt R, Corcoran M. Matrix metalloproteinases and tumor invasion: from correlation and causality to the clinic. Semin Cancer Biol 1996; 7:147–154.
89. Hyashi T, Stetler-Stevenson WG, Fleming MV, Fishback N, Koss MN, Liotta LA, Ferrans VJ, Travis WD. Immunohistochemical study of metalloproteinases and their tissue inhibitors in the lungs of patients with diffuse alveolar damage and idiopathic pulmonary fibrosis. Am J Pathol 1996; 149:1241–1256.
90. Hayashi T, Fleming MV, Stetler-Stevenson WG, Liotta LA, Moss J, Ferrans VJ, Travis WD. Immunohistochemical study of matrix metalloproteinases (MMPs) and their tissue inhibitors (TIMPs) in pulmonary lymphangioleiomyomatosis (LAM). Hum Pathol 1997; 28:1071–1078.
91. Scadding JG, Hinson KFW. Diffuse fibrosing alveolitis (diffuse interstitial fibrosis of the lungs). Thorax 1967; 22:291–304.
92. Kay JM, Kahana LM, Rihal C. Diffuse smooth muscle proliferation of the lungs with severe pulmonary hypertension. Hum Pathol 1996; 27:969–974.
93. Takemura G, Takastsu Y, Kaitani K, Ono M, Ando F, Tanada S, Niwa H, Tankawa

H, Fujiwara T, Yamabe H. Metastasizing uterine leiomyoma. A case with cardiac and pulmonary metastasis. Pathol Res Pract 1996; 192:622–629.
94. Parenti DJ, Morley TF, Giudice JC. Benign metastasizing leiomyoma. A case report and review of the literature. Respiration 1992; 59:347–350.
95. Uchida T, Tokumaru T, Kojima H, Nakagawaji K, Imaizumi M, Abe T. A case of multiple leiomyomatous lesions of the lung: an analysis of flow cytometry and hormone receptors. Surg Today 1992; 22:265–268.
96. Sprio RH, McPeak CJ. On the so-called metastasizing leiomyoma. Cancer 1966; 19:544–548.
97. Bachman D, Wolff M. Pulmonary metastases from benign-appearing smooth muscle tumors of the uterus. Am J Roentgenol 1976; 127:441–446.
98. Mehzad M. Leiomyosarcoma of the uterus presenting with pneumothorax. Br J Dis Chest 1977; 71:132–134.
99. Wolff M, Silva F, Kaye G. Pulmonary metastases (with admixed epithelial elements) from smooth muscle neoplasia. Report of nine cases, including three males. Am J Surg Pathol 1979; 3:325–342.
100. Gerst PH, Levy J, Swaminathan K, Kshettry V, Albu E. Metastatic leiomyosarcoma of the uterus: unusual presentation of a case with late endobronchial and small bowel metastases. Gynecol Oncol 1993; 49:271–275.
101. Ford JM, Pang J, Coutts J, Evans BD. Metastasizing leiomyoma of the uterus. Aust NZ J Obstet Gynecol 1988; 28:154–155.
102. Pocock E, Craig JR, Bullock WK. Metastatic uterine leiomyomata. A case report. Cancer 1976; 38:2096–2100.
103. Stephenson CA, Henley FT, Goldstein AR. Benign metastasizing leiomyoma. Ala J Med Sci 1984; 21:78–81.
104. Winkler TR, Burr LH, Robinson CL. Benign metastasizing leiomyoma. Ann Thorac Surg 1987; 43:100–101.
105. Shin MS, Fulmer JD, Ho KJ. Unusual computed topographic manifestations of benign metastasizing leiomyomas as cavitary nodular lesions or interstitial lung disease. Clin Imaging 1996; 20:45–49.
106. Jautzke G, Muller-Ruchholtz E, Thalmann U. Immunohistological detection of estrogen and progesterone receptors in multiple and well differentiated leiomyomatous lung tumors in women with uterine leiomyomas (so-called benign metastasizing leiomyomas). A report on 5 cases. Pathol Res Pract 1996; 192:215–223.
107. Tazelaar HD, Kerr D, Yousem SA, Saldana MJ, Langston C, Colby TV. Diffuse pulmonary lymphangiomatosis. Hum Pathol 1993; 24:1313–1322.
108. Colby TV, Koss MN, Travis WD. Tumors of the Lower Respiratory Tract; Armed Forces Institute of Pathology Fascicle, Third Series. Washington, DC: Armed Forces Institute of Pathology, 1995.
109. Korobowicz E, Sierocinska-Sawa J. Pulmonary lymphangioleiomyomatosis—a case report. Pol J Pathol 1996; 47:83–86.
110. Kang HW, Kim CJ, Kang SK, Lee KS, Lee CS, Kim YH. Pulmonary lymphangioleiomyomatosis in a male. J Korean Med Sci 1991; 6:83–85.
111. Kerr LA, Blute ML, Ryu JH, Swensen SJ, Malek RS. Renal angiomyolipoma in

association with pulmonary lymphangioleiomyomatosis: forme fruste of tuberous sclerosis? Urology 1993; 41:440–444.
112. Pachter MR, Lattes R. Mesenchymal tumors of the mediastinum. III. Tumors of lymph vascular origin. Cancer 1963; 16:108–117.
113. Bachman D, Wolff M. Pulmonary metastases from benign-appearing smooth muscle tumors of the uterus. Am J Roentgenol 1976; 127:441–446.
114. Boehler A, Speich R, Russi EW, Weder W. Lung transplantation for lymphangioleiomyomatosis. N Engl J Med 1996; 335:1275–1280.
115. Rawson AJ, Patton GW, Brooks JS. Lymphangiomyomatosis in the Atlantic bottlenose dolphin (*Tursiops truncatus*). J Wildl Dis 1992; 28:323–325.

12

Ultrastructural Pathology of Pulmonary Lymphangioleiomyomatosis

YUH FUKUDA

Nippon Medical School
Tokyo, Japan

I. Introduction

Lymphangioleiomyomatosis (LAM) is a disease occurring exclusively in women of childbearing age. Abnormal overproduction of smooth muscle cells in the lungs and in the systemic lymphatic tissue occurs in LAM. Chest x-rays, computed tomography, and macroscopic examination of the lungs of LAM patients reveal multiple dilated cystic lesions resembling those observed in emphysematous or honeycombing lungs (1–3). In general, the morphogenesis of these cystic lesions in pulmonary LAM (PLAM) is thought to be mediated by airtrapping due to bronchiolar obstruction by proliferating smooth muscle cells (4,5). In this chapter, the ultrastructure of LAM-affected lungs is described and a possible mechanism of pulmonary structural remodeling in PLAM is discussed.

PLAM is characterized mainly by abnormal accumulation of smooth muscle cells in an area of the pulmonary lymphatic system. These smooth muscle cells are located in peribronchial, peribronchiolar, and perivascular areas, the pleurae, and occasionally alveolar walls. Lymph vessels are not normally detected in peripheral alveolar walls themselves, but the stroma of the alveolar walls is a pathway of fluid flow to the opened system of lymphatic tissue. Therefore, it is considered that smooth muscle cells that accumulate in alveolar walls are also associated with the lymphatic system. Cystic dilated lymph vessels containing fluid are frequently found in the area of smooth muscle cell accumulation, especially in the pleurae and peribronchial area where the large lymph vessels are normally located in LAM-affected lungs.

The main active clinical signs of PLAM are hemoptysis, pneumothorax, and pleural effusion. In histopathological specimens of the lungs of patients with these active signs, the accumulated smooth muscle cells are large and the stroma and intra-alveolar spaces are edematous and occasionally hemorrhagic. In such specimens of the lungs of patients with few of these clinical signs, the smooth muscle cells are small and the stroma is not edematous but compact and shows mild fibrous change. Thus, the microscopic lesions may be divided into early lesions and late lesions (6). Estrogen and/or progesterone receptors are known to be present in the abnormal smooth muscle cells in PLAM, (7,8). The symptoms of PLAM worsen during estrogen administration, pregnancy, and even menses (9–11). The cells in an early PLAM lesion may be activated by estrogen. Analysis of the histopathological changes with a focus on the differences between early and late lesions is useful for understanding the mechanism of pulmonary structural remodeling in PLAM. The differences between early and late lesions are described in this chapter.

II. Ultrastructure of Cells in PLAM

A. Smooth Muscle Cells in Early Lesions

The accumulated abnormal cells in PLAM resemble smooth muscle cells ultrastructurally (4,6,12–17), although they contain a well-developed rough endoplasmic reticulum, which is characteristic of myofibroblasts. The abnormal smooth muscle cells in PLAM are morphologically different from the normal smooth muscle cells in bronchial, alveolar duct, and vascular walls. Normal smooth muscle cells are homogeneous in size and shape; they are elongated, spindle-shaped, arranged in parallel and form bundles, and contain elongated and oval nucleus, and cytoplasm which contains parallel-arranged myofilaments.

The abnormal smooth muscle cells in PLAM, especially those in early and active lesions, are large and almost plump but irregular in shape and somewhat irregularly arranged, compared to normal smooth muscle cells (Fig. 1). The nucleus is convoluted and contains an abundance of euchromatin and a large round nucleolus (12). These findings indicate that the cells are metabolically active. The cytoplasm contains numerous actin microfilaments, which are randomly arranged and frequently form dense bodies (Fig. 2). Moreover, the cytoplasm contains an abundance of α-smooth muscle actin. Actin microfilaments aggregate and form dense bodies at the cytoplasmic side of the cell membrane, and the cells adhere to the extracellular matrix (ECM). At the sites of direct con-

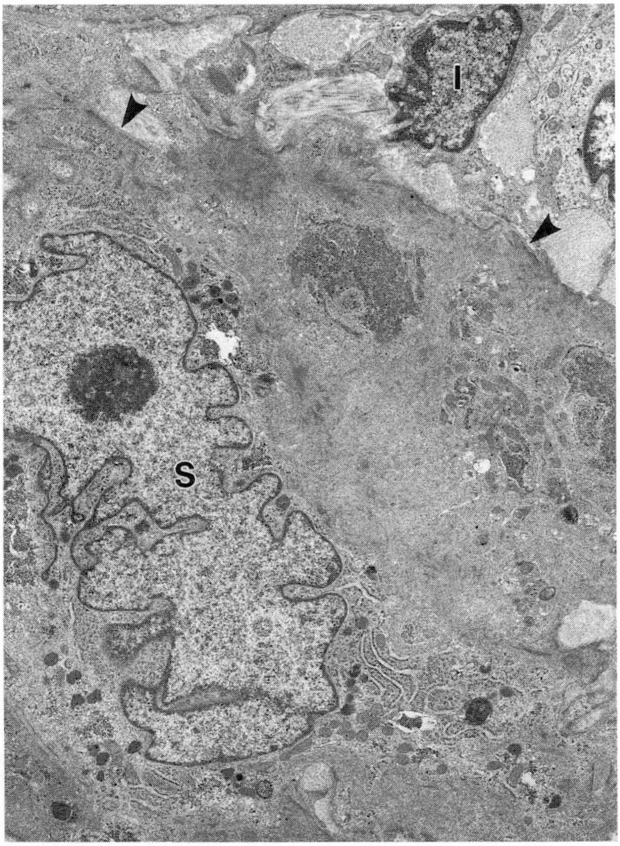

Figure 1 Early PLAM lesion. Accumulated smooth muscle cell (S) is much larger than the adjacent interstitial cells (I). The cell contains convoluted nucleus, large nucleolus, and bundles of actin microfilaments and glycogen granules in its cytoplasm. Rough endoplasmic reticulum, electron-dense small granules are prominent close to the nucleus. Discontinuous basement membrane (arrowheads) is noted. The cytoplasm of right side interstitial cell is slightly swollen. (×6000.) (From Ref. 6.)

tact between these smooth muscle cells, adherent junctions and gap junctions are frequently observed without basement membrane. Prominent intermediate filaments are also found mixed with actin microfilaments in the cytoplasm (Fig. 2). They are composed mainly of desmin and some vimentin, as determined by immunohistochemical study. On the cytoplasmic side of cell membrane, some pinocytotic and coated vesicles are observed (Fig. 2). These vesicles are irregularly distributed and fewer in number than those in normal smooth muscle cells. Glycogen granules are abundant in the cytoplasm (Fig. 2), so the cytoplasm of these

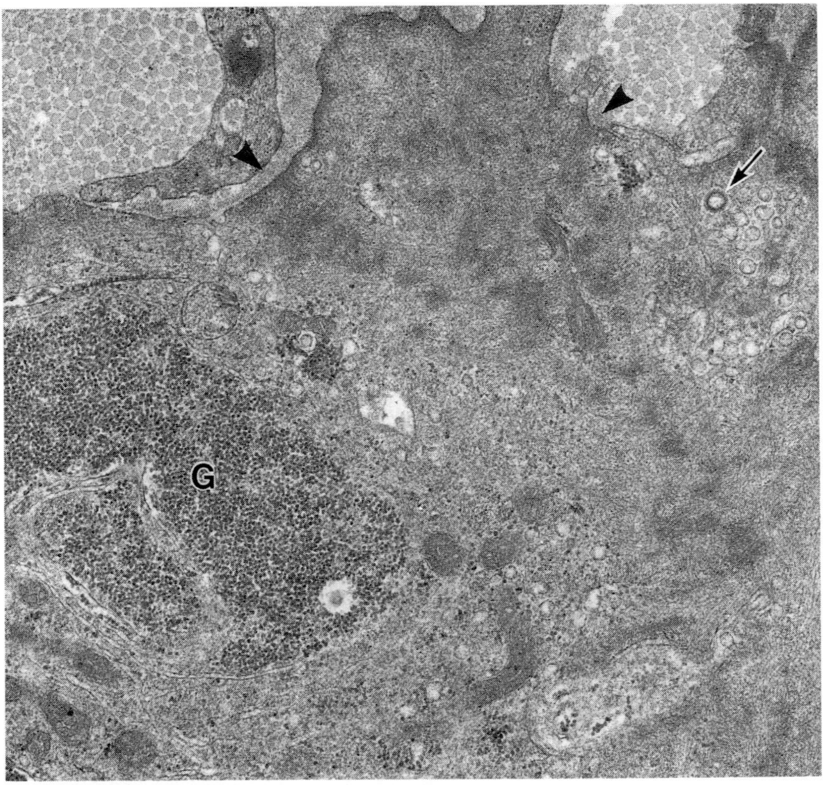

Figure 2 Early lesion of PLAM. In the cytoplasm of smooth muscle cell, aggregated glycogen granules (G), dense bodies composed of accumulated actin microfilaments, and intermediate filaments are conspicuous. Dense bodies on cell membrane associated with discontinuous basement membrane (arrowheads) are found. Pinocytotic vesicle and coated vesicle (arrow) are not well developed. (×30,000.)

cells appears partially clear in light microscopic observation (15). In terms of the above findings, the cells resemble immature and blastic cells. Mitochondria and rough endoplasmic reticulum are well developed compared to those in normal smooth muscle cells (Fig. 2) (12,14,15). The rough endoplasmic reticulum in some cells is dilated. The Golgi apparatus is also well developed in the abnormal smooth muscle cells in PLAM (Fig. 3). Electron-dense granules, measuring 100–500 nm in diameter, are numerous adjacent to the Golgi apparatus in the cells (Fig. 1-4) (6,12,14). The mitochondria, rough endoplasmic reticulum, Golgi apparatus, and electron-dense granules are located close to the nucleus, whereas the cytoskeletal components are located at the periphery of the cells. The well-de-

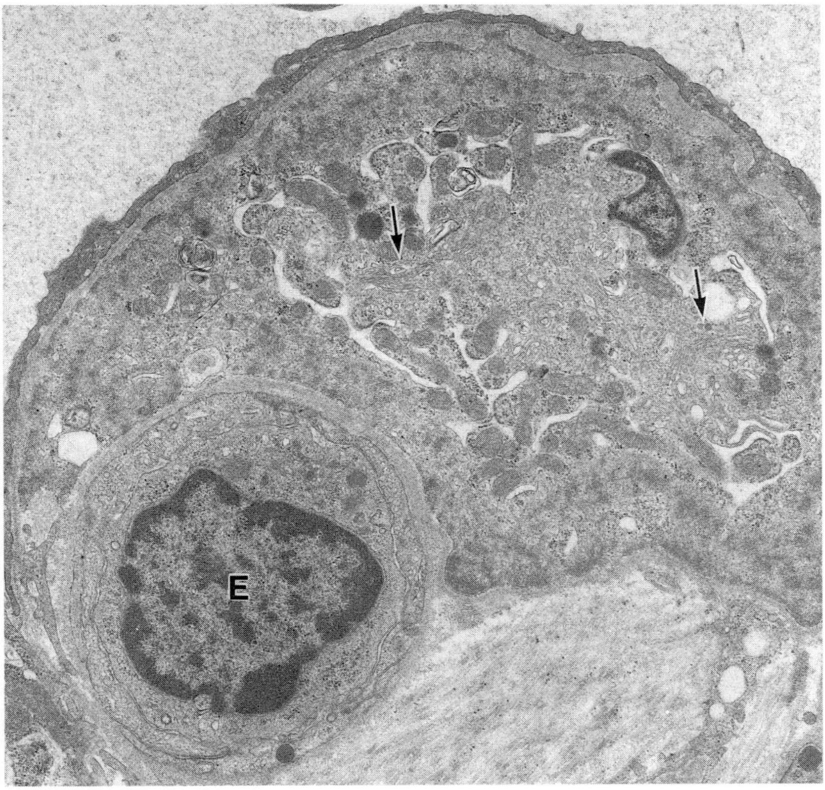

Figure 3 Early lesion of PLAM. Smooth muscle cell is located in peripheral alveolar wall. This cell shows well developed Golgi apparatus (arrows) and electron-dense granules. Mitochondria are relatively predominant. (×20,000.)

veloped features of these organelles indicate that these cells produce protein and suggest that they store it in granules and secrete the contents. As observed under high magnification, some granules have crystal-like lamellar structures and are surrounded by unit membranes (Fig. 4) (6,14). The periodicity of these lamellar structures is 6–10 nm. Other electron-dense granules are homogeneous in appearance, and some of them have fingerprint-like structures (Fig. 4).

The presence of cytoplasmic granules having crystal-like lamellar structures is characteristic of the abnormal smooth muscle cells in PLAM; normal smooth muscle cells do not have these granules. Similar granules consisting of crystal-like lamellar structures and surrounded by unit membranes have been detected in the cytoplasm of many types of cells: hemangioma and hemangioblastoma cells (18,19), alveolar soft part sarcoma cells (20), juxtaglomerular cell tumor cells

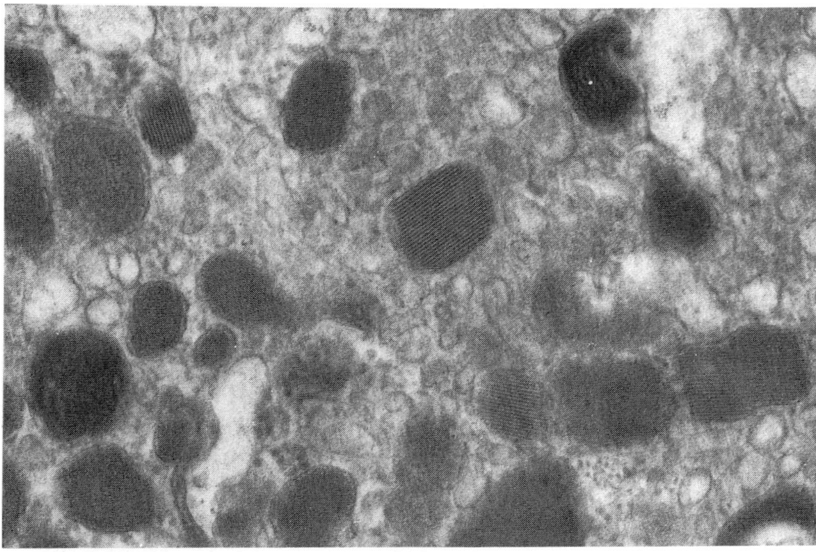

Figure 4 Early lesion of PLAM. High magnification of electron-dense granules of smooth muscle cell. Granules measuring up to 500 nm in diameter show lamellar structures having periodicity of 6–10 nm. Some granules show finger print-like structure (×54,000.) (From Ref. 6.)

(21), histiocytes associated with lymphoplasmacytic lymphoma (22), paraganglioma cells (23), oligodendroglioma cells (24), neuroepithelioma cells (25), and subependymal giant cell tumor cells of a patient with tuberous sclerosis (26). Even under a light microscope, large periodic acid Schiff stain–positive crystalloids are detected in these cells (20). However, the crystalloids in the abnormal smooth muscle cells of PLAM are usually too small to be detected by light microscopy. The proteins in some non–PLAM-cell cytoplasmic granules having crystalloids have been identified, such as renin in juxtaglomerular cell tumor cells (21) and immunoglobulin in histiocytes associated with lymphoplasmacytic lymphoma (22). It has been suggested that these proteins are stored and crystalized in the granules and show the lamellar structures in the granules. It is not known which proteins are stored in the granules in the abnormal smooth muscle cells in PLAM. Elastase is suspected to be present in these granules, because the elastic fibers exclusively located in the nests of abnormal smooth muscle cells in PLAM are degraded (6). Moreover, the abnormal smooth muscle cells in PLAM are positive for melanoma related marker HMB-45 (27). HMB-45 has not been detected in other smooth muscle cells and therefore is considered to be a good immunohistochemical marker for the cells of PLAM as well as melanoma cells (27,28). It has been suggested that the granules of PLAM are antigenically similar to premelanosomes, because in melanocytes HMB-45 is present in melanosome (29). HMB-45 has also been detected immunohistochemically in cells in PLAM-like lesions in tuberous sclerosis. In addition, ultrastructural crystalloid granules have been detected in the smooth muscle cells in uterine LAM-like lesions in tuberous sclerosis (30). The PLAM-like lesions associated with tuberous sclerosis are similar to PLAM lesions, and it is considered impossible to differentiate these two types of lesions in histological specimens of the lung (2,12,13).

Furthermore, numerous deposits of electron-dense granular material are present in the cytoplasm of some of the abnormal smooth muscle cells in PLAM. These deposits are especially numerous in such cells in early lesions, and they vary in size. They are surrounded by unit membranes and appear to have been phagocytosed by the cells. Energy dispersive x-ray microanalysis and light microscopic iron staining reveal the presence of iron in these deposits. These deposits are considered to be deposits of hemosiderin, which was phagocytosed by the cells.

B. Smooth Muscle Cells in Late Lesions

The smooth muscle cells in late and stable PLAM lesions are smaller and more compactly arranged than those in early PLAM lesions (Fig. 5) (6). The nucleus is small and convoluted, and the nucleolus is also small. The cytoplasm appears more dense, because the cell organelles are less conspicuous than those of the smooth muscle cells in early lesions. Actin microfilaments and intermediate filaments are compactly arranged, and dense bodies are frequently found. The mitochondria, Golgi apparatus, and rough endoplasmic reticulum are less well developed and the electron-dense granules are fewer in these cells than in early lesions (Fig. 5). However, crystal-like lamellar structures are found in some electron-dense granules in late PLAM lesions. Glycogen granules are also found in the abnormal smooth muscle cells in these lesions.

C. Other Cell Changes Associated with Accumulated Smooth Muscle Cells

Dilated vascular systems are found in association with accumulation of abnormal smooth muscle cells in PLAM. The endothelial cells of these vessels have less developed junctional structures and rest on an inconstant and discontinuous basement membrane because these vessels are part of the lymphatic system. The cytoplasm of the endothelial cells of these lymphatic vessels contains lipid droplets (12). The type I alveolar epithelial cells adjacent to the accumulated smooth muscle cells in early PLAM lesions are occasionally exfoliated. Type II alveolar epithelial cells are increased in number on the alveolar walls adjacent to the accumulated smooth muscle cells. Some capillary endothelial cells and interstitial cells locationally involved in the accumulation of smooth muscle cells in early

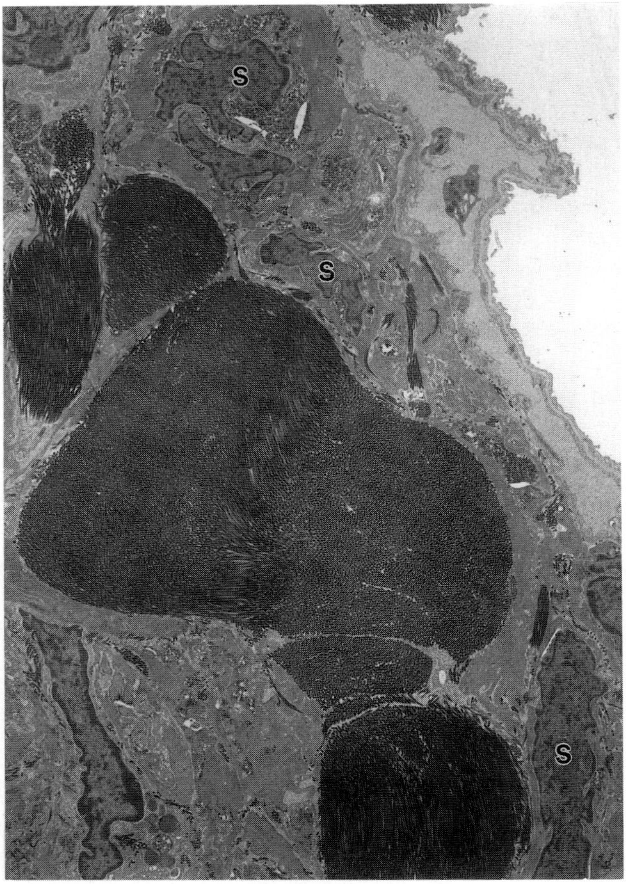

Figure 5 Late lesion of PLAM. Relatively small-sized smooth muscle cells (S) are found in an alveolar wall. Compare to the cell of an early lesion (Fig. 1). The cytoplasm appears more dense because cell organelles are less conspicuous compared to those of cells in the early lesion. Compactly accumulated collagen fibrils make thick bundles. (Tannic acid and double stain, ×4500.) (From Ref. 6.)

PLAM lesions are swollen (Fig. 1). Macrophages are increased in number and large and located not only in the alveolar spaces but also occasionally in the interstitium of alveolar walls. The cytoplasm of these macrophages contains a large amount of very electron-dense granular material, which has been confirmed with light microscopic iron staining and energy dispersive x-ray microanalysis to be hemosiderin. Multinucleated giant cells are occasionally found to be phagocytosing calcified and ferruginous elastic fibers in both early and late lesions.

III. Ultrastructure of ECM in PLAM

A. ECM in Early Lesions

The ECM of the lung is composed of basement membrane, collagen fibers, elastic fibers, other glycoproteins, and glycosaminoglycans. The main components of the basement membrane are type IV collagen, laminin, heparan sulfate glycosaminoglycan, and entactin. Basement membrane is present in alveolar walls, where it forms an air/blood blood barrier in cooperation with thin type I alveolar epithelial cells and capillary endothelial cells. Basement membrane is also present in basal layers of other epithelial cells, endothelial cells, mesothelial cells, and surrounding smooth muscle cells. Normally, the smooth muscle cells in bronchial, alveolar, and vascular walls are covered almost entirely by basement membrane. On the other hand, the basement membrane surrounding the abnormal smooth muscle cell in PLAM is discontinuous (Figs. 1,2). In some areas of smooth muscle cell accumulation in early lesions, the epithelial basement membrane is damaged and absent and contains fibrin deposits. Occasionally numerous electron-dense variously sized granules are present in the epithelial basement membrane and basement membrane–associated microfibrils (Figs. 6,7) (6,14). Energy dispersive

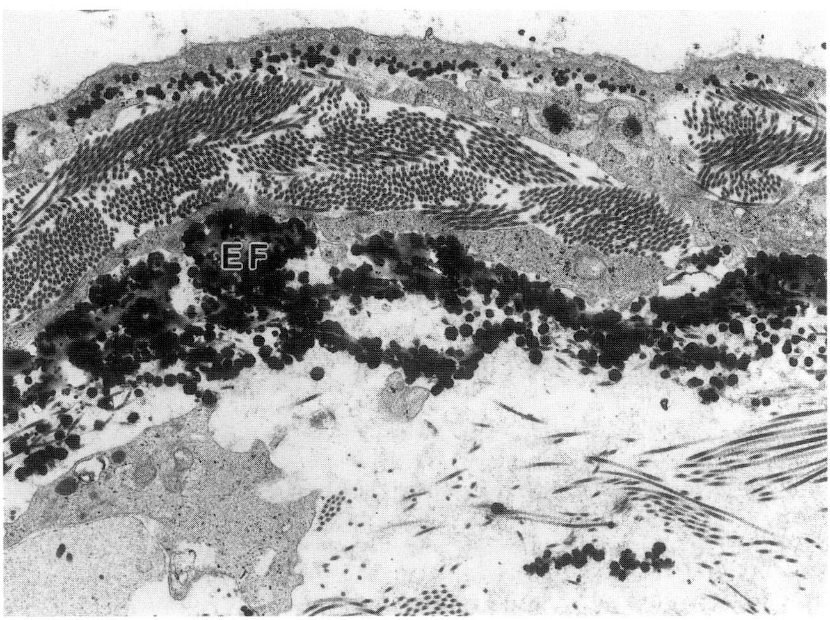

Figure 6 Early lesion of PLAM. Extracellular electron-dense materials deposit on epithelial basement membrane, basement membrane–associated microfibrils, elastic fibers (EF), and collagen fibrils in the edematous stroma, which is adjacent to the accumulated smooth muscle cells. (Tannic acid and double stain, ×6000.)

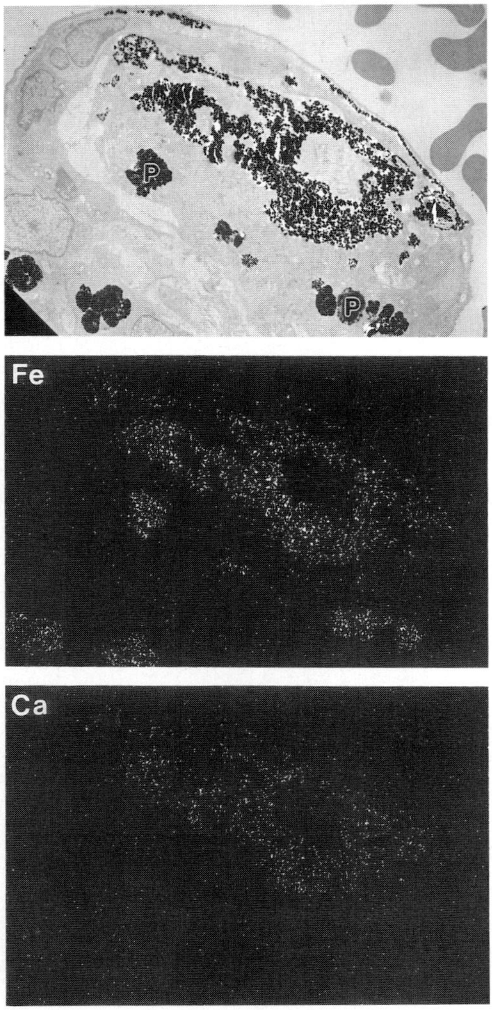

Figure 7 Early lesion of PLAM. Energy dispersive x-ray microanalysis. (Top) Electron microscopic picture without staining. (Middle) Fe: The existence of iron in the same ultrathin specimen is shown. Electron-dense materials on basement membrane and elastic fibers and intracellular phagocytosed materials (P) of smooth muscle cell are positive for iron. (Bottom) Ca: The existence of calcium in the same ultrathin specimen is shown. Dense deposits located on basement membrane and elastic fibers are positive for calcium, but intracellular phagocytosed materials (P) are negative for calcium. (×1500.)

x-ray microanalysis reveals the presence of calcium, iron, and phosphorus in these deposits (Fig. 7) (6). It has been suggested that the partial degradation of the basement membrane is responsible for the deposition of these granules.

In normal lungs, collagen fibers are present in bronchial, bronchiolar, alveolar, and vascular walls and the pleurae in association with or without elastic fibers. They are ultrastructurally composed of compactly arranged bundles of collagen fibrils. The presence of collagen fibers in the lung is important in that they provide resistance to mechanical tension. In PLAM, some collagen fibrils adjacent to accumulated smooth muscle cells are associated with electron-dense granules, which are similar to those present in the basement membrane (Fig. 6). Some collagen fibrils located close to the smooth muscle cells show spiraling in longitudinal sections and collagen flowers in cross sections (Fig. 8) (6,14). These collagen fibrils do not form bundles, but are randomly and loosely arranged. The pattern of cross-striation in the spiraling collagen fibrils is normal. Similar abnormal collagen fibrils have been detected in some hereditable connective tissue disorders in which the skin is hyperextensible and fragile, and in many other

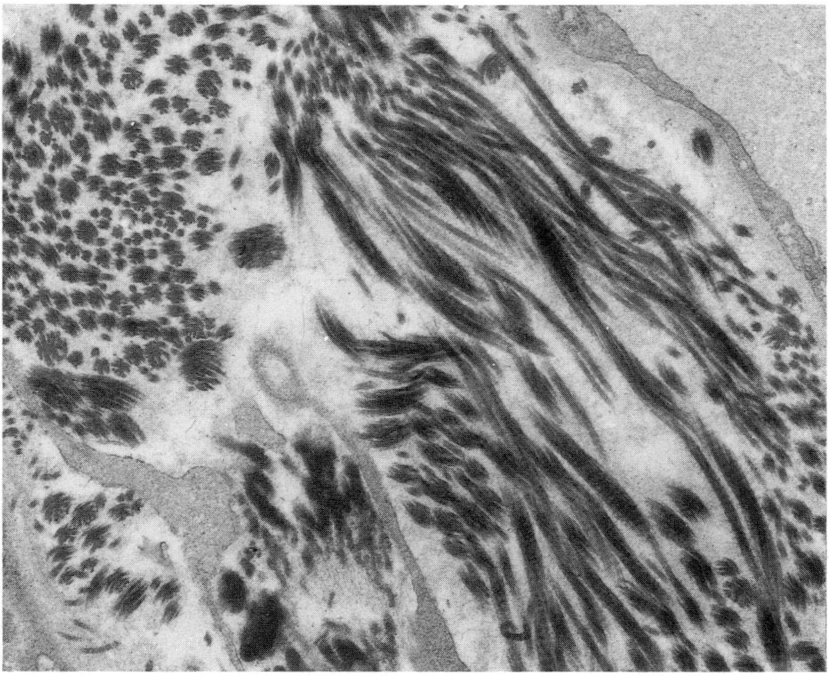

Figure 8 Early lesion of PLAM. Collagen fibrils adjacent to the accumulated smooth muscle cells show spiraling in longitudinal sections and collagen flowers in cross sections. (Tannic acid and double stain, ×25,000.)

conditions (32). In the lungs, such fibrils have been observed in experimentally induced emphysema (33) and pulmonary fibrosis (34) and in human emphysema (35) and idiopathic pulmonary fibrosis (36). It has been suggested that the partial degradation of the collagen fibrils is responsible for the formation of the spiraling fibrils. These abnormal collagen fibrils likely function insufficiently to prevent the mechanical tension of the alveolar walls.

Elastic fibers are present in areas subjected to mechanical stretching in normal lungs. They are normally present in association with collagen fibers and smooth muscle cells in bronchial and bronchiolar walls, alveolar ducts, tips of alveolar septa, and vascular walls. Elastic fibers are ultrastructurally composed of amorphous components and microfibrils. The amorphous components are biochemically polymerized elastin, and the microfibrils are composed of fibrillin and microfibril-associated proteins (37). The elastic fibers in early PLAM lesions are decreased in numbers, small, and aggregated in areas of smooth muscle cell accumulation. These fibers are surely not enough to provide elasticity in the lungs of LAM. They are irregularly outlined and frequently present in association with very electron-dense deposits (Figs. 6, 7) (6). Such electron-dense deposits are observed not only in alveolar wall elastic fibers but also in those in vascular walls adjacent to accumulated smooth muscle cells. These deposits have been found by energy dispersive x-ray microanalysis to be composed of calcium, iron, and phosphorus (Fig. 7) (6). Moreover, they are morphologically identical to the deposits observed in the basement membrane and collagen fibrils (Figs. 6,7). However, the deposits are more numerous in the elastic fibers than in the basement membrane and collagen fibrils. Calcium and calcium-like material deposition in elastic fibers has also been detected in emphysematous dilated alveolar walls in cases of experimental paraquat toxicity (34) and human emphysematous lungs (38). These deposits are well known to be present in the elastic laminae of arteriosclerotic vascular walls. It is easy to imagine that these fibers containing deposits of granular materials are not functionally elastic. The importance of elastic fiber degradation in the pulmonary structural remodeling in PLAM is discussed later.

B. ECM in Late Lesions

In late PLAM lesions, the accumulated smooth muscle cells are associated with fibrotic change. Ultrastructurally, large numbers of normal collagen fibrils form thick bundles, which are associated with the smooth muscle cell accumulation (Fig. 5). These collagen fibrils are thought to be newly formed in the disease process. Alveolar walls adjacent to the accumulated smooth muscle cells contain still spiraling collagen fibrils. Some of the collagen fibrils and epithelial basement membrane contain electron-dense deposits, though these deposits are fewer in the late than in the early lesions.

Elastic fibers are rarely found in areas of smooth muscle cell accumulation, and they are not long but short, round, and aggregated. Some elastic fibers in late PLAM lesions also contain deposits. Occasionally small amorphous components are found in association with accumulated smooth muscle cells (Fig. 9). These amorphous components are almost round and not associated with microfibrils. Some of the amorphous components are located at the cytoplasmic infoldings of smooth muscle cells. Such amorphous components without microfibrils have been observed in alveolar walls in emphysema (38) and experimental arteriosclerosis (39) and in the extracellular areas of the cultured pulmonary fibroblasts treated with lysyl oxidase inhibitor (40). In normal elastogenesis, secreted elastin and microfibril components together form elastic fibers adjacent to the cells from which they are secreted (37). Elastin deposition on microfibrils results in formation of a bundle of microfibrils, and mature amorphous components are formed at the center of such a bundle (40). It is suspected that these amorphous components without microfibrils are formed under some pathological conditions, for

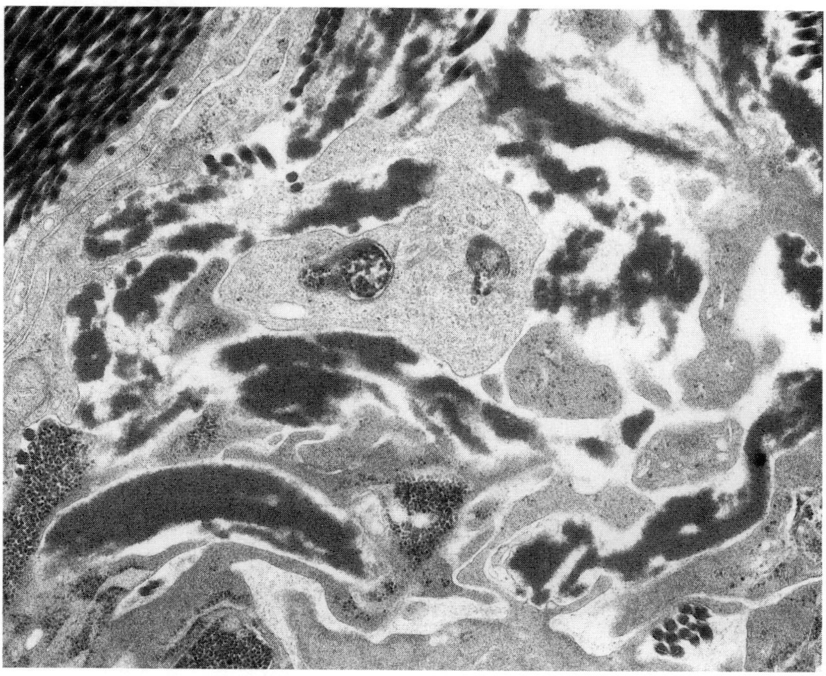

Figure 9 Late lesion of PLAM. Small-sized amorphous components of elastic fiber are located adjacent to the cytoplasmic infoldings of smooth muscle cells. These amorphous components are not associated with microfibrils. (Tannic acid and double stain, ×20,000.)

example, in cases of elastin and microfibril protein production imbalance. These amorphous components may not be able to display elasticity in the lung, because they are not located in a correct and effective area of the lung and are not fibrous but present as small and round masses.

IV. Pulmonary Structural Remodeling in PLAM

The LAM lung is known to contain multiple cysts and show signs of emphysematous change or honeycombing (1–3). However, the peripheral alveolar sacs in lobules in PLAM are not obliterated but are usually well preserved. Thus, the pulmonary structure of PLAM is not real honeycombing, but is very similar to centriacinar emphysema. Blebs and cystic dilated lymph vessels on the pleurae are also characteristic findings of PLAM. In ultrastructural and immunohis-

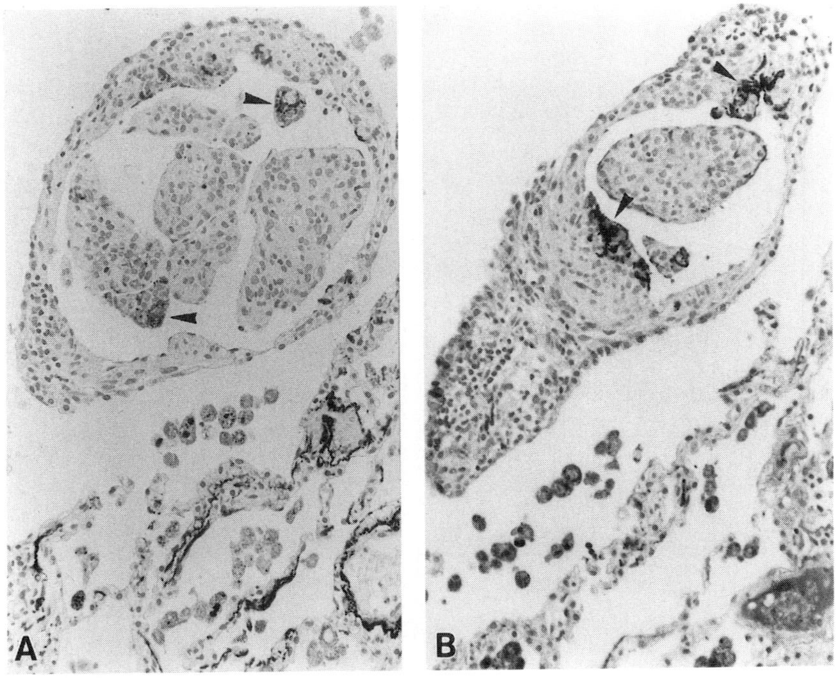

Figure 10 Light microscopic immunoperoxidase study of a late lesion of PLAM. (A) Anti-elastin antibody reacts with elastic fibers of alveolar walls and vessels. Elastic fibers (arrowheads) in the areas of smooth muscle cell accumulation are decreased, disrupted, and granular in appearance. (B) Serially sectioned specimen of Figure 10A. Elastic fibers (arrowheads) exclusively located in the areas of smooth muscle cell accumulation react with anti-α_1-antitrypsin antibody. (×200.) (From Ref. 6.)

tochemical studies involving detection of elastin and α_1-antitrypsin, the change of elastic fibers in PLAM has been found to be similar to emphysematous changes, blebs, and bullae in the lungs (38,41,42). The elastic fibers in areas of smooth muscle cell accumulation are not fibrous, but small and aggregated (Fig. 10). In electron microscopic pre-embedding immunohistochemical studies, some amorphous components of elastic fibers in areas of smooth muscle cell accumulation react with anti-elastin antibody (Fig. 11). The amorphous components of normal mature elastic fibers in alveolar walls far from the accumulated smooth muscle cells react evenly with anti-elastin antibody only at their periphery (Fig. 11). This finding is similar to that of normal lungs. It does not mean that the antigenicity of the central area of the amorphous components is lost; in fact, the cut end surface of such amorphous components reacts strongly with anti-elastin antibody. Moreover, in postembedding immunohistochemical studies, the amorphous

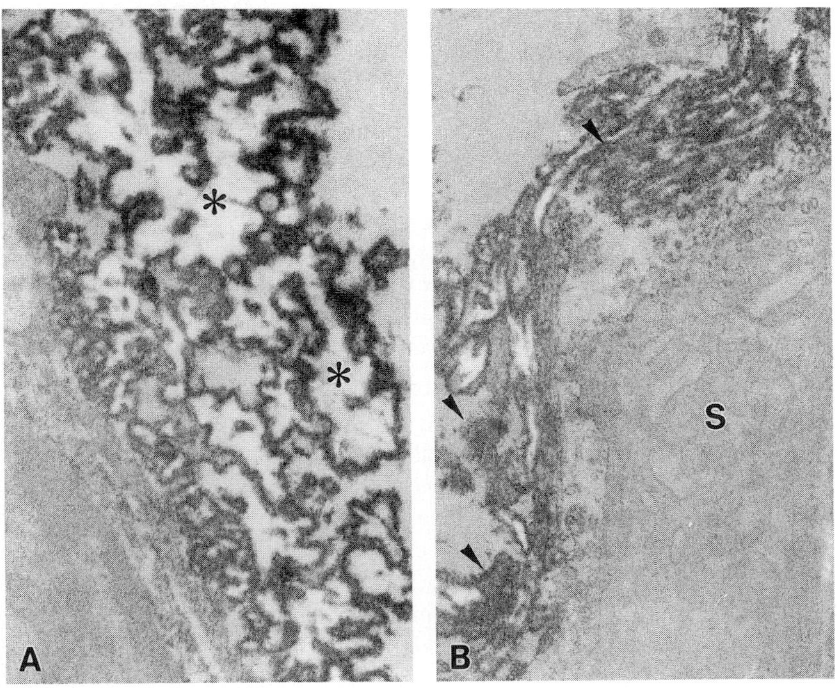

Figure 11 Electron microscopic immunoperoxidase study of an early lesion of PLAM. (A) Anti-elastin antibody reacts with elastic fibers of alveolar wall, which are distant from the area of smooth muscle cell accumulation, in the outer zones of amorphous components (asterisks). (B) Elastic fibers located in the area of smooth muscle cell (S) accumulation react evenly in their amorphous components (arrowheads) with anti-elastin antibody. (×20,000.) (From Ref. 6.)

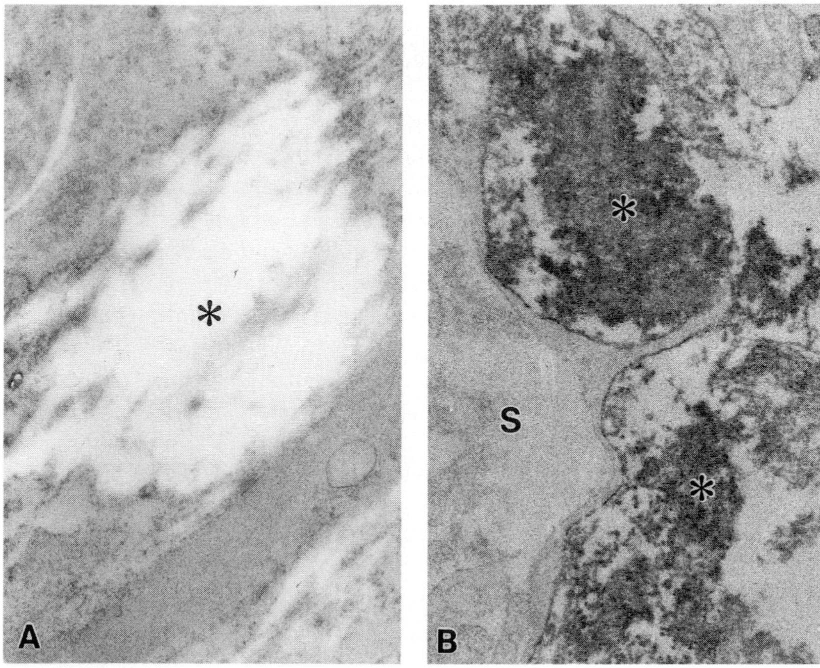

Figure 12 Electron microscopic immunoperoxidase study of an early lesion of PLAM. (A) Anti-α_1-antitrypsin antibody reacts poorly with elastic fiber (asterisk) distant from the area of smooth muscle cell accumulation. (×35,000.) (B) Amorphous components (asterisks) of elastic fibers in the area of smooth muscle cell (S) accumulation react evenly with anti-α_1-antitrypsin antibody. (×30,000.) (From Ref. 6.)

components of mature elastic fibers have been found to react evenly with anti-elastin antibody (43). It has been speculated that the antibody cannot penetrate into the mature amorphous components in pre-embedding methods (44,45). Amorphous components which are evenly stained with anti-elastin antibody are thought to be immature and somewhat cross-linked fibers in developing organs (44,45) or hydrolytic and degraded fibers in emphysematous lungs, blebs, and bullae (38,41,42). Elastic fibers containing amorphous components which are evenly stained with anti-elastin antibody in early PLAM lesions are probably degraded fibers (6). Calcium deposition in elastic fibers may be a consequence of damage to elastic fibers. It has been proposed that the elastic fibers are degraded in an early stage of PLAM when the patient shows severe clinical symptoms. At some point in the treatment of PLAM, the activity of the disease must be controlled. Although the structural changes of the lungs in PLAM associated with the degradation of ECM may be irreversible, the progress of the disease must be suppressed by appropriate therapy.

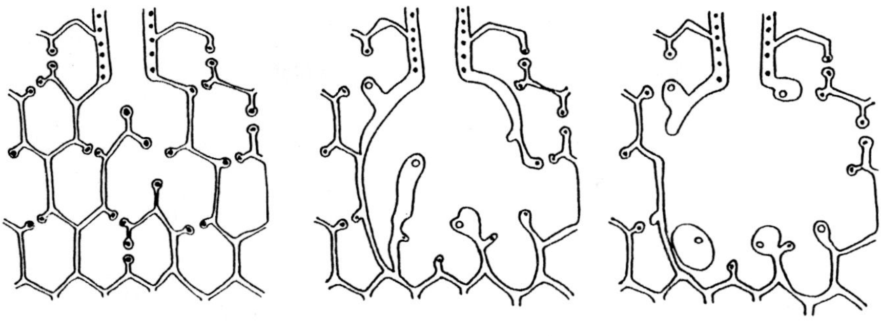

Figure 13 Diagram of pulmonary structural remodeling of PLAM. (A) Control lung. Elastic fibers (●) are located in alveolar walls and bronchial wall and keep the normal pulmonary structures. (B) Early stage of PLAM. Abnormal smooth muscle cell accumulations associated with degraded elastic fibers (○) are found in and around the emphysema-like lesion. These degraded elastic fibers react with ant- α_1-antitrypsin antibody. (C) Late stage of PLAM. Abnormal smooth muscle cells and increased collagen fibers make nodular structures around the emphysema-like lesion. Elastic fibers (○) in the areas of smooth muscle cell accumulation are also degraded and react with ant- α_1-antitrypsin antibody. (From Ref. 6.)

The abnormal elastic fibers in areas of smooth muscle cell accumulation react exclusively with anti–α_1-antitrypsin antibody in both early and late PLAM lesions (Fig. 10) (6). In addition, macrophages in intraalveolar spaces and serum in vessels react with anti–α_1-antitrypsin antibody. Moreover, in electron microscopic pre-embedding immunohistochemical studies, anti–α_1-antitrypsin antibody has been found to react evenly with amorphous components of elastic fibers (Fig. 12) (6). Normal elastic fibers in alveolar walls far from the accumulated smooth muscle cells do not react with anti–α_1-antitrypsin antibody (Fig. 12). These findings mean that α_1-antitrypsin is deposited exclusively in the morphologically abnormal elastic fibers. α_1-Antitrypsin is known to be a very strong inhibitor of serine proteinases including neutrophil elastase. Matrix metalloproteinases, which are important ECM proteinases, may also be involved in the pulmonary structural remodeling in PLAM. The function of these proteinases and antiproteinases is described in detail in other chapters of this book. Elastic fiber degradation by elastase due to an imbalance of elastase/α_1-antitrypsin is thought to be one of the mechanisms of development of emphysema (46). Abnormal elastic fibers in centriacinar emphysema, blebs, and bullae react evenly with anti–α_1-antitrypsin antibody (41,42). Although we do not have direct evidence of a correlation between elastase activity and the degradation of elastic fibers in PLAM, it has been suggested that both α_1-antitrypsin and elastase are present in the abnormal elastic fibers located in areas of smooth muscle cell accumulation in PLAM and are involved in degradation of elastic fibers. It has been reported that the elastase/α_1-antitrypsin complex exhibits elastolytic activity in vitro (47). Figure 13 shows a schematic of the process of pulmonary structural remodeling in PLAM. It has been proposed that the formation of emphysema-like lesions in PLAM is mediated by the degradation of elastic fibers and that this elastic fiber degradation is related to an imbalance of the elastase/α_1-antitrypsin system, similar to the probable pathogenesis of emphysema.

References

1. Dail DH. Uncommon tumors. In: DH Dail, Hammar SP, eds. Pulmonary Pathology. New York: Springer-Verlag, 1994:1279–1461.
2. Colby TV, Carrington CB. Interstitial lung disease. In: WM Thurlbeck, Churg AM, ed. Pathology of the Lung. New York: Thiem Medical Publishers, Inc., 1995:589–737.
3. Hasleton PS. Benign lung tumors and their malignant counterparts. In: Hasleton PS, ed. Spencer's Pathology of the Lung. New York: McGraw-Hill, 1996:875–986.
4. Corrin B, Leibow AA, Friedman PJ. Pulmonary lymphangiomyomatosis. A review. Am J Pathol 1975; 79:348–382.
5. Carrington CB, Cugell DW, Gaensler EA, Marks A, Redding RA, Schaff JT, Tomasian A. Lymphangioleiomyomatosis. Physiologic-pathologic-radiologic correlations. Am Rev Respir Dis 1977; 116:977–995.
6. Fukuda Y, Kawamoto M, Yamamoto A, Ishizaki M, Basset F, Masugi Y. Role of elastic fiber degradation in emphysema-like lesions of pulmonary lymphangiomyomatosis. Human Pathol 1990; 21:1252–1261.
7. Brentani MM, Carvalho CR, Saldiva PH, Pacheco MM, Oshima CT. Steroid receptors in pulmonary lymphangiomyomatosis. Chest 1984; 85:96–99.
8. Colley MH, Geppert E, Franklin WA. Immunohistochemical detection of steroid receptors in a case of pulmonary lymphangioleiomyomatosis. Am J Surg Pathol 1989; 13:803–807.
9. Banner AS, Carrington CB, Emory WB, Kittle F, Leonard G, Ringus J, Taylor P, Addington WW. Efficacy of oophorectomy in lymphangioleiomyomatosis and benign metastasizing leiomyoma. N Engl J Med 1981; 305:204–209.
10. Yockey CC, Riepe RE, Ryan K. Pulmonary lymphangioleiomyomatosis complicated by pregnancy. Kansas Med 1986; 87:277–278.
11. Sobonya RE, Quan SF, Fleishman JS. Pulmonary lymphangioleiomyomatosis: quantitative analysis of lesions producing airflow limitation. Human Pathol 1985, 16:1122–1128.
12. Wolff M. Lymphangiomyoma: clinicopathologic study and ultrastructural confirmation of its histogenesis. Cancer 1973; 31:988–1007.
13. Vazquez JJ, Fernandez-Cuervo L, Fidalgo B. Lymphangiomyomatosis: morphogenetic study and ultrastructural confirmation of the histogenesis of the lung lesion. Cancer 1976; 37:2321–2328.

14. Basset F, Soler P, Marsac J, Corrin B. Pulmonary lymphangiomyomatosis: three new cases studied with electron microscopy. Cancer 1976; 38:2357–2366.
15. Kane PB, Lane BP, Cordice JW, Greenberg GM. Ultrastructure of the proliferating cells in pulmonary lymphangiomyomatosis. Arch Pathol Lab Med 1978; 102:618–622.
16. Schiaffino E, Tavani E, Dellafiore L, Schmid C. Pulmonary lymphangiomyomatosis. Report of a case with immunohistochemical and ultrastructural findings. Appl Pathol 1989; 7:265–272.
17. Peyrol S, Gindre D, Cordier JF, Loire R, Grimaud JA. Characterization of the smooth muscle cell infiltrate and associated connective matrix of lymphangiomyomatosis. Immunohistochemical and ultrastructural study of two cases. J Pathol 1992; 168:387–395.
18. Ho KL. Ultrastructure of cerebellar capillary hemangioblastoma. III. Crystalloid bodies in endothelial cells. Acta Neuropathol 1985; 66:117–126.
19. Pasyk KA, Grabb WC, Cherry GW. Cellular haemangioma. Light and electron microscopic studies of two cases. Virchows Arch Pathol Anat Histol 1982; 396:103–126.
20. Mukai M, Torikata C, Iri H, Mikata A, Sakamoto T, Hanaoka H, Shinohara C, Baba N, Kanaya K, Kageyama K. Alveolar soft part sarcoma. An elaboration of a three-dimensional configuration of the crystalloids by digital image processing. Am J Pathol 1984; 116:398–406.
21. Camilleri JP, Hinglais N, Bruneval P, Bariety J, Tricottet V, Rouchon M, Mancilla-Jiminez R, Corvol P, Menard J. Renin storage and cell differentiation in juxtaglomerular cell tumors: an immunohistochemical and ultrastructural study of three cases. Human Pathol 1984; 15:1069–1079.
22. Harada M, Shimada M, Fukayama M, Kaneko T, Kitazume K, Weiss SW. Crystal-storing histiocytosis associated with lymphoplasmacytic lymphoma mimicking Weber-Christian disease: immunohistochemical, ultrastructural, and gene-rearrangement studies. Human Pathol 1996; 27:84–87.
23. Kyriacou K, Shipkey FH, Loewen R. Crystalloid structures in retroperitoneal paragangliomas: a light and electron microscopic study. Ultrastruct Pathol 1991; 15:57–67.
24. Sarasa JL, Ramon y Cajal Agueras S, Burzaco J. Crystals in an oligodendroglioma: an optical, histochemical, and ultrastructural study. Ultrastruct Pathol 1990; 14:151–159.
25. Torikata C, Mukai M, Kageyama K. Spontaneous olfacatory neuroepithelioma in a domestic medaka (*Oryzias latipes*). Cancer Res 1989; 49:2994–2998.
26. Jay V, Edwards V, Rutka JT. Crystalline inclusions in a subependymal giant cell tumor in a patient with tuberous sclerosis. Ultrastruct Pathol 1993; 17:503–513.
27. Bonetti F, Chiodera PL, Pea M, Martignoni G, Bosi F, Zamboni G, Mariuzzi GM. Transbronchial biopsy in lymphangiomyomatosis of the lung. HMB45 for diagnosis. Am J Surg Pathol 1993; 17:1092–1102.
28. Tanaka H, Imada A, Morikawa T, Shibusa T, Satoh M, Sekine K, Abe S. Diagnosis of pulmonary lymphangioleiomyomatosis by HMB45 in surgically treated spontaneous pneumothorax. Eur Respir J 1995; 8:1879–1882.
29. Bonetti F, Pea M, Martignoni G, Zamboni G, Iuzzolino P. Cellular heterogeneity in

lymphangiomyomatosis of the lung [letter; comment]. Human Pathol 1991; 22:727–728.
30. Kimura O, Watanabe M, F. D, Kitamoto T, Nakura H. An autopsy case of tuberous sclerosis complicated with pulmonary lymphangiomyomatosis, renal and hepatic angiomyolipoma and uterine adenomyosis. 42nd Annual Meeting of The Japanese Society of Pathology, Nov 7-8, 1996.
31. Capron F, Ameille J, Leclerc P, Morent P, Barbagellata M, Reynes M, Rochemaure J. Pulmonary lymphangioleiomyomatosis and Bourneville's tuberous sclerosis with pulmonary involvement: the same disease? Cancer 1983; 52:851–855.
32. Ghadially FN. Extracellular matrix (extracellular components). In: Ghadially FN, ed. Ultrastructural Pathology of the Cell and Matrix. London: Butterworths, 1982:881–947.
33. Stephens RJ, Freeman G, Evans MJ. Ultrastructural changes in connective tissue in lungs of rats exposed to NO_2. Arch Intern Med 1971; 127:873–883.
34. Fukuda Y, Ferrans VJ, Schoenberger CI, Rennard SI, Crystal RG. Patterns of pulmonary structural remodeling after experimental paraquat toxicity. The morphogenesis of intraalveolar fibrosis. Am J Pathol 1985; 118:452–475.
35. Belton JC, Crise N, McLaughlin RF, Jr., Tueller EE. Ultrastructural alterations in collagen associated with microscopic foci of human emphysema. Human Pathol 1977; 8:669–677.
36. Crystal RG, Fulmer JD, Baum BJ, Bernardo J, Bradley KH, Bruel SD, Elson NA, Fells GA, Ferrans VJ, Gadek JE, Hunninghake GW, Kawanami O, Kelman JA, Line BR, McDonald JA, McLees BD, Roberts WC, Rosenberg DM, Tolstoshev P, Von Gal E, Weinberger SE. Cells, collagen and idiopathic pulmonary fibrosis. Lung 1978; 155:199–224.
37. Mecham RP, Prosser IW, Fukuda Y. Elastic fibers. In: Crystal RG, West JB, Barnes PJ, Cherniack NS, Weibel ER, eds. The Lung: Scientific Foundations. New York: Raven Press, Ltd., 1991:389–398.
38. Fukuda Y, Masuda Y, Ishizaki M, Masugi Y, Ferrans VJ. Morphogenesis of abnormal elastic fibers in lungs of patients with panacinar and centriacinar emphysema. Human Pathol 1989; 20:652–659.
39. Katsuda S, Kajikawa K. Elastogenesis in experimental arteriosclerosis of rabbits. J Electron Microsc 1977; 26:111–119.
40. Fukuda Y, Nakazawa N, Yamanaka N. Interactions of elastin and microfibrils in elastogenesis of human pulmonary fibroblasts in culture. Connect Tiss Res 1993; 29:301–310.
41. Haraguchi S, Fukuda Y. Histogenesis of abnormal elastic fibers in blebs and bullae of patients with spontaneous pneumothorax: ultrastructural and immunohistochemical studies. Acta Pathol Jpn 1993; 43:709–722.
42. Fukuda Y, Ishizaki M, Masugi Y. Distribution of elastin and alpha-1 antitrypsin in emphysematous lungs. Connect Tiss (Tokyo) 1990; 21:27–28.
43. Damiano VV, Tsang A, Christner P, Rosenbloom J, Weinbaum G. Immunologic localization of elastin by electron microscopy. Am J Pathol 1979; 96:439–455.
44. Fukuda Y, Ferrans VJ. The electron microscopic immunohistochemistry of elastase-treated aorta and nuchal ligament of fetal and postnatal sheep. J Histochem Cytochem 1984; 32:747–756.

45. Fukuda Y, Ferrans VJ, Crystal RG. Development of elastic fibers of nuchal ligament, aorta, and lung of fetal and postnatal sheep: an ultrastructural and electron microscopic immunohistochemical study. Am J Anat 1984; 170:597–629.
46. Gadek JE, Hunninghake GW, Fells GA, Zimmerman RL, Keogh BA, Crystal RG. Evaluation of the protease-antiprotease theory of human destructive lung disease. Bull Eur Physiopathol Respir 1980; 16:27–40.
47. Martin WJ, Taylor JC. Abnormal interaction of alpha$_1$-antitrypsin and leukocyte elastolytic activity in patients with chronic obstructive pulmonary disease. Am Rev Respir Dis 1979; 120:411–419.

13

Regulation of Cell Cycle Progression in Vascular Smooth Muscle Cells

Breaking the Cycle

HENRICUS J. DUCKERS, MANFRED BÖHM, ZHI YONG YANG, and ELIZABETH G. NABEL

University of Michigan Medical Center
Ann Arbor, Michigan

I. Cell Cycle Control: Introduction

Acute and chronic arterial injuries generate a complex process of proliferative, inflammatory and thrombotic responses in vascular cells, which contribute to vascular pathologies, such as atherosclerosis and restenosis. This process of vascular smooth muscle cell (VSMC) migration and proliferation is also the major delimiter of the long-term success of peripheral and coronary artery percutaneous interventions. In 25–50% of atherosclerotic coronary lesions treated by percutaneous intervention, restenosis occurs irrespective of the device employed (balloon angioplasty, atherectomy, or laser angioplasty) (1). The neointima formation after arterial injury is characterized by a regulated series of events including intimal VSMC migration and proliferation, subsequent extracellular matrix synthesis and deposition, followed by cell replication inhibition and connective tissue remodeling (2). In this chapter, we provide an overview of the regulatory mechanisms involved in VSMC growth, which play an eminent role in these vascular diseases. While the mechanisms that stimulate VSMC proliferation are well described, the mechanisms that limit formation of the neointima are not well understood.

Considerable progress has been made recently in the identification of cell cycle inhibitory proteins. Originally defined in budding yeast, the cyclin-dependent kinase inhibitors (CKIs) have mammalian homologs, which have been shown to inhibit the interaction of cyclins and cyclin-dependent kinase in different stages of the cell cycle (3). Mutations and homologous deletions in a number of these cell cycle proteins have been associated with primary tumors, including hereditary melanoma and Wilms' tumor (4). The cyclin-dependent kinase inhibitors are also involved in the pathogenesis of vascular proliferative diseases, such as angiogenesis, atherosclerosis, and restenosis. These CKIs are of considerable interest as genetic treatments for vascular proliferative disorders. In this chapter, we will summarize the advances made in the vascular gene therapies targeting cell cycle regulatory pathways in human vascular proliferative diseases.

II. The Mammalian Cell Cycle Clock

Cell cycle progression and senescence is controlled by a regulatory mechanism composed of multiple cyclins, their cyclin-dependent kinase (CDK) counterparts, and regulatory kinases and phosphatases (5). In the first phase (G_1) of the cell cycle, the cell is susceptible to growth factor stimulation, which triggers intracellular signaling cascades that initiate the cell cycle. Once the cell has passed the G_1/S checkpoint, the cell becomes refractory to growth factor–induced signaling and is committed to complete the S/G_2 and M phase of the cycle. Cyclin-dependent kinase complexes are composed of a catalytic CDK subunit and a positive regulatory subunit, the cyclin. The differential expression and relative affinities of the cyclins to the CDKs and their rapid proteolysis allows for sequential complex formation of the CDKs to the cyclins D, E, A, and B through G_1 and G_2 phases of the cell cycle (6).

In mammalian cells, progression through the early G_1 phase is dependent on cyclin D–CDK4 and 6 complex formation, whereas cyclin E and A–CDK2 complexes are thought to be essential for the late G_1-S phase progression. The retinoblastoma gene product inhibits cell cycle progression from G_1 into S phase by sequestering and inactivating a set of cellular transcription factors, including E2F and Elf-1 (7). After cell cycle activation, Rb is rapidly phosphorylated and the Rb–E2F and Rb–Elf-1 complexes are thereby disrupted. The release of these transcription factors is associated with progression through the G_1/S checkpoint of the cell cycle and DNA synthesis in the S phase. The complex formed between cyclin B and cdc2 kinase is required for progression from G_2 through the M phases. Degradation of cyclin B allows the cell to proceed through the M phase. The enzymatic activity of CDK2 in association with either cyclin E or A, necessary for G_1 progression, is controlled posttranscriptionally by threonine and tyrosine phosphorylation, mediated by regulatory kinases (CDK-activating kinases) and phosphatases (CDK inhibitors) (6,8).

III. Cell Cycle Inhibitory Proteins: Breaking the Cycle

Several models of G_1 cell cycle arrest have been explored in mammalian cells including the effects on DNA damage by ionizing radiation, growth inhibitory factors (TGF-β), cytostatic drugs (lovastatin, rapamycin), cell-cell contact, and mitogen deprivation. These studies demonstrate that the primary mechanisms of cell cycle control in response to a variety of cyclin-dependent signals is mediated at the level of CKIs that inhibit CDK activities via stoichiometric binding and inactivation (4).

The p53 tumor suppressor gene was the first cell cycle regulatory protein identified and is the most commonly mutated gene in human neoplasia. Following DNA damage, p53 delays the G_1 phase progression to allow DNA repair before entry into S and M phase (9). The ability of p53 to either reversibly arrest G_1 cell cycle progression or induce apoptosis is partly due to its capacity to bind specific DNA sequences and to transactivate target genes such as p21 $^{CIP1/WAF1}$ and Gadd45 (10), although both of these genes can be induced by other pathways. Both apoptosis and G_1 arrest are physiological mechanisms for regulating cell growth. Jacks and coworkers showed that tumors devoid of the p53 tumor suppressor gene were resistant to radiation or chemotherapeutic therapy but found relapse in p53-expressing tumors, demonstrating a p53-dependent signal transduction pathway linking DNA damage to cell cycle control and apoptosis. p53 knockout mice and humans carrying mutant p53 genes (Li Fraumeni syndrome) develop normally except for a predisposition to malignant tumors (11). Recently, a relative of p53 has been identified, designated p73, which appears not only to resemble p53 structurally but also may have similar functions (12). p73 activates the transcription of p53-responsive genes and inhibit cell growth in a p53-like manner by inducing apoptosis. p73 has been mapped on the short arm of chromosome 1, a site thought to harbor tumor suppressor genes.

The CKIs modulate the phosphorylation state and enzymatic activity of cyclin–CDK complexes necessary for G_1 progression. The CKIs can be divided into two families based on protein sequence homology and their putative CDK targets: the KIP/CIP family and the INK family. Three members of the KIP/CIP family have been identified thus far: p21$^{CIP1/WAF1}$, p27^{KIP1}, and p57^{KIP2}, named after their apparent molecular mass on SDS electrophoresis gels. These proteins contain distinct CDK and cyclin-binding domains near the amino terminus, which share sequence homology. In contrast to the INK family proteins, the KIP/CIP family binds to and inhibits most of the cyclin–CDK complexes. p21$^{CIP1/WAF1}$, also known as WAF1, CIP1, SDI1, is a downstream target of the p53 tumor suppressor gene and directly inhibits the kinase activities of several G_1 cyclin–CDK complexes. Induction of p53 in response to DNA damage results in G_1 prolongation, at which point DNA repair is accomplished prior to DNA replication in S phase. $p21^{CIP1/WAF1}$ also inhibits PCNA-dependent DNA replication and repair in the absence of a cyclin/CDK (13). Recently, facilitation of transcriptional activation of NF-κb by $p21^{CIP1/WAF1}$ was described, providing a mechanism whereby $p21^{CIP1/WAF1}$ also alters the expression of genes involved in cellular adhesion and differentiation (14). Overexpression of $p21^{CIP1/WAF1}$ in vitro results in cell cycle exit and terminal differentiation, but no apoptosis, in normal and transformed malignant cell lines (15). Deletion of the $p21^{CIP1/WAF1}$ locus is associated with enhanced proliferation, but has no effect on differentiation. $p21^{CIP1/WAF1}$-null mice undergo normal development . and are fully fertile, suggesting that $p21^{CIP1/WAF1}$ is not required for normal cell cycle function or that $p21^{CIP1/WAF1}$ function during embryogenesis has an abundant functional redundancy (16).

The $p27^{KIP1}$ gene encodes for an inducible CDK2 inhibitor and has been implicated in G_1 arrest in response to TGF-β, cell-cell contact, agents that elevate cAMP, and the growth-inhibitory drug rapamycin (17,18). $p27^{KIP1}$ binds to and inhibits complexes formed by cyclin E–CDK2 and cyclin A–CDK2. Regulation of $p27^{KIP1}$ activity occurs mainly by degradation in the ubiquitin-proteasome pathway (19). Clurman et al. recently showed in NIH 3T3 cell cultures that $p27^{KIP1}$ functions primarily as a CDK inhibitor at low ATP concentrations (20). However, at ATP concentrations approaching physiological levels, $p27^{KIP1}$ is directly phosphorylated by cyclin E–CDK2, resulting in a rapid elimination of the CKI from the cell and transition of the cells from G_1 to S phase. This suggests that $p27^{KIP1}$ is a substrate rather than an inhibitor of the kinase complex. Furthermore, the presence of other CKIs (in particular, $p15^{INK4b}$, which competes for cyclin D–CDK4 binding with $p27^{KIP1}$ in vivo and in vitro (21), the localization of $p27^{KIP1}$ in the cell (22), and $p27^{KIP1}$ concentration relative to the cyclin D and E content (4) all seem to affect $p27^{KIP1}$ activity. Disruption of the $p27^{KIP1}$ gene in mice results in an increase in animal size and cellularity of many adult organs and a predisposition to develop pituitary tumors (23,24). The increased size is attributed to benign hyperplasia leading to enlargement of tissues that normally express $p27^{KIP1}$ at high levels. Female $p27^{KIP1}$-deficient mice are sterile due to an impaired luteal cell differentiation and a disordered estrogen cycle. Cell cycle arrest induced by TGF-β, rapamycin, or contact inhibition is unaffected in $p27^{KIP1}$-/- cells, suggesting that $p27^{KIP1}$ is not essential in these pathways. The lack of gross developmental defects in $p21^{CIP1/WAF1}$-null and $p27^{KIP1}$-null mice suggests the existence of compensatory mechanisms during embryogenesis that rescue the phenotype of these CKI-deficient mice.

$p57^{KIP2}$ is a potent inhibitor of all G_1 and S phase CDKs, including cyclin E-ck2, cyclin D2-CDK4, and cyclin A-CDK2 (25,26). The gene encoding for

$p57^{KIP2}$ is paternally imprinted in humans and mice and is located at chromosome 11p15.5, a site implicated in human cancers including breast, bladder, lung, ovary, kidney, and testicle (25). Rearrangements at 11pl5 and $p57^{KIP2}$ mutations have also been described in patients with Beckwith Wiedemann syndrome, a cancer-predisposing syndrome (27). In mammalian cells, $p57^{KIP2}$ is localized in the nucleus and, when overexpressed, causes cell cycle arrest in G_1 phase. $p57^{KIP2}$ can be distinguished from $p21^{CIPl/WAF1}$ and $p27^{KIP1}$ by its unique domain structure. In humans, $p57^{KIP2}$ consists of three structurally distinct domains following a heterogeneous amino-terminal region: an aminoterminal CDK-inhibitory domain with similarity to $p21^{CIP1/Waf1}$ and $p27^{KIP1}$; a region containing alternating proline-alanine repeats (papa repeats); and a carboxy-terminal nuclear-targeting domain that contains a putative CDK phosphorylation site (25,26). The $p57^{KIP2}$ carboxy-terminal domain (QT domain) has sequence conservation with the carboxy terminus of $p27^{KIP1}$ but not $p21^{CIP1/WAF1}$. It likely functions in protein–protein interactions. Structure-activity studies, however, indicate that the murine QT domain and the internal domains have no effect on cell cycle distribution in vitro. Alternative splicing at the amino-terminus of $p57^{KIP2}$ generates heterogenicity of the translational initiation and results in at least three different splice forms of human $p57^{KIP2}$ (28). In contrast to widespread expression of $p21^{CIP1/WAF1}$ and $p27^{KIP1}$ in human tissue, $p57^{KIP2}$ is expressed in a tissue-specific manner in the placenta, skeletal muscle, brain, eye, kidney, and heart (25,28). The unique properties of $p57^{KIP2}$ within the KIP/CIP family is also underscored by observations made in $p57^{KIP2}$ knockout mice. While disruption of $p21^{CIP1/WAF1}$ or $p27^{KIP1}$ does not lead to gross developmental defects, deletion in the $p57^{KIP2}$ locus of mice is lethal, in part in utero and in part postnatal. These $p57^{KIP2}$-null animals have major defects in the formation of the palate, lens, intestine, and endochondral bone formation (29). Histological examination of the tissue demonstrates a significant increase in apoptotic cells in the palate, gastrointestinal smooth muscle cells, and lens fiber cells, as well as impaired terminal differentiation of chondrocytes and increased cell numbers in the epiphysial zone due to inappropriate cell proliferation.

The INK4 family members—$p15^{INK4B}$, $p16^{INK4A}$, $p18^{INK4C}$, and $p19^{INK4D}$—all contain four copies of sequences resembling ankyrin repeats and specifically inhibit CDK4 and CDK6, thereby controlling Rb phosphorylation and release of the E2F transcription factor (4). In addition, they have also been shown to compete with cyclin D for binding to CDK4 and 6 and thus disrupt cyclin D–CDK association and prevent the formation of the active kinase complexes (30).

The $pl6^{INK4A}$ is the gene product of the multiple tumor suppressor gene 1 (MTS-1), mapped to chromosome 9p21-22 (31). It is frequently deleted and inactivated by nonsense mutations in a wide spectrum of human cancers, including hereditary melanoma and pancreatic cancer (32). $p16^{INK4A}$ specifically binds to and inactivates a quaternary complex consisting of CDK4, cyclin D, and Rb.

In vivo and in vitro, p16^{INK4A} associates with CDK4 and CDK6 to form stable binary complexes lacking cyclin Dl (30). Mice carrying a targeted deletion of p16^{INK4A} show no gross congenital defects but are prone to spontaneous tumorigenesis, suggesting that INK4A is not essential for viability or organogenesis (33). pl6 -/- mice do display features consistent with abnormal extramedullary hematopoiesis, implicating pl6^{INK4A} as a regulator of proliferation of some hematopoietic lineages or their progenitors. Considering that Rb is the main target of pl6^{INK4A} function, these observations are consistent with the various hematological abnormalities seen in Rb -/- mice (34,35).

The MTS2 gene is located in the vicinity of MTS1 (9p2l-22) and encodes a 15 kDa protein, p15^{INK4B}, which inhibits cyclin D–CDK6 and cyclin D–CDK4 kinase activity (36). This recently characterized regulatory gene product shares homology with pl6^{INK4A}. Since high titers of pl5^{INK4B} are induced following exposure to TGF-β, it is speculated that pl5^{INK4B} may be an effector of TGF-β-induced cell cycle arrest at the G_1/S transition through CDK4 and CDK6 kinase inhibition. Alternatively, P15^{INK4B} competes with p27^{KIP1} for binding to the cyclin D–dependent kinases (21). Since pl5^{INK4B} has prior access to the CDK4 complex in the cytoplasm, p27^{KIP1} binding to these CDK complexes in the cell nucleus is prevented, and p27^{KIP1} binds and inhibits cyclin–CDK2 (22). Since TGF-β induces pl5^{INK4B} mRNA, p15^{INK4B} activity appears to be regulated at the transcriptional level.

pl8^{INK4C} encodes for a protein with structural and functional homology to pl6^{INK4A} (30,37). It binds strongly to CDK6 and to a lesser degree CDK4 to form binary inactive kinase complexes. The pl8^{INK4C} gene has been mapped to chromosome 1p32, which is known for deletions in several tumors. However, despite the apparent structural and functional similarities with p16^{INK4A}, screening of different malignant cell lines and primary tumors does not show pl8^{INK4C} gene inactivation (30). Furthermore, unlike pl6^{INK4A}, p18^{INK4C} expression is largely independent of Rb status, and no relationship seems to exist between the expression of pl6^{INK4A} and pl8^{INK4C}. In humans, pl8^{INK4C} is mainly expressed in skeletal muscle, pancreas, and heart. pl9^{INK4D} binds and inactivates CDK4 and CDK6 and is expressed ubiquitous in normal tissue (38). Like pl8^{INK4C}, transcription of pl9^{INK4D} mRNA is rapidly upregulated as the cells approach the G_1/S transition.

IV. Cell Cycle Control in Vascular Proliferative Disorders

In vascular diseases, such as restenosis and atherosclerosis, neointimal VSMC proliferation plays a central role. Vascular smooth muscle cells are predominantly located in the tunica media of the arterial wall and are normally maintained in a nonproliferative, differentiated state in vivo. Unlike skeletal muscle cells, VSMC reenter the cell cycle upon injury or growth factor stimulation. Arterial injury results in the migration of VSMC into the intima, where smooth muscle cells proliferate and synthesize extracellular matrix components (2,39). These processes cause the intima to expand and gradually encroach on the arterial lumen.

While many vascular studies have focused on identification of growth factors and cytokine genes that stimulate vascular cell proliferation, attention has now shifted to analysis of regulatory pathways which govern cell cycle progression, senescence, and differentiation. The use of gene transfer and the ability to manipulate mouse genetics have proven to be powerful tools to identify the role of different genes in the pathogenesis of vascular proliferative diseases in vivo, including the mechanisms by which cell proliferation contributes to the formation of neointima.

Primary smooth muscle cell cultures express $p21^{CIP1/WAF1}$ when arrested in G_1 by serum deprivation, and recombinant $p21^{CIP1/WAF1}$ gene expression inhibit endothelial and VSMC growth in vitro (15,40). $p21^{CIP1/WAF1}$ is not constitutively expressed in normal quiescent arteries, but is induced after arterial balloon injury in porcine iliofemoral arteries. In the pig model, intimal VSMC proliferation typically is detected in the neointima as early as 2 days after injury (41). Intimal VSMC proliferation peaks at 7 days, with 15–20% of cells dividing, and returns to basal values (2%) by day 14. The expression pattern of endogenous $p21^{CIP1/WAF1}$ gene product inversely correlates with the kinetics and localization of VSMC proliferation (42). $p21^{CIP1/WAF1}$ protein was expressed at increased levels at 7–21 days after injury in VSMC, when intimal cell proliferation is declining. $p21^{CIP1/WAF1}$ immunostaining was most prominent in the lower region of the neointima adjacent to the internal elastic lamina. This region does not contain detectable proliferating cells and is associated with TGF-β expression and procollagen synthesis (43). These findings suggest that the $p21^{CIP1/WAF1}$ gene product might limit intimal smooth muscle proliferation after arterial injury by inducing G_1/G_0 arrest in VSMC, possibly in conjunction with other TGF-β–inducible CKIs, such as $p27^{KIP1}$. The expression pattern of $p21^{CIP1/WAF1}$ can be explained by upregulation of $p21^{CIP1/WAF1}$ and $p27^{KIP1}$ expression after cell-matrix contact with type I fibrillar collagen mediated by integrin signaling, as recently shown by studies of Ross and coworkers (44). Vascular smooth muscle cells may migrate into the neointima and interact with the neointimal matrix through specific membrane receptors of the integrin family, leading to activation of intracellular signaling pathways, decrease in focal adhesion sites, upregulation of CKIs, and eventually inhibition of migration, cell cycle withdrawal, and cell differentiation. In vivo, ADV-$p21^{CIP1/WAF1}$ infection of porcine arteries following balloon injury reduces BrdU incorporation by 35% and I/M area ratio by 37% (42). These studies indicate that direct gene transfer of a CDK inhibitor can reduce VSMC growth and thereby reduce intimal hyperplasia. Similar findings were described in the rat carotid artery model of restenosis where adenovirus-mediated $p21^{CIP1/WAF1}$ infection reduced the extent of intimal hyperplasia (40).

The retinoblastoma gene product (Rb) inhibits cell cycle progression in many mammalian cell types by sequestering transcription factors required for G_1/S transition (7). The effects of many cyclin–CDK and CKI interactions are mediated through their effect on the phosphorylation status and therefore activity of Rb. Chang et al. suggested that Rb also plays a critical role in regulating the proliferation of VSMC, both in response to growth factor stimulation in vitro and to injury in vivo (45). Localized infection of porcine endothelial cells and VSMC with ADV-ΔRb, an unphosphorylatable, constitutively active Rb, results in a significant reduction in cell proliferation, yet cells remain viable, suggesting that ADV-ΔRb–infected cells represents cell cycle arrest as opposed to cell death. Likewise, ADV-ΔRb infection inhibits [^{3}H]thymidine incorporation, supporting the hypothesis that ΔRb gene expression arrests VSMC proliferation before entry into the S phase. In the rat carotid artery injury as well as in the pig balloon injury model, transgenic ΔRb expression results in a 42–47% decrease in the neointima/media area ratio relative to control arteries. The degree of inhibition of cell proliferation and intimal hyperplasia by the ADV-ΔRb gene transfer is comparable to that achieved by $p21^{CIP1/WAF1}$ or $p27^{KIP1}$.

Other genetic interventions addressing cell cycle regulatory proteins in the cardiovascular system comprise the use of antisense oligonucleotides against PCNA and cdc2 kinase in rabbit autologous vein grafts (46). In this study, the effects of cell cycle inhibition on endothelial function were also evaluated. Treatment results in inhibited neointimal hyperplasia and diet-induced, accelerated graft atherosclerosis. Moreover, endothelial function is preserved in this animal model as indicated by the findings that rabbit vein grafts treated with the antisense generate more nitric oxide and exhibit enhanced vasoreactivity as compared to control grafts, resulting in a reduction of superoxide radical generation, VCAM-1 expression, and monocyte binding in grafts. Since dysfunction of the endothelium may arise from mechanical or biochemical activation of endothelial cells, blockade of the cell cycle might prevent endothelial cell activation directly or indirectly by altering the activation of VSMC and therefore preventing cytokine and growth factor release by these cells.

Alternatively, inhibition of the cell cycle in human vein grafts with ex vivo treatment of E2F decoy oligodeoxynucleotide reduces not only the graft susceptibility to accelerated atherosclerosis, but also reduces neointimal hyperplasia and enhances medial hypertrophy, which renders the graft more resistant to the increased hemodynamic stress and might prolong the life span of the venous grafts (47). Moreover, since endothelial function was preserved in oligodeoxynucleotide–treated grafts, they were more resistant to graft-associated atherosclerosis.

The prevention and treatment of cell proliferation in arteries after percutaneous intervention represents an attractive target for gene therapy proposals. Selective targeting of cell cycle regulatory proteins might inhibit cell proliferation and migration, induce withdrawal from the cell cycle, and promote cell differentiation and senescence, rather than apoptosis. Furthermore, recent studies demonstrate that cell cycle arrest not only prevents smooth muscle cell proliferation and migration but also prevents dysfunction of the endothelium as shown by improved vasoreactivity and nitric oxide production, rendering the vessel less susceptible to inflammatory infiltration and free radical formation. Studies in several animal models demonstrate that these genetic approaches are feasible and effective in limiting cell proliferation, migration, and extracellular matrix deposition. Furthermore, these studies show that despite the multiplicity of the atherosclerotic or restenotic lesion, local ectopic expression of a single critical regulatory gene is sufficient to abrogate lesion formation in different animal models for human vascular proliferative disease.

V. Summary and Conclusions

Since vascular smooth muscle cell proliferation is important in the neointimal formation following arterial injury, the role of these cell cycle control proteins has become a subject of increased interest in molecular cardiovascular research. D- and E-cyclins, in conjunction with CDK2, CDK4, and CDK6, have been implicated in controlling passage through the G_1 checkpoint, after which cells become committed to a round of cell division. Progression through the cell cycle is negatively regulated by CKIs, which bind to and inactive these CDK–cyclin complexes. Two families of CKIs have thus far been identified: the KIP/CIP family, which inactivates most of the CDKs involved in G_1 progression with little specificity, and the INK family, which binds specifically to CDK4 and 6. The KIP/CIP family members can inactivate the cyclin/CDK complexes directly and therefore will prevent Rb phosphorylation, which is necessary for G_1/S transition. In contrast, INK family members inactivate CDK 4/6 by competing with cyclin D for binding to CDK4/6 to form stable binary complexes lacking cyclin Dl. Expression of CDKs results in G_1/G_0 cell cycle arrest, resulting in inhibition of cell proliferation and migration and promotion of cell differentiation and senescence.

Recent studies show that the KIP/CIP family members function as regulators of neointimal cell proliferation in vitro and in vivo following arterial injury and in atherosclerotic lesions, whereas the INK family does not seem to be involved in the regulation of VSMC proliferation. Targeting cell cycle regulatory pathways by modification of gene expression in endothelial and smooth muscle cells within the vessel wall is feasible and effective. The alternative programs of gene expression induced by these regulatory genes resulted in a significant attenuation of intimal hyperplasia and preservation of the endothelial function. Given these observations in different animal models, these gene therapy approaches merit further investigation to understand the molecular mechanisms of cell cycle control in the pathogenesis of vascular diseases and to develop new treatments to limit cellular proliferation in these disorders.

Acknowledgments

H.D. is sponsored by the Dutch Scientific Organisation (N.W.O.); M.B. is sponsored by the Deutsche Forschungsgemeinschaft (D.F.G.). E.G.N. is an Established Investigator of the American Heart Association.

References

1. Herrman JP, Hermans WR, Vos J, Serruys PW. Pharmacological approaches to the prevention of restenosis following angioplasty. The search for the Holy Grail? (Part 1). Drugs 1993; 46:18–52.
2. Ip JH, Fuster V, Badimon L, Badimon J, Taubman MB, Chesebro JH. Syndromes of accelerated atherosclerosis: role of vascular injury and smooth muscle cell proliferation. J Am Coll Cardiol 1990; 15:1667–1687.
3. Harper JW, Elledge SJ. Cdk inhibitors in development and cancer. Curr Opin Genet Dev 1996; 6:56–64.
4. Sherr CJ, Roberts JM. Inhibitors of mammalian G_1 cyclin-dependent kinases. Genes Dev 1997; 9:1149–1163.
5. Sherr CJ. G1 phase progression: cycling on cue. Cell 1994; 79:551–555.
6. Sherr CJ. Mammalian G_1 cyclins. Cell 1993; 73:1059–1065.
7. Weinberg RA. The retinoblastoma protein and cell cycle control. Cell 1995; 81:323–330.
8. Koff A, Giordano A, Desai D, Yamashita K, Harper JW, Elledge S, et al. Formation and activation of a cyclin E-cdk2 complex during the Gl phase of the human cell cycle. Science 1992; 257:1689–1694.
9. Levine AJ. p53, the cellular gatekeeper for growth and division. Cell 1997; 88:323–331.
10. Smith ML, Chen TI, Zhan Q, Bae I, Chen CY, Gilmer TM, et al. Interaction of the p53-regulated protein Gadd45 with proliferating cell nuclear antigen. Science 1994; 266:1376–1380.
11. Donehower LA, Harvey M, Slagle BL, McArthur ML, Montgomery CA Jr, Butel JS, et al. Mice deficient of p53 are developmentally normal but susceptible to spontaneous tumours. Nature 1992; 356:215–221.
12. Jost CA, Marin MC, Kaelin WCJ. p73 is a human p53-related protein that can induce apoptosis. Nature 1997; 389:191.
13. Luo Y, Hurwitz J, Massague J. Cell-cycle inhibition by independent CDK and PCNA binding domains in p2lCipl. Nature 1995; 375:159–161.
14. Perkins ND, Felzien LK, Betts JC, Leung K, Beach DH, Nabel GJ. Regulation of NF-kappaB by cyclin-dependent kinases associated with the p300 coactivator. Science 1997; 275:523–527.

15. Yang ZY, Perkins ND, Ohno T, Nabel EG, Nabel GJ. The p2l cyclin-dependent kinase inhibitor suppresses tumorigenicity in vivo. Nature Med 1995; 1:1052–1056.
16. Deng C, Zhang P, Harper JW, Elledge SJ, Leder P. Mice lacking p2lClPl/WAF1 undergo normal development, but are defective in Gl checkpoint control. Cell 1995; 82:675–684.
17. Toyoshima H, Hunter T. p27, a novel inhibitor of Gl cyclin-Cdk protein kinase activity, is related to p2l. Cell 1994; 78:67–74.
18. Coats S, Flanagan WM, Nourse J, Roberts JM. Requirement of p27Kipl for restriction point control of the fibroblast cell cycle. Science 1996; 272:877–880.
19. Pagano M, Tam SW, Theodoras AM, Beer-Romero P, Del SG, Chau V, et al. Role of the ubiquitin-proteasome pathway in regulating abundance of the cyclin-dependent kinase inhibitor p27. Science 1995; 269:682–685.
20. Sheaff RJ, Groudine M, Gordon M, Roberts JM, Clurman BE. Cyclin E-CDK2 is a regulator of p27Kipl. Genes Dev 1997; 11:1464–1478.
21. Reynisdottir I, Polyak K, Iavarone A, Massague J. Kip/Cip and Ink4 Cdk inhibitors cooperate to induce cell cycle arrest in response to TGF-beta. Genes Dev 1995; 9:1831–1845.
22. Reynisdottir I, Massague J. The subcellular locations of pl5(ink4b) and p27(Kipl) coordinate their inhibitory interactions with cdk4 and cdk2. Genes Dev 1997; 11:492–503.
23. Fero ML, Rivkin M, Tasch M, Porter P, Carow CE, Firpo E, et al. A syndrome of multiorgan hyperplasia with the features of gigantism, tumorigenesis and female sterility in $p27^{Kip1}$-deficient mice. Cell 1996; 85:733–744.
24. Kiyokawa H, Kineman RD, Manova-Todorova KO, Soares VC, Hoffman ES, Ono, et al. Enhanced growth of mice lacking the cyclin-dependent kinase inhibitor function of p27(Kipl). Cell 1996; 85:721–732.
25. Matsuoka S, Edwards MC, Bai C, Parker S, Zhang P, Baldini A, et al. p57KIP2, a structurally distinct member of the p2lClPl Cdk inhibitor family, is a candidate tumor suppressor gene. Genes Dev 1995; 9:650–662.
26. Lee MH, Reynisdottir I, Massague J. Cloning of p57KIP2, a cyclin-dependent kinase inhibitor with unique domain structure and tissue distribution. Genes Dev 1995; 9:639–649.
27. Hatada I, Ohashi H, Fukushima Y, Kaneko Y, Inoue M, Komoto Y, et al. An imprinted gene $p57^{kip2}$ is mutated in Beckwith-Wiedemann syndrome. Nature Gen 1996; 14:171–173.
28. Tokina T, Urano T, Furuhata T, Matsushima M, Miyatsu T, Sasaki S, et al. Characterization of the human $p57^{kip2}$ gene: alternative splicing, insertion/deletion polymorphisms in VNTR sequences in the coding resion, and mutational analysis. Genes Dev 1996; 97:625–631.
29. Zhang P, Wong C, Finegold M, Hou H, Thompson JC, Silverman A, et al. Altered cell differentiation and proliferation in mice lacking $p57^{kip2}$ indicates a role in Beckwith-Wiedemann syndrome. Nature 1997; 387:151–158.
30. Ragione FD, Russo GL, Oliva A, Mercurio C, Mastropietro S, Pietra VD, et al. Biochemical characterization of $pl6^{Ink4}$ and pl8 containing complexes in human cell lines. J Biol Chem l996; 271:15942–15949.

31. Quelle DE, Ashmun RA, Hannon GJ, Rehberger PA, Trono D, Richter KH, et al. Cloning and characterization of murine pl6INK4a and pl5INK4b genes. Oncogene 1995; 11:635–645.
32. Nobori T, Miura K, Wu DJ, Lois A, Takabayashi K, Carson DA. Deletions of the cyclin-dependent kinase-4 inhibitor gene in multiple human cancers. Nature 1994; 368:753–756.
33. Serrano M, Lee HW, Chin L, Cordon-Cardo C, Beach DH, DePinho RA. Role of the INK4a locus in tumor suppression and cell mortality. Cell 1996; 85:27–37.
34. Jacks T, Fazeli A, Schmitt EM, Bronson RT, Goodell MA, Weinberg RA. Effects of an Rb mutation in the mouse. Nature 1992; 359:295–300.
35. Lee EYHP, Chang CY, Hu N, Wang YCJ, Lai CC, Herrup K, et al. Mice deficient for Rb are nonviable and show defects in neurogenesis and haematopoiesis. Nature 1992; 359:288–294.
36. Hannon GJ, Beach DH. $pl5^{INK4B}$ is a potential effector of TGFβ induced cell cycle arrest. Nature 1994; 371:257–261.
37. Guan KL, Jenkins CW, Li Y, Nichols MA, Wu X, O'Keefe CL, et al. Growth suppression by $p16^{INK4/MTS1}$ and $p14^{INK4B/MTS2}$-related CDK6 inhibitor, correlates with wild-type pRb function. Genes Dev 1994; 8:2939–2952.
38. Chan FKM, Zhang J, Cheng L, Shapiro DN, Winoto A. Identification of human and mouse pl9, a novel CDK4 and CDK6 inhibitor with homology to $pl6^{INK4}$. Mol Cell Biol 995; 15:2682–2688.
39. Schwartz SM, Ross R. Cellular proliferation in atherosclerosis and hypertension. Prog Cardiovasc Dis 1984; 26:355–372.
40. Chang MW, Barr E, Lu MM, Barton K, Leiden JM. Adenovirus-mediated overexpression of the cyclin/cyclin-dependent kinase inhibitor, p21 inhibits vascular smooth muscle cell proliferation and neointima formation in the rat carotid artery model of balloon angioplasty. J Clin Invest 1995; 96:2260–2268.
41. Ohno T, Gordon D, San H, Pompili VJ, Imperiale MJ, Nabel GJ, et al. Gene therapy for vascular smooth muscle cell proliferation after arterial injury. Science 1994; 265:781–784.
42. Yang ZY, Simari RD, Perkins ND, San H, Gordon D, Nabel, et al. Role of the p2l cyclin-dependent kinase inhibitor in limiting intimal cell proliferation in response to arterial injury. Proc Natl Acad Sci USA 1996; 93:7905–7910.
43. Clowes AW, Reidy MA, Clowes MM. Kinetics of cellular proliferation after arterial injury. I. Smooth muscle growth in the absence of endothelium. Lab Invest 1983; 49:327–333.
44. Koyama H, Raines EW, Bornfeldt KE, Roberts JM, Ross R. Fibrillar collagen inhibits arterial smooth muscle proliferation through regulation of Cdk2 inhibitors. Cell 1996; 87:1069–1078.
45. Chang MW, Barr E, Seltzer J, Jiang YQ, Nabel GJ, Nabel EG, et al. Cytostatic gene therapy for vascular proliferative disorders with a constitutively active form of the retinoblastoma gene product. Science 1995; 267:518–522.
46. Chen D, Krasinski K, Sylvester A, Chen J, Nisen PD, Andres V. Downregulation of cyclin-dependent kinase 2 activity and cyclin A promoter activity in vascular

smooth muscle cells by p27(KIPl), an inhibitor of neointima formation in the rat carotid artery. J Clin Invest 1997; 99:2334–2341.

47. Mann JM, Whittemore AD, Donaldson MC, Belkin MA, Orav EJ, Polak J, et al. Preliminary clinical experience with genetic engineering in human vein grafts: evidence for target gene inhibition (abstr). Circulation 1997; 96:4.

14

Smooth Muscle Cells and Restenosis

GEORGE SOPKO

National Heart, Lung and Blood Institute
National Institutes of Health
Bethesda, Maryland

I. Introduction

Coronary revascularization by percutaneous transluminal coronary angioplasty (PTCA) as a treatment for coronary heart disease (CHD), the leading cause of mortality in the United States, has progressed significantly over the past several decades. The first PTCA was done in 1977, and by 1994 approximately 408,000 PTCAs had been performed; since 1990 it has been the dominant mode of coronary revascularization (1). Many new catheter-based revascularization approaches have been developed since the first PTCA. Typically, the procedures aim at reducing luminal obstruction and improving coronary flow by (1) dilation of the vessel, (2) removing the obstruction (debulking) with a targeted energy (laser) or ablating it mechanically (atherectomy, rotablade, drill), or (3) stenting, providing an intravascular scaffolding to facilitate and to maintain patency. The revascularization strategy may involve a combination of many of these approaches to provide optimal results. Regardless of the technique, all of the catheter-based procedures cause arterial wall injury. As a matter of fact, minimal wall injury may indicate less than adequate procedure. The unavoidable injury leads to a significant disruption of endothelial and vessel wall integrity, setting in motion a number of molecular and cellular responses initiating a healing process, which in some patients leads to hyperplastic response compromising lumen, a process called restenosis.

Despite the continuous evolution in catheter technology, restenosis remains the major limitation of catheter-based revascularization techniques. Approximately one-third of the patients have clinically evident restenosis usually requiring additional treatment. Reported restenosis rates range from 12% to nearly 60%, peaking 1–3 months after the procedure (2,3). The National Heart, Lung and Blood Institute (NHLBI) has fostered innovative research on the mechanisms(s) of restenosis to develop a rational therapy(ies) and ultimately to prevent this complication and in 1990 released a Request for Application (RFA NIH 91-HL-02-H) focusing on multidisciplinary basic and clinical research directed at fundamental mechanisms of restenosis. In addition, the Institute has supported a number of research projects directly and indirectly related to restenosis, including PTCA Registry I and II and New Application Coronary Intervention (NACI) Registry, which have provided the most comprehensive contemporary reports on the success and complications of catheter-based coronary revascularization techniques (4–6).

Over the past decade a number of empiric approaches and large amounts of nonfederal monies were spent testing various pharmacologic agents to prevent clinical restenosis without significant success. A number of important observations and experimental approaches to unravel the pathophysiology have been made. However, the understanding of restenosis continues to pose a challenge (7).

II. Pathobiology

Injury disrupts an atherosclerotic plaque with a number of different cells activated at as well as directed to the site of injury involving platelets, endothelial and vascular smooth muscle cells, growth factors, and immune responses. Platelets adhering to an injured site are among the first cellular elements recruited followed by smooth muscle cells and other cells. As a result, a number of mitogens/multiple growth factors are released, which play a principal role in intimal hyperplasia. Intimal hyperplasia is the dominant cellular response at the site of injury and in restenosis. Restenosis specimens obtained by atherectomy reveal an abundance of what appears to be a smooth muscle cell with a substantial amount of extracellular neomatrix, particularly collagens (8–10). Compared to primary lesions, smooth muscle cells from restenotic lesions are two to three times more active (11). Smooth muscle cells migrate from surrounding structures to injured intima and proliferate at the site of injury with the formation of an extracellular matrix (12). Restenotic lesions showed significantly higher and earlier occurring smooth muscle cell growth/migratory kinetics compared with primary (atherosclerotic) lesions (13,14). Furthermore, compared with normal cells, smooth muscle cells from restenotic lesions appear to be much less sensitive to heparin, a major physiological inhibitor of smooth muscle cell growth (15). However, the extent of smooth muscle cell proliferation and the relevance of findings from in vitro and in vivo experiments to human restenosis have recently been questioned (16).

III. Humoral Events

Injury induces platelet-derived growth factor (PDGF)-β receptor expression at the smooth muscle cell proliferation site. PDGF, produced by platelets and also by endothelial cells, stimulates smooth muscle cell migration and exhibits chemotaxis for smooth muscle cells, leukocytes, and fibroblasts, attracting them to subendothelial space (17–19). Through this "paracrine" action, PDGF may mediate subendothelial tissue responses. Basic fibroblast growth factors (b-FGF) are potent smooth muscle cell mitogens, also stimulating angiogenesis and regulating components of an extracellular matrix (20–23). As with other growth factors, there is an increased expression of FGF receptors with injury (20). A systemic infusion of b-FGF increases smooth muscle cell proliferation (21). In general, FGF is an important component of signal transduction complex participating in mitogenesis of smooth muscle cells. Transforming growth factor-beta 1 (TGF-β) is a regulatory cytokine released from platelets with chemotaxis for macrophages and monocytes and induction of angiogenesis (24). Experimental data show that TGF-β is a potent wound-healing factor inhibiting the growth of normal smooth muscle cells. In contrast to normal cells, it stimulates the growth of cells from atherosclerotic lesions as well as increasing collagen synthesis (25). TGF-β can also induce its own production, potentially initiating a vicious and chronic cycle participating in restenosis (26–27). However, the precise role of TGF-β in restenosis remains to be clarified.

Thromboxane A_2 is a potent platelet aggregator and mitogen facilitating smooth muscle cell proliferation. Serotonin, a potent vasoconstrictor released from platelets, has mitogenic and chemotactic effects on smooth muscle cells (28). In injury, serotonin is upregulated (via phospholipase C coupling) rendering the injured site more sensitive to vasoconstrictors and growth factors. Endothelins are peptides modulating vasomotor tone, cell proliferation, and hormone production. A number of factors, such as stress and growth factors (TGF, bFGF, IGF) induce transcription of endothelin-1 mRNA leading to increased intravascular secretion of endothelin-1, which binds to smooth muscle cell receptors, causing vasoconstriction (29–30). Endothelin-1 in turn may mediate effects of several vasoactive peptides and growth hormones, including an important interaction with angiotensin II (31). In their growth-promoting effects it appears that endothelin-1 and angiotensin II may share intracellular signal pathways (32). The impact could be potentiated by the impaired production of nitric oxide, substance-mitigating endothelin-induced vasoconstriction, and growth-promoting effects. An insulin-like growth factor (IGF-I) is an omnipresent polypeptide, structurally similar to insulin produced by smooth muscle cells. IGF-I is needed for cells to go through the cell division cycle and it may allow cells to continue to grow after induction by PDGF (33). Although a weaker mitogen than PDGF, it is a potent migration stimulator, perhaps directing chemotaxis (34). It is possible that injury-induced local accumulation of IGF-I contributes to neointimal proliferation (35).

With the exposure of subendothelial space there is a release of pro-coagulant factors and rapid thrombus formation. Thrombin, a potent mitogen, remains elevated for several weeks after injury (36). It activates growth-related gene expression in smooth muscle cells, signaling to produce other growth factors, stimulates proliferation via proteolytic activation of its receptor, and stimulates chemotaxis of inflammatory cells (effects similar to those of PDGF) (37–40). Certain plasminogen activators, such as tissue (t-PA) and urokinase (u-PA), control fibrinolysis by converting plasminogen to the active proteolytic enzyme plasmin (41–42) and are involved in activities regulating matrix turnover. Furthermore, t-PA and u-PA are also considered mitogens. Plasmin facilitates smooth muscle cell migration and proliferation, can activate latent forms of certain growth factors, such as TGF-β and can directly or indirectly degrade a number of extracellular matrix proteins (43). Plasminogen activator inhibitor type 1 (PAI-1) may inhibit some of these processes. The importance of the fibrinolytic system was confirmed in a knockout mice model. Neointima formation was reduced in u-PA knockout mice, unchanged in t-PA knockout mice, and increased in PAI knockout mice (44–47). Fibrin and fibronectin facilitate the migration and attachment of smooth muscle cells.

One elegant theory, supported by a growing body of data, indicates that immunologic and inflammatory mechanisms play an important role in restenosis (48). Injury leads to a generation of cytokines with subsequent activation of growth factors, providing an opportunity for a self-stimulatory, autocrine, and paracrine feedback loop that amplifies and sustains smooth muscle cell proliferation. For example, stress and the inflammatory cytokinases interleukin-1-beta (IL-1β) and a tumor necrosis factor alpha (TNF-α) can activate transcription nuclear factor kappa B (NF-κ-B), which then induces transcription of E-selectin and the vascular adhesion molecule-1 (VCAM). These molecules promote local recruitment of leukocytes by rendering endothelium hyperadhesive to leukocytes and promoting their transendothelial migration. Oxidized LDL and cytokines induce expression of VCAM-1, a condition which could also recruit leukocytes and accompanying platelets to the injury site (49,50). Oxidized LDL is cytotoxic: it interferes with endothelium-dependent relaxation by inactivating EDRF, it augments agonist-induced vasoconstriction (51,52), and it can affect counter-regulatory factors. For example, oxidized lipids can suppress TGF-β-1, an antiproteolytic factor (53). TGF-β-l inhibits smooth muscle proliferation while b-FGF enhances proteolysis, and the inhibitory action of the TGF-β-1 may ultimately signal the end of proliferatory response (54). Leukotriene B_4 also up-regulates surface leukocyte adherence receptors (55), mediating leukocyte adhesion and transendothelial migration.

IV. Apoptosis

It is also likely that multiple mechanisms, in addition to those related to smooth muscle cells, are involved in restenosis (56). Not all restenotic lesions contain hypercellular responses. Current theories on restenosis include a late loss of patency implicating wall remodeling, a process independent of cellular hyper-proliferative responses. The role of apoptosis in modulating the cellularity of lesions has been proposed. Apoptosis, genetically programmed cell death, was observed most frequently in the hypercellular tissue of restenotic specimens (57). It is possible that apoptosis, a process that maintains a stable cell number in tissues with varying proliferative activity, is disturbed in restenotic lesions.

An extracellular matrix is also thought to play an important role in intimal hyperplasia (58). The bulk of the stent-related restenotic lesions was dominated by extracellular (acellular) matrix (59). Extracellular matrix binds and serves as a reservoir outgrowth factors responsible for cellular proliferation (b-FGF, TGF-β1). The major components of an extracellular matrix include collagen types II–IV, elastin, fibronectin (an adhesive protein), tenascin (with both adhesive and counteradhesive properties), thrombospondin, biglycan, decorin, and ground substance (which contains several types of proteoglycans). Cell adhesion molecules play an important role in the interaction between cells as well as with extracellular matrix, ultimately modulating the intimal cytoskeleton (60). Injury-induced extracellular matrix remodeling may involve both induction of proteolytic enzymes and their respective inhibitors along with the release of stored growth factors (61), potentially modifying cell behavior and migration. For example, fibronectin and laminin, two extracellular matrix proteins, have opposite effects on smooth muscle cell phenotypic expression: fibronectin promotes transformation to the secretory state while laminin maintains the contractile state (62). Both tenascin and thrombospondin play a similar role, facilitating the phenotypic transformation of smooth muscle cells. Among mitogens, endothelin-1 stimulates collagen type I synthesis while angiotensin-II stimulates collagen type III synthesis by smooth muscle cells, each differentially and synergistically affecting vascular structure after injury (63). With injury, smooth muscle cells may selectively express matrix-degrading metalloproteinases, enabling them to migrate through the matrix network. Neointimal cells generate a number of matrix proteins (64,65).

V. Adventitia

Injury to adventitia can lead to fibrosis and to intercellular and transmural communications and to interactions contributing to intimal hyperplasia and restenosis with a subsequent cellular invasion by myofibroblasts. The data suggest that perivascular manipulation, leading to injury to adventitia, is accompanied by induction of regulatory genes, such as angiotensinogen and tissue factor, and by vascular lesion formation in rats (66–69). Endoluminal balloon injury to a normal vessel leads to adventitial remodeling accompanied by both transformation of fibroblasts into alpha-smooth muscle actin–expressing myofibroblasts and their migration toward the lumen, contributing to neointima formation (70,71). These activated adventitial myofibroblasts expressing cytoskeletal protein markers can lead to spatial adventitial remodeling and constrictive fibrosis/scar formation, another contribution to restenosis (72,73). The adventitial fibrosis then can contribute to negative vessel remodeling, eventually leading to a constriction of lumen and restenosis.

VI. Molecular Events

Injury initiates a cascade of molecular events with both direct and indirect effects, such as downregulation of some growth-inhibiting mechanisms and upregulation of growth factors facilitating smooth muscle cell proliferation and migration.

Release and activation of various cellular-bound mitogens leads to altered transduction and expression of primary response genes, which in turn leads to altered cellular responses and to neoproliferation. For example, mitogens such as PDGF, angiotensin II, endothelin, and thrombin activate protein kinase inducing nuclear proto-oncogene (c-myb, c-fos, and c-myc) expression, KC and JE gene (product protein) expression, and smooth muscle cell proliferation (74–83). In turn, KC and JE could then recruit neutrophils and monocytes to the site of injury with JE facilitating smooth muscle cell migration. Oxidized LDL and cytokines activate oxidant-responsive NF-κB transcriptional pathway leading to VCAM-1 expression, an endothelial adhesion molecule (49). On the other hand, activation of protein kinase C pathway leads also to antiproliferative response mediated by TGF-β having a net effect of favoring cellular hypertrophy rather than hyperplasia (84,85). Restenotic human lesions showed TGF-β 1 overexpression with a decrease in type II receptor. This receptor-variant cell dysfunction could allow slow but uncontrolled cell growth accompanied by an overproduction of extracellular matrix components (25). Induction of response (nuclear proto-oncogenes) genes, such as an immediate early gene group (i.e., c-myc) and the delayed early gene group (i.e., osteopontin), may possibly represent a final common pathway of the signal transduction activated by various mitogens, mediating a time-dependent new protein synthesis and smooth muscle cell behavior (86). Recent data suggest that smooth muscle cell migration and proliferation have distinct signaling pathways (35).

Normal cell growth is the result of regulatory activities promoting proliferation of cells counterbalanced by their apoptotic death. Transcriptional regulations by inducing regulatory genes are considered necessary for cell growth. For example, E2F transcription factors induce genes, such as c-myc, regulating the S phase of the cell cycle and apoptosis (87). Overexpression of E2F-1 can cause oncogenesis (88,89). Studies with E2F-1–deficient mice showed that E2F-1 positively regulates apoptosis and suppresses cell proliferation and is not critical for cells to enter the S phase (90). These data suggest that a single gene in response to other cellular events can regulate proliferation as well as suppress cell activities.

A recent report suggested another intriguing mechanism, a viral infection, for restenosis. One-third of the patients with restenosis had lesions containing cytomegalovirus DNA sequence. Smooth muscle cells infected with the virus expressed an early protein that bound to a p53 tumor-suppressor gene and inhibited its function. Inhibition of p53 then can set the stage for an escape leading to cellular proliferation. Cytomegalovirus is also known to activate the transcriptional factor NF-κB, which modulates a number of genes involved in inflammatory and immune responses, including expression of adhesion molecules (91,92). Thus, injury can reactivate latent cytomegalovirus locally, setting in motion regulatory events that facilitate intimal hyperplasia or suppress apoptosis, either of which can contribute to restenosis (93,94). Interestingly, a mutant p53 gene is also involved in controlling tumor angiogenesis by increasing protein kinase C production and enhancing vascular endothelial growth factor (VEGF) expression (95). Other infectious agents have also been implicated in neointimal hyperplasia.

The role of a genetic predisposition to restenosis has also been raised. The proposed mechanism includes the insertion/deletion ACE gene polymorphism, which affects ACE plasma levels (96–98). Angiotensin II interacts with the G protein–coupled receptor and cross-talk with a tyrosine kinase signaling cascade, potentially leading to anti-apoptotic response and vascular lesion formation. The role of genetic defects in platelet function in restenosis is not known. However, recent data provide a linkage between genetic defects in platelets and coronary disease. This defect was related to polymorphism in glycoprotein IIIa, which is expressed in both platelets and endothelial cells, possibly altering the binding of this polypeptide with other proteins participating in thrombosis (99). Since thrombosis appears to play a key role in neointimal formation, it is possible that those patients who have genetic defect(s) in platelet function predisposing them to thrombosis may also be at high risk for restenosis.

VII. Smooth Muscle Cell Transformation

Intimal hyperplasia involves phenotypic transformation of smooth muscle cells from the normal contractile state, characterized by presence of myosin and lack of response to mitogens, to a synthetic state, characterized by migration and proliferation. Extracellular matrix components play an important role in this process (62). This transformation enables smooth muscle cells to migrate and proliferate into neointima and is accompanied by increased sensitivity to mitogens, growth stimuli, and vasoconstrictors. The shift in the phenotype can be stimulated by leukotrienes LTB4, LTC4, LTD4, which also facilitates proliferative response to mitogens (100,101) as well as by other factors, such as PDGF. Smooth muscle cells from angioplasty lesions and from human atheroma lesions produced PDGF-like mitogen and expressed PDGF-A chain mRNA. (102) The expression of PDGF-A gene and PDGF alpha and beta receptor mRNA increases with transformation from contractile to a synthetic phenotype (75,76,103,104). Angiotensin II and TGF-β increase expression of PDGF-A mRNA and PDGF-like mitogens (105,106). Furthermore, smooth muscle cells can proliferate independently of extracellular PDGF and exogenous growth factors, perhaps due to endogenous PDGF-like mitogen(s) and TGF-β produced by the regenerating smooth muscle cells (23,106).

VIII. Strategies to Combat Restenosis

A number of approaches and various agents have been studied to thwart the hyperproliferative response of smooth muscle cells. Many of these were empirical, while others tested specific hypotheses. Conceptually, the approaches here will be divided into empirical strategies, strategies targeting either smooth muscle cells or their mitogens, thus altering their ability to proliferate, or strategies focusing on endothelialization, thus indirectly inhibiting smooth muscle cell proliferation. Each of these strategies has its own set of issues and challenges.

A. Empirical Strategies

Over the years a number of pharmacologic agents thought to have the potential to prevent restenosis have been tested. Based on in vitro studies showing some growth-inhibiting effects or on the notion of certain drugs appearing conceptually very appealing, numerous agents were tested with a hope for a quick commercial return. For example, calcium channel blockers with their antiremodeling effects on a vessel wall were conceptually appealing. However, just about all of these agents, including several different class agents, such as ACE-inhibitors, trapidil (a PDGF antagonist), lovastatin (a HMG-CoA reductase inhibitor), high-dose steroid therapy, antiplatelet agents, and other anticoagulants have not prevented restenosis. For example, lipid-modification strategies failed despite adequate lipid lowering (107–114). However, in one small randomized trial of hypertriglyceridemic patients undergoing angioplasty, triglyceride lowering with bezafibrate yielded lower restenosis rate compared to no therapy (115). A decrease in triglycerides and plasminogen activator inhibitor type 1 were independently related to prevention of restenosis (116). This preventive effect may be related to the fact that hypertriglyceridemia, via increased formation of plasminogen activator inhibitor type 1, is associated with decreased fibrinolytic activity. Probucol, known to prevent LDL oxidation, has also been reported to decrease angiographic restenosis (117).

B. Antimitogenic Strategies

Based on the notion that vascular injury leads to an upregulation of the mitogens, a number of chemotherapeutic agents such as colchicin, vincristine, and actinomycin-D have been tested but failed to prevent restenosis (118). Heparin was one of the agents studied early with promising results obtained in in vitro and vivo experimental (119). In vitro, heparin inhibits rat, bovine, baboon, and human smooth muscle cell proliferation. It has numerous inhibitory effects, such as inhibition of mitogen-induced protein kinase activation with subsequent prevention of c-fos and c-myc of proto-oncogene expression, selective inhibition of proteases involved in extracellular matrix degradation, and potentiation of inhibitory effects of b-FGF. (120,121). The complexity of multiple and at times diverse effects of drugs can be illustrated by the effect of heparin. In addition to the above illustrated antiproliferative properties, heparin also stimulates the expression of b-FGF, a potent smooth muscle cell mitogen (122). Contrary to other animal models, low molecular weight heparin failed to inhibit intimal hyperplasia in a baboon angioplasty model (123). ACE inhibitors suppress intimal hyperplasia in a rat (124). However, as with other agents showing promising results in vitro as well as in a specific animal model, it had no significant impact in humans (125). Discrepancies in results observed in different animal models may be due to the fact that different animal species have different pathways leading to interspecies differences in smooth muscle cell response (123). Specific antibodies to b-FGF, a potent mitogen for smooth muscle cell proliferation, inhibited smooth muscle cell proliferation (126). Blocking antibody to PDGF suppressed local accumulation of smooth muscle cells but not their proliferation (127). Recent data suggested that trapidil, which competitively blocks PDGF receptors and also inhibits thromboxane A_2, can reduce restenosis (128). Although prostaglandins PGE1, PGE2, and PGI2 inhibit smooth muscle cell growth in vitro, prostaglandin inhibitors have not prevented clinical restenosis. Administration of endothelin-receptor blocker to rats reduced neointimal formation by 50% (129). There are no data on its impact in humans. Since thrombin appears to play a significant role in restenosis, a number of antithrombin strategies have been pursued. Experimentally, hirudin blocks the thrombin activation of fibrinogen, retards platelet aggregation, inhibits thrombin-induced mitogenesis, blocks thrombin-induced monocyte chemotactic activity, and has shown promising results inhibiting restenosis after angioplasty in animals (130–135).

Targeting platelets to reduce restenosis has been an attractive but until recently a rather disappointing experience. New agents aim at blocking glycoprotein IIb/IIIa, one of the adhesion receptors on the surface of platelets involved in binding fibrinogen and platelet adhesion/aggregation. Systemic administration of a monoclonal antibody fragment (Reo ProR) to platelet glycoprotein Gp-IIb/IIIa has been recently shown to reduce both acute clinical events and clinical restenosis (136). However, the administration of this agent carries a risk of significant bleeding and thrombocytopenia (137).

A number of other approaches have been tried, including analogs of somatostatin, a polypeptide, that inhibits cellular proliferation and secretion of other peptides and hormones. Lanreotide, an analog of somatostatin, prevents a local accumulation of IGF-I with experimental endothelial injury (35). Angiopeptin, synthetic analog of somatostatin has been show to inhibit experimental smooth muscle cell proliferation (138–140). However, several clinical trials have provided inconclusive results; although clinical events were reduced no significant change in restenosis was found (141,142). One of the major challenges of the therapies has been to effectively target specific factor(s), which would then inhibit smooth muscle cells without being counteracted by neutralizing antibodies on repeat exposure. An intriguing alternative approach would be to selectively obliterate the proliferating subpopulation of smooth muscle cells (143).

C. Cytotoxic and Cytostatic Strategies

These strategies deliver a toxin into a cell employing various delivery systems (144). Antineoplastic agents cytarabine, doxorubicin, and vincristine inhibited, in a dose-response fashion, smooth muscle proliferation altering cytoskeletal elements, such as actin, microtubules, and vimentin. (145). In vitro, colchicin inhibited proliferative and migratory smooth muscle activity accompanied by destruction of cytoplasmic structure (12). In rats, both local and systemic delivery of diphtheria toxin recombinantly modified to target the epidermal growth factor receptor virtually inhibits neointimal hyperplasia. Local delivery, however, avoids systemic toxicity (146). Chimeric toxin, created by genetically fusing the gene encoding TGF-α to the gene encoding *Pseudomonas* exotoxin, targeted to receptors on smooth muscle cells achieved cytolysis, killing rapidly proliferating cells (147). Another approach employs a transfer of growth regulatory genes into a cell using viral vectors. Local transfection with the herpes simplex virus thymidine kinase gene accompanied by systemic administration of prodrug ganciclovir inhibited neointima formation (148).

A less traumatic approach, avoiding tissue damage due to cytotoxic therapy, aims at inhibiting the cell cycle by suppressing the translation of a specific gene leading to downregulation of the corresponding protein. Gene transfer or manipulation of gene expression has been investigated and presents a very appealing approach to controlling the restenosis process (149,150). Using retroviral infection and liposome-mediated transfection, a reporter gene can be directly transferred into denuded endothelium of a normal artery, with both endothelial and smooth muscle cells expressing the gene. Transfection with recombinant adenovirus can also be used to selectively target neointimal cells for gene transfer (151). Another approach is the antisense technique, where short segments of synthetic RNA or DNA complement and bind segments of native messenger RNA to block translation or transcription, resulting in a specific protein synthesis decrease. This technique allows the targeting of specific elements such as smooth muscle cells and their activity (152). A dose-dependent antiproliferative effect was observed with downregulation of a human c-myc gene by antisense oligonucleotide in vitro and after local catheter-based delivery (153,154). Similarly, c-myb antisense oligonucleotide induced inhibition of neointimal formation in vitro (155,156). Another targeted approach involves human adenoviruses, which can infect many vascular cells, including endothelium. A successful transfer of recombinant adenoviral vector expressing cell regulatory gene has been reported (157–159). Targeting genes expressed early after activation by growth factors such as c-myc using antisense oliogonucleotides prevents neointimal formation in rat and porcine models. Inhibition of c-myc also independently inhibits biosynthesis of collagen type 1 and 2, the two major constituents of an extracellular matrix (160). Reduction in neointimal formation was also observed after targeting late G1 genes, such as c-myb proto-oncogene, which is required for DNA synthesis in the S phase (153,154). Another approach to reducing neointimal formation is to enhance cell cycle inhibitory genes, such as p21 (161). In a rat angioplasty model, localized infection with p2l-encoding adenovirus inhibits growth factor–stimulated smooth muscle cell proliferation by arresting the G1 phase of the cell cycle and reduces neointima formation (162). One of the attractive features of gene therapy is the direct application to the site of angioplasty, thus potentially avoiding systemic effects. As promising as these approaches are, however, many questions need to be answered. These include the bioavailability and therapeutic efficacy of gene transfer strategy, selection of the best method of delivery, the duration and concentration or dose necessary to inhibit smooth muscle cell proliferation, the long-term effects of gene manipulation, and whether sites distant from the targeted area may be adversely affected.

D. Endothelial Repair Strategies

Endothelial cells receive and process signals from endovascular (luminal) space and regulate underlying smooth muscle cell behavior (163). The intact endothelium is the only biological nonthrombogenic surface exhibiting many functions pivotal for the prevention of intimal hyperproliferation (164). In response to various physical and hormonal *stimuli*, intact endothelium actively regulates vascular tone either through releasing vasodilating substances, such as endothelial-derived relaxing factor (EDRF), prostacyclin, adenosine di- and triphosphate, or vasoconstricting factors, such as endothelin, thromboxane A_2, superoxide anion, and endothelium-derived constricting factor (165–167). Injured endothelium is thought to produce a number of growth factors affecting smooth muscle cell activity counterbalanced by endothelium-derived growth inhibitors, namely, heparin/heparan sulfate, TGF-β, and nitric oxide (168). EDRF has properties similar to nitric oxide (NO) while inhibiting platelet adhesion and aggregation (169). In vascular injury, atherosclerosis, and hypertension there is an impaired formation of EDRF leading to a disturbed vasoactive function (170). Recent data suggest that formation of NO affects intimal hyperplasia; administration of L-arginine, a precursor of NO, inhibited intimal hyperplasia by 39% (171).

With the understanding that many endothelial functions are pivotal for the prevention of intimal hyperproliferation, a novel concept of accelerated regeneration of endothelium has been devised and tested. In contrast to other vascular mitogens, vascular endothelial growth factor (VEGF) is both a potent endothelial cell mitogen in vitro and permeability mediator and a unique angiogenic factor because of its specific affinity to bind to receptors (tyrosine-kinases KDR and flt-1), which are found only on endothelial cells (172–175). Expression of VEGF is increased in hypoxia-related angiogenesis, such as with wound healing, proliferative retinopathy, revascularization ischemia, and tumor progression (176,177). Through hypoxia-induced paracrine mechanisms inducing/mobilizing KDR receptors, this VEGF upregulation expression is thought to promote local neovascularization (178). Local administration of VEGF results in profound acceleration of endothelial regeneration after balloon injury in rats. There was an inverse relationship between endothelial regeneration and intimal hyperplasia supporting the concept that rapid endothelial regeneration limits intimal hyperplasia (179). It is also possible that by its suppressive effect on smooth muscle cell proliferation, VEGF would subsequently reduce extracellular matrix formation, thus also limiting restenosis (180). Interestingly, regenerating endothelial cells show impaired vasomotor reactivity response, which raises several questions, such as what role the restoration of intimal structural integrity may play in affecting restenosis, and whether certain endothelial functions play an equal role in preventing restenosis. What is the downside of this approach? What are the effects on cancer angiogenesis? Since VEGF is proinflammatory and may require multiple administrations, what are the late/long-term sequelae?

E. Stenting

Stents provide structural support against wall collapse leaving the final lumen diameter generally larger than any other catheter-based revascularization (181,182). Numerous designs have been tested, but few have yielded desirable results. Initially used as a bailout procedure, the use of stents has so rapidly increased that in some centers it accounts for nearly two-thirds of all catheter-based revascularizations. Several major trials have recently shown that restenosis is significantly reduced after stenting, to as low as 13% and to an average about 20–25% (183,184). Obviously such low restenosis rates are very appealing to practitioners. However, it is not known whether such low rates are related, in part, to the selection of patient who had an ideal profile, stenting de novo discrete lesions in a segment with a large lumen. A recent study also raised the interesting issue of possibly different mechanism contributing to restenosis with stents. In their porcine model, neointimal formation was related largely to intimal injury, but contribution of thrombus formation to this process was considered minimal (185). Long-term patency of currently employed stents is not known. It could be speculated that stents, as a "full metal jacket" of foreign material, may induce neointimal proliferation through perhaps an inflammatory cascade, rather than thrombin activation pathways. Whether this process could be chronic low intensity and leading to a new expression of cellular response is not known. Even stents are not without their problems (186–188). The need for anticoagulation or antiplatelet therapy carries associated morbidity as well as cost. Alternative strategies include coating stents with a biologically active material (heparin, beta-emitting isotopes, gene transfer), being irradiated, or being constructed from biodegradable material, to reduce thrombogenicity and to reduce hyperproliferative response (189–193). Some have been tested with promising results, and apparently several ongoing studies are testing new approaches on a larger scale (193).

F. Radiotherapy

Radiation effects on a host of cells have been known for decades. Low doses (<20 cGy) of gamma radiation have been used to inhibit keloid formation (194) and hyperplastic bone response after hip surgery. However, it is a relatively new field with little knowledge about complications if used as the primary cardiovascular therapy. Radiotherapy is based on the concept that quiescent cells are relatively resistant to its effects, while it is cytotoxic for proliferating cells, such as those induced by injury (195). It can be delivered endovascularly (called brachytherapy) via catheter or stent or externally in a single dose or multifraction (192,193). The multifraction approach can locally deliver a high dose in brief bursts while minimizing the exposure of surrounding tissues. Ionizing radiation modulates gene expression (196), including possibly activating growth delay genes (197). In cell culture, gamma radiation inhibited smooth muscle cell proliferation but did not affect their migration (198,199). Irradiation of intima reduced the neointimal proliferation in stented porcine model (192). Generally, there is a dose-response relationship. Different sources of radiation have been used, such as irridium-192 and strontium/yttrium-90, which allow deeper tissue penetration. As with other types of injury, it has broad-range effects, including inducing an expression of b-FGF, a growth facilitator, and possible acceleration or induction of atherosclerosis (200,201). High doses (>2500 cGy) of gamma radiation injure elastic membrane, leading to intimal thickening and fibrosis. The injury to vasa vasorum has been proposed as a mechanism leading to the above pathology (195,202,203). Interestingly, radiation injury (with doses <5000 sGy) appears to be largely confined to small vessels, with large vessels, such as carotids, being relatively spared (204,205). In view of powerful cell ablation with radiotherapy delivered during acute injury period, there has been concern about the weak healing response and late aneurysmal formation. Data from the cancer field indicate that there is a latency period of more than 10 years after exposure before seeing cardiovascular complications, and the risks increase after a dose of 40 cGy. Most of the late complications of (high-dose) radiation therapy directed at mediastinum for Hodgkin's disease or breast cancer were primarily related to pericardium, but also to coronary artery disease (206–208).

A low-dose, primarily beta, radiation has been shown to inhibit hyperproliferative response in different animal models (209–212). Since a beta isotope has low penetration (<4 mm) and is absorbed by the immediate tissue, it minimizes the radiation exposure of both the patient as well as the operator. Recent clinical data suggest that low-dose intravascular radiation is a feasible approach to controlling the neointimal proliferation with little acute toxicity (213,214). An intravascular approach is invasive and associated with morbidity and hospital-related cost. A targeted (focused) external radiation approach is intuitively appealing and is obviously less traumatic, but is largely untested for cardiovascular applications. However, delayed low single dose (8 cGy) or multifraction (16 cGy) radiation in rabbit not only failed to inhibit but actually accelerated neointimal proliferation after stent implantation (215). Compared to beta radiation, gamma radiation offers more uniform dose delivery approach. It is currently thought that radiation upregulates inhibitory systems of smooth muscle cell proliferation, including an induction of apoptosis. Many challenges lie ahead. We need to address a number of issues, such as: which cell is the target, the optimal time and dose window, the effect on other cells, single fraction or multifraction delivery, and whether beta and gamma sources are equally effective in preventing neointimal proliferation. We also need to know how to calculate dosimetry, how to deliver effective (uniform) dose for eccentric lesions, whether there are any negative interactions between radiation and cardiovascular and other drugs, and the late risks of radiotherapy, particularly for young patients. Since it takes years to experience late complications, we may have to select specific intermediate endpoints in order to monitor for safety. It is possible that one of the best indicators of radiation injury is adventitia thickening, assessed by intravascular ultrasound.

IX. Summary

In summary, catheter-based revascularization techniques invariably result in injury, accompanied by varying degrees of thrombosis, inflammation, and hyperplastic responses ultimately leading to neointima formation. Many endogenous substances with mitogenic properties, proposed to play significant roles in neointima formation and proliferation, are released with injury leading to activation of various pathways and interactions leading to the transcription and posttranscription of intracellular events involving multiple growth factors, cellular receptors, and gene induction. Smooth muscle cells play an important role in neointimal hyperplasia, but other cells such as fibroblasts, and possibly macrophages, can undergo phenotypic transformation and contribute to hyperplasia. These complex biochemical interactions involve activation of multiple systems involved in regulation of many cells behavior, which ultimately govern prothrombotic and proliferative activities. With multiple systems involved frequently contributing independently to neointima formation, they also provide an opportunity for (dys)regulatory redundancies, therefore posing a challenge for therapeutic interventions directed toward a single target. Although several new approaches, such as stents and radiation therapy, are very promising and offer alternative strategies dealing with restenosis, they are not without their own problems and challenges. What might the future directions be? Perhaps the development of a molecular angioscopy will allow us to identify the status of vascular wall components, including presence or absence of endothelium, inflammatory and other cells thought to participate in neointima proliferation. As much progress as has been made, we still fall short of combating the problem. We need a better understanding of the mechanisms and interactions involved in neointimal formation; this step is pivotal for the development of effective interventions in preventing restenosis and in reducing the morbidity and cost associated with repeated revascularization.

References

1. National Hospital Discharge Survey. National Center for Health Statistics, personal communication.
2. Liu MW, Roubin GS, King SB. Restenosis after coronary angioplasty: potential biologic determinants and role of intimal hyperplasia. Circulation 1989; 79:1374–1387.
3. Topol EJ, Leya F, Pinkerton CA, Whitlow PL, Hofling B, Simonton CA, for the CAVEAT study group. A comparison of directional atherectomy with coronary angioplasty in patients with coronary artery disease. N Engl J Med 1993; 329:221–227.
4. Proceedings of the National Heart, Lung, and Blood Institute Workshop on the Outcome of Percutaneous Transluminal Angioplasty. Am J Cardiol 1994; 53:1c–146c.
5. Detre KM, Holubkov R, Kelsey SF, Cowley M, Kent KM, Williams D, Myler R, Faxon DP, Holmes D, Bourassa M, Block P, Gosselin A, Bentivoglio L, Leatherman L, Dorros G, King S, Galichia J, Al-Bassan M, Leon M, Robertson T, Passamani E. Percutaneous transluminal coronary angioplasty in 1985–1986 and 1977–1981. The National Heart Lung and Blood Institute Registry. N Engl J Med 1988; 318:265–270.
6. Holmes DR Jr, Myler R, Kent K, Williams DO, Faxon D, King SB III, Bentivoglio L, Cowley M, Dorros G, Galichia J, Gosselin A, Al-Bassam M, Block P, Bourassa M, Leatherman L, Desvigne-Nickens P, Steenkiste A, Kelsey K, Detre K. National Heart, Lung and Blood Institute percutaneous transluminal coronary angioplasty registry as a standard for comparison new devices. When should we use it, and what should we compare? Circulation 1991; 84:1828–1830.
7. Glagow S. Intimal hyperplasia, vascular modeling, and the restenosis problem. Circulation 1994; 89:2888–2891.
8. Safian RD, Gelbfish JS, Erny RD, Schnitt SJ, Schmidt DA, Baim DS. Coronary atherectomy: clinical, angiographic, and histologic findings and observations regarding potential mechanisms. Circulation 1990; 82:69–79.
9. Garratt KN, Holmes DR, Bell MR Jr, Bresnahan JF, Kaufmann UP, Vlietstra RE, Edwards W. Differences between primary atheromatous and restenosis lesions and influence of subintimal tissue resection. J Am Coll Cardiol 1991; 17:442–448.
10. Wilcox JN, Scott N, Lumsden AB, Subramamian RR, Rodriguez JC, Kelly A. Onset of cell proliferation and growth factor expression after clinical angioplasty of primate vascular lesions (abstr). Circulation 1993; 88:2526.
11. Hofling B, Welsch U, Heimer J, Gonschior P, Bauriedel G. Analysis of atherectomy specimens. Am J Cardiol 1993; 72:96E–107E.
12. Clowes AW: Pathologic intimal hyperplasia as a response to vascular injury and reconstruction. In: Rutherford RB, ed. Vascular Surgery. 3rd ed. Philadelphia: WB Saunders Co, 1989:266–275.

13. Isner JM, Kearney M, Bortman S, Pickering JG, Riessen R, Topol EJ, for CAVEAT Investigators. A sequential biopsy of human atheromata in vivo: longitudinal analysis of atheromatous coronary arterial walls in 11 patients treated for primary and restenosis lesions with directional atherectomy (abstr). J Am Coll Cardiol 1993; 21:74.
14. Chan P, Munro E, Patel M, Betteridge L, Schachter M, Sever P, Wolfe J. Cellular biology of human intimal hyperplastic stenosis. Eur J Vasc Surg 1993; 7:129–135.
15. Bauriedel G, Winstetter U, DeMaio SJ, Kandolf R, Hofling B. Migratory activity of human smooth muscle cells cultivated from coronary and peripheral primary and restenotic lesions removed by percutaneous atherectomy. Circulation 1992; 85:554–564.
16. O'Brien ER, Alpers CE, Stewart DK, Fergusson M, Tran N, Gordon D, Benditt EP, Hinohara T, Simpson JB, Schwartz SM. Proliferation of primary and restenotic coronary artery tissue. Implications for antiproliferative therapy. Circ Res 1993; 73:223–231.
17. Jawien A, Bowen-Pope DF, Lindner V, Schwartz SM, Clowes A. Platelet-derived growth factor promotes smooth muscle migration and intimal thickening in a rat model of balloon angioplasty. J Clin Invest 1992; 89:507–611.
18. Ross R, Raines EW, Bowen-Pope DF. The biology of platelet-derived growth factor. Cell 1986; 46:155–169.
19. Thyberg J, Hedin U, Sjolund M, Palmberg L, Bottger B. Regulation of differentiated properties and proliferation of arterial smooth muscle cells. Arteriosclerosis 1990; 10:966–969.
20. Klagsburn M, D'Amore PA. Regulators of angiogenesis. Annu Rev Physiol 1991; 53:217–239.
21. Casscells W, Lappi DA, Olwin BB, Wai C, Siegman M, Speir EH, Sasse J, Baird A. Elimination of smooth muscle cells in experimental restenosis: targeting of fibroblast growth factor receptors. Proc Natl Acad Sci USA 1992; 89:7159–7163.
22. Lindner V, Lappi DA, Baird A, Majack RA, Reidy MA. Role of basic fibroblast growth factor in vascular lesion formation. Circ Res 1991; 68:106–113.
23. Majevsky MW, Lindner V, Twardzik DR, Schwartz SM, Reidy MA. Production of transforming growth factor beta during repair of arterial injury. J Clin Invest 1991; 88:904–910.
24. Border WA, Ruoslahti E. Transforming growth factor-beta in disease: the dark side of tissue repair. J Clin Invest 1992; 90:1–7.
25. McCaffrey TA, Consigli S, Du B, Falcone DJ, Sanborn TA, Spokojny AM, Bush HL Jr. Decreased type II/type I TGF-beta receptor ratio in cells derived from human atherosclerotic lesions. Conversion from an antiproliferative to profibrotic response to TGF-beta 1. J Clin Invest 1995; 96:2667–2675.
26. van Obberghen-Schilling E, Roche NS, Flanders KC, Sporn MB, Roberts AB. Transforming growth factor-beta 1 positively regulates its own expression in normal and transformed cells. J Biol Chem 1988; 263:7741–7746.
27. Das SK, White AC, Fanburg BL. Modulation of transforming growth factor-beta1 antiproliferative effects on endothelial cells by cysteine, cystine, and N-acetylcysteine. J Clin Invest 1992; 90:1649–1656.

28. Nemecek GM, Coughlin SR, Handley DA, Moskowitz MA. Stimulation of aortic smooth muscle cells mitogenesis by serotonin. Proc Natl Acad Sci 1986; 83:674–678.
29. Bobik A, Grooms A, Millar JA, Mitchell A, Grinpukel S. Growth factor activity of endothelin on vascular smooth muscle. Am J Physiol 1990; 258:C408–415.
30. Hirata Y, Takagi Y, Fukuda Y, Marumo F. Endothelin is a potent mitogen for rat vascular smooth muscle cells. Atherosclerosis 1989; 78:225–228.
31. Ito H, Hirata Y, Adachi S, Tanaka M, Tsujino M, Koike A, Nogami A, Murumo F, Hiroe M. Endothelin-1 is an autocrine/paracrine factor in the mechanism of angiotensin-induced hypertrophy in cultured rat cardiomyocytes. J Clin Invest 1993; 92:398–403.
32. Weber H, Webb ML, Serafino R, Taylor DS, Moreland S, Norman J, Molloy CJ. Endothelin-1 and angiotensin-II stimulate delayed mitogenesis in cultured rat aortic smooth muscle cells: evidence for common signaling mechanism. Mol Endocrinol 1994; 8:148–158.
33. Khorsani MJ, Fagin JA, Giannella-Neto D, Forrester JS, Cercek B. Regulation of insulin-like growth factor-I and its receptor in rat aorta after balloon denudation. Evidence for local bioactivity. J Clin Invest 1992; 90:1926–1931.
34. Bornfeldt KE, Raines EW, Nakano T, Graves LM, Krebs EG, Ross R. Insulin-like growth factor-I and platelet-derived factor-BB induce directed migration of human arterial smooth muscle cells via signaling pathways that are distinct from those of proliferation. J Clin Invest 1994; 93:1266–1274.
35. Howell M, Orskov H, Frystyk J, Flyvbjerg A, Gronbaek H, Foegh M. Lanreotide, a somatostatin analogue, reduces insulin-like growth factor I accumulation in proliferating aortic tissue in rabbits in vivo. A preliminary study. Eur J Endocrinol 1994; 130:422–425.
36. Hatton MSW, Moar SL, Richardson M. Deendothelialization in vivo initiates a thrombogenic reaction at the rabbit aorta surface. Correlation of uptake of fibrinogen and antithrombin III with thrombin generation by the exposed endothelium. Am J Pathol 1989; 135:499–508.
37. McNamara CAI, Sarembock IJ, Gimple LW, Fenton III JW, Coughlin SR, Owens GK. Thrombin stimulates proliferation of cultured rat aortic smooth muscle cells by a proteolytically activated receptor. J Clin Invest 1993; 91:94–98.
38. Carney DH, Mann R, Redin WR, Pernia SD, Berry D, Heggers JP, Hayward PG, Robson MC, Christie J, Annable C. Enhancement of incisional wound healing and neovascularization in normal rats by thrombin and synthetic thrombin receptor-activating peptides. J Clin Invest 1992; 89:1469–1477.
39. Bar-Shavit R, Benezra M, Eldor A, HY-Am E, Fenton III JW, Wilner GD, Vlodavsky I. Thrombin immobilized to extracellular matrix is a potent mitogen for vascular smooth muscle cells: nonenzymatic mode of action. Cell Regul 1990; 1:453–463.
40. Crowley ST, Ray CJ, Nawaz D, Majack RA, Horwitz LD. Multiple growth factors are released from mechanically injured vascular smooth muscle cells. Am J Physiol 1995; 269 (5 Pt 2) :H1641–H1647.
41. Vassalli J-D, Sappino A-P, Belin D. The plasminogen activator/plasmin system. J Clin Invest 1991; 88:1067–1072.

42. Andrade-Gordon P, Strickland S. Interaction of heparin with plasminogen activators and plasminogen: effects on the activation of plasminogen. Biochemistry 1986; 25:4033–4040.
43. Rifkin DB, Moscatelli D, Bizik J, Quarto N, Blei F, Dennis P, Falumenhaft R, Mignatti P. Growth factor control of extracellular proteolysis. Cell Diff Dev 1990; 32:313–318.
44. Carmeliet P, Kieckens L, Schoonjans L, Ream B, van Nuffelen A, Prendergast G, Cole M, Bronson R, Collen D, Mulligan RCM. Plasminogen activator inhibitor-1 gene-defficient mice. I. Generation by homologous recombination and characterization. J Clin Invest 1993; 92:2746–2255.
45. Carmeliet P, Stassen JM, Schoonjans L, Ream B, van den Oord JJ, De Mol M, Mulligan RCM, Collen D. Plasminogen activator inhibitor-I gene-defficient mice. II. Effects on hemostasis, thrombosis and thrombolysis. J Clin Invest 1993; 92:2756–2760.
46. Carmeliet P, Schoonjans L, Kieckens L, Ream B, Degen J, Bronson R, De Vos R, van den Oord JJ, Collen D, Mulligan RCM. Physiological consequences of loss of plasminogen activator gene function in mice. Nature 1994; 368:419–424.
47. Carmeliet P, Stassen JM, De Mol M, Declercq C, Bouche A, Collen D. Arterial neointima formation after trauma in mice with inactivation of the t-PA, u-PA or PAI genes (abstr). Fibrinolysis 1994; 8:280.
48. Libby P, Schwartz D, Brogi E, Tanaka H, Clinton SK. A cascade model for restenosis. A special case of atherosclerosis progression. Circulation 1992; 86(III):47–52.
49. Marui N, Offermen MK, Swerlick R, Kunsch C, Rosen CA, Ahmad A, Alexander RW, Medford RM. Vascular cell adhesion molecule-1 (VACM-1) gene transcription and expression are regulated through an anti-oxidant-sensitive mechanism in human vascular endothelial cells. J Clin Invest 1993; 92:1866–1874.
50. Quinn MT, Parthasarathy S, Fong LG, Steinberg D. Oxidatively modified low density lipoproteins: a potential role in recruitment and retention of monocyte/macrophages during atherogenesis. Proc Natl Acad Sci USA 1987; 84:2995–2998.
51. Simon BC, Cunningham LD, Cohen RA. Oxidized low density lipoproteins cause contraction and inhibit endothelium-dependent relaxation in pig coronary artery. J Clin Invest 1990; 86:75–79.
52. Berliner JA, Territo MC, Sevanian A, Ramin S, Kim JA, Bamshad B, Esterson M, Fogelman AM. Minimally modified low density lipoprotein stimulate monocyte endothelial interactions. J Clin Invest 1990; 85:1260–1266.
53. Chin JH, Azhar S, Hoffman BB. Inactivation of endothelial derived relaxing factor by oxidized lipoproteins. J Clin Invest 1992; 89:10–18.
54. Pepper MS, Belin D, Montesano R, Orci L, Vassali J-D. Transforming growth factor-beta 1 modulates basic fibroblast growth factor-induced proteolytic and angiogenic properties of endothelial cells in vitro. J Cell Biol 1990; 111:743–755.
55. Lindstrom P, Lerner R, Palmblad J, Patarroyo M. Rapid adhesive responses of endothelial cells and of neutrophils induced by leukotriene B4 are mediated by leukocytic adhesion protein CD18. Scand J Immunol 1990; 31:737–744.
56. Holifield B, Helgason T, Jemelka S, Taylor A, Navran S, Allen J, Seidel C. Dif-

ferentiated vascular myocytes: are they involved in neointimal formation? J Clin Invest 1996; 97:814–825.
57. Isner JM, Kearney M, Bortman S, Passeri J. Apoptosis in human atherosclerosis and restenosis. Circulation 1995; 91:2703–2711.
58. Riessen R, Isner JM, Blessing E, Loushin C, Nikol S, Wight TN. Regional differences in the distribution of the proteoglycans biglycan and decorin in the extracellular matrix of atherosclerotic and restenotic human arteries. Am J Pathol 1994; 144:962–974.
59. Chung I-M, Reidy MA, Schwartz SM, Wight TN, Gold HK. Enhanced extracellular matrix synthesis may be important for restenosis of arteries after stent deployment (abstr). Circulation 1996; 94:2034.
60. Strauss BH, Chisholm RJ, Keely FW, Gotlieb AI, Logan RA, Armstrong PW. Extracellular matrix remodeling after balloon angioplasty injury in a rabbit model of restenosis. Circ Res 1994; 75:650–658.
61. Moscatelli D, Rifkin DB. Membrane and matrix localization of proteinases: a common theme in tumor invasion and angiogenesis. Biochem Biophys Acta 1989; 948:67–85.
62. Hedin U, Bottger BA, Forsberg E. Diverse effects of fibronectin and laminin on phenotypic properties of cultured arterial smooth muscle cells. J Cell Biol 1988; 107:307–319.
63. Rizvi MA, Katwa L, Spadone DP, Myers PR. The effect of endothelin-1 on collagen type-I and type-III synthesis in cultured porcine coronary artery vascular smooth muscle cells. J Mol Cell Cardiol 1996; 28:243–252.
64. Saksela O, Rifkin DB. Release of fibroblast growth factor-heparin sulfate complexes from endothelial cells by plasminogen activator mediated proteolytic activity. J Cell Biol 1990; 110:767–775.
65. Sato Y, Tsuboi R, Moses H, Rifkin DB. Characterization of the activation of latent TGF-β1 by co-cultures of endothelial and pericytes or smooth muscle cells: a self regulating system. J Cell Biol 1990; 111:757–763.
66. Webster WS, Bidhop SP, Geer JC. Experimental aortic intimal thickening. Am J Pathol 1974; 76:245–264.
67. Chignier E, Eloy R. Adventitial resection of small artery provokes endothelial loss and intimal hyperplasia. Surg Gynecol Obst 1986; 163:327–334.
68. Barker SG, Tilling CC, Miller GC, Beesley JE, Fleetwood G, Stavri GT, Baskerville PA, Martin JF. The adventitia and atherogenesis: removal initiates intimal proliferation in the rabbit which regresses on generation of a "neoadventitia." Atherosclerosis 1994; 105:131–144.
69. Booth RF, Martin JF, Honey AC, Hassal DG, Beesley JE, Moncada S. Rapid development of atherosclerotic lesions in the rabbit carotid artery induced by perivascular manipulation. Atherosclerosis 1989; 76:257–268.
70. Shi Y, Pieniek M, Fard A, O'Brien J, Mannion JD, Zalewski A. Adventitial remodeling following coronary arterial injury. Circulation 1996; 93:340–348.
71. Shi Y, O'Brien JE, Fard A, Mannion JD, Wang D, Zalewski A. Adventitial myofibroblasts contribute to neointimal formation in injured porcine coronary arteries. Circulation 1996; 94:1655–1664.

72. Skalli O, Schurch W, Seemayer T, Lagace R, Montandon D, Pittet B, Gabbiani G. Myofibroblasts from diverse pathologic settings are heterogeneous in their content of actin isoforms and intermediate filament proteins. Lab Invest 1989; 60:275–285.
73. Darby I, Skalli 0, Gabbiani G. Alpha-smooth muscle actin is transiently expressed by myofibroblasts during experimental wound healing. Lab Invest 1990; 63:12–29.
74. Poon M, Marmur JD, Rosenfield C-L, Rollins BJ, Taubman MB. The KC gene is induced in vivo by vascular injury and in smooth muscle culture by growth factors (abstr). Circulation 1990; 82:827.
75. Naftilan AJ, Pratt RE, Dzau VJ. Angiotensin II induces c-fos expression in smooth muscle via transcriptional control. Hypertension 1989; 13:706–711.
76. Naftilan AJ, Pratt RE, Dzau VJ. Induction of PDGF A-chain and c-myc gene expression by angiotensin II in cultured rat vascular smooth muscle cells. J Clin Invest 1989; 83:1419–1424.
77. Miller AD, Curran T, Verma IM. C-fos protein can induce cellular transformation: A novel mechanism of activation of cellular oncogene. Cell 1984; 35:51–60.
78. Marmur JD, Friedrich VL, Rossikhina M, Rollins BJ, Taubman MB. The JE gene encodes a smooth muscle chemotactic factor that is induced by vascular injury (abstr). Circulation 1990; 82:2774.
79. Nilsson J, von Euler AM, Dalsgaard C-J. Stimulation of connective tissue cell growth by substance P and substance K. Nature 1985; 315:61–63.
80. Nilsson J, Sejersen T, Hultgardh-Nilsson A, Dalsgaard C-J. DNA synthesis induced by the neuropeptide substance K correlates to the level of myc-gene transcripts. Biochem Biophys Res Commun 1986; 137:167–174.
81. Kindy MS, Sonenshein GE. Regulation of oncogene expression in cultured aortic smooth muscle cells. J Biol Chem 1986; 261:12856–12868.
82. Brown KE, Kindy MS, Sonenshein GE. Expression of the c-myb pro-oncogene in bovine vascular smooth muscle cells. J Biol Chem 1992; 267:4625–4630.
83. Miano JM, Tota RR, Vlasic N, Danishefsky KJ, Stemerman MB. Early protooncogene expression in rat aortic smooth muscle cells following endothelial removal. Am J Pathol 1990; 137:761–765.
84. Gibons GH, Pratt RE, Dzau VJ. Vascular smooth muscle cell hypertrophy vs. hyperplasia: autocrine transforming growth factor-beta expression determines growth response to angiotensin II. J Clin Invest 1992; 90:456–461.
85. Gibons GH, Pratt RE, Dzau VJ. Angiotensin II is a bifunctional modulator of vascular smooth muscle cell growth: interaction with basic fibroblast growth factor (abstract). Hypertension 1989; 14:358.
86. Gadeau AP, Campan M, Millet D, Candresse T, Desranges C. Osteopontin overexpression is associated with arterial smooth muscle cell proliferation in vitro. Arterioscl Thromb 1993; 13:120–125.
87. Thalmeier K, Synovzik H, Mertz R, Winnacker EL, Lipp M. Nuclear factor E2F mediates basic transcription and transactivation by E1a of the human MYC promoter. Genes Dev 1989; 3:527–536.
88. Yang XH, Sladek TL. Overexpression of the E2F-1 transcription factor gene mediates cell transformation. Gene Expr 1995; 4:195–204.

89. Xu G, Livingston DM, Krek W. Multiple members of the E2F transcription factor family are the products of oncogenes. Proc Natl Acad Sci USA 1995; 92:1357–1361.
90. Filed SJ, Tsai FY, Kuo F, Zubiaga AM, Kaelin WG, Livingston DM, Orkin SH, Greenberg ME. E2F-1 functions in mice to promote apoptosis and suppress proliferation. Cell 1995; 85:549–561.
91. Kowalik TE, Wing B, Haskill JS, Azizkhan JC, Baldwin AS Jr, Huang ES. Multiple mechanisms are implicated in the regulation of NF-kappa B activity during human cytomegalovirus infection. Immunology 1993; 78:405–412.
92. Grundy JE, Downes KL. Up-regulation of LFA-3 and ICAM-1 on the surface fibroblasts infected with cytomegalovirus. Immunology 1993; 78:405–412.
93. Zhou YF, Leon MB, Waclawiw MA, Popma JJ, Yu ZX, Finkel T, Epstein SE. Association between prior cytomegalovirus infection and the risk of restenosis after coronary atherectomy. N Engl J Med 1996; 335:624–630.
94. Zhu H, Shen Y, Shenk T. Human cytomegalovirus IE1 and IE2 proteins block apoptosis. J Virol 1995; 69:7960–7970.
95. Keiser A, Weich HA, Brandner G, Marmae D, Kolch W. Mutant p53 potentiates protein kinase C induction of vascular endothelial growth factor expression. Oncogene 1994; 9:963–969.
96. Rigat B, Huberet C, Alhenc-Gelas F, Cambien F, Forvol P, Soubrier F. An insertion-deletion polymorphism in the angiotensin I-converting enzyme gene accounting for half variances of serum levels. J Clin Invest 1990; 86:1343–1346.
97. Ohishi M, Fujii K, Minamino T, Higaki J, Kamitani A, Raguki H, Zhao Y, Mikami H, Miki T, Ogihara T. A potent genetic risk factor for restenosis. Nat Genet 1993; 5:324–325.
98. Kaski JC, Zhang Y, Calvino R, Vazquez-Rodriguez JM, Castro-Beiras A, Jeffery S, Carter N. Angiotensin-converting enzyme insertion/deletion polymorphism and restenosis after coronary angioplasty in unstable angina pectoris. Am J Cardiol 1996; 77:875–877.
99. Weiss EJ, Bary PF, Tayback M, Schulman SP, Kickler TS, Becker LC, Weiss JL, Gerstenblith G, Goldschmidt-Clermont PJ. A polymorphism of a platelet glycoprotein receptor as an inherited risk factor for coronary thrombosis. N Engl J Med 1996; 334:1090–1094.
100. Palmberg L, Claesson H-E, Thyberg J. Effects of leukotrienes on phenotypic properties and growth of arterial smooth muscle cells. J Cell Sci 1989; 93:403–408.
101. Palmberg L, Claesson HE, Thyberg J. Leukotrienes stimulate initiation of DNA synthesis in cultured arterial smooth muscle cells. J Cell Sci 1987; 88:151–159.
102. Libby P, Warner SJC, Salomon RN, Birinyi LK. Production of platelet-derived growth factor-like mitogen by smooth muscle cells from human atheroma. N Engl J Med 1988; 318:1493–1498.
103. Sjolund, Hedin U, Sejersen T, Heldin C-H, Thyberg J. Arterial smooth muscle cells express platelet derived growth factor (PDGF) A chain mRNA, secrete a PDGF-like mitogen, and bind exogenous PDGF in a phenotype- and growth state dependent manner. J Cell Biol 1988; 106:403–413.
104. Walker LN, Bowen-Pope DF, Ross R, Reidy MA. Production of platelet-derived

growth factor-like molecules by cultured arterial smooth muscle cells accompanies proliferation after arterial injury. Proc Natl Acad Sci USA 1986; 83:7311–7315.
105. Majack RA, Majesky MW, Goodman LV. Role of PDGF-A expression in the control of vascular smooth muscle cell growth by transforming growth factor-beta. J Cell Biol 1990; 111:239–247.
106. Schwartz SM, Foy L, Bowen-Pope DF, Ross R. Derivation and properties of platelet-derived growth factor-independent rat smooth muscle cells. Am J Pathol 1990; 136:1417–1428.
107. Corcos T, David PR, Bal PG, Renkin J, Dangoisse V, Rapold HG, Bourassa MG. Failure of diltiazem to prevent restenosis after percutaneous transluminal coronary angioplasty. Am Heart J 1985; 109:926–931.
108. Whitworth HB, Roubin GS, Hollman J, Meier B, Leimgruber PP, Douglas JS Jr, King SB III, Gruentzig AR. Effect of nifedipine on recurrent stenosis after percutaneous transluminal coronary angioplasty. J Am Coll Card 1986; 8:1271–1276.
109. Weintraub WS, Boccuzzi SJ, Klein JL, Kosinski AS, King SB, Ivanhoe R, Cedarholm JC, Stillabower ME, Talley JD, DeMaio SJ, O'Neill WW, Frazier JE, Cohen-Bernstein CL, Robbins DC, Brown CL, Alexander RW, and the Lovastatin Restenosis Trial Study Group. Lack of effect of lovastatin on restenosis after angioplasty. N Engl J Med 1994; 331:1331–1337.
110. O'Keefe JH, Stone GW, McAllister BD Jr, Maddex CH, Ligon R, Kacich RL, Kahn J, Cavero PG, Hartzler GO. Lovastatin plus robucol for prevention of restenosis after percutaneous transluminal coronary angioplasty. Am J Cardiol 1996; 77:649–652.
111. Schwartz L, Bourassa MG, Lesperance J. Aldridge HE, Kazim F, Salvatori VA, Henderson M, Bonan R, David PR. Aspirin and dipyridamole in the prevention of restenosis after percutaneous transluminal coronary angioplasty. N Engl J Med 1988; 318:1714–1719.
112. Thornton MA, Gruentzig AR, Hollman J, King SB III, Douglas JS. Coumadin and aspirin in prevention of recurrence after transluminal coronary angioplasty: a randomized study. Circulation 1984; 69:721–727.
113. Pepine CJ, Hirschfeld JW, Macdonald RG, Henderson MA, Bass TA, Goldberg S, Savage MP, Vetrovec G, Cowley M, Taussig AS, Whitworth HB, Margolis JR, Hill JA, Bove AA, Jugo R. A controlled trial of corticosteroids to prevent restenosis after coronary angioplasty. Circulation 1990; 81:1753–1761.
114. Serruys PW, Rutsch W, Heyndrickx GR, Danchin N, Mast G, Wijns W, Rensing BJ, Vos J, Stibbe J. Prevention of restenosis after percutaneous transluminal coronary angioplasty with thromboxane A2-receptor blockade. A randomized, double-blind, placebo-controlled trial. Circulation 1991; 84:1568–1580.
115. Ishiwata S, Nakanishi S, Nishiyama S, Seki A. Prevention of restenosis by bezafibrate after successful coronary angioplasty. Coron Artery Dis 1995; 6:883–889.
116. Vague P, Juhan-Vague I, Aillaud MF, Badier C, Viard R, Alessi MC. Correlation between fibrinolytic activity, plasminogen activator inhibitor level, plasma insulin level, and relative body weight in normal and obese subjects. Metabolism 1986; 35:250–253.

117. Yokoi H, Kubawa Y, Yamaguchi H. The PART group. One year follow-up results of the probucol angioplasty restenosis trial (PART) (abstr). Circulation 1996; 94:0523.
118. Freed MS, Safian MA, Safian RD, Jones DE, O'Neil WW, Grines CL. An intensive poly-pharmaceutical approach to the prevention of restenosis: the mevacor, ACE inhibitor, colchicine (BIG-MAC) pilot trial (abstr). J Am Coll Cardiol 1993; 21:33.
119. Lindner V, Olson NE, Clowes AW, Reidy MA. Inhibition of smooth muscle cell proliferation in injured rat arteries. J Clin Invest 1992; 90:2044–2049.
120. Ottlinger ME, Pukac LA, Karnovsky MJ. Heparin inhibits mitogen-activated protein kinase activation in intact rat vascular smooth muscle cells. J Biol Chem 1993; 268:19173–19176.
121. Pukac LA, Castellot JJ Jr, Wright TC Jr, Caleb BL, Karnovsky MJ. Heparin inhibits c-fos and c-myc mRNA expression in vascular smooth muscle cells. Cell Regul 1990; 1:435–443.
122. Skaletz-Rorowski A, Schmidt A, Breithardt G, Buddecke E. Heparin-induced overexpression of basic fibroblast growth factor, basic fibroblast growth factor receptor, and cell associated proteoheparan sulfate in cultured coronary smooth muscle cells. Arterioscler Thromb Vasc Biol 1996; 16:1063–1069.
123. Geary RL, Koyama N, Wang TW, Vergei S, Clowes AW. Failure of heparin to inhibit intimal hyperplasia in injured baboon arteries. The role of heparin-sensitive and -insensitive pathways in the stimulation of smooth muscle cell migration and proliferation. Circulation 1995; 91:2972–2981.
124. Powell JS, Clozel JP, Muller RKM, Kuhn H, Hefti F, Hosang M, Baumgartner HR. Inhibitors of angiotensin-converting enzyme prevent myointimal proliferation after vascular injury. Science 1989; 245:186–188.
125. MERCATOR Study Group. Does new angiotensin-converting enzyme inhibitor cilazapril prevent restenosis after percutaneous transluminal angioplasty? Results of the MERCATOR Study: a multicenter, randomized, double-blind placebo controlled trial. Circulation 1992; 86:100–110.
126. Lindner V, Reidy MA. Proliferation of smooth muscle cells after vascular injury is inhibited by an antibody against basic fibroblast growth factor. Proc Natl Acad Sci USA 1991; 88:3739–3743.
127. Ferns GAA, Raines EW, Sprugel KH, Montani AS, Reidy MA, Ross R. Inhibition of neointimal smooth muscle cell accumulation after angioplasty by an antibody to PDGF. Science 1991; 253:1129–1132.
128. Maresta A, Balducelli M, Cantini L, Casari A, Chioin R, Fabbri M, Fontanelli A, Preti PAM, Repetto S, DeServi S, Varani E, for the STARC investigators. Trapidil (triazolopyrimidine), a platelet-derived growth factor antagonist, reduces restenosis after percutaneous transluminal angioplasty. Results of the randomized, double blind STARC study. Circulation 1994; 90:2710–2715.
129. Douglas SA, Louden C, Vickery-Clark LM, Storer BL, Hart T, Feurestein GL, Elliott JD, Ohstein EM. A role for endogenous endothelin-1 in neointimal formation after rat carotid artery balloon angioplasty: protective effects of the novel nonpeptide endothelin receptor antagonist SB 209670. Circ Res 1994; 75:190–197.

130. Markwardt F. Pharmacology of hirudin: one hundred years after the first report of the anticoagulant agent in medicinal leeches. Biomed Biochem Acta 1985; 44:1007–1013.
131. Heras M, Chesebro JH, Webster MWI, Mruk JS, Grill DE, Peeny WJ, Bowie EJW, Badimon L, Fuster V. Hirudin, heparin and placebo during deep arterial injury in the pig: the in vivo role of thrombin in platelet-mediated thrombosis. Circulation 1990; 82:1476–1484.
132. Cannon CP, Maraganore JM, Loscalzo J, McAllister A, Eddings K, George D, Selwyn AP, Adelman B, Fox I, Braunwald E, Ganz P. Anticoagulant effects of Hirulog, a novel thrombin inhibitor, in patients with coronary artery disease. Am J Cardiol 1993; 71:778–782.
133. Wenzel UO, Fouqueray B, Grandaliano G, Kim YS, Karamitsos C, Valente AJ, Abboud HE. Thrombin regulates expression of monocyte chemoattractant protein-1 in vascular smooth muscle cells. Circ Res 1995; 77:503–509.
134. Utenberg C, Sandrock D, Nebendahl K, Buchwald AB. Reduced acute thrombus formation results in decreased neointimal proliferation after coronary angioplasty. J Am Coll Cardiol 1995; 26:1747–1754.
135. Ragosta M, Barry WL, Gimple LW, Gertz SD, McCoy KW, Stouffer GA, McNamara CA, Powers ER, Owens GK, Sarembock IJ. Effect of thrombin inhibition with desulfatohirudin on early kinetics of cellular proliferation after balloon angioplasty in atherosclerotic rabbits. Circulation 1996; 93:1194–1200.
136. EPIC Investigators. Use of monoclonal antibody directed against the platelet glycoprotein IIb/IIIa receptor in high-risk coronary angioplasty. N Engl J Med 1994; 330:956–961.
137. Kereiakes DJ, Essel JH, Abbottsmith CW, Broderick TM, Runyon P. Abciximab-associated profound thrombocytopenia: therapy with immunoglobulin and platelet transfusion. Am J Cardiol 1996; 78:1161–1163.
138. Mooradian DL, Fernandes B, Diglio CA, Lester BR. Angiopeptin (BIM23014C) inhibits vascular smooth muscle cell migration in vitro through a G-protein-mediated pathways and is associated with inhibition of adenyl cyclase and cyclic AMP accumulation. J Cardiovasc Pharmacol 1995; 25:611–618.
139. Foegh ML, Asotra S, Conte JV, Howell M, Kagan E, Verma K, Ramwell PW. Early inhibition of myointimal proliferation by angiopeptin after balloon catheter injury in rabbit. J Vasc Surg 1994; 19:1084–1091.
140. Lundergan C, Foegh ML, Vargas R, Eufemio M, Bormes GW, Kot PA, Ramwell PW. Inhibition of myointimal proliferation of the rat carotid artery by the peptides, angiopeptin and BIM 23034. Atherosclerosis 1989; 80:49–55.
141. Eriksen UH, Bagger JP, Emanuelsson H, Foegh M, Henningsen P, Saunamaki K, Schaeffer M, Thayssen P, Orskov H. Randomized double-blind Scandinavian trial of angiopeptin versus placebo for the prevention of clinical events and restenosis after coronary balloon angioplasty. Am Heart J 1995; 130:1–8.
142. Emanuelsson H, Beatt KJ, Bagger JP, Balcon R, Heikkila J, Piessens J, Schaeffer M, Suryapranata H, Foegh M. Long-term effects of angiopeptin treatment in coronary angioplasty. Reduction in clinical events but not angiographic restenosis. European Angiopeptin Study Group. Circulation 1995; 91:1689–1696.

143. Powell JS, Clozel JP, Muller RK, Kuhn H, Hefti F, Hosang M, Baumgartner HR. Inhibitors of angiotensin-converting enzyme prevent myointimal proliferation after vascular injury. Science 1989; 245:186–188.
144. Epstein SE, Speir E, Unger EF, Guzman RJ, Finkel T. The basis of molecular strategies for treating restenosis after angioplasty. J Am Coll Cardiol 1994; 23:1278–1288.
145. Voisard R, Dartsch PC, Seitzer U, Hannekum A, Roth D, Kochs M, Hombach V. The in-vitro efect of antineoplastic agents on proliferative activity and cytoskeletal components of plaque-derived smooth muscle cells from human coronary arteries. Coron Artery Dis 1993; 4:935–942.
146. Pastore CJ, Isner JM, Bacha PA, Kearney M Pickering JG. Epidermal growth factor receptor-targeted cytotoxin inhibits neointimal hyperplasia in vivo. Results of local versus systemic delivery administration. Circ Res 1995; 77:519–529.
147. Fu YM, Mesri EA, Yu ZX, Kreitman RJ, Pastan I, Epstein SE. Cytotoxic effects of vascular smooth muscle cells of the chimeric toxin, heparin binding TGF alpha-Pseudomonas exotoxin. Cardiovasc Res 1993; 27:1691–1697.
148. Chang MW, Ohno T, Gordon D, Lu MM, Nabel GJ, Nabel EG, Leiden JM. Adenovirus-mediated transfer of the herpes simplex virus thymidine kinase gene inhibits vascular smooth muscle cell proliferation and neointima formation following balloon angioplasty of the rat carotid artery. Mol Med 1995; 1:172–181.
149. Lim CS, Chapman GD, Gammon RS, Muhlestein JB, Bauman RP, Stack RS, Swain JL. Direct in vivo gene transfer into the coronary and peripheral vasculature of the intact dog. Circulation 1991; 83:2007–2011.
150. Nabel EG, Plautz G, Nabel GJ. Site-specific gene expression in vivo by direct gene transfer into the arterial wall. Science 1990; 249:1285–1288.
151. Guzman RJ, Lemarchant P, Crystal RG, Epstein SE, Finkel T. Efficient and selective adenovirus-mediated gene tranfer into neovascular intima. Circulation 1993; 88:2838–2848.
152. Speir E, Epstein SE. Inhibition of smooth muscle cell proliferation by antisense oligonucleotide targeting the messenger RNA encoding proliferating cell nuclear antigen. Circulation 1992; 86:538–547.
153. Shi Y, Hutchinson HG, Hall DJ, Zalewski A. Downregulation of c-myc expression by antisense oligonucleotides inhibits proliferation of human smooth muscle cells. Circulation 1993; 88:1190–1195.
154. Shi Y, Yard A, Galeo A, Hutchinsosn HG, Vermani P, Dodge GR, Hall DJ, Shaheen F, Zalewski A. Transcatheter delivery of c-myc antisense oligomers reduces neointimal formation in a porcine model of coronary artery balloon injury. Circulation 1994; 90:944–951.
155. Simons M, Rosenberg RD. Antisense nonmuscle myosin heavy chain and c-myb oligonucleotides suppress smooth muscle cell proliferation in vitro. Circ Res 1992; 70:835–843.
156. Simons M, Edelman ER, DeKeyser J-L, Langer R, Rosenberg. Antisense c-myb oligonucleotides inhibit intimal arterial smooth muscle cell accumulation in vivo. Nature 1992; 359:67–80.
157. March KL, Madison JE, Trapnell BC. Pharmacokinetics of adenoviral vector-

mediated gene delivery to vascular smooth muscle cells: modulation by polyxamer 407 and implications for cardiovascular gene therapy. Hum Gene Ther 1995; 6:41–53.

158. March KL, Bauriedel G, Trapnell BC. Gene therapy to block restenosis following percutaneous transluminal coronary angioplasty: feasibility of strategies to target smooth muscle cells using adenoviral vectors (abstr). Circulation 1993; 88:1990.
159. Morishita R, Gibbons GH, Ellison KE, Von der Leyen H, Zhang L, Kaneda Y, Dzau VJ. A viral-mediated antisense oligonucleotide delivery system to prevent restenosis (abstr). Circulation 1993; 88:1991.
160. Shi Y, Fard A, Galeo A, Hutchinson HG, Vermani P, Dodge GR, Hall DJ, Zalewski A. Transcatheter delivery of c-myc antisense oligomers reduces neointimal formation in a porcine model. Circulation 1994; 90:944–951.
161. Chang MW, Barr E, Seltzer J, Jiang Y-Q, Nabel GJ, Nabel EG, Parmacek MS, Leiden JM. Cytostatic gene therapy for vascular proliferative disorders with constitutively active form of the retinoblastoma gene product. Science 1995; 267:518–521.
162. Chang MW, Barr E, Lu MM, Barton K, Leiden JM. Adenovirus-mediated overexpression of the cyclin/cyclin-dependent kinase inhibitor, p2l inhibits vascular smooth muscle cell proliferation and neointima formation in the rat carotid artery model of balloon angioplasty. J Clin Invest 1995; 96:2260–2268.
163. Daniel TO, Ives HE. Endothelial control of vascular function. News Physiol Sci 1989; 4:139–142.
164. Ross R. Atherosclerosis: a defense mechanism gone awry. Am J Pathol 1993; 143:985–1002.
165. Marshall JJ, Kontos HA. Endothelium-derived relaxing factors: a perspective from in vivo data. Hypertension 1990; 16:371–386.
166. Castellot JJ Jr, Favreau LV, Karnovsky Mi, Rosenberg RD. Inhibition of vascular smooth muscle cell growth by endothelial cell-derived heparin: possible role of platelet endoglycosidase. J Biol Chem 1982; 257:11256–11260.
167. Fritze LMS, Reilly CF, Rosenberg RDA. Antiproliferative heparan sulfate species produced by post confluent smooth muscle cells. J Cell Biol 1985; 100:1041–1049.
168. Scott-Burden T, Vanhoutte PM. Regulation of smooth muscle celll growth by endothelium-derived factors. Tex Heart Inst J 1994; 21:91–97.
169. Furchgott RF, Zawadzki JV. Obligatory role of endothelial cells in the relaxation of arterial smooth muscle by acetylcholine. Nat Lond 1980; 288:373–376.
170. Luscher TF, Yang Z, Diedrich,D, Buhler FR. Endothelium derived vasoactive substances: potential role in hypertension, atherosclerosis and vascular occlusion. J Cardiovasc Pharmacol 1989; 14(suppl) 6:S63–69.
171. McNamara DB, Ignarro LJ, Akers DL. L-Arginine inhibits balloon catheter-induced intimal hyperplasia without improving neoendothelial-dependent acetylcholine-induced relaxation (abstr). Circulation 1993; 88:1993.
172. Connoly DT, Heuvelman DM, Nelson R, Olander JV, Eppley BL, Delfino JJ, Siegel NR, Leimgruber RM, Feder J. Tumor vascular permeability factor stimulates endothelial cell growth and angiogenesis. J Clin Invest 1989; 84:1470–1478.

173. Leung D, Cachianes W, Kuang W, Goeddel D, Ferrara N. Vascular endothelial growth factor is a secreted angiogenic mitogen. Science 1989; 246:1306–1312.
174. Brown LF, Berse B, Jackman RW, Tognazzi K, Guidi AJ, Dvorak HF, Senger DR, Connoly JL, Schnitt SJ. Expression of vascular permeability factor (vascular endothelial growth factor) and its receptors in breast cancer. Hum Pathol 1995; 26:86–91.
175. Hatva E, Kaipainen A, Mentula P, Jaaskelainen J, Paetau A, Haltia M, Alitalo K. Expression of endothelial-specific receptor tyrosine kinases and growth factors in human brain tumors. Am J Pathol 1995; 146:368–378.
176. Hashimoto E, Ogita T, Nakaoka T, Matsuoka R, Takao A, Kira Y. Rapid induction of vascular endothelial growth factor by transient ischemia in rat heart. Am J Physiol 1994; 267:H1948–1954.
177. Banai S, Shweiki D, Pinson A, Chandra M, Lazarovici G, Keshet E. Upregulation of vascular endothelial growth factor expression induced by myocardial ischemia: implication for coronary angiogenesis. Cardiovasc Res 1994; 28:1176–1179.
178. Brogi E, Schatteman G, Wu T, Kim EA, Varticovski L, Keyt B, Isner JM. Hypoxia-induced paracrine regulation of vascular endothelial growth factor receptor expression. J Clin Invest 1996; 97:469–476.
179. Asahar T, Bauters Ch, Pastore Ch, Kearney M, Rossow S, Bunting S, Ferrara N, Symes J, Isner JM. Local delivery of vascular endothelial growth factor accelerates re-endothelialization and attenuates intimal hyperplasia in balloon-injured rat carotid artery. Circulation 1995; 91:2793–2801.
180. Wight TN, Ross R. Proteoglycans in primate arteries. II: synthesis and secretion of glycosaminoglycans by arterial smooth muscle cells in culture. J Cell Biol 1975; 67:675–686.
181. Serruys PW, de Jaegere P, Kiememeij C, Macaya H, Rutsch W, Heyndrickx G, Emanuelsson G, Marco J, Legrand V, Materne P, Belardi J, Sigwart U, Colombo A, Goy JJ, van den Heuvel P, Delcan J, Morel M-A, for the Benestent study group. A comparison of balloon-expandable stent implantation with balloon angioplasty in patients with coronary artery disease. N Engl J Med 1994; 331: 489–495.
182. Fischman DL, Leon MB, Baim DS, Schatz RA, Savage MP, Penn I, Detre K, Veltri L, Rieci DR, Nobuyoshi M. A randomized comparison of coronary stent placement and balloon angioplasty in the treatment of coronary artery disease. (The STRESS Study). N Engl J Med 1994; 331:496–501.
183. Colombo A, Hall P, Nakamura S, Almagor Y, Maiello L, Martini G, Gaglione A, Goldberg SL, Tobis JM. Intracoronary stenting without anticoagulation accomplished with intravascular ultrasound guidance. Circulation 1995; 91:1676–1688.
184. Kuntz RE, Gibson M, Nobuyoshi M, Baim DS. Generalized model of restenosis after conventional balloon angioplasty, stenting and directional atherectomy. J Am Coll Cardiol 1993; 21:15–25.
185. Carter AJ, Laird JR, Farb A, Kufs W, Wortham DC, Virmani R. Morphologic characteristics of lesion formation and time course of smooth muscle cell proliferation in porcine proliferative restenosis model. J Am Coll Cardiol 1994; 24:1398–1405.
186. Serruys PW, Di Mario C. Who was thrombogenic: the stent or the doctor. Circulation 1995; 91:1891–1893.

187. Topol EJ. The stentor and the sea change. Am J Cardiol 1995; 76:307–308.
188. Williams DO. Dressing up the Palmaz-Schatz stent. Circulation 1996; 93:400–402.
189. Lincoff AM, Topol EJ. Local drug delivery for the prevention of restenosis. Fact, fancy, and future. Circulation 1994; 90: 2070–2084.
190. Cox D, Anderson P, Roubin G, Chou C, Agrawal S, Cavender J. Effect of local delivery of heparin and methotrexate on neointimal proliferation in stented porcine coronary arteries. Coron Art Dis 1992; 3:237–248.
191. Serruys PW, Emanuelsson H, van der Giessen W, Lunn AC, Kiemeney F, Macaya C, Rutsch W, Heyndrickx G, Suryapranata H, Legrand V, Goy JJ, Materne P, Bonnier H, Morice M-C, Fajadet J, Belardi J, Colombo A, Garcia E, Ruygrok P, de Jaegere P, Morel M-A, on the behalf of Benestent-II study. Heparin-coated Palmaz-Schatz stents in human coronary arteries. Early outcome of the Benestent-II pilot study. Circulation 1996; 93:412–422.
192. Waksman R, Robinson KA, Crocker IR, Gravanis MB, Palmer SJ, Wang C, Cipolla GD, King SB 3rd. Intracoronary radiation before stent implantation inhibits neointima formation in stented porcine coronary arteries. Circulation 1995; 92:1383–1386.
193. Laird JR, Carter AJ, Kufs WM, Hoopes TG, Farb A, Nott SH, Fischell RE, Fischell DR, Virmani R, Fischell TA. Inhibition of neointimal proliferation with low-does radiation from a beta-particle-emitting stent. Circulation 1996; 93:529–536.
194. Lo TC, Seckel BR, Salzman FA, Wright KA. Single-dose electron beam irradiation in treatment and prevention of keloids and hypertrophic scars. Radiother Oncol 1990; 19:267–272.
195. Rubin P, Casarett GW. Clinical radiation pathology. Philadelphia: WB Saunders, 1968:43–51.
196. Weichselbaum R, Hallahan D, Sukhatme V, Dritschilo A, Sherman M, Kufe D. Biological consequences of gene regulation after ionizing radiation exposure. J Natl Cancer Inst 1991; 83:480–484.
197. Fornace A Jr. Mammalian genes induced by radiation; activation of genes associated with growth control. Annu Rev Genet 1992; 26:507–526.
198. Fischer-Dzoga K, Dmitrievich GS, Griem ML. Radiosensitivity of vascular tissue. II. Differential radiosensitivity of aortic cells in vitro. Radiat Res 1984; 99:536–546.
199. Fischer-Dzoga K, Dmitrievich GS, Schaffner T. Effect of hyperlipemic serum and irradiation on wound healing in primary quiescent cultures of vascular cells. Exp Mol Pathol 1989; 52:1–12.
200. Haimovitz-Friedman A, Vlodavsky I, Chaudhuri A, Witte L, Fuks Z. Autocrine effects of fibroblast growth factor in repair of radiation damage in endothelial cells. Cancer Res 1991; 51:2552–2558.
201. Schwartz RS, Koval TM, Edwards WD, Camrud A, Bailey KR, Browne K, Vlietstra RE, Holmes DR Jr. Effect of external beam irradiation on neointimal hyperplasia after experimental coronary artery injury. J Am Coll Cardiol 1992; 19:1106–1113.
202. Gold H. Production of arteriosclerosis in rat: Effects of X-ray and a high-fat diet. Arch Pathol Lab Med 1961; 71:268–273.

203. Lindsay S, Kohn HI, Dakin FA. Aortic arteriosclerosis in the dog after localized aortic X-ray irradiation. Circ Res 1962; 10:51–60.
204. Farjardo LF. Morphologic patterns of radiation injury. Front Radiat Ther Oncol 1989; 23:75–84.
205. Murros KE, Toole JF. The effect of radiation of carotid arteries. Arch Neurol 1989; 46:449–455.
206. Boivin JF, Hutchinson GB, Lubin JH, Mauch P. Coronary artery disease mortality in patients tretated for Hodgkins disease. Cancer 1992; 69:1241–1247.
207. Glanzmann C, Huguenin P, Lutolf UM, Maire R, Jenni R, Gumppenberg V. Cardiac lesions after mediastinal irradiation for Hodgkin's disease. Radiother Oncol 1994; 30:43–54.
208. Gottdiener JS, Katin MJ, Borer JS, Bacharach SL, Green MV. Late cardiac effects of therapeutic mediastinal radiation. N Engl J Med 1983; 308:569–572.
209. Bottcher HD, Schopohl B, Lierman D, Kollath J, Adamietz IA. Endovascular irradiation—a new method to avoid recurrent stenosis after stent implantation in peripheral arteries: technique and preliminary results. J Int Rad Oncol Biol Phys 1994; 29:183–186.
210. Urban P, Verin V, Popowski Y, Schwager M, Papirov I, Chatelain P, Kurtz JM, Rutishauser W. Clinical feasibility and safety of intraluminal beta irradiation to prevent restenosis after coronary balloon angioplasty (abstr). Circulation 1996; 8:1221.
212. Rivard A, Leclerc G, Bouchard M, Janicki C, Roorda S, Beaudoin G, Carrier R. Low-dose beta-emitting radioactive stents inhibit neointimal hyperplasia in porcine coronary arteries: an IVUS assessment (abstr). Circulation 1996; 8:1223.
212. Waksman R, Robinson KA, Crocker IR, Seung K-B, Cipolla G, Gravanis MB, King SB. Intracoronary radiation decreases new additional intimal hyperplasia in a repeat balloon angioplasty swine model of restenosis (abstr). Circulation 1996; 8:1217.
213. Terstein P, Masullo V, Jani S, Popma JJ, Mintz GS, Russo RJ, Schatz RA, Steuterman S, Morris NB, Guarneri EM. Radiation therapy following coronary stenting-6 month follow-up of a randomized trial (abstr). Circulation 1996; 8:1222.
214. Condado JA, Gurdiel OG, Espinosa R, Gonzales J, Burger B, Villoria G, Acquatella H, Crocker IR, Seung K-B, Liprie SF, Waksman R. Long-term angiographic and clinical outcome following balloon angioplasty and intracoronary radiation therapy in humans (abstr). Circulation 1996; 8:1218.
215. Herhlein C, Kaiser S, Kollum M, Kinscherf R, Metz J, Fritz P. External beam radiation fails to inhibit neointima formation in stented rabbit arteries (abstr). Circulation 1996; 8:1219.

and 23 controls, the area of epithelium, submucosa, and muscle in asthmatic airway walls were found to be increased in membranous bronchi with an internal perimeter > 2 mm and in all cartilaginous bronchi as compared to controls (7). Although baseline airway resistance was only slightly increased by the airway wall thickening, when the percent muscle shortening required to cause airway closure was calculated, significantly less muscle shortening was required by asthmatic as compared to nonasthmatic airways. Since airways resistance is inversely proportional to the fourth power of the airway radius, any increase in airway wall thickness results in geometric increases in airway resistance for a given level of airway muscle shortening and may contribute substantially to airway hyperresponsiveness (3,8).

Several studies have utilized models of airway wall structure to assess the role of airway smooth muscle thickening in bronchial hyperresponsiveness. A computational model has compared the relative importance of submucosal thickening, adventitial thickening, and increases in smooth muscle mass in the hyperresponsiveness of asthma and chronic obstructive pulmonary disease (10). This study concluded that increases in muscle mass may be the most important factor responsible for the increased airway resistance in response to bronchoconstricting stimuli (10). The authors suggest that the increased muscle thickness allowed for increased smooth muscle shortening and increased tension, resulting in greater constriction of the airway lumen. Similarly, another model based upon the elastic properties, wall component thickness, and lung parenchymal shear modulus of a 2-mm outer diameter canine bronchus has been utilized to analyze the interrelationships between load, smooth muscle contraction, and airway wall thickening on airway narrowing (11,12). This model suggested that the amount of smooth muscle is an important determinant of the maximal degree of airway narrowing at high lung volumes when the loads on airway smooth muscle are large, while the amount of smooth muscle is relatively unimportant at small volumes when loads are small relative to the maximum length-tension curve. Furthermore, this model suggested that small volumes and loads predispose to an increase in residual volume and gas trapping, while at high volumes and loads increasing smooth muscle contractility might lead to increased airway resistance and a decrease in FEV_1/FVC ratio without increases in gas trapping (12,13). This prediction of a dissociation in the FEV_1/FVC ratio and gas trapping has been substantiated in a companion study assessing spirometric responses to histamine challenge in patients with mild asthma where individual asthmatics were noted to have a predominant fall in the FEV_1/FVC ratio, while other individuals had a predominant fall in FVC consistent with an increase in residual volume and gas trapping (13).

It is uncertain, however, whether increased muscle thickness corresponds in vivo to increased contractile responses (14). For example, an in vitro study has demonstrated greater passive tension and diminished maximal active shortening of human bronchial smooth muscle as compared to porcine trachealis, which was attributed to a parallel elastic connective tissue component within human airway tissue, which must be overcome for shortening to occur (15). In addition, morphometric analysis of an animal model of bronchoconstriction has suggested that a thickened mucosal membrane represents an increased load that may limit airway smooth muscle shortening and attenuate excessive airway narrowing (16). Therefore, these studies would be consistent with the hypothesis that increases in airway mucosal and submucosal thickness might result in increased elastance and decreased muscle shortening. However, other studies have suggested that inflammatory changes might decrease the elastance in asthmatic airways resulting in increased muscle shortening. For example, human bronchial smooth muscle strips treated in vitro with collagenase were found to have decreases in passive tension and increased shortening and force generation in response to electrical field stimulation and histamine challenge (17). The authors suggest that collagenase production by inflammatory cells recruited to asthmatic airways might result in the degradation of the extracellular matrix, thereby allowing excessive bronchoconstriction by decreasing the resistive load that airway smooth muscle must overcome to shorten. It has also been suggested that asthmatic airway smooth muscle is unloaded in asthma due to the presence of fewer mucosal folds (18). The number of mucosal folds may determine the collapse pressure of the airway since these folds serve as a load on airway smooth muscle. It has also been suggested that bronchoconstriction and increased lung volumes in the setting of airway inflammation might produce a flow of inflammatory exudate from the submucosa across the smooth muscle (12). This might then diminish the elastic load on airway smooth muscle by expanding the peribronchial space and thereby unlinking the airway from the parenchyma (12). This suggests that gas trapping in asthmatic airways reflects the degree to which smooth muscle is unloaded by peribronchial inflammation. Therefore, gas trapping may serve as a direct measure of excessive bronchoconstriction (12).

Last, although increases in airway smooth muscle may have both structural and physiological consequences which are important in the pathogenesis of airway hyperresponsiveness in asthma, it is unclear whether airway smooth muscle thickening is reversible with currently available treatments (14). Further studies are required to more clearly define the clinical significance of airway smooth muscle thickening in asthma, as well as interventions that can reverse this process (14).

III. The Role of Airway Smooth Muscle in Asthmatic Airway Hyperresponsiveness

Airway hyperresponsiveness to a wide variety of bronchoconstricting stimuli is a characteristic feature of asthmatic airways and can be mediated by either exogenous stimuli, such as allergens, excercise (dry air), sulfur dioxide, hypotonic or hypertonic aerosols, or by endogenous mediators, such as acetylcholine, histamine, methacholine, leukotrienes (LTC_4, LTD_4, LTE_4), prostaglandins (PGD_2, $PGF_{2\alpha}$), thromboxanes (TXA_2), platelet activating factor, endothelin, tachykinins (substance P, neurokinin A), and bradykinin (19–25). Chronic airway inflammation may represent the basis for airway hyperresponsiveness, as evidenced by the association of inflammatory cellular infiltration and altered airway function (26). The contribution of airway smooth muscle to asthmatic airway hyperresponsiveness remains an area of active investigation, with both excessive contractility and impaired relaxation representing possible mechanisms. However, other consequences of airway inflammation, such as increased release of bronchoconstricting stimuli, increased epithelial or endothelial permeability, sensitization of airway sensory nerves, enhanced cholinergic reflex mechanisms, and neurogenic inflammation, may also play important roles in the pathogenesis of airway hyperresponsiveness in asthma (23,25).

Signal transduction pathways leading to smooth muscle contraction involves the phospholipase C–mediated generation of inositol 1,4,5-triphosphate (IP_3), Ca^{2+} release from intracellular stores, activation of myosin light chain kinase by the Ca^{2+}-calmodulin complex, phosphorylation of the 20,000 dalton subunit of myosin, and cross-bridge cycling of actomyosin with subsequent smooth muscle contraction (27–29). Relaxation is mediated by dephosphorylation of myosin (27,28). It has been suggested that intrinsic abnormatlities in airway smooth muscle cell Ca^{2+}/calmodulin/myosin light chain kinase pathways may exist, which mediate increased contractility in asthma. For example, it has been hypothesized that airway smooth muscle might be exposed to physical stress as a consequence of increased airway pressures in asthma, with consequent increases in contractile enzyme activity (27). When airway smooth muscle cells from canine trachealis muscle were subjected to mechanical strain in vitro, increases in myosin light chain kinase (MLCK)–mediated myosin light chain phosphorylation activity and actomyosin ATPase activity, as well as increases in the cellular content of MLCK and myosin were detected, which could potentially result in increases in cell contractility by increasing maximum force development (27). Similarly, the mechanical stress–induced increases in myosin might contribute to the smooth muscle hypertrophy present in some asthmatic airways. In addition, decreased rates of phosphatase-dependent myosin dephosphorylation were noted, which might result in increases in myosin phosphorylation and smooth muscle contraction. Increases in MLCK have also been reported in a canine model of rag weed pollen–sensitized airway hyperresponsiveness (29,30). Sensitized tracheal and bronchial smooth muscles demonstrated significant increases in actomyosin ATPase activity, 20 kDa myosin light chain phosphorylation, and MLCK activity, which were a consequence of increases in MLCK quantity. In contrast to the mechanical strain model, this model did not demonstrate a difference in myosin phosphatase activity between crude tracheal smooth muscle tissue homogenates from control and sensitized animals, suggesting that increased myosin light chain phosphorylation is a consequence of increased MLCK activity rather than decreased smooth muscle phosphatase activity (31).

It has also been hypothesized that abnormalities in protein kinase C (PKC) expression or activation may contribute to increased airway smooth muscle contractility in asthma (14). Multiple isoforms of PKC have been detected in canine airway smooth muscle, including PKC βI and βII, which are conventional, calcium-dependent isoforms, PKC ε and θ, which are novel, calcium-independent forms, and PKC ξ, an atypical, calcium- and phospholipid-independent isoform (14,32). Studies performed in animal models have suggested that PKC activation is involved in the maintenance of airway smooth muscle tone and is dependent on voltage-dependent calcium channels and extracellular calcium (33). PKC activation by phorbol ester has been reported to induce increases in resting membrane potential and the isometric force generated by guinea pig airway smooth muscle, which were comparable to changes induced by passive sensitization with IgG_1(34). In a guinea pig model of passive sensitization, pretreatment with PKC inhibitors (H7 and NA-0345) attenuated ovalbumin-induced depolarization, as well as inital and sustained increases in isometric force generated by airway smooth muscle cells, suggesting that sensitization activates PKC (35). Similarly, pretreatment with staurosporine attenuated sensitization– and specific antigen–induced changes in membrane potential and isometric tone (36). In isolated human bronchial smooth muscle, PKC activation by phorbol 12,13-dibutyrate (PDB) induces slowly developing but sustained contractions, which were attenuated by the nonspecific PKC inhibitor staurosporine, by PKC downregulation secondary to prolonged exposure to PDB, by removal of extracellular calcium, and by the calcium channel antagonist verapamil (33). This suggests that PKC activation induces prolonged human airway smooth muscle contraction, which is dependent on extracellular calcium. In addition, passive desensitization by overnight incubation in serum from asthmatic patients decreased the maximal response to PDB, suggesting that decreases in PKC activity might be involved in altered airway smooth muscle function. Additional studies are required to further define the role of PKC activation in airway smooth muscle contractility in asthma.

Experiments utilizing passive sensitization of airway smooth muscle in vitro via prolonged exposure to serum from atopic individuals have served as models to study the effects of high IgE concentrations on increased contractility (14,37). Passive sensitization of human bronchial tissue to serum with high RAST titers to *Dermatophagoides* species has been reported to enhance contractile responses to histamine via mobilization of extracellular calcium and to increase the involvement of calcium voltage-dependent channels in KCL-mediated contractions

(21,38). However, passive sensitization decreased human bronchial tissue contractility to the cholinergic agonist carbachol (21). Furthermore, passive sensitization of human bronchial smooth muscle to serum with high IgE concentrations has been reported to enhance both maximal shortening velocity (V_{max}) and maximal shortening (ΔL_{max}) in the absence of either specific or nonspecific antigen challenge (37). These studies suggest that passive sensitization of human bronchi may have a direct effect on asthmatic bronchial hyperresponsiveness via enhancement of airway smooth muscle contractility. Passive sensitization may also enhance the contractile response of airway smooth muscle to neuropeptides (14). Passive sensitization of human bronchi has been reported to increase the amplitude of contractile responses to substance P and neurokinin A, which were independent of decreases in neutral endopeptidase activity since the changes persisted in the presence of the neutral endopeptidase inhibitor phosphoramidon (39).

Although airway hyperresponsiveness to a variety of nonatopic, nonsensitizing stimuli is a characteristic feature of individuals with asthma, conflicting results have been reported regarding the presence of abnormal contractile responses to bronchoconstricting stimuli in vitro by human asthmatic airway smooth muscle cells (14,40). Several studies have failed to document a correlation between bronchial smooth muscle responsiveness in vitro and responsiveness to histamine or metacholine challenges in vivo (41–45). In addition, two series have suggested that human bronchial smooth muscle from asthmatics exhibit decreased sensitivity to histamine and carbachol (41,46,47). However, other studies have suggested increased contractile responses by asthmatic airway smooth muscle cells. In a study of seven patients with fatal asthma, in vitro contractile responses of isolated tracheal strips to histamine, cholinergic electrical field stimulation, and acetylcholine were greater in asthmatics than in controls (19). However, no differences in contractile responses to acetylcholine, histamine, and cholinergic nerve stimulation were present in fourth generation bronchial spirals obtained from these asthmatics and controls (48). Enhanced contractile responses of asthmatic bronchi to indirect bronchoconstricting stimuli have also been reported (14,41). In a study comparing 19 bronchial strips from six asthmatic patients and 21 bronchial strips from seven controls, hyperresponsiveness to adenosine was detected in the asthmatic bronchi, which could be attenuated by combined histamine and leukotriene antagonism, suggesting that adenosine acted indirectly via release of histamine and leukotrienes, possibly from mast cells (41). The authors suggest that the adenosine hyperresponsiveness in isolated bronchi from asthmatic patients correlates with airway hyperreactivity that is characteristic of asthma.

Several lines of evidence exist which suggest that airway smooth muscle relaxation is impaired in asthma and may contribute to airway hyperresponsiveness in this setting. A recent study has tested the hypothesis that asthmatic hyperresponsiveness is a result of the inability of inspiration to stretch airway smooth muscle (49). This was studied by performing methacholine challenges on a cohort of 10 asthmatics and 10 normal controls who were prohibited from taking deep inspirations. When deep inspiration was prohibited, the response to methacholine was similar between asthmatics and normals. In addition, 6 of the 10 normal subjects developed asthmatic responses. This suggests that the bronchodilating effect of deep inspiration was impaired in asthmatic airways. In contrast, deep inspiration had a bronchodilating effect in normal controls possibly mediated by smooth muscle stretching with subsequent stress relaxation. The authors suggest that this differential response to deep inspiration may be important in the pathogenesis of airway hyperresponsiveness in asthma.

Defective β-adrenergic receptor function has also been identified as a possible mechanism underlying impaired airway smooth muscle relaxation in asthma (14). In a canine model of nonspecific airway hyperreactivity, impaired β-adrenergic responses have been demonstrated with decreased cAMP generation in response to isoproterenol (50). In this model, β-adrenergic receptors were increased in number, but had decreased affinity for ^{125}I-cyanopindolol. In bronchial smooth muscle isolated from a canine ragweed pollen–sensitization model, isotonic relaxation subserved by early recruited (<2 sec) normally cycling crossbridges was prolonged, while late-phase isotonic relaxation was unchanged (51). Similarly, isolated rabbit tracheal smooth muscle passively sensitized with serum from atopic asthmatics was demonstrated to have significantly attenuated maximal relaxation and sensitivity to isoproterenol or PGE_2, which was associated with decreased cAMP generation (52). In addition, these attenuated responses could be blocked by pretreatment with muscarinic M_2 receptor antagonists or pertussis toxin, which ADP ribosylates the inhibitory G protein (G_i). Increases in $G_{i\alpha 3}$ subunit protein were also documented in sensitized tissue. These authors suggest that impaired β-adrenergic receptor function in atopic sensitized airways is due to increased muscarinic M_2 receptor/G_i protein-coupled inhibition of adenyl cyclase activity.

Conflicting results regarding β-adrenergic receptor dysfunction in smooth muscle from human asthmatic airways have been reported (14,53). While two studies have failed to demonstrate in vivo or in vitro defects in β-adrenergic receptor function, other studies have demonstrated impaired relaxant responses to β-adrenergic agonists, which may correlate with the severity of asthma (14,19,46–48,53,54). Furthermore, two studies that assessed β-adrenergic receptor numbers via ^{125}I-cyanopindolol binding to asthmatic airway smooth muscle have reported increases in receptor numbers, which were associated with increased receptor affinity for isoproterenol but attenuated responsiveness to β-adrenergic agonists (53,55). These studies suggest an uncoupling of β-adrenergic receptor density and postreceptor effects in asthmatic airways (14,55). In a separate study, however, β-adrenergic receptor numbers and binding of ^{125}I-cyanopindolol in four patients with fatal asthma were not different from controls with bronchial carcinoma (56). Lastly, β_2-adrenergic receptor autoantibodies have been detected in the serum of approximately 40% of asthmatic patients as compared to approximately 5% of normal subjects (57). These β_2-adrenergic receptor autoantibodies are directed against an extracellular or transmembrane spanning domain of the protein and may act as functional receptor antagonists or mediate the downregulation of receptor numbers.

Proinflammatory cytokines may also be important in the modulation of β-adrenergic receptor dysfunction in asthma (14). Pretreatment with proinflammatory cytokines, such as TNF-α and IL-1β, have been reported to produce significant reductions in isoproterenol-mediated maximal relaxation in isolated tracheas from a guinea pig antigen challenge model of asthma (58). In support of this is evidence from a AD12-SV40 transformed human airway epithelial cell line where IL-1β induced increases in β-adrenergic receptor density and decreases in cAMP responses to isoproterenol (59). These studies suggest that proinflammatory cytokines may play an important role in the uncoupling of β-adrenergic receptors in asthmatic airway smooth muscle cells. Last, activation of PKC by the phorbol ester PMA has been reported to reduce both β-adrenergic receptor density and cAMP responsiveness to isoproterenol in bovine airway smooth muscle (60).

Passive sensitization experiments have also provided evidence for impaired relaxation in asthmatic airway smooth muscle cells. Passive sensitization of human bronchial rings significantly attenuated the relaxant responses mediated by ion channels, such as those in response to a calcium channel blocker and a potassium channel opener (61). However, relaxant responses mediated via activation of β-adrenergic receptors were not impaired, suggesting that receptor activation and signal transduction remained coupled. Passive sensitization of human isolated bronchial smooth muscle has also been reported to significantly attenuate the relaxant responses of vasoactive intestinal peptide (VIP), a neuropeptide that mediates inhibitory nonadrenergic noncholinergic bronchodilator responses (25,39). However, the role of VIP-mediated inhibitory nonadrenergic noncholinergic responses in human airways remains incompletely defined (25). While decreases in VIP immunoreactive nerves have been documented in patients dying from asthma, no decreases in VIP immunoreactivity or the number of VIP-immunoreactive nerves have been documented in studies of bronchial biopsies of asthmatic patients (25,62–64).

Nitric oxide (NO) has also been hypothesized to modulate both airway smooth muscle tone and responsiveness in asthma. The effect of NO is mediated via activation of soluble guanylate cyclase, with resultant increases in intracellular cGMP (65). NO also functions as an inhibitory nonadrenergic noncholinergic bronchodilator, which modulates cholinergic neural responses in human airways in vitro via the functional antagonism of acetylcholine (25,66). NO has been demonstrated to mediate bronchodilatation in a guinea pig model where NO-attenuated methacholine induced bronchoconstriction (67). In another guinea pig model, inhibition of nitric oxide synthesis has been reported to augment increases in basal tone, as well as increases in airway contractility in response to histamine, carbachol, and methacholine (68). In addition, epithelium denudation resulted in an upward shift of the histamine response curve, suggesting that NO release by airway epithelium acts as a negative feedback system on histamine-induced contractions and airway hyperresponsiveness. NO inhibition has also been reported to augment bronchial hyperresponsiveness to inhaled bradykinin, but not acetylcholine in a Brown-Norway rat model (69). Last, deficient NO generation has been proposed as a mechanism underlying virus-induced airway hyperreactivity. In a guinea pig model of parainfluenza type 3 viral infection, NO release was markedly decreased from animals with enhanced contractile responses, while preincubation with the NO precursor, L-arginine, completely prevented the enhanced contraction and restored NO production to control levels (70).

IV. Mechanisms of Increased Smooth Muscle Mass in the Asthmatic Airway

A. Airway Smooth Muscle Hypertrophy

Smooth muscle hypertrophy may occur as a consequence of recurrent muscular contraction and may be related to four mechanisms. First, the asthmatic airway may be exposed to frequent stimulation by neurohormones, neuropeptides, and locally produced mediators of inflammation, which induce smooth muscle contraction (71). Increased parasympathetic activity might also be related to a reduction in M2 muscarinic suppressor activity in the parasympathetic ganglion. Decreased M2 receptor function has been noted in airways of experimental animals after viral infection and may also represent a cause of airway hyperresponsiveness in humans (72). Moreover, two mediators present in the inflamed airway, TNF-α and interleukin-1β, may act synergistically to induce transcriptional down regulation of muscarinic M2 receptors (73). In addition, increased parasympathetic tone may be due to the augmentation of the cholinergic effect due to costimulation with serotonin or TNF. Second, smooth muscle hypertrophy may occur in the asthmatic airway in response to repeated episodes of airway smooth muscle contraction manifested clinically as bronchospasm. Third, cytokine mediators of airway inflammation may result in an alteration of receptor expression in airway smooth muscle resulting in a decreased response to endogenous counterregulatory stimuli. For example, interleukin 1-β may cause downregulation of β_2 receptor function in airway smooth muscle cells (14,58). The result of this downregulation of smooth muscle relaxation might be an unopposed contractile stimulus. Finally, the damage to or the loss of the airway epithelium in asthmatic airways may result in (1) the loss of epithelium-derived relaxant factors, (2) the loss of epithelial barrier functions, thereby exposing the submucosa to mediators in the airway lumen that stimulate muscle contraction, and (3) the loss of epithelial-derived products such as soluble TNF receptors, which would modulate inflammatory mediator effects (74). The loss of these inhibitory and counterregulatory mechanisms may also result in unopposed myocyte contractile stimulation.

B. Mechanisms of Airway Smooth Muscle Hyperplasia

The increase in airway smooth muscle (ASM) mass noted in asthma also may be due to a proliferative response of airway smooth muscle cells. A variety of competence and progression factors produced in the asthmatic airway may have an effect on smooth muscle proliferation. Much work in this area has been performed in vitro in cultured experimental animal and human airway smooth muscle systems (reviewed in Ref. 75). Some of the conditions and mediators present in the asthmatic airway that may induce smooth muscle proliferation are presented in Table 1.

Table 1 Mediators that May Induce Airway Smooth Muscle Proliferation in Asthma

Factor	Ref.
Allergen stimulation	76
Strain	77
Mast cell products	
Histamine	78
Mast cell tryptase	79
Thromboxane	81
Leukotriene D4	82
Adrenergic receptor stimulation	83
Peptides	
Tachykinins	84
Endothelin	85–88
Cytokines and growth factors	
Tumor necrosis factor-α	89,90
Platelet-derived growth factor	91,92
Insulin-like growth factor	93
Epidermal growth factor	86
Serum	94
α-Thrombin	87,95

C. Allergen Stimulation and Smooth Muscle Strain

Allergic asthma may be characterized by the presence of recurrent exposure to allergens, the recurrence of bronchospasm, and the local release of both stored and newly synthesized mast cell–derived mediators. The effect of repeated allergen stimulation on ASM proliferation was studied in a rat model actively sensitized to ovalbumin. In this in vivo model, allergen challenge resulted in 9- to 25-fold increases in DNA synthesis in ASM in large, medium, and in small airways (76). In a model using canine ASM cells in culture, the effect of strain on ASM proliferation was studied. In this system, cyclic stretching of the cells approximately doubled the growth rate of subconfluent cultures compared to control cells (77).

D. Mast Cell Products

Airway mast cells release upon activation a variety of preformed stored and newly synthesized mediators. Among the preformed constituents of mast cell granules are histamine and mast cell tryptase. Both of these potent stored mast cell mediators have been studied for their potential to stimulate ASM proliferation. Histamine has been studied in a canine ASM culture system. In that system, histamine in micromolar concentrations increased radiolabeled thymidine incorporation by ASM cells up to twofold in a dose-related manner (78). One of the most abundant proteins in mast cell granules is the neutral serine proteinase tryptase (79). This enzyme has a variety of effects in the lung. It is a potent mitogen for lung fibroblasts (80). In an in vitro model using cultured canine airway smooth muscle cells, mast cell tryptase in nanomolar concentrations increased ASM numbers two- to threefold over 2–4 days of culture (79). Therefore, two of the most abundant mast cell granule products are capable of stimulating ASM proliferation.

In addition to the release of preformed mediators, mast cells may generate eicosanoid mediators upon activation. Two products of eicosanoid metabolism by mast cells and by other lung cells have been studied for proliferative effects on ASM cultures. Thromboxane A_2 is a potent proinflammatory eicosanoid. Because of the short half-life of thromboxane A_2, more stable congeners of this eicosanoid have been studied. Two thromboxane A_2 mimetics have been studied in vitro in a cultured rabbit ASM cell system. Both carbocyclic thromboxane A_2(CTA_2) and U-46619 in nanomolar concentrations were capable of inducing 50% increases in cell counts by day 4 of culture. This effect of CTA_2 was inhibited by treatment with quinacrine and by nordihydroguairetic acid implying that activation of phospholipase A_2 and subsequent production of other eicosanoids may be involved in induction of this proliferative response (81). Further, CTA_2 treatment of ASM cells induces the release of leukotriene D_4, which alone is able to induce a modest effect on ASM proliferation. A more profound effect of leukotriene D_4 on ASM cell proliferation may be through the modulation of the effect of insulin-like growth factor on ASM cell proliferation. Leukotriene D_4 treatment of ASM cells dramatically enhances the proliferative response of cultured rabbit ASM cells to insulin-like growth factor (82). This effect of leukotriene D_4 is mediated through the induction of a protease that metabolizes insulin-like growth factor binding protein-2(IGFBP-2). The reduction IGFBP-2 in the extracellular fluid allows for an augmented response of ASM to insulin-like growth factor by decreasing binding to the binding protein and allowing more free factor for binding to cellular receptors (82).

E. Adrenergic Agents and Neuropeptides

Adrenergic agents and neuropeptides and their receptors may also be involved in the perpetuation or modulation of airway inflammation in asthma. The effect of adrenergic agents which activate either α- or β-adrenergic receptors has been studied in in vitro systems using cultured rabbit ASM cells. The α_1-adrenergic receptor agonists phenylephrine and methoxamine in micromolar concentrations induce increases of up to 40% in ASM cell counts above untreated controls. The α_2-receptor agonist clonidine induces similar changes in ASM cell numbers (83). These effects are blocked by pretreatment of the cells with pertussis toxin which ADP-ribosylates G proteins which inhibit adenylate cyclase activation. The effect of β-adrenergic agents on ASM proliferation is discussed below.

F. Neuropeptides

A variety of peptides of the nonadrenergic noncholinergic nervous system may also participate in the perpetuation of airway inflammation either due to the release of sensory neuropeptides in the airway mucosa or due to the loss of epithelial cell–produced enzymes, such as neutral endopeptidase, which metabolize and inactivate these peptides. Other peptides such as the endothelins may be produced by a variety of cells in the airway including epithelial cells, endothelial cells, muscle cells, and perhaps also neuronal cells. The tachykinin family of neuropeptides includes substance P, neurokinin A, and neurokinin B. These neuropeptides may interact with three distinct receptors designated NK_1, NK_2, and NK_3. Substance P in micromolar and nanomolar concentrations stimulates proliferation of cultured rabbit ASM cells, while neurokinin A and neurokinin B have little effect. The effect of substance P on ASM proliferation is inhibited by the NK_1 selective receptor antagonist GR,82,334 (84). Thus, substance P acting via an NK_1 receptor is capable of inducing ASM cell proliferation.

The endothelins including ET- 1 and ET-3 are present in significant quantities in the lung and may be present in increased concentrations in asthmatic airways. These peptides may interact with at least two endothelin receptors designated ET_A and ET_B. In a study of cultured rabbit ASM cells, endothelin-1 in nanomolar concentrations induced cellular proliferation. This effect of endothelin was blocked by cotreatment of the ASM cells with an inhibitor of phospholipase A_2 or with an inhibitor of cyclooxygenase, implying that the proliferative effect of endothelin is mediated via activation of phopholipase A_2 and the subsequent production of eicosanoids (85). In a study of cultured ovine ASM cells, ET-1 in nanomolar and picomolar concentrations bound to cellular receptors activated expression of c-fos and induced a doubling of the number of cultured cells at 24 hours (86). In a similar study of cultured rat ASM cells, ET-1 was shown to increase DNA synthesis by 50% and to activate the MAP kinase pathway via a Raf-1–independent mechanism (87). However, a study of cultured human tracheal smooth muscle cells suggests that the effect of ET- 1 alone on ASM cell DNA synthesis is modest. On the other hand, ET-1 in nanomolar concentrations substantially augmented the proliferative response of ASM cells to epidermal growth factor (88). ET-3 and the selective ET_B receptor agonist sarafotoxin had no effect. Therefore, ET-1 presumably acting via an ET_A receptor appears to be capable alone or in concert with growth factors of inducing the proliferation of ASM.

G. Cytokines and Growth Factors

Cytokines and growth factors present in the asthmatic airway have been reported to activate both resident airway cells and migratory inflammatory cells. The effect of tumor necrosis factor alpha (TNF-α) on human ASM cell proliferation has been reported in two studies. Stewart et al. (89) reported studies of cultured human airway smooth muscle cells in which TNF at low concentrations (3–30 pM) caused an increase in [^{3}H]-thymidine incorporation at 48 hours. However, TNF at higher doses did not cause a proliferative response and even prevented the proliferative response to other stimuli such as thrombin, epidermal growth factor, and fetal calf serum. On the other hand, Amrani et al. (90) reported that stimulation of cultured human airway smooth muscle cells with TNF in concentrations up to 1 nM resulted in increases in cell number. Further, this effect was mimicked by a recombinant TNF protein, which specifically activates the 55 kDa TNF receptor and by an activating anti-p55 antibody but not by a recombinant TNF protein, which activates only the 75 kDa TNF receptor. The effect was not blocked by a TNFRp75-blocking antibody. Therefore, TNF in picomolar concentrations acting via TNFRp55 receptors appears to be capable of stimulation of human smooth muscle proliferation (90).

Platelet-derived growth factor (PDGF) is a dimer that may exist in three isoforms designated AA, BB, and AB. Using cultured rabbit airway smooth muscle cells, PDGF-AB in concentrations of 1–50 ng/ml was found to increase ASM cell counts up to threefold after 4 days (91). In studies of cultured human ASM cells, all three isoforms of PDGF were tested in the presence and absence of fetal calf serum. In the absence of fetal calf serum, human ASM cells proliferate in response to stimulation with PDGF-AB or PDGF-BB and much less so in response to PDGF-AA. In the presence of fetal calf serum, all three isoforms stimulate ASM proliferation. It is assumed that the effect of PDGF-AB and PDGF-BB isoforms is mediated via PDGFRβ, which is expressed on these cells in the presence or in the absence of fetal calf serum (92).

Insulin-like growth factors (IGF), insulin-like growth factor receptors, and IGF-binding proteins are capable of regulating growth in a variety of cell systems. IGFs have been studied in cultured rabbit ASM cells. In rabbit ASM cell membrane preparations, IGF-I and IGF-II bind to IGF receptors. IGF type I and type II receptors are present on rabbit ASM cells. IGF-binding protein-2, which may regulate the availability of IGF to bind with membrane receptors, is produced by ASM cells and released into the culture media. Treatment of rabbit ASM cell cultures with either IGF-I or IGF-2 in ng/ml concentrations increases ASM cell counts at day 4 by up to 230% (93).

The effect of epidermal growth factor on ASM cell proliferation has been studied in human ASM cells. Treatment of human ASM cells for 18 hours with epidermal growth factor in pM concentrations induces a 20- to 40-fold increase in [^{3}H]-thymidine incorporation compared to untreated cells. As noted earlier, cotreatment of these ASM cells with epidermal growth factor and with endothelin-1 has a synergistic effect on cellular proliferation greater than that of epidermal growth factor alone (88).

H. Serum Factors

The addition of fetal calf serum, in concentrations of up to 10%, results in a two- to three-fold increase in ASM cell counts by day 4 in both rabbit and human ASM cell culture systems (91). The mechanism of this effect has been studied in rabbit ASM cell cultures by the treatment of cells with selective inhibitors of protein kinase C activity (Ro-31-8220 and Ro-31-7549) or with an inhibitor of protein tyrosine kinase activity (ST638). Ro3l-8220 pretreatment of rabbit ASM cells resulted a dose-related (1 nM to 1 μM) inhibition (up to 100%) of the fetal calf serum induced proliferation in cells measured from 2 to 7 days. Similarly, Ro-31-7549 pretreatment of rabbit ASM cells resulted in a dose-related (10 nM to 10 μM) inhibition (up to 100%) of fetal calf serum–induced proliferation of cell counts from days 2 to 7. Similarly, depletion of protein kinase C activity by pretreatment with phorbol ester inhibits the proliferative response of rabbit ASM cells to fetal calf serum over 2–4 days. Therefore, inhibition of protein kinase C activity appears to block the proliferative response of ASM cells to fetal calf serum. It is of interest that inhibition of protein tyrosine kinase activity with ST638 (100 nM to 100 μM) also inhibits this proliferative response. One possible conclusion is that the proliferative response to serum requires a second messenger system, which includes both protein kinase C and tyrosine kinase activation (94).

One serum product that may be activated and present in the airway during airway inflammation is thrombin. Thrombin in a concentration of 1.0 U/ml stimulates proliferation of cultured human ASM cells to a degree similar to epidermal growth factor or 10% fetal calf serum. This effect is inhibited by the thrombin antagonist hirudin (95). This effect appears to be mediated via activation of a seven transmembrane thrombin receptor, which results in the mitogen-activated protein kinase activation via a Raf-1–independent mechanism. Activation of this pathway and the proliferative response to thrombin are inhabitable by prior activation of cyclic AMP–dependent protein kinase (87).

V. Inhibition of Smooth Muscle Proliferation

A variety of factors potentially present in asthmatic airway tissue may serve to inhibit the proliferative response of airway smooth muscle. Some of these factors are listed in Table 2, including some that increase intracellular cAMP levels and therefore protein kinase A activity, as well as glucocorticosteroid therapy, heparin, and inhibition of protein kinase C and of tyrosine kinases.

A. Factors That Increase cAMP-Dependent Protein Kinase Activity

The effect of the selective β_2-adrenergic agonist salbutamol has been studied in a human airway smooth muscle cell culture system with and without stimulation with thrombin. While thrombin (0.3 U/ml) increased [^{3}H]-thymidine incorporation in ASM cells eightfold, preincubation with salbutamol inhibited this response. Pretreatment with the phosphodiesterase inhibitor 3-isobutyl-l-methylxanthine (IBMX) with salbutamol resulted in a synergistic inhibition of thrombin-induced increases in [^{3}H]-thymidine incorporation (96). In a separate study

Table 2 Factors that May Inhibit Airway Smooth Muscle Proliferation in Asthma

Factor	Ref.
β-Adrenergic receptor stimulation	96,98
Prostaglandin E_2	97
Vasoactive intestinal peptide	100
Glucocorticoid treatment	97,98
Heparin	97
Inhibition of protein kinase C	94
Inhibition of tyrosine kinase	94

utilizing cultured bovine ASM cells, both salbutamol (0.1–10 μM) and salmeterol (0.01–10 μM) treatment inhibited increases in [^{3}H]-thymidine incorporation and increases in cell number induced by treatment with 3% fetal bovine serum (97). Similarly, the β-adrenergic receptor agonist isoproterenol in nM concentrations is capable of inhibiting leukotriene D_4-induced proliferation of rabbit ASM cells in culture. This inhibition of leukotriene D_4–induced proliferation by isoproterenol was blocked by pretreatment of the cells with the cAMP antagonist Rp-cAMPS (98).

The effect of prostaglandin E_2 (PGE_2) treatment on fetal bovine serum or platelet-derived growth factor–induced ASM cell proliferation has been studied in human ASM cells in culture. While fetal bovine serum increased the incorporation of [^{3}H]-thymidine 4- to 5.5-fold over control cells, PGE_2 in concentrations of 10^{-8}–10^{-6}M inhibited, in a dose-dependent manner, the proliferative response of human ASM cells to 2.5–10% fetal bovine serum. Similarly, PGE_2 in concentrations of 10^{-8}–10^{-6} M inhibited by up to 50% the increase in [^{3}H]-thymidine incorporation in cultured ASM cells induced by platelet-derived growth factor (50 ng/ml) (99).

Vasoactive intestinal peptide (VIP) is a neuropeptide present in the airway which is also known to activate adenylate cyclase. In a human ASM cell culture system, VIP in concentrations of 1.0 nM to 1.0 μM reduced baseline growth of ASM cells. In this system, histamine (100 nM–100 μM) increased ASM cell counts by 66%, while VIP pretreatment reduced the proliferative response to histamine by over 50%. Pretreatment of ASM cells with a selective protein kinase A inhibitor abolished the effect of VIP (100). Therefore, the inhibitory effect of VIP also appears to be mediated by increases in cAMP levels.

B. Glucocorticoid Treatment

Glucocorticosteroid therapy may have a variety of therapeutic effects on the asthmatic airway. Therefore, it was of interest to study the effects of glucocorticosteroids on ASM cell proliferation. In a bovine ASM cell culture system, both cortisol in nM concentrations and beclomethasone in nM concentrations inhibit by 40% the increases in incorporation of [^{3}H]-thymidine induced by 3% fetal bovine serum (97). Similarly, treatment of rabbit ASM cells in culture with methylprednisolone, in concentrations of 0.1–10 μM, inhibits the proliferative response of these cells to leukotriene D_4. The effect of glucocorticoid treatment is additive to that of β-adrenergic treatment suggesting separate mechanisms for the effects of β-adrenergic therapy and glucocorticoid therapy (98).

C. Heparin

Heparin is stored in mast cell granules and released on mast cell activation. In studies of human ASM cell cultures, heparin, in concentrations of 10–100 U/ml inhibited cell proliferation in response to 5 or 10% fetal bovine serum. The mechanism of this effect of heparin is not clear but may relate to its negative charge or to its ability to inhibit growth factor binding to cells (99).

D. Inhibition of Other Intracellular Signaling Pathways

As was suggested in the discussion of the proliferative effect of serum factors on ASM cells, the effect of serum on cellular proliferation is blocked by inhibitors of protein kinase C and tyrosine kinases (94). The protein kinase C inhibitors Ro-31-8220 and Ro-31-7549 inhibit the proliferative response of rabbit ASM cells to 10% fetal bovine serum. Similarly, the protein tyrosine kinase inhibitor ST638 inhibits the proliferative response to the same stimulus. The inhibition of both protein kinase C with Ro-31-8220 and protein tyrosine kinases with ST638 results in an additive inhibition of proliferation of rabbit ASM cells in response to fetal bovine serum (94).

VI. Summary

It is clear that a variety of mast cell products, neuropeptides, cytokines, growth factors, and other serum factors may be involved in the response of airway smooth muscle to the airway inflammation characteristic of asthma. The balance of the endogenous proliferative stimuli and antiproliferative factors in the airway may determine the extent of airway remodeling in this inflammatory setting. The therapeutic challenge may be not only to reduce the inflammatory response but also to understand and modulate the extent of airway remodeling occurring in response to these inflammatory stimuli.

References

1. Carroll N, Elliot J, Morton A, James A. The structure of large and small airways in nonfatal and fatal asthma. Am Rev Respir Dis 1993; 147:405–410.
2. Saetta M, DiStefano A, Rosina C, Thiene G, Fabbri L. Quantitative structural analysis of peripheral airways and arteries in sudden fatal asthma. Am Rev Respir Dis 1991; 143:138–143.
3. Wiggs BR, Bosken C, Paré PD, James A, Hogg J. A model of airway narrowing in asthma and in chronic obstructive pulmonary disease. Am Rev Respir Dis 1992; 145:1251–1258.
4. Dunnill MS, Massarella GR, and Anderson JA. A comparison of the quantitative anatomy of the bronchi in normal subjects, in status asthmaticus, in chronic bronchitis and in emphysema. Thorax 1969; 24:176–179.
5. Ebina M, Yaegashi H, Chiba R, Takahashi T, Motomiy M, Tanemura M. Hyper-

reactive site in the airway tree of asthmatic patients revealed by thickening of bronchial muscles. Am Rev Respir Dis 1990; 141:1327–1332.
6. Heard BE, Hossain S. Hyperplasia of bronchial muscle in asthma. J Pathol 1973; 110:319–331.
7. James AL, Paré PD, Hogg JC. The mechanics of airway narrowing in asthma. Am Rev Respir Dis 1989; 139:242–246.
8. Knox AJ. Airway re-modelling in asthma: role of airway smooth muscle. Clin Sci 1994; 86:647–652.
9. Ebina M, Takahasi T, Chiba T, Motomiya M. Cellular hypertrophy and hyperplasia of airway smooth muscles underlying bronchial asthma: a 3-D morphometric study. Am Rev Respir Dis 1993; 148:720–726.
10. Lambert RK, Wiggs BR, Kuwano K, Hogg J, Pare P. Functional significance of increased airway smooth muscle in asthma and COPD. J Appl Physiol 1993; 74:2771–2781.
11. Macklem PT. Theoretical basis of airway instability. Chest 1995; 107:87S–88S.
12. Macklem PT. A theoretical analysis of the effect of airway smooth muscle load on airway narrowing. Am J Respir Crit Care Med 1996; 153:83–89.
13. Gibbons WJ, Sharma A, Lougheed D, Macklem PT. Detection of excessive bronchoconstriction in asthma. Am J Respir Crit Care Med 1996; 153:582–589.
14. Black JL. Role of airway smooth muscle. Am J Respir Crit Care Med 1996; 153:S2–S4.
15. Ishida K, Paré PD, Hards J, Schellenberg R. Mechanical properties of human bronchial smooth muscle in vitro. J Appl Physiol 1992; 73:1481–1485.
16. Okazawa M, Wang L, Lambert RK, Verburgt L, Vedal S, Bert JL, Pinder KL, Pare PD. Mucosal folding and airway smooth muscle shortening. Chest 1995; 107:88S.
17. Bramley AM, Roberts CR, Schellenberg RR. Collagenase increases shortening of human bronchial smooth muscle in vitro. Am J Respir Crit Care Med 1995; 152:1513–1517.
18. Hogg JC. Airway behavior and its regulation: How do structural changes affect airway behavior? Am J Respir Crit Care Med 1996; 153:S16–S18.
19. Bai TR. Abnormalities in airway smooth muscle in fatal asthma. Am Rev Respir Dis 1990; 141:552–557.
20. Barnes PJ, Rodger IW, Thomson NC. Pathogenesis of asthma. In: Barnes PJ, Rodger IW, Thomson NC, eds. Asthma: Basic Mechanisms and Clinical Management. 2nd ed. London: Academic Press, 1992:391–411.
21. Black JL, Marthan R, Armour CL, Johnson P. Sensitization alters contractile responses and calcium influx in human airway smooth muscle. J Allergy Clin Immunol 1989; 84:440–447.
22. Hay DWP, Lutmann P, Hubbard WC, et al. Endothelin receptor subtypes in human and guinea-pig pulmonary tissues. Br J Pharmacol 1993; 110:1175–1183.
23. Sheppard D. Airway hyperresponsiveness. Mechanisms in experimental models. Chest 1993; 96:1165–1168.
24. Stewart AG, Tomlinson PR, Wilson J. Airway wall remodelling in asthma: a novel target for the development of anti-asthma drugs. Trends Pharmacol Sci 1993; 14:275–279.

25. Barnes PJ. What is the role of nerves in chronic asthma and symptoms? Am J Respir Crit Care Med 1996; 153:S5–S8.
26. Denburg JA. The inflammatory response. Am J Respir Crit Care Med 1996; 153:S11–S13.
27. Smith PG, Tokui T, Ikebe M. Mechanical strain increases contractile enzyme activity in cultured airway smooth muscle cells. Am J Physiol 1995; 268:L999–L1005.
28. deLarnerolle P. Airway smooth muscle and asthma. Am J Respir Cell Mol Biol 1992; 7:565–566.
29. Jiang H, Rao K, Liu X, Halayhko A, Liu G, Stephens N. Early changes in airway smooth muscle hyperresponsiveness. Can J Physiol Pharmacol 1994; 72:1440–1447.
30. Jiang H, Rao K, Halayko A, Liu X, Stephens N. Ragweed sensitization-induced increase of myosin light chain kinase content in canine airway smooth muscle. Am J Respir Cell Mol Biol 1992; 7:567–573.
31. Liu X, Halayko AJ, Liu G, Rao K, Jian H, Stephens N. Myosin light chain phosphatase activity in ragweed pollen-sensitized canine tracheal smooth muscle. Am J Respir Cell Mol Biol 1994; 11:676–681.
32. Donnelly RK, Yang K, Omary MB, Azhar S, Black J. Expression of multiple isoenzymes of protein kinase C in airway smooth muscle. Am J Respir Cell Mol Biol 1995; 13:253–256.
33. Rossetti M, Savineau JP, Crevel H, Marthan R. Role of protein kinase C in nonsensitized and passively sensitized human isolated bronchial smooth muscle. Am J Physiol 1995; 268:L966–L971.
34. Souhrada M, Souhrada JF. Sodium and calcium influx induced by phorbol esters in airway smooth muscle cells. Am Rev Respir Dis 1989; 139:927–1032.
35. Souhrada M, Souhrada JF. The role of protein kinase-C in sensitization and antigen response of airway smooth muscle. Am Rev Respir Dis 1989; 140:1567–1572.
36. Souhrada M, Souhrada JF. Inhibitory effect of staurosporine on protein kinase C stimulation of airway smooth muscle cells. Am Rev Respir Dis 1993; 148:425–430.
37. Mitchell RW, Ruhlmann E, Magnussen H, Leff A, Rabe K. Passive sensitization of human bronchi augments smooth muscle shortening velocity and capacity. Am J Physiol 1994; 267:L218–L222.
38. Marthan R, Crevel H, Guénard H, Savineau J. Responsiveness to histamine in human sensitized airway smooth muscle. Respir Physiol 1992; 90:239–250.
39. Ben-Jebria A, Marthan R, Rossetti M, Savineau J. Effect of passive sensitization on the mechanical activity of human isolated bronchial smooth muscle induced by substance P, neurokinin A and VIP. Br J Pharmacol 1993; 109:131–136.
40. Colusurdo GN, Larsen GL. Airway hyperresponsiveness. In: Busse WW, Holgate ST, eds. Asthma and Rhinitis. Boston: Blackwell Scientific Publications, 1995:1044–1056.
41. Bjorck T, Gustafsson LE, Dahlén SE. Isolated bronchi from asthmatics are hyperresponsive to adenosine, which apparently acts indirectly by liberation of leukotrienes and histamine. Am Rev Respir Dis 1992; 145:1087–1091.
42. Armour CL, Lazar NL, Schellenberg RR, Taylor SM, Chan N, Hogg JC, Pare PD.

A comparison of in vivo and in vitro human airway reactivity to histamine. Am Rev Respir Dis 1984; 129:907–910.
43. Cerrina J, Le Roy Ladurie M, Labat C, Raffestin B, Bayol A, Brink C. Comparison of human bronchial muscle responses to histamine in vivo with histamine and isoproterenol agonists in vitro. Am Rev Respir Dis 1986; 134:57–61
44. Roberts JA, Raeburn D, Rodger IW, Thomson NC. Comparison of in vivo airway responsiveness and in vitro smooth muscle sensitivity to methacholine in man. Thorax 1984; 39:837–843.
45. Vincenc KS, Black JL, Yan K, Armour CL, Donnelly PD, Woolcock AJ. Comparison of in vivo and in vitro responses to histamine in human airways. Am Rev Respir Dis 1983; 128:875–879.
46. Goldie RG, Spina D, Henry PJ, Lulich K, Paterson J. In vitro responsiveness of human asthmatic bronchus to carbachol, histamine, β-adrenoreceptor agonists and theophylline. Br J Clin Pharmacol 22:669–676.
47. Whicker SD, CL Armour, and JL Black. Responsiveness of bronchial smooth muscle from asthmatic patients to relaxant and contractile agonists. Pulmon Pharmacol 1988; 1:25–31.
48. Bai TR. Abnormalities in airway smooth muscle in fatal asthma. Am Rev Respir Dis 1991; 143:441–443.
49. Skloot G, Permutt S, and Togias A. Airway hyperresponsiveness in asthma: a problem of limited smooth muscle relaxation with inspiration. J Clin Invest 1995; 96:2393–2403.
50. Emala C, Black C, Curry C, Levine M, Hirshman C. Impaired β-adrenergic receptor activation of adenylyl cyclase in airway smooth muscle in the basenji-greyhound dog model of airway hyperresponsiveness. Am J Respir Cell Mol Biol 1993; 8:668–675.
51. Stephens NL, Jiang H. Relaxation of smooth muscle. Can J Physiol Pharmacol 1993; 72:1345–1350.
52. Hakonarson H, Herrick DJ, Grunstein MM. Mechanism of impaired β-adrenoceptor responsiveness in atopic sensitized airway smooth muscle tissue. Am J Physiol 1995; 269:L645–L652.
53. Bai TR, Mak JCW, Barnes PJ. A comparison of β-adrenrgic receptors and in vitro relaxant responses to isoproterenol in asthmatic airway smooth muscle. Am J Respir Cell Mol Biol 1992; 6:647–651.
54. Svedmyr NL, Larsson SA, Thiringer GK. Development of resistance in beta-adrenergic receptors of asthmatic patients. Chest 1976; 69:479–483.
55. Spina D, Rigby PJ, Paterson JW, Goldie R. Autoradiographic localization of β-adrenoceptors in asthmatic human lung. Am Rev Respir Dis 1989; 140:1410–1415.
56. Sharma RK, Jeffery PK. Airway β-adrenoceptor number in cystic fibrosis and asthma. Clin Sci 1990; 78:409–417.
57. Turki J, Liggett SB. Receptor-specific functional properties of β2-adrenergic receptor autoantibodies in asthma. Am J Respir Cell Mol Biol 1995;12:531–539.
58. Wills-Karp M, Uchida Y, Lee JY, Jinot J, Hirata A, Hirata F. Organ culture with proinflammatory cytokines reproduces impairment of the β-adrenoceptor-mediated relaxation in tracheas of a guinea pig antigen model. Am J Respir Cell Mol Biol 1993; 8:153–159.

59. Anakwe O, Zhou S, Benovic J, Askoy M, Kelsen SG. Interleukins impair beta-adrnergic receptor adenylated cyclase system function in human airway epithelial cells. Chest 1995; 107:138S–139S.
60. Grandordy BM, Mak JCW, Barnes PJ. Modulation of airway smooth muscle β-adrenoceptor function by a muscarinic agonist. Life Sci 1993; 54:185–191.
61. Villanove X, Marthan R, Tunon de Lara JM, Johnson P, Savineau J-P, McKay K, Alouan L, Armour C, Black J.. Sensitization decreases relaxation in human isolated airways. Am Rev Respir Dis 1993; 148:107–112.
62. Ollerenshaw S, Jarvis D, Woolcock A, Sullivan C, Scheibner T. Absence of immunoreactive vasoactive intestinal peptide in tissue from lungs of patients with asthma. N Engl J Med 1989; 320:1244–1248.
63. Lilly CM, Bai TR, Shore SA, Hall A, Drazen JM. Neuropeptide content of lungs from asthmatic and nonasthmatic patients. Am J Respir Crit Care Med 1995; 151:548–553.
64. Howarth PH, Springall DR, Redington AE, Djukanovic R, Holgate S, Polak JM. Neuropeptide-containing nerves in bronchial biopsies from asthmatic and nonasthmatic subjects. Am J Respir Cell Mol Biol 1995; 13:288–296.
65. Nijkamp FP and Folkerts G. Nitric oxide and bronchial hyperresponsiveness. Arch Int Pharmacodyn 1995; 329:81–96.
66. Ward JK, Belvisi MG, Fox AJ, Miura M, Tadjkarimi S, Yacoub MH, Barnes PJ. Modulation of cholinergic neural bronchoconstriction by endogenous nitric oxide and vasoactive intestinal peptide in human airways in vitro. J Clin Invest 1993; 92:736–743.
67. Dupuy PM, Shore SA, Drazen JM, Frostell C, Hill WA, Zapol WM. Bronchodilator action of inhaled nitric oxide in guinea pigs. J Clin Invest 1992; 90:421–428.
68. Nijkamp FP, van der Linde HJ, Folkerts G. Nitric oxide synthesis inhibitors induce airway hyperresponsiveness in the guinea pig in vivo and in vitro: role of the epithelium. Am Rev Respir Dis 1993; 148:727–734.
69. Tsukagoshi H, Robbins RA, Barnes PJ Chung KF. Role of nitric oxide and superoxide anions in interleukin-1 beta-induced airway hyperresponsiveness to bradykinin. Am J Respir Crit Care Med 1994; 150:1019–1025.
70. Folkerts G, van der Linde HJ, Nijkamp FP. Virus-induced airway hyperresponsiveness in ginea pigs is related to a deficiency in nitric oxide. J Clin Invest 1995; 95:26–30.
71. Richardson J. Airways smooth muscle. J Allergy Clin Immunol 1987; 80:409–411.
72. Jacoby DB. Viral respiratory infection: a mechanism for the induction of airway inflammation and airway hyperreactivity. Ann Intern Med 1995; 123:288–304.
73. Haddad E, Rousell J, Lindsay M, Barnes P. Synergy between tumor necrosis factor α and interleukin 1β in inducing transcriptional downregulation of muscarinic M2 receptor gene expression. J Biol Chem 1996; 271:32586–32592.
74. Laitinen A, Laitinen L. Cellular infiltrates in asthma and in chronic obstructive pulmonary disease. Am Rev Respir Dis 1991; 143:1159–1160.
75. Hirst S, Twort C. The proliferative response of airway smooth muscle. Clin Exp Allergy 1992; 22:907–915.
76. Panettieri R, Murray R, Bilgen G, Eszterhas A, Martin J. Repeated allergen inha-

lations induce DNA synthesis in airway smooth muscle and epithelial cells in vivo. Chest 1995; 107:93S–95S.
77. Smith P, Janiga K, Bruce M. Strain increases airway smooth muscle cell proliferation. Am J Respir Cell Mol Biol 1994; 10:85–90.
78. Panettieri, RA Yadish PA, Rubinstein VA, Kelly AM, Kotlikoff ML. Histamine induces proliferation and c-fos transcription in cultured airway smooth muscle. Am J Physiol 1990; 259:L365–L371.
79. Brown JK, Tyler CL, Jones CA, Ruoss SJ, Hartmann T, Caughey GH. Tryptase, the dominant secretary granular protein in human mast cells, is a potent mitogen for cultured dog tracheal smooth muscle cells. Am J Respir Cell Mol Biol 1995; 13:227–236.
80. Rouss S, Hartmann T, Caughey G. Mast cell tryptase is a mitogen for cultured fibroblasts. J Clin Invest 1991; 88:493–499.
81. Noveral JP, Grunstein MM. Role and mechanism of thromboxane-induced proliferation of cultured airway smooth muscle cells. Am J Physiol 1992; 263:L555–561.
82. Cohen P, Noveral JP, Bhala A, Nunn SE, Herrick DJ, Grunstein MM. Leukotriene D4 facilitates airway smooth muscle cell proliferation via modulation of the IGF axis. Am J Physiol 1995;269:L151–7.
83. Noveral JP, Grunstein MM. Adrenergic receptor mediated regulation of cultured rabbit airway smooth muscle proliferation. Am J Physiol 1994; 11:L291–L299.
84. Noveral JP, Grunstein MM. Tachykinin regulation of airway smooth muscle cell proliferation. Am J Physiol 1995;269:L339–43.
85. Noveral JP Rosenberg SM Anbar RA, Pawlowski NA, Grunstein MM. role of endothelin-1 in regulating proliferation of cultured rabbit ASM cells. Am J Physiol 992;263:L317–L324.
86. Glassberg M, Ergul A, Wanner A, Puett D. Endothelin-1 promotes mitogenesis in airway smooth muscle cells. Am J Respir Cell Mol Biol 1994; 10:316–321.
87. Shapiro P, Evans J, Davis R, Posada J. The seven-transmembrane-spanning receptors for Endothelin and Thrombin cause proliferation of airway wmooth muscle cells and activation of the extracellular regulated kinase and c-Jun NH2-terminal kinase groups of mitogen-activated protein kinases. J Biol Chem 1996;271:5450–5457.
88. Panettieri R, Goldie R Rigby P, Eszterhas A, Hay D. Endothelin-1-induced potentiation of human sirway smooth muscle proliferation: an ET_A receptor -mediated phenomenon. Br J Pharmacol 1996; 118:191–197.
89. Stewart A, Tomlinson P, Fernandes D, Wilson J, Harris T. Tumor necrosis factor-α modulates mitogen responses of human cultured airway smooth muscle. Am J Respir Cell Mol Biol 1995; 12:110–119.
90. Amrani Y, Panettiei R, Frossard N, Bronner C. Activation of the TNFα-p55 receptor induces myocyte proliferation and modulates agonist-evoked calcium transients in cultured human tracheal smooth muscle cells. Am J Respir Cell Mol Biol 1996; 15:55–63.
91. Hirst SJ, Barnes PJ, Twort CH. Quantifying proliferation of cultured human and rabbit airway smooth muscle cells in response to serum and platelet-derived growth factor. Am J Respir Cell Mol Biol 1992; 7:574–581.

92. Hirst SJ, Barnes PJ, Twort CH. PDGF isoform-induced proliferation and receptor expression in human cultured airway smooth muscle cells. Am J Physiol 1996; 270:L415–428.
93. Noveral JP, Bhala A, Hintz RL, Grunstein MM, Cohen P. Insulin-like growth factor axis in airway smooth muscle cells. Am J Physiol 1994; 267:L761–765.
94. Hirst SJ, Webb BJ, Giembycz MA, Barnes PJ, Twort CH. Inhibition of fetal calf serum stimulated proliferation of rabbit cultured tracheal smooth muscle cells by selective inhibitors of protein kinase C and protein tyrosine kinase. Am J Respir Crit Care Med 1995; 12:149–161.
95. Panettieri R, Hall I, Maki C, Murray R. a-Thrombin increases cytosolic calsium and induces human airway smooth muscle cell proliferation. Am J Respir Cell Mol Biol 1995; 13:205–216.
96. Thomlinson PR, Wilson J, Stewart AG. Inhibition by salbutamol of the proliferation of airway smooth muscle cells grown in culture. Br J Pharmacol 1994; 111:641–647.
97. Young PG, Skinner JM, Black PN. Effect of glucocorticoids and β-adrenoreceptor agonists on the proliferation of airway smooth muscle. Eur J Pharmacol 1995; 273:137–144.
98. Schramm CM, Omlor GJ, Quinn LM, Noveral JP. Methylprednisolone and isoproterenol inhibit airway smooth muscle proliferation by separate and additive mechanisms. Life Sci 1996; 59:PL9–14.
99. Johnson PR, Carey D, Armour CL, Black JL. PGE2 and heparin are antiproliferative mediators for human airway smooth muscle cells in culture. Am J Physiol 1995; 13:L514–L519.
100. Maruno K, Absood A, Said S. VIP inhibits basal and histamine-stimulated proliferation of human airway smooth muscle cells. Am J Physiol 1995; 12:L1047–L1051.

16

The Role of Smooth Muscle Cells in Primary Pulmonary Hypertension

MITCHELL D. BOTNEY

Washington University School of Medicine
St. Louis, Missouri

I. Introduction

Primary pulmonary hypertension (PPH) is a disease characterized by a progressive increase in pulmonary artery impedance, ultimately producing right ventricular failure and death. PPH can occur at any age and in both genders. The mean age of patients enrolled in the NIH Registry on Primary Pulmonary Hypertension was 36 years, although 9% of the registrees were more than 60 years old (1). The ratio of women to men was 1.7:1. The importance of a genetic predisposition or susceptibility is suggested by the presence of familial forms of PPH (2) and by the relatively few people developing pulmonary hypertension (with identical pathology to PPH) following widespread ingestion of the anorexic agent aminorex fumurate (3). Dyspnea is the cardinal symptom of PPH, occurring in more than 95% of patients in the NIH series (1), although the severity of dyspnea does not always correlate with the elevation in pulmonary arterial pressures. Pharmacologic therapies have improved, but results are still unsatisfactory. Transplantation is an alternative therapy but is not without problems.

At the time most patients with PPH present to clinical attention, pathological lesions include pulmonary artery medial hypertrophy, intimal proliferation, and adventitial thickening. The pathogenesis of these lesions is poorly understood and, by definition, the inciting event is unknown. On the basis of animal studies, and by analogy to systemic arteries, it seems likely endothelial injury is required. Whether injury occurs secondary to infection, ingestion of a toxin, exposure to an environmental toxin, or simply reflects a spontaneous modulation of cellular phenotype remains unclear. A pulmonary artery "response to injury" may be similar to the "response to injury" hypothesis described for systemic arteries (4), with differences between pulmonary and systemic artery patterns of remodeling reflecting the influence of hemodynamic factors. Whereas injury to the endothelial cell may initiate the response, the smooth muscle cell (SMC) mediates the response. Indeed, one pathologic characteristic of PPH is the presence of SMC in vessels or vascular compartments normally devoid of SMC. Although the definition of SMC is becoming more complex (5), with evidence for multiple subpopulations of SMC within blood vessels and phenotype plasticity, the SMC mediates the vasoconstriction and vascular remodeling characteristic of PPH. Understanding the role of SMC in vasoconstriction and vascular remodeling is of central importance to understanding the pathophysiology and pathogenesis of PPH.

II. Smooth Muscle Cells in the Normal Pulmonary Artery

Pulmonary arteries consist of three basic compartments. All have a thin intimal layer, composed of a single layer of endothelial cells and basement membrane, lining the blood vessel lumen. The outermost layer of the vessel is the adventitia, composed of fibroblasts and connective tissue enriched in collagen. Between the intima and adventitia is the medial layer comprised of SMC (or their precursors) and connective tissue. Though all three compartments are present in different segments of the pulmonary artery, the structure of the vessel varies depending upon location.

The structure of the normal pulmonary artery reflects the physical properties required of a particular vascular segment (6,7). The hilar vessels, extending from the pulmonary trunk through branches as small as 1000 mm in diameter, are most directly exposed to the pulsatile pressures of the right ventricle. Elastin, the elastic protein of the body, is abundant in these segments and contributes to their distensibility. Elastin fibers are organized into concentric cylindrical lamellae connected by radially oriented elastin fibers, which serve to transmit luminal pressures evenly throughout the vessel wall (8,9). An emerging model of the vasculature is one in which all structural components of the vessel are mechanically and functionally connected. Pulmonary artery compliance is determined by the passive mechanical properties of the connective tissue scaffold and the active regulation of SMC tone.

A transition from elastic to muscular artery occurs between 1000 and 500 μm diameter as fewer medial elastin fibers distinguish the normal muscular artery from the more proximal elastic artery. Vessels between 500 μm and approximately 70 μm diameter have a thin layer of circumferentially oriented medial SMC limited by internal and external elastic laminae. A transition between the true muscular artery and pulmonary arterioles occurs as the muscular artery gradually loses its muscular media. Arteriole segments have a spiral arrangement so that, on cross section, medial SMC appear to alternate with segments lacking a medial layer. Poorly characterized contractile "intermediate" and "pericyte" cells are found in the nonmuscular part of the vessel wall (10). These cells may proliferate and differentiate into SMC under appropriate conditions. Eventually, the arterioles form capillaries that consist of a single layer of endothelial cells only.

Although vascular SMC may appear homogeneous by classic cytochemical criteria, recent observations demonstrate several SMC subpopulations in the vascular wall. At least four phenotypes, based on immunoreactivity to several contractile and cytoskeletal proteins, cell morphology and elastic lamellar arrangements were observed in the medial layer of the mature bovine main pulmonary artery (11). In addition, each cell population expresses these contractile and cytoskeletal proteins at different times during development, consistent with the hypothesis that multiple distinct SMC lineages exist simultaneously within the vascular wall.

The SMC performs two important functions in the normal pulmonary artery. First it originates and maintains the structural integrity of the vasculature by synthesizing the extracellular matrix of the pulmonary artery. Second, the SMC maintains the vascular tone required to optimally match pulmonary perfusion to ventilation.

The synthesis and deposition of elastin and collagen by SMC in the pulmonary arteries is a highly ordered process beginning in late fetal and early neonatal periods and ending by maturity. For example, tropoelastin exhibits a complex biphasic pattern of expression in the developing bovine pulmonary artery (12). In early gestation, tropoelastin expression is homogeneous throughout the entire pulmonary artery wall; at midgestation, expression is markedly decreased in the outer wall but maintained in the inner media; in late gestation, as pulmonary artery pressure increases prior to birth, a heterogeneous pattern of reexpression is observed throughout the entire pulmonary artery. This suggests tropoelastin expression is modulated by mechanical as well as nonmechanical factors during gestation.

Pulmonary vascular resistance or compliance in the normal pulmonary artery is maintained by factors that either contract or relax the vascular smooth musculature (Fig. 1). In general, the effects of these mediators on pulmonary

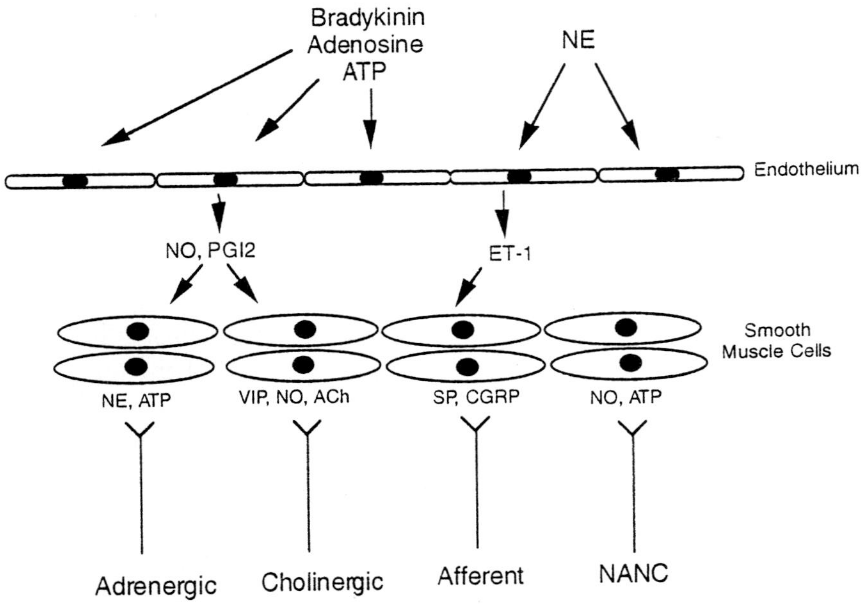

Figure 1 Regulation of pulmonary vascular tone. Pulmonary vascular tone is regulated by autonomic nerves and mediators released from inflammatory cells and endothelial cells.

vascular tone vary with species, age, and preexisting tone. (For a comprehensive discussion of the regulation of pulmonary tone, which is beyond the scope of this review, see Ref. 13.) These factors include the autonomic nervous system as well as nonneural factors. Increases in pulmonary vascular resistance and decreases in pulmonary vascular compliance can be induced by sympathetic nerve stimulation mediated by α-adrenoceptors (13). The role of cholinergic nerves in regulating vascular tone is less certain, but recent studies indicate a role for nonadrenergic, noncholinergic mechanisms. The neuronal form of nitric oxide synthase has been localized to nerves innervating smooth muscle of pulmonary vessels (14), consistent with a role for neurally derived nitric oxide regulation of vascular tone (15).

The pulmonary vascular SMC also responds to many nonneural factors. Angiotensin II constricts isolated pulmonary artery rings (16,17) and increases pulmonary artery resistance in vivo following intravenous administration (18). Endothelins (19), prostacyclin, and thromboxane (20) as well as several factors also regulate pulmonary vascular tone via the vascular SMC (13). Thus, the SMC relaxes or contracts in response to both neural and nonneural mechanisms to maintain appropriate pulmonary vascular resistance and compliance.

In summary, the SMC has an important function in the normal pulmonary artery. It synthesizes and assembles much of the extracellular matrix found in the pulmonary artery and responds to signals originating from other sources, such as the endothelium or autonomic nervous system, to maintain appropriate vascular tone.

III. Smooth Muscle Cells in Primary Pulmonary Hypertension

Hypotheses proposed for the pathogenesis of PPH have changed in the last four decades. Initially considered a problem of vasoconstriction (21,22), later studies demonstrated the importance of vascular remodeling as an important component in the pathophysiology of PPH (23). Today it remains unknown whether the vasoconstriction and remodeling characteristic of PPH reflect two separate pathophysiologic processes, whether remodeling is a consequence of vasoconstriction, or whether vasoconstriction and remodeling are simply different facets of a common underlying pathophysiology. Nevertheless, the vascular SMC again participates by mediating the increased vascular tone observed in PPH as well as by contributing to the structural remodeling in primary pulmonary hypertension.

The hypothesis that PPH was a disease characterized by abnormal vasoconstriction was based on observations that vasodilators lowered pulmonary artery pressures in patients with PPH (21,22,24,25). While considerable progress has been made in determining the mechanism of abnormal vasoconstriction and improving vasodilators, only about 30% of patients respond to vasodilator therapy (26–30). Because patients can "lose" their responsiveness to vasodilators over time, a response to vasodilators may be an early feature of PPH, which is eventually lost as the pulmonary arteries remodel (30). However, these clinical observations do not provide information on the pathophysiologic relationship between vasoconstriction and remodeling.

Pathologic studies demonstrate extension of SMC peripherally into partially muscularized or nonmuscularized arterioles, neointima formation, and increased deposition of connective tissue proteins, such as elastin and collagen, in hypertensive pulmonary arteries from patients with PPH (31–34). Although these early cytochemical studies could not determine whether remodeling persisted late in the course of disease, subsequent studies demonstrated that SMC in pulmonary arteries from patients with PPH are actively expressing and synthesizing extracellular matrix proteins in the neointima of elastic pulmonary arteries (35) and in both the media and neointima of small muscular pulmonary arteries (36) (Fig. 2).

Putative factors mediating remodeling in PPH are only now being determined. Interestingly, many factors that can induce changes in vascular tone can also stimulate remodeling. For example, immunoreactive nitric oxide synthase

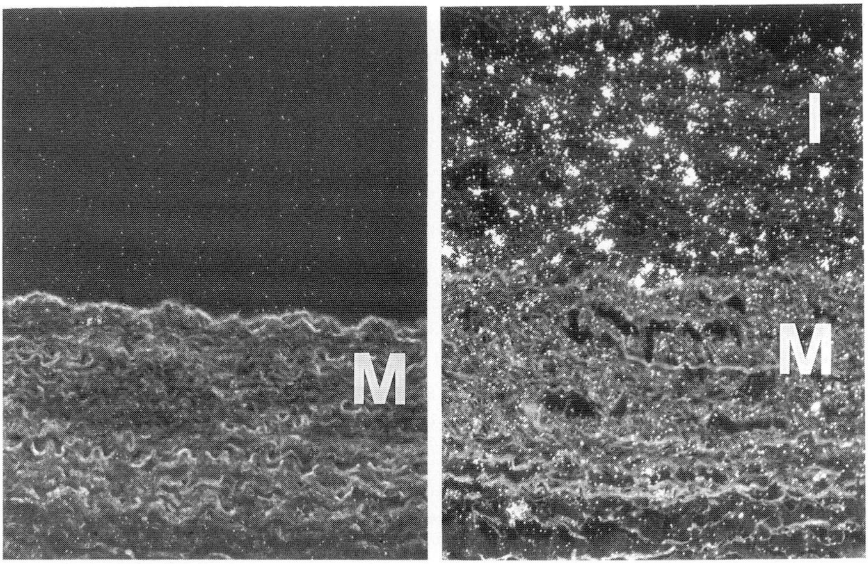

Figure 2 Pulmonary vascular remodeling persists in severe PPH. Human right main pulmonary artery in situ hybridization for tropoelastin. Persistent elastin synthesis in the neointima is suggested by the presence of tropoelastin mRNA associated with neointimal cells of hypertensive vessels (right). No tropoelastin mRNA is observed in normal vessels (left). I, neointima; M, media. (From Ref. 36.)

and urinary 6-keto-prostaglandin $F_{1\alpha}$ (a stable metabolite of prostacyclin) are decreased (37,38), whereas immunoreactive endothelin and urinary 11-dehydro-thromboxane B_2 (a stable metabolite of thromboxane A_2) are increased (38,39) in patients with PPH compared to normal. Expression of angiotensin-converting enzyme (ACE) is increased in both the endothelium and in the neointima of hypertensive pulmonary arteries compared to normal arteries (40). Immunohistochemistry with isoform-specific antibodies demonstrated TGF-β2 and TGF-β3 in nearly all hypertensive small muscular pulmonary arteries, in close proximity to areas of procollagen immunoreactivity (41). Sequential immunohistochemistry—in situ hybridization of large elastic arteries showed neointimal nonfoamy macrophages close to neointimal SMC expressing fibronectin and type I collagen (42) and that "active" TGF-β1 was associated with these nonfoamy neointimal macrophages (43).

These observations, based on the few human tissue studies available, can be organized into a working hypothesis in which vasoconstriction and remodeling are different facets of a common underlying pathophysiology (Fig. 3). As vascular ACE activity increases, the potent vasodilators nitric oxide (NO) and prostacyclin (PGI_2) decrease. Decreases in these two factors release from inhi-

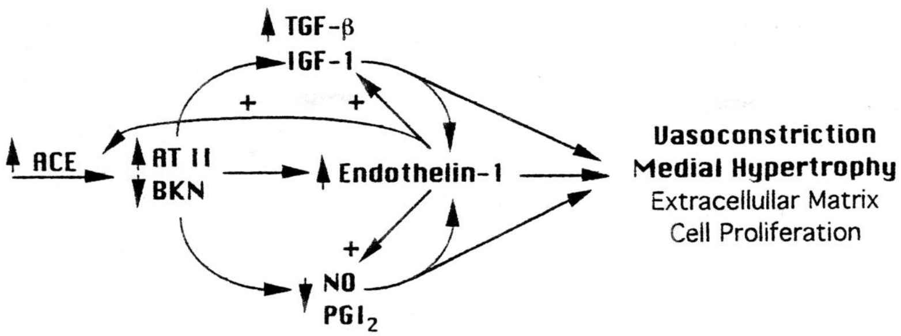

Figure 3 A working hypothesis of the pathophysiology of PPH. Increased vascular ACE activity leads to increased tissue angiotensin II, TGF-β, and endothelin-1 production. Both TCF-β and endothelin induce vascular smooth muscle cell matrix formation. Increased ACE activity reduces bradykinin levels, NO, and PGI_2. NO and PGI_2 inhibit the production of endothelin-1 and shorten the duration of endothelin-1 activity. Decreased in NO and PGI_2 will augment endothelin-1 production. Consistent with this scheme, ACE, TGF-β, endothelin-1, and matrix production are increased in pulmonary arteries of patients with primary pulmonary hypertension, whereas NO synthase and PGI_2 are decreased. Although an ACE-dependent mechanism is depicted in this figure, an ACE-independent mechanism is not excluded. This ACE-independent mechanism may also involve changes in NO, PGI_2, TGF-β, and endothelin-1 as well as other factors.

bition the production and activity of endothelin-1, a potent vasoconstrictor. Together, the increase in endothelin-1 and decreases in NO and PGI_2 lead to vasoconstriction. At the same time increased ACE activity is associated with increases in angiotensin II, TGFβ, and endothelin-1 production. These factors induce extracellular matrix production. Thus, according to this hypothesis, both vasoconstriction and remodeling result from modulation of the same factors.

ACE inhibitors interfere with TGF-β and endothelin production by inhibiting angiotensin II production (44). Increased bradykinin levels, for example after ACE inhibition, will stimulate NO and PGI_2 production (45–47). ACE inhibition, therefore, should have profound effects on extracellular matrix production as well as on vasoconstriction. However, endothelin-1 also modulates PGI_2 (48), NO (49), TGF-β (50), and ACE (51), indicating a complex regulation of these mediators. Undoubtedly there are also ACE-independent mechanisms of remodeling as well as ACE-dependent mechanisms of remodeling.

IV. Smooth Muscle Cells in Animal Models of Pulmonary Vascular Remodeling

The presence of ECM protein synthesis as a component of vascular remodeling has been demonstrated in several animal models of pulmonary hypertension including chronic alveolar hypoxia in the rat (52) and newborn calf (53, 54), monocrotaline (MCT) intoxication in rat (55), and chronic air emboli in sheep (56).

The morphologic pattern of increased elastin synthesis in the hypoxic neonatal calf displays a complex pattern (54). Low levels of tropoelastin mRNA are detected using the technique of in situ hybridization in SMC associated with elastic lamellae of the inner medial layer of normal animals. In contrast, higher levels of tropoelastin mRNA are seen in SMC lying between the elastic lamellae of the outer media. Furthermore, broad circumferential bands of SMC in normal vessels and nodular foci in hypertensive vessels have no detectable tropoelastin mRNA. Type I procollagen mRNA is dispersed throughout the medial layer of normal vessels while the pattern in hypertensive vessels more closely resembles the pattern seen with tropoelastin. Thus, extracellular matrix may not be synthesized by all SMC subpopulations found in the vascular wall (57).

What stimulates vascular SMC extracellular matrix production in pulmonary hypertension is not known. Interestingly, hypoxia per se does not appear responsible for increased tropoelastin production in the neonatal calf model of pulmonary hypertension (58). However, vascular remodeling in hypoxic rats is markedly attenuated when pressure and flow are reduced by coarctation of the left pulmonary artery (59). These experiments suggest that mechanical forces, such as increased wall tension, play an important role in vascular remodeling. Several experiments in vitro support this hypothesis. For example, pulsatile stretch rapidly induced collagen synthesis in cultured vascular SMC (60), and mechanical stretch of isolated pulmonary rings rapidly induced tropoelastin and procollagen mRNA expression (61). In addition, intact endothelium is necessary for increased tropoelastin and procollagen mRNA expression (61), suggesting that important interactions occur between the different compartments of the blood vessel.

While the role of growth factors in patients with primary pulmonary hypertension can only be inferred, the presence of several growth factors has been described in animal models, allowing the expectation that the role of these growth factors in pulmonary vascular remodeling will be experimentally determined in the future. For example, continuous air embolization into the pulmonary arterial circulation of sheep induces pulmonary hypertension accompanied by the appearance of SMC in normally nonmuscular arteries, medial thickening of muscular arteries, and intimal hyperplasia (56). An early but transient increase in TGF-β_1 (62) and a slightly later but more sustained increase in insulin-like growth factor (IGF) is observed in lung lymph from hypertensive sheep (63). IGF immunoreactivity is present in neointimal cells, but not adjacent medial smooth muscle cells, of remodeling small muscular arteries. In vitro studies are consistent with the in vivo descriptive studies since IGF induces the synthesis of tropoelastin in chick embryonic aortae in organ culture (64,65) and cultured bovine pulmonary artery SMC (66) and stimulates the synthesis of proteoglycans by cultured bovine pulmonary artery endothelial cells (67). Other studies suggest that IGF- 1 participates in systemic vascular remodeling since steady-state levels of aorta IGF-1 mRNA are increased and immunohistochemical studies detect IGF-1 in the neointima but not media of mechanically injured aortae (68,69).

A role for TGF-β is suggested by studies in the monocrotaline (MCT) model of pulmonary vascular remodeling. Rat pulmonary arteries rapidly remodel after a single injection of MCT (70,71). Early pathological changes include pulmonary artery endothelial swelling and blebbing (55) and inflammatory infiltrates (72,73). Later changes include increased vascular tropoelastin and type I procollagen synthesis and deposition (55,74). In situ hybridization demonstrates that matrix gene expression begins as early as 7 days following MCT injection, before any physiologic changes are detected (75). Total lung TGF-β is increased following MCT injury, with MCT gene expression colocalizing to areas of tropoelastin but not procollagen gene expression. TGF-β_1 stimulates production of fibronectin (76,77), collagen (78,79), and tropoelastin (80,81). TGF-β_1 also stimulates smooth muscle cell migration (82) and replication in vitro (83,84) and in vivo (85). TGF-β_1 mRNA and protein are also detected in remodeling carotid arteries following mechanical injury (85).

Medial SMC in both normotensive and hypertensive vessels are the major source of TGF-β_1 in the hypoxic neonatal calf model of remodeling (86). A progressive, age-dependent increase in normal pulmonary artery TGF-β_1 mRNA follows birth, whereas no increase occurs in hypertensive pulmonary arteries. Since TGF-β inhibits neonatal vascular SMC growth, increasing TGF-β in the normal neonatal pulmonary artery may regulate normal developmental regulation and cessation of proliferation, whereas the absence of TGF-β could contribute to the excessive or continued proliferation observed in this model of pulmonary vascular remodeling.

Platelet-derived growth factor (PDGF) mRNA is increased in lungs of chronically hypoxic rats (87), and PDGF-B and its receptor are increased in the hyperoxic model of pulmonary vascular remodeling (88). PDGF promotes SMC migration (89,90) and cell growth (83,91) and stimulates the production of several extracellular matrix components (92–94). PDGF is produced by vascular SMC (95,96), endothelial cells (97,98), and macrophages (99,100). PDGF mRNA and protein are increased in rat carotid arteries after mechanical injury (101,102) and is found in human carotid atherosclerotic lesions (103–105).

Lung vascular endothelial growth factor (VEGF) gene expression and protein increase in the hypoxic model of pulmonary vascular remodeling (106). VEGF stimulates endothelial cell migration and replication (107). The biological activities of VEGF are mediated by two transmembrane receptor kinases, flt-

1 and flk-1/KDR, that are expressed predominantly on vascular endothelial cells. The expression of both VEGF receptors is also upregulated by hypoxia (106).

Consistent with the immunohistochemistry localizing ACE to areas of active remodeling in hypertensive pulmonary arteries obtained from patients with PPH, emerging experimental evidence indicates that ACE participates in pulmonary vascular remodeling and matrix synthesis. ACE protein and mRNA expression are focally increased in small rat pulmonary arteries during chronic hypoxia even though total lung ACE decreases (108). In addition, ACE inhibitors, as well as antagonists of type I angiotensin II receptors, attenuate the development of pulmonary hypertension in the monocrotaline (109,110) and hypoxia models (111). Inhibition of remodeling may account for this attenuation in pulmonary artery hypertension and right ventricular hypertrophy since MCT-induced SMC tropoelastin and type I collagen expression is decreased by ACE inhibition. ACE inhibition also attenuates SMC replication and decreases muscular pulmonary artery thickness during exposure to prolonged hypoxia (112).

The presence of these growth factors in pulmonary arteries from several different animal models of pulmonary hypertension strongly suggests that they induce or maintain pulmonary vascular remodeling. Many, but not all, of these growth factors have been identified in remodeling pulmonary arteries from patients with PPH. Undoubtedly, there are other factors involved in pulmonary vascular remodeling. Putative factors initially detected in pulmonary arteries from patients with PPH will require subsequent confirmation of their participation in pulmonary vascular remodeling through experimental studies in animal models. Conversely, the clinical relevance of factors identified in animal models will require confirmation that they are present in human hypertensive pulmonary arteries. This underscores the importance of further studies with human tissues as well as the judicious use of animal models of remodeling.

V. Interactions Between Pulmonary Vascular Hemodynamics and Remodeling

The histologic pattern of vascular remodeling in animal models does not resemble the pathology seen with PPH. Neointimal formation is prominent in PPH but is not found in animal models of pulmonary vascular remodeling. One explanation for this difference is based on the clinical observation that the large elastic arteries of the normal pulmonary vasculature remain relatively free of neointimal hyperplasia in the elderly (113) or in the presence of diabetes, tobacco smoking, or hypercholesterolemia (114). The absence of neointimal hyperplasia despite risk factors for atherosclerosis probably reflects the substantially lower blood pressures present in pulmonary arteries (114) since neointimal changes are uniformly and characteristically found in the presence of pulmonary hypertension (115,116).

Therefore, to examine the influence of increased pressure on pulmonary vascular remodeling in the rat, the left subclavian artery was anastomosed to the left pulmonary artery 7 days after MCT injury. Histologic studies demonstrated that the left main pulmonary arteries from all animals receiving monocrotaline + shunt developed an extensive but patchy neointima (Fig. 4) (117). Remodeling was not induced by shunt alone, demonstrating the importance of injury as there was no evidence of remodeling, histologically or by in situ hybridization, up to 6 months following surgery. Type I procollagen, tropoelastin, and TGF-β gene expression was observed only in the neointima following MCT + shunt (Fig. 5), similar to remodeling human pulmonary arteries. A role for SMC is again suggested since immunohistochemistry showed that nearly all neointimal cells were SMC with less than 2% macrophages present. The likely explanation is that hemodynamic changes secondary to the shunt modified the pattern of remodeling that occurred in response to injury.

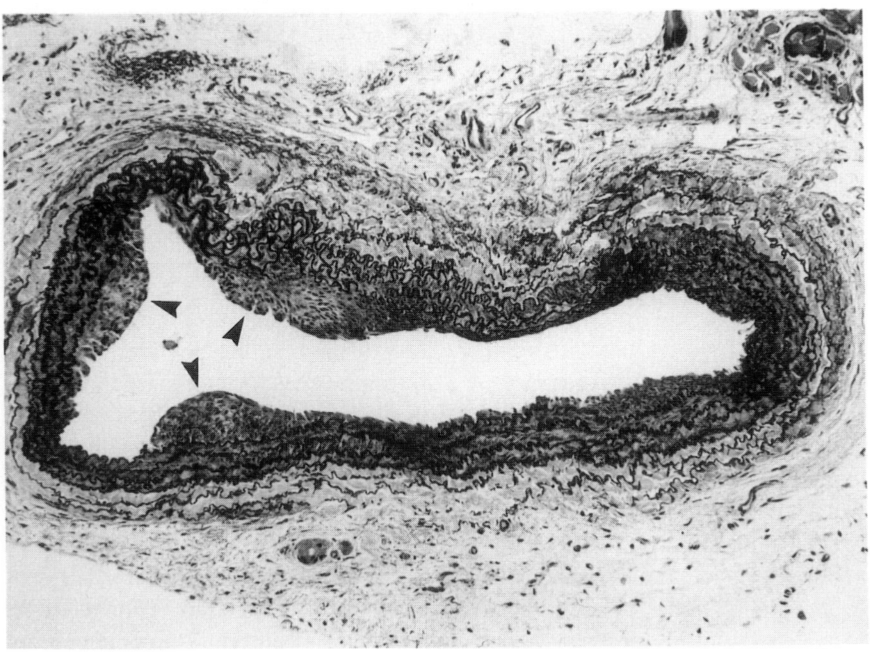

Figure 4 Systemic pressures modify the pulmonary arterial response to injury. Neointima (arrowheads) is present 28 days after monocrotaline-injured pulmonary arteries subjected to systemic-like hemodynamics via subclavian-pulmonary artery anastomosis. The neointima in this elastic pulmonary artery is present diffusely but varies in thickness (Verhoeff-van Gieson stain ×40). (From Ref. 117.)

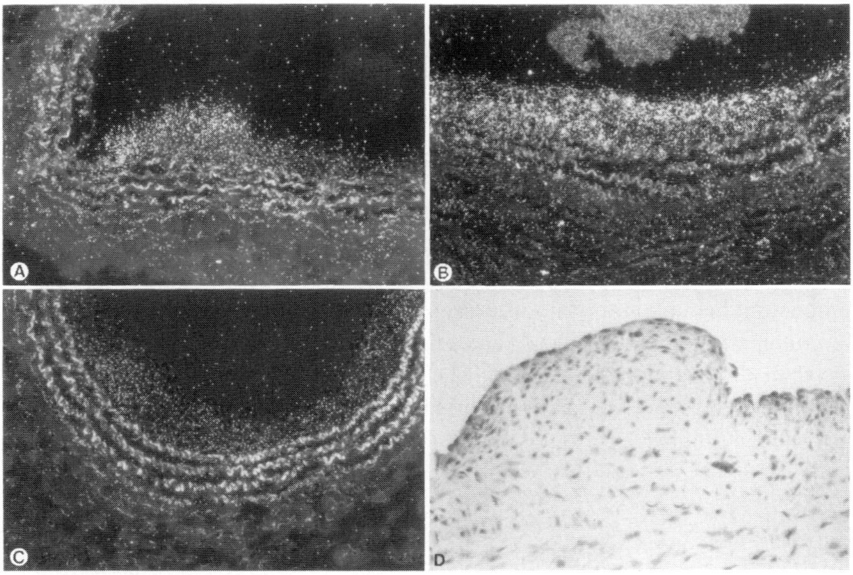

Figure 5 Type I procollagen (A), tropoelastin (B), and TGF-β1 (C) gene expression is confined to the neointima in monocrotaline-injured pulmonary arteries subjected to systemic hemodynamics. TGF-β1. and TGF-β3 gene expression was also confined to the neointima (not shown) similar to TGF-β1. No type I procollagen gene expression was seen at the medial-advertitial border, in contrast to monocrotaline alone. No signal was seen with sense control probes. ACE immunoreactivity is associated with endothelial cells and neointimal smooth muscle cells closest to the lumen (D). No immunoreactivity was seen with control rabbit serum. (From Ref. 117.)

It is unclear what is responsible for neointimal formation in the monocrotaline + shunt model of pulmonary vascular remodeling. Mechanical forces, such as increased stretch, can modulate matrix protein synthesis. Pulsatile stretch rapidly induced collagen synthesis in cultured vascular smooth muscle cells (60), and mechanical stretch of isolated pulmonary artery rings rapidly induced tropoelastin and procollagen mRNA expression (61). Intact endothelium was necessary for increased tropoelastin and procollagen mRNA expression, suggesting that important interactions occur between the different compartments of the blood vessel. More recently, medial smooth muscle cell type I procollagen immunoreactivity and total pulmonary artery collagen and elastin synthesis were found to increase with increasing stretch in rabbit pulmonary artery strips maintained in organ culture (118). It is unclear, however, whether the increased collagen and elastin synthesis observed in these in vitro studies is related to mechanical forces alone or related to the combination of stretch plus injury incurred during dissection of the vessel. The absence of remodeling in animals with shunt alone suggests that mechanical stretch alone does not induce matrix synthesis in vivo but that accompanying endothelial or smooth muscle cell injury is necessary.

Shear stress is another component of the mechanical forces acting upon the vascular wall. Systemic arteries tend to normalize to a wall shear stress value of approximately 15 dynes/cm^2 (119,120). Neointimal formation is thought to be one mechanism by which the vessel is able to maintain an appropriate mechanical environment. Shear stress is linearly proportional to the flow rate through the vessel and inversely proportional to the third power of the vessel diameter. The diameter of the postanastomotic pulmonary artery ballooned to roughly twice its normal size in all animals. In the absence of any change in blood flow, the shear stress in the postanastomotic pulmonary artery would be reduced to one-eighth the normal vessel shear stress. Although pulmonary artery blood flow undoubtedly increased as the result of the systemic-pulmonic shunt, thereby increasing shear stress, we hypothesize that the net effect is decreased shear stress since shear stress will be more affected by changes in diameter than changes in flow. Thus, one explanation for the absence of pulmonary artery neointimal formation in animal models of pulmonary hypertension despite endothelial injury is the absence of increased mechanical stretch or decreased wall shear stress. The contribution of mechanical forces to pulmonary vascular remodeling, however, has not been systematically studied in animal models.

VI. Primary Pulmonary Hypertension: Unifying Vasoconstriction and Vascular Remodeling

The studies described above suggest a hypothesis that defines the relationship between vasoconstriction and remodeling as two different manifestations of a common pathophysiology. The hypothesis also explains the difference in the pattern of remodeling between animal models and patients. The initial response to vascular injury, occurring in the presence of normal pulmonary artery hemodynamics, is SMC-mediated vasocontraction. This is due to early changes in ACE, TGF-β, endothelin-1, NO, PGI_2 as well as probable decreases and increases in other vasodilators and vasocontractors, respectively. Changes in these same factors participate in initiating and maintaining SMC-mediated medial remodeling. If the vascular injury is limited, remodeling may cease with some residual fibrosis or even complete resolution. However, if injury or remodeling persists, medial hypertrophy develops secondary to smooth muscle hypertrophy and hyperplasia and deposition of extracellular matrix proteins. As a result, hemodynamics in those vessels changes and neointima formation is induced. This process continues until remodeling throughout the entire vascular tree is characterized pathologically by both medial hypertrophy and neointima (34–36,113,114). Thus, the natural history of remodeling in primary pulmonary hypertension may be that the pattern of vascular remodeling changes with time as the pulmonary hemodynamic conditions change.

Is there evidence that the pattern of remodeling in patients with primary pulmonary hypertension has changed over time? At the time of lung transplantation, remodeling in large elastic pulmonary arteries is localized to the neointima. To determine whether there was evidence of previous remodeling in the medial layer, we examined the indigestable elastin "skeleton" remaining after a single normal and hypertensive pulmonary artery were digested with formic acid (121). Since elastin is characteristically synthesized when vessels remodel, the extremely stable elastin skeleton indirectly provides an "historical" record of the pattern of vascular remodeling. Increased numbers of thickened elastin strands in the medial elastin skeleton are demonstrated in the hypertensive artery compared to the normal vessel consistent with previous remodeling. This suggests that the pattern of vascular remodeling changes with time in primary pulmonary hypertension since only neointimal remodeling is observed at the time of lung transplantation.

VII. Future Directions

Progress is being made in understanding the pathogenesis of PPH. Studies that were not feasible with cadaveric tissue are being performed by several groups with human hypertensive lungs obtained at the time of transplantation. As a result, new insights into the pathogenesis of PPH are emerging. Nevertheless, knowledge about the factors present in hypertensive human pulmonary arteries remains limited, underscoring the need for additional studies with human tissues.

An animal model of PPH that replicates the human disease may be unachievable since the initiating factors are not known, and early events are difficult to define because patients with PPH remain asymptomatic until relatively late in the course of their disease. Nevertheless, animal models of pulmonary hypertension retain their usefulness. For example, right ventricular hypertrophy or hypertrophy of the arterial medial layer are common indices of pulmonary hypertension. Both indices are useful since they reflect a physiologically relevant response to pulmonary vascular injury. However, these morphological changes are cumulative and indirect reflections of more immediate responses to injury, such as matrix synthesis and degradation, smooth muscle replication, and migration within the pulmonary artery. Using animal models to define the mechanism(s) of matrix synthesis and degradation, smooth muscle replication, and migration in response to pulmonary vascular injury may yield important insights into the pathogenesis of PPH.

It is becoming apparent from both animal and human tissue studies that pulmonary vascular remodeling resembles systemic vascular remodeling. Many of the same mediators are present, smooth muscle cell replication and migration occurs, and extracellular matrix is synthesized and deposited in both pulmonary and systemic vascular remodeling, although hemodynamic conditions unique to the systemic vasculature may influence its pattern of remodeling. A better understanding of the similarities and differences between pulmonary and systemic vascular remodeling may provide important insights into both pulmonary and systemic vascular remodeling.

Many of the same factors modulating pulmonary vascular tone are putative mediators of pulmonary vascular remodeling. Whether the vasoconstriction and remodeling associated with PPH reflect two separate pathophysiologic processes is unknown, as is whether remodeling is a consequence of vasoconstriction or whether vasoconstriction and remodeling are simply different facets of a common underlying pathophysiology. Defining the relationship between vasoconstriction and vascular remodeling may provide important insights into the pathogenesis of PPH.

Many recent in vitro studies demonstrate the influence of pulsatile stretch and shear stress on vascular cells. The synthesis of several growth factors as well as vasoregulatory factors are regulated by these hemodynamic factors. Nevertheless, very little is still known about how hemodynamics influence vascular cells in vivo. Animal models in which pulmonary hemodynamics can be manipulated to resemble systemic hemodynamics provide a unique opportunity to study the influence of blood pressure and flow on vascular cells in vivo, particularly their response to injury.

Primary pulmonary hypertension is characterized by progressively increasing pulmonary vascular impedance inducing right ventricular hypertrophy and, eventually, right heart failure and death. Pulmonary vascular resistance (PVR) is only one component of pulmonary vascular impedance, which also includes pulmonary artery compliance and reflected flow and pressure waves, thereby underestimating the actual impedance to right ventricular outflow (122). Most clinical trials use PVR to determine the efficacy of therapeutic interventions because measurements of pulmonary vascular impedance are difficult to obtain, but all three components of impedance are abnormal in patients with PPH (123) and in animal models of pulmonary hypertension (124,125). Therapeutic trials that use PVR rather than pulmonary vascular impedance as a hemodynamic endpoint may be misleading. How pulmonary vasoconstriction and vascular remodeling leads to increased pulmonary vascular impedance is poorly defined. Experimental studies using animal models with histologic changes resembling the pathology of PPH should provide valuable information on the coupling between the pulmonary artery and right ventricle and potentially provide diagnostically and prognostically useful insights.

References

1. Rich S, Dantzker DR, Ayres SM, Bergofsky EH, Brundage BH, Detre KM, Fishman AP, Goldring RM, Groves BM, Koerner SK, Levy BC, Reid LM, Vreim CE, Williams GM. Primary pulmonary hypertension. A national prospective study. Ann Intern Med 1987; 107:216–223.
2. Loyd JE, Primm RK, Newman JH. Familial primary pulmonary hypertension: clinical patterns. Am Rev Respir Dir 1984; 129:194–197.
3. Widgren S. Pulmonary hypertension related to Aminorex intake. Springer 1977; 64:1–64.
4. Ross R. Atherosclerosis: a defense mechanism gone awry. Am J Pathol 1993; 143:987–1002.
5. Schwartz SM, Mecham RP. The Vascular Smooth Muscle Cell-Molecular and Biological Responses to the Extracellular Matrix. New York: Academic Press, 1996.
6. Wagenvort CA, Wagenvoort N. Pathology of Pulmonary Hypertension. New York: J. Wiley & Sons, 1977.
7. Harris P, Heath D. The Human Pulmonary Circulation. Its Form and Function in Health and Disease. 3rd ed. Edinburgh: Churchill Livingstone, 1986.
8. Wolinsky H, Glagov S. Structural basis for the static mechanical properties of the aortic media. Circ Res 1963; 14:400–413.
9. Clark JM, Glagov S. 1985. Transmural organization of the arterial media. The lamellar unit revisited. Arteriosclerosis 1985; 5:19–34.
10. Meyrick B, Reid L. The effect of continued hypoxia on rat pulmonary arterial circulation. An ultrastructural study. Lab Invest 1978; 38:188–200.
11. Frid MG, Moiseeva EP, Stenmark KR. Multiple phenotypically distinct smooth muscle cell populations exist in the adult and developing bovine pulmonary arterial media in vivo. Circ Res 1994; 75:669–681.
12. Durmowicz AG, Frid MG, Wohrley JD, Stenmark KR. Expression and localization of tropoelastin mRNA in the developing bovine pulmonary artery is dependent on vascular cell phenotype. Am J Respir Cell Mol Biol 1996; 14:569–576.
13. Barnes PJ, Liu SF. Regulation of pulmonary vascular tone. Pharmacol Rev 1995; 47:87–131.
14. Klimaschewki K, Kummer W, Mayer B, Courad JY, Preissler U, Philippin B, Heym C. Nitric oxide synthase in cardiac nerve fibers and neurons of rat and guinea pig heart. Circ Res 1992; 71:1533–1537.
15. Liu SF, Crawlet DE, Rohde JAL, Evans TW, Barnes PJ. Role of nitrix oxide and guanosine 3′-, 5′-cyclic monophosphate in mediating nonadrenergic noncholinergic neural relaxation in guinea-pig pulmonary arteries. Br J Pharmacol 1992; 107:861–866.
16. Chand N, Altura BM. Acetylcholine and bradykinin relax intrapulmonary arteries by acting on endothelial cells: role in lung vascular diseases. Science 1981; 213:1376–1379.

17. Boe J, Simonsson BG. Effects of angiotensin II and bradykinin on isolated human pulmonary arteries. Eur J Respir Dis 1981; 61:95–101.
18. Goll HM, Nyhan DP, Geller HS, Murray PA. Pulmonary vascular responses to angiotensin II and captopril in conscious dogs. J Appl Physiol 1986; 61:1552–1559.
19. Michael JR, Markewitz BA. Endothelins and the lung. Am Rev Respir Crit Care Med 1996; 154:555–581.
20. Barnard JW, Ward RA, Adkins WK, Taylor AE. Characterization of thromboxane and prostacyclin effects on pulmonary vascular resistance. J Appl Physiol 1992; 72:1845–53.
21. Dresdale DT, Schultz M, Michtom RH. Primary pulmonary hypertension: I. Clinical and hemodynamic study. Am J Med 1951; 11:686–705.
22. Wood P. Pulmonary hypertension with special reference to the vasoconstrictive factor. Br Heart J 1959; 21:557–570.
23. Reid L. Vascular remodeling. In: Fishman AP, ed. The Pulmonary Circulation: Normal and Abnormal. Philadelphia: University of Pennsylvania Press, 1990: 259–282.
24. Reeves JT, Groves BM, Turkevich D. The case for treatment of selected patients with primary pulmonary hypertension. Am Rev Respir Dis 1986; 134:342–346.
25. Rich S, Brundage BH. High-dose calcium channel blocking therapy for primary pulmonary hypertension: evidence for long-term reduction in pulmonary arterial pressure and regression of right ventricular hypertrophy. Circulation 1987; 76:135–141.
26. Dantzker D, D'Alonzo GE, Gianotti L, Fuentes F, Nickeson D, Emerson M. Vasodilators and primary pulmonary hypertension. Chest 1989; 95:1185–1189.
27. Palevsky HI, Schloo BL, Pietra GG, Weber KT, Janicki JS, Rubin E, Fishman AP. Primary pulmonary hypertension: vascular structure, morphometry, and responsiveness to vasodilator agents. Circulation 1989; 80:1207–1221.
28. Rich S, Brundage BH, Levy PS. The effect of vasodilator therapy on the clinical outcome of patients with primary pulmonary hypertension. Circulation 1985; 71:1191–1196.
29. Weir EK, Rubin LJ, Ayres SM, Bergofsky EH, Brundage BH, Detre KM, Elliott CG, Fishman AP, Goldring RM, Groves BM, Kernis JT, Koerner SK, Levy PS, Pietra GG, Reid LM, Rich S, Vreim CE, Williams GW, Wu M. The acute administration of vasodilators in primary pulmonary hypertension. Am Rev Respir Dis 1989; 140:1623–1630.
30. Weir EK. Acute vasodilator testing and pharmacological teatment of primary pulmonary hypertension. In: Fishman P, ed. The Pulmonary Circulation: Normal and Abnormal. Philadelphia: University of Pennsylvania Press, 1990:259–282.
31. Heath D, Edwards JE. The pathology of hypertensive pulmonary vascular disease. A description of six grades of structural changes in the pulmonary arteries with special reference to congeital cardiac septal defects. Circulation 1985; 18:533–547.
32. Wagenvoort CA, Wagenvoort N. Primary pulmonary hypertension: a pathologic study of the lung vessels in 156 clinically diagnosed cases. Circulation 1970; 42:1163–1184.
33. Bjornsson J, Edwards WD. Primary pulmonary hypertension: a histopathologic study of 80 cases. Mayo Clin Proc 1985; 60:16–25.

34. Pietra GG, Edwards WD, Kay JM, Rich S, Kernis J, Schloo B, Ayres SM, Bergofsky EH, Brundage BH, Detre KM, Fishman AP, Goldring RM, Groves BM, Levy PS, Reid LM, Vreim CE, Williams GW. Histopathology of primary pulmonary hypertension: a qualitative and quantitative study of pulmonary blood vessels from 58 patients in the National Heart, Lung and Blood Institute, primary pulmonary hypertension registry. Circulation 1989; 80:1198–1206.
35. Botney MD, Kaiser LR, Cooper JD, Mecham RP, Roby J, Parks WC. Extracellular matrix protein gene expression in atherosclerotic pulmonary arteries. Am J Pathol 1992; 140:357–364.
36. Botney MD, Liptay MJ, Kaiser LR, Cooper JD, Parks WC, Mecham RP. Active collagen synthesis by pulmonary arteries in human primary pulmonary hypertension. Am J Pathol 1993; 143:121–129.
37. Giaid A, Saleh D. Reduced expression of endothelial nitric oxide synthase in the lungs of patients with pulmonary hypertension. N Engl J Med 1995; 333:214–221.
38. Christman BW, McPherson CD, Newman JH, King GA, Bernard GR, Groves BM, Loyd JE. An imbalance bewteen the extraction of thromboxane and prostacyclin metabolites in pulmonary hypertension. N Engl J Med 1992; 327:70–75.
39. Giaid A, Yanagisawa M, Langleben D. Expression of endothelin-1 in the lungs of patients with pulmonary hypertension. N Engl J Med 1993; 328:1732–1739.
40. Schuster DP, Crouch EC, Parks WC, Johnson T, Botney MD. Angiotensin converting enzyme expression in primary pulmonary hypertension. Am J Respir Crit Care Med 1996; 154:1087–1091.
41. Botney MD, Bahadori L, Gold LI. Vascular remodeling in primary pulmonary hypertension: potential role for transforming growth factor-β. Am J Pathol 1994; 144:286–295.
42. Liptay MJ, Parks WC, Mecham RP, Roby J, Kaiser LR, Cooper JD, Botney MD. Neointimal macrophages co-localize with extracellular matrix gene expression in human atherosclerotic pulmonary arteries. J Clin Invest 1993; 91:588–594.
43. Bahadori L, Milder J, Gold LI, Botney MD. Active macrophage-associated TGF-β colocalizes with type I procollaen gene expression in atherosclerotic human hypertensive pulmonary arteries. Am J Pathol 1995; 146:1140–1149.
44. Ito H, Hirata, Adachi S, Tanaka M, Tsujino M, Koike A, Nogami A, Murumo F, Hiroe M. Endothelin-1 is an autocrine/paracrine factor in the mechanism of angiotension II-induced hypertrophy in cultured rat cardiomyocytes. J Clin Invest 1993; 92:398–403.
45. Wiemer G, Scholkens BA, Becker RHA, Busse R. Ramiprilat endhances endothelial autacoid formation by inhibiting breakdown of endothelium-derived bradykinin. Hypertension 1991; 18:558–563.
46. Wiemer G, Popp R, Scholkens BA, Gogelein H. Enhancement of cytosolic calcium, prostacyclin and nitric oxide by bradykinin and the ACE inhibitor ramiprilat in porcine brain capillary endothelial cells. Brain Res 1994; 638:261–266.
47. Cherry PD, Furchgott RF, Zawadzki JV, Jothianandan D. Role of endothial cells in relaxation of isolated arteries by bradykinin. Proc Natl Acad Sci USA 1982; 79:2106–2110.
48. Miura K, Yukimura T, Yamashita Y, Shimmen T, Okumura M, Yamanaka S,

Imanishi M, Yamamoto K. Renal and femoral vascular responses to endothelin-1 in dogs: role of prostaglandins. J Pharmacol Exp Ther 1991; 256:11–17.
49. Warner TD, Mitchell JA, de Nucci G, Vane JR. Endothelin-1 and endothelin-3 release EDRF from isolated perfused arterial vessels of the rat and rabbit. J Cardiovasc Pharm 1989; 13:S85–S88.
50. Hahn AW, Resink TJ, Bernhardt J, Ferracin F, Buhler FR. Stimulation of autocrine platelet–derived growth factor AA-homodimer and transforming growth factor beta in vascular smooth muscle cells. Biochem Biophys Res Commun 1991; 178:1451–1458.
51. Kawaguchi H, Sawa H, Yasuda H. Endothelin stimulates angiotensin I to angiotensin II conversion in cultured pulmonary artery endothelial cells. J Mol Cell Card 1990; 22:839–842.
52. Poiani GJ, Tozzi CA, Yohn SE, Pierce RA, Belsky SA, Berg RA, Yu SY, Deak SB, Riley DJ. Collagen and elastin metabolism in hypertensive pulmonary arteries of rats. Circ Res 1990; 66:968–978.
53. Stenmark KR, Fasules J, Hyde DM, Voelkel NF, Henson J, Tucker A, Wilson H, Reeves JT. Severe pulmonary hypertension and arterial adventitial changes in newborn calves at 4,300 m. Am J Physiol 1987; 62:821–830.
54. Prosser IW, Stenmark KR, Suthar M, Crouch EC, Mecham RP, Parks WC. Regional heterogeneity of elastin and collagen gene expression in intralobar arteries in response to hypoxic pulmonary hypertension as demonstrated by in situ hybridization. Am J Pathol 1989; 135:1073–1087.
55. Todorovich-Hunter L, Johnson DJ, Ranger P, Keeley FW, Rabinovitch M. Altered elastin and collagen synthesis associated with progressive pulmonary hypertension induced by monocrotaline: a biochemical and ultrastructural study. Lab Invest 1988; 58:184–195.
56. Perkett EA, Brigham KL, Meyrick B. COntinuous air embolization into sheep causes sustained pulmonary hypertension and increased pulmonary vasoreactivity. Am J Pathol 1988; 132:444–454.
57. Wohrley JD, Frid MG, Moiseeva EP, Orton EC, Belknap JK, Stenmark KR. Hypoxia selectively induces proliferation in a specific subpopulation of smooth muscle cells in the bovine neonatal pulmonary arterial media. J Clin Invest 1995; 96:273–281.
58. Durmowicz AG, Badesch DB, Parks WC, Mecham RP, Stenmark KR. Hypoxia-iduced inhibition of tropoelastin synthesis by neonatal calf pulmonary artery smooth muscle cells. Am J Respir Cell Mol Biol 1991; 5:464–469.
59. Rabinovitch M, Konstram MA, Gamble WJ, Papanicolau N, Aronovitz AJ, Treves S, Reid LM. Changes in pulmonary blood flow affect vascular response to chronic hypoxia in rats. Circ Res 1983; 54:432–441.
60. Leung DYM, Glagov S, Mathews MB. A new in vitro system for studying cell response to mechanical stimulation. Exp Cell Res 1977; 109:285–298.
61. Tozzi CA, Poiani GJ, Harangozo AM, Boyd CD, Riley DJ. Pressure-induced connective tissue synthesis in pulmonary artery segments is dependent on intact endothelium. J Clin Invest 1989; 84:1005–1012.
62. Perkett EA, Lyons RM, Moses AL, Brigham KL, Meyrick B. Transforming growth

factor-β activity in sheep lung lymph during the development of pulmonary hypertension. J Clin Invest 1990; 86:1459–1464.
63. Perkett EA, Badesch DB, Roessler MK, Stenmark KR, Meyrick B. Insulin-like growth factor I and pulmonary hypertension induced by continuous air embolization in sheep. Am J Respir Cell Mol Biol 1992; 6:82–87.
64. Foster J, Rich CB, Florini JR. Insulin-like growth fator I, somatomedin C, induces the synthesis of tropoelastin in aortic tissue. Collagen Rel Res 1987; 7:161–169.
65. Foster JA, Miller ML, Benedict MR, Richman RA, Rich CB. Evidence for insulin-like growth factor-I regulation of chick aortic elastogenesis. Matrix 1989; 9:328–335.
66. Badesch D, Lee PD, Parks WC, Stenmark KR. Insulin-like growth factor I stimulates elastin sythesis by bovine pulmonary arterial smooth muscle cells. Biochem Biophys Res Commun 1989; 160:382–387.
67. Bar RS, Dake BL, Stueck S. Stimulation of proteoglycans by IGF I and II in mirovessel and large vessel endothelial cells. Am J Physiol 1987; 253:E21–27.
68. Hansson H-A, Jennische E, Skottner A. Regenerating endothelial cells express insulin-like growth factor-I immunoreactivity after arterial injury. Cell Tissue Res 1987; 250:499–505.
69. Cercek B, Fishbein MC, Forrester JS, Helfant RH, Fagin JA. Induction of insulin-like growth factor-I messenger RNA in rat aorta after balloon denudation. Circ Res 1990; 66:1755–1760.
70. Hayashi Y, Lalich JJ. Prodution of cor pulmonale in rats by single injection of monocrotaline. Am J Pathol 1967; 48:35.
71. Hayashi Y, Hussa JF, Lalich JJ. Cor pulmonale in rats. Lab Invest 1967; 16:875–881.
72. Stenmark KR, Morganroth ML, Remigio LK, Voelkel NF, Murphy RC, Henson PM, Mathias MM, Reeves JT. Alevolar inflammation and arachidonate metabolism in monocrotaline-induced pulmonary hypertension. Am J Physiol 1985; 248:H859–H866.
73. Wilson DW, Segall HJ, Pan LCW, Dunston SK. Progressive inflammatory and structural changes in the pulmonary vasculature of monocrotaline-treated rats. Microvasc Res 1989; 38:57–80.
74. Kameji K, Otsuka H, Hayashi Y. Increase of collagen synthesis in pulmonary arteries of monocrotaline-treated rats. Experientia 1980; 36:441–442.
75. Tanaka Y, Bernstein ML, Mecham RP, Patterson GA, Cooper JD, Botney MD. Site-specific responses to monocrotaline-induced vascular injury: evidence for two distinct mechanisms of remodeling. Am J Respir Cell Mol Biol 1996; 15:390–397.
76. Ignotz RA, Endo T, Massague J. Regulation of fibronectin and type I collagen mRNA levels by transforming growth factor-β. J Biol Chem 1987; 262:6443–6446.
77. Ignotz RA, Massague J. Transforming growth factor-β stimulates the expression of fibronectin and collagen and their incorporation into the extracellular matrix. J Biol Chem 1986; 26:4337–4345.
78. Penttinen RP, Kobayashi S, Bornstein P. Transforming growth factor β increases mRNA for matrix proteins both in the presence and in the absence of changes in mRNA stability. Proc Natl Acad Sci USA 1988; 85:1105–1108.

79. Fine A, Goldstein RH. The effect of transforming growth factor-β on cell proliferation and collagen formation by lung fibroblasts. J Biol Chem 1987; 262:3897–3902.
80. Liu JM, Davidson JM. The elastogenic effect of recombinant transforming growth factor-beta on porcine aortic smooth muscle cells. Biochem Biophys Res Commun 1988; 154:895–901.
81. McGowan SE, McNamer R. Transforming growth factor-β increases elastin production by neonatal rat lung fibroblasts. Am J Respir Cell Mol Biol 1990; 3:369–376.
82. Bell L, Madri JA. Effect of platelet factors on migration of cultured bovine aortic endothelial and smooth muscle cells. Circ Res 1989; 65:1057–1065.
83. Majack RA, Majesky MW, Goodman LV. Role of PDGF-A expression in the control of vascular smooth muscle cell growth by transforming growth factor-β. J Cell Biol 1990; 111:239–247.
84. Assoian RK, Sporn MB. Type-β transforming growth factor in human platelets: release during platelet degranulation and action on vascular smooth muscle cells. J Cell Biol 1986; 102:1217–1223.
85. Majesky MW, Lindner V, Twardzik DR, Schwartz SM, Reidy MA. Production of transforming growth factor β1 during repair of arterial injury. J Clin Invest 1991; 88:904–910.
86. Botney MD, Parks WC, Crouch EC, Stenmark K, Mecham PR. TGF-β1 is decreased in remodeling hypertensive bovine pulmonary arteries. J Clin Invest 1992; 89:1629–1635.
87. Katayos D. Increased expression of PDGF A- and B-chain genes in rat lungs with hypoxic pulmonary hypertension. Am J Physiol 1993; 264:L100–106.
88. Powell PP, Wang CC, Jones R. Differential regulation of the genes incoding platelet-derived growth factor receptor and its ligand in rat lung during microvascular and alveolar wall remodeling in hyperoxia. Am J Respir Cell Mol Biol 1992; 7:278–285.
89. Grotendorst GR, Seppa HEJ, Kleinman HK, Martin GR. Attachment of smooth muscle cells to collagen and their migration toward platelet-derived growth factor. Proc Natl Acad Sci USA 1981; 78:3669–3672.
90. Grotendorst GR, Chang T, Seppa HEJ, Kleinman HK, Martin GR. Platelet-derived growth factor is a chemoattractant for vascular smooth muscle cells. J Cell Physiol 1982; 113:261–266.
91. Ross R, Glomset J, Kariya B, Harker L. A platelet-dependent serum factor that stimulates the proliferation of arterial smoooth muscle cells in vitro. Proc Natl Acad Sci USA 1974; 71:1207–1210.
92. Blatti SP, Foster DN, Ranganathan G, Moses HL, Getz MJ. Induction of fibronectin gene transcription and mRNA is a primary response to growth-factor stimulation of AKR-2B cells. Proc Natl Acad Sci 1988; 85:1119–1123.
93. Majack RA, Cook SC, Bornstein P. Platelet-derived growth factor and heparin-like glycosaminoglycans regulate thrombospondin synthesis and deposition in the matrix by smooth muscle cells. J Cell Biol 1985; 101:1059–1070.

94. Schonherr E, Jarvelainen HT, Sandell LJ, Wight TN. Effects of platelet-derived growth factor and transforming frowth factor-β1 on the synthesis of a large versican-like chondroitin sulfate proteoglycan by arterial smooth muscle cells. J Biol Chem 1991; 266:17640–17647.
95. Sjolund M, Hedin U, Sejersen T, Heldin C-H, Thyberg J. Arterial smooth muscle cells express platelet-derived growth factor (PDGF) A chain mRNA, secrete a PDGF-like mitogen, and bind exogenous PDGF in a phenotype- and growth state-dependent manner. J Cell Biol 1988; 106:403–413.
96. Majesky MW, Benditt ED, Schwartz SM. Expression and developmental control of platelet-derived growth factor A-chain and B-chains/sis genes in rat aortic smooth muscle cells. Proc Natl Acad Sci USA 1988; 85:1524–1528.
97. Barrett TB, Gajdusek CM, Schwartz SM, McDougall JK, Benditt EP. Expression of the sis gene by endothelial cells in culture and in vivo. Proc Natl Acad Sci USA 1984; 81:6772–6774.
98. Albelda SM, Elias JA, Levine EM, Kern JA. Endotoxin stimulates platelet-derived growth factor production from cultured human pulmonary endothelial cells. Am J Physiol 1989; 257:L65–70.
99. Shimokado K, Raines EW, Madtes DK, Barrett TB, Benditt EP, Ross R. A significant part of macrophage-derived growth factor consists of at least two forms of PDGF. Cell 1985; 43:277–286.
100. Ross R, Masuda J, Raines EW, Gown AM, Katsuda S, Sasahara M, Malden LT, Masuko H, Sato H. Localization of PDGF-B protein in macrophages in all phases of atherogenesis. Science 1990; 248:1009–1012.
101. Walker LN, Bowen-Pope DF, Ross R, Reidy MA. Production of platelet-derived growth factor-like molecules by cultured arterial smooth muscle cells accompaies proliferation after arterial injury. Proc Natl Acad Sci USA 1986; 83:7311–7315.
102. Majesky MW, Reidy MA, Bowen-Pope DF, Hart CE, Wilcox JN, Schwartz SM. PDGF ligand and receptor gene expression during repair of arterial injury. J Cell Biol 1990; 111:2149–2158.
103. Barrett TB, Benditt EP. sis (Platelet-derived growth factor B chain) gene tanscript levels are elevated in human atherosclerotic lesions compared to normal artery. Proc Natl Acad Sci USA 1987; 84:1099–1103.
104. Barrett TB, Benditt EP. Platelet-derived growth factor gene expression in human atherosclerotic plaques and normal artery wall. Proc Natl Acad Sci USA 1988; 85:2810–2814.
105. Wilcox JN, Smith KM, Williams LT, Schwartz SM, Gordon D. Platelet-derived growth factor mRNA detection in human atherosclerotic plaques by in situ hybridization. J Clin Invest 1988; 82:1404–1408.
106. Tuder RM, Flook BE, Voelkel NF. Increased gene expression for VEGF and the VEGF receptors KDR/Flk and Flt in lungs exposed to acute or to chronic hypoxia. Modulation of gene expression by nitric oxide. J Clin Invest 1995; 95:1798–1807.
107. Ferrara N, Houck K, Jakeman LL. Molecular and biological properties of the vascular endothelial growth factor family of proteins. Endocrinol Rev 1992; 13:18–32.
108. Morrell NW, Atochina EN, Morris KG, Danilov SM, Stenmark KR. Angiotensin

converting enzyme expression is increased in small pulmonary arteries of rats with hypoxia-induced pulmonary hypertension. J Clin Invest 1995; 96:1823–1833.
109. Molteni A, Ward WF, Ts'ao C, Solliday NH. Monocrotaline-induced pulmonary fibrosis in rats: amelioration by Captopril and penicillamine. Proc Soc Exp Biol Med 1985; 180:112–120.
110. Molteni A, Ward WF, Ts'ao CH, Solliday NH. Monocrotaline-induced cardiopulmonary damage in rats: amelioration by the angiotensin-converting enzyme inhibitor CL242817. Proc Soc Exp Biol Med 1986; 182:483–493.
111. Morrell NW, Morris KG, Stenmark KR. Role of angiotensin-converting enzyme and angiotensin II in development of hypoxic pulmonary hypertension. Am J Physiol 1995; 269:H1186–H1194.
112. Nong Z, Stassen JM, Moons L, Collen D, Janssens S. Inhibition of tissue angiotensin-converting enzyme with Quinapril reduces hypoxic pulmonary hypertension and pulmonary vascular remodeling. Circulation 1996; 94:1941–1947.
113. Heath D, Wood E, Dushane J, Edwards JE. The structure of the pulmonary trunk at different ages and in cases of pulmonary hypertension and pulmonary stenosis. J Pathol Bacteriol 1959; 77:443.
114. Heath D, Wood EH, DuShane JW, Edwards JE. The relatoin of age and blood pressure to atheroma in the pulmonary arteries and thoracic aorta in congential heart disease. Lab Invest 1960; 9:259–272.
115. Glagov S, Ozoa AK. Significance of the relatively low incidence of atherosclerosis in the pulmonary, renal, and mesenteric arteries. Ann NY Acad Sci 1968; 149:940–955.
116. Wissler RW, Vesselinovitch D. Atherogenesis in the pulmonary artery. In: Fishman AP, ed. The Pulmonary Circulation: Normal and Abnormal. Philadelphia: University of Pennsylvania Press 1990:245–255.
117. Tanaka Y, Schuster DP, Davis EC, Patterson GA, Botney MD. The role of vascular injury and hemodynamics in pulmonary artery remodeling. J Clin Invest 1996; 98:434–442.
118. Kolpakov V, Rekhter MD, Gordon D, Wang WH, Kulik TJ. Effect of mechanical forces on growth and matrix protein synthesis in the in vitro pulmonary artery. Circ Res 1995; 77:823–831.
119. Ku DN, Zhu C. The mechanical environmental of the artery. In: Sumpio B, ed. Hemodynamic Forces and Vascular Cell Biology. Austin: R.G. Landes, 1993:1–23.
120. Davies PF. Flow-mediated endothelial mechanotransduction. Physiol Rev 1995; 75:519–560.
121. Crissman RS. SEM observations of the elastic networks in canine femoral artery. Am J Anat 1986; 175:481–492.
122. Piene H. Pulmonary arterial impedance and right ventricular function. Physiol Rev 1986; 66:606–652.
123. Laskey WK, Ferrari VA, Palevsky HI, Kussmaul WG. Pulmonary artery hemodynamics in primary pulmonary hypertension. J Am Coll Card 1993; 21:406–412.

124. Fourie PR, Coetzee AR, Bolliger CT. Pulmonary artery compliance: its role in right ventricular-arterial coupling. Cardiovasc Res 1992; 26:839–844.
125. Ha B, Lucas L, Henry GW, Frantz EG, Ferreiro JI, Wilcox BR. Effects of chronically elevated pulmonary arterial pressure and flow on right ventricular afterload. Am J Physiol 1994;

17

Effects of Nitric Oxide and Cyclic GMP on Smooth Muscle Proliferation

RAED A. DWEIK and SERPIL C. ERZURUM

The Cleveland Clinic Foundation
Cleveland, Ohio

I. Introduction

Since the finding that endothelium-derived relaxing factor (EDRF) is nitric oxide (NO) (1,2), NO has been found to be a multifunctional molecule that mediates a number of physiological processes in almost all vertebrate organ systems, including such diverse functions as smooth muscle relaxation, platelet inhibition, central and autonomic neurotransmission, tumor cell lysis, bacterial killing, and stimulation of hormonal release (3–5). While the number of newly discovered potential targets of NO is continually expanding, the majority of NO effects under physiologic conditions still appear to be mediated primarily by the activation of the intracellular NO receptor guanylyl cyclase and consequently increasing the level of guanosine 3′,5′-cyclic monophosphate [cyclic GMP (cGMP)] (4,6). Cyclic GMP plays a central role as a second messenger in regulation of smooth muscle cells, platelet function, and ion transport (7). In this chapter we will focus on the current knowledge of NO and cGMP-mediated signaling as it pertains to smooth muscle and their potential role in the pathogenesis of lymphangioleiomyomatosis (LAM).

II. Nitric Oxide Synthase Enzymes

Nitric oxide is a diffusible gas that is produced by a group of enzymes known collectively as nitric oxide synthases (NOS; EC 1.14.13.39). These enzymes convert the amino acid L-arginine to NO and L-citrulline in the presence of oxygen and NADPH as cosubstrates, a reaction that requires several cofactors including FAD, FMN, tetrahydrobiopterin and calmodulin (Fig. 1) (8). NOS enzymes share homology with cytochrome P450 reductase (8). NO is relatively unstable and is rapidly oxidized in solution to the stable metabolic end products nitrite (NO_2^-) and nitrate (NO_3^-), which can be used as indirect indicators to monitor NO formation (8). Three isoforms of NOS, which are the products of individual genes (8,9), have been identified, including two constitutive forms [neuronal (nNOS or NOS I) and endothelial (eNOS or NOS III)] and an inducible form (iNOS or NOS II) (Table 1) (3,5,8). In general, NOS I and III are continuously expressed in neuronal and endothelial cells, respectively, and are dependent on increases in

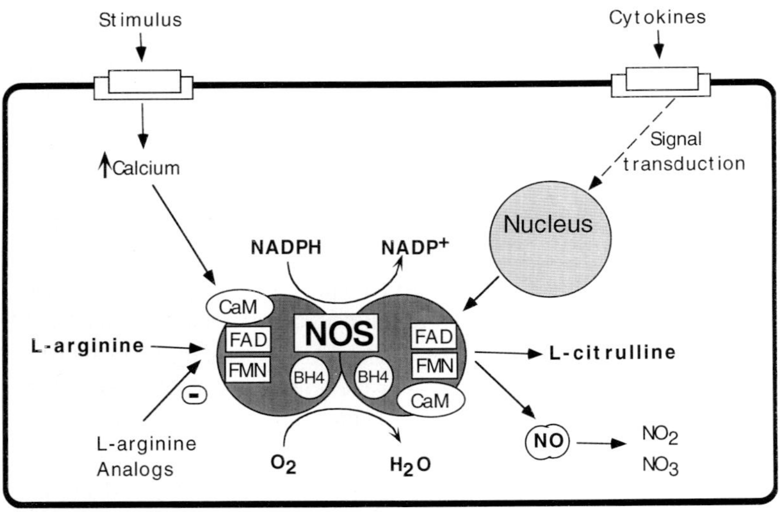

Figure 1 The formation of nitric oxide (NO) by nitric oxide synthase (NOS). NOS converts L-arginine to citrulline and NO in the presence of NADPH and molecular oxygen as cosubstrates. The reaction also requires the presence of flavoproteins (FAD, FMN) and tetrahydrobiopterin (BH_4) as cofactors. The nitrogen in NO is provided by L-arginine, while the oxygen is from molecular oxygen. NO is an unstable diffusible gas and is rapidly (3–5 sec) oxidized in solution to nitrate (NO_3^-) and nitrite (NO_2^-). The constitutive forms of NOS (types I and III) are activated by calcium influx into the cell, while the inducible form of NOS (type II) is activated by cytokines through signal transduction and gene induction. All NOS can be competitively inhibited by arginine analogs (see text).

Table 1 Nitric Oxide Synthase Enzymes

NOS isoforms	Type	Regulation	Size (kDa)	Chromosomal location (human)
Constitutive				
bNOS	I	Calcium/Calmodulin	155	12q24.2
eNOS	III	Calcium/Calmodulin	135	7q35-36
Inducible				
iNOS	II	Induced by cytokines, endotoxin, and oxidants	125	17cen-q12

intracellular calcium to bind calmodulin, which results in enzyme activation leading to picomolar levels of NO production (Fig. 1) (8). NOS I is also found at relatively abundant levels in skeletal muscle (10). NOS II is regulated at the level of transcription and mRNA stability and is expressed after exposure of cells to specific cytokines and endotoxin (4,5,7,8). NOS II is calcium independent, avidly binding calmodulin even at low calcium concentrations intracellularly, and produces nanomolar levels of NO (8). NOS II has been described in epithelial, endothelial, and smooth muscle cells, and in macrophages, fibroblasts, and neutrophils. Regulation of expression of NOS II varies in different cell types, but typically is increased by cytokines such as TNF-α, interferon-γ (IFN-γ), and interleukin-1β (IL-1β). NOS II expression is decreased by glucocorticoids, transforming growth factor beta (TGF-β), platelet-derived growth factor, epidermal growth factor, insulin-like growth factor 1, and thrombin (5,11–13). Regulation of NOS III at the level of transcription is less well studied, but the gene is induced by oxygen tension, shear stress, and IFN-γ (11,12,14,15). Both NOS I and III mRNA are increased by estrogens (see below). NOS III, unlike I and II, is membrane associated due to myristoylation of its amino-terminal end (9).

A. NOS and NO Production by Smooth Muscle

Smooth muscle cells are able to produce NO (16). When stimulated by the appropriate cytokines, vascular smooth muscle cells can express NOS II (17–19). Furthermore, NOS II has been cloned from IFN-γ-stimulated vascular smooth muscle cells and is similar to NOS II cloned from other cells, suggesting that it is highly conserved (20). NOS II is also induced in vascular smooth muscle cells during endotoxemia and inflammation and by flow shear stress (21). In rat pulmonary artery smooth muscle cells, NOS II mRNA expression is undetectable under basal conditions, but it can be induced by endotoxin and cytokines (IL-1β, IFN-γ, and TNF-α) (19). Upon stimulation of these cells, NOS II mRNA becomes detectable at 4 hours and continues to increase at 24 hours (19,22), a response similar to that seen in hepatocytes from rat and human (22). The half-life of NOS II mRNA in vascular smooth muscle cells can be prolonged by cycloheximide, implying that NOS II activity in these cells can also be regulated at the posttranscriptional level (23). Vascular smooth muscle cells have the ability to regenerate the essential substrate L-arginine for NOS by the synthesis of argininosuccinate from citrulline and aspartate, a two-step reaction catalyzed by argininosuccinate synthase (co-induced in these cells when NOS II is induced) and argininosuccinate lyase, which is constitutively expressed in vascular smooth muscle cells (24). Although a transcriptionally regulated "arginine-citrulline cycle" has been suggested in vascular smooth muscle cells (24), other work has shown that NO synthesis by NOS II in vascular smooth muscle is dependent on the presence of extracellular L-arginine (17). NO production by NOS II in smooth muscle cells is also dependent on the de novo biosynthesis of tetrahydrobiopterin, an essential cofactor for NOS (22,25). Cytokine induction of NOS II expression in vascular smooth muscle cells can be inhibited by corticosteroids (26) and retinoids (27).

The role of NO produced by vascular smooth muscle cells is currently under investigation. It is possible that the endogenous production of NO caused by NOS II in injured vascular smooth muscle cells contributes to prevention of vasospasm and inhibition of smooth muscle proliferation (28). In addition, induction of NOS II in vascular smooth muscle cells may have an autocrine function. Once NOS II is activated in vascular smooth muscle cells, it may regulate energy metabolism in these cells (switching to anaerobic glycolysis) (29), inhibit proliferation (30,31), and even induce cell death (32,33). NO produced by vascular smooth muscle cells may also lead to toxic effects on adjacent endothelial cells (34) or stimulate their proliferation (33) and can induce apoptotic death in leukemic cell lines (35). These effects of NO produced by NOS II in vascular smoooth muscle cells have been postulated to be contributing factors in acute lung injury (34), neovascularization in atherosclerotic plaques (33), restoration of smooth muscle growth quiescence after endothelial injury (31), host defense against cancer (35), and the pathogenesis of inflammatory disease (30).

B. NOS Inhibitors and NO Generators

Studies utilizing NOS inhibitors and/or NO generators have contributed to our understanding of the various functions of NO. Analogs of L-arginine that act as false substrates for NOS can be used as inhibitors of endogenous NO synthesis. Several inhibitors are available, including *N*-monomethyl-L-arginine (L-NMMA), *N*-nitro-L-arginine, *N*-iminoethyl-L-ornithine, L-*N*-nitroarginine-*p*-nitroanilide, and *N*-nitro-L-arginine methyl ester (L-NAME), which can inhibit both the constitutive and the inducible forms of NOS (8). L-Aminoguanidine is reported to be a more selective inhibitor (10- to 100-fold more selective) of NOS II compared to NOS I or III (3,18). Several compounds can also release NO (NO generators) and include: diethylamine NONOate, S-nitrosogluthathione, spermine NONOate, sodium nitroprusside, glyceryl trinitrite, molsidomine (3-morpholino-sydnonimimine), isosorbide dinitrite, and S-nitroso-*N*-acetylpenicillamine.

III. NO as a Signal Molecule

NO is highly diffusible and may act within the cell in which it is generated or in adjacent cells. Thus, NO can function as an intra- or intercellular messenger that participates in signal transduction (5,7,36). The diffusion of NO may be most limited by its many possible chemical reactions. NO combines readily with superoxide anion (O_2^-) to form peroxynitrite ($ONOO^-$), a potent oxidant that may mediate free radical induced injury (3,4,8,11). NO can also exert biological effects through several biochemical interactions. Major interactions of NO are through its binding to iron centers in hemoglobin, other heme proteins, iron-sulfur centers, or to the thiol groups of proteins (3,6,11). For example, NO may lead to the S-nitrosylation of thiol groups, thus resulting in modulation of protein and receptor function (37). For the most part, interactions of NO with enzymes leads to inactivation of the enzyme, with the notable exception of guanylyl cyclase, which is stimulated by NO (4,7). The reaction of NO with reduced thiol yields S-nitrosothiols, which are more stable than NO itself and may act by slow, prolonged release of NO (3,18,38). Thus, some effects of NO may be mediated via low molecular weight S-nitrosothiol intermediates (3,18,38). In this context, NO is known to react with a sulfhydryl group on albumin to form S-nitrosoalbumin (38). Whether nitrosoalbumin acts as a significant reservoir of NO in vivo to prolong its bioactivity as a circulating hormone or EDRF is unclear (3,18,38). In addition, NO has a direct activating effect on cyclooxygenase (39) but an inhibitory effect on various enzyme activities involved in growth regulation including ribonucleotide reductase (40), thymidine kinase (41), and the mitochondrial enzyme aconitase (42). NO can deaminate purine and pyrimidine bases in DNA, resulting in increased mutagenesis and in DNA strand breaks, which may possibly induce cell apoptosis (32,43). These diverse mechanisms may explain the multiple actions of NO that span alsmost all organ systems.

IV. NO and cGMP

While the number of newly discovered potential targets of NO is continually expanding, the majority of NO effects under physiologic conditions still appear to be mediated primarily by the activation of the intracellular NO receptor guanylyl cyclase and consequently increasing the level of the cyclic nucleotide cGMP (4,6,7).

Two major families of guanylyl cyclase are known: the particulate-associated enzymes, which are transmembrane receptors that contain guanylyl cyclase in their intracellular domains, and the soluble type, which is activated by nitric oxide (6). Soluble guanylyl cyclase is an $\alpha\beta$ heterodimer, and each subunit contains catalytic and heme-binding domains (7). The enzyme has a basal cyclase activity, which is stimulated up to 200-fold by NO (44). NO appears to exert its effect by binding to the heme iron of soluble guanylate cyclase (7,26,45). Activation of guanylyl cyclase leads to an increase in intracellular cGMP concentration, which then mediates physiologic responses in the cell through its effects on cGMP gated ion channels, cGMP-regulated phosphodiesterases, or cGMP-dependent protein kinases (7). Activation of specific cyclic nucleotide target proteins is believed to underlie the differential effects of cGMP in cells (46). cGMP-dependent kinases or G-kinases (GK) may be either soluble or membrane bound. GKI is found in smooth muscle cells and is comprised of an α and a β subunit, which are produced through alternative splicing of a single gene (7,46,47). In addition, there is evidence suggesting that cGMP may also activate cAMP-dependent kinases (A-kinases) (7,48). cGMP also regulates cation channels, probably through phosphorylation of channels mediated by cGMP sensitive kinases (7,46,49). Furthermore, cGMP is able to regulate certain classes of cyclic nucleotide phosphodiesterases. Phosphodiesterases have been classified into six general families based upon primary protein and cDNA sequences (7). The phosphodiesterases also exert part of the cellular control over the levels and duration of action of cAMP and cGMP and are differentially regulated. Phosphodiesterases in families II, III, V, and VI are regulated by cGMP (7). For example, in the case of family II, cGMP stimulates cAMP hydrolysis by the phosphodiesterases, while in family III, the cAMP hydrolyzing cGI-PDE is inhibited by cGMP (7) (Fig. 2).

V. Effect of NO on Smooth Muscle

NO inhibits smooth muscle tone and smooth muscle cell proliferation and migration (50,51) (Fig. 2). Although there is mounting evidence in the literature for NO as an inhibitor of smooth muscle proliferation, there is some evidence suggesting that NO may have a biphasic effect, with stimulation of smooth muscle proliferation at lower (picomolar) levels and inhibition at higher levels (52).

A. NO-Induced Smooth Muscle Relaxation

NO causes relaxation of smooth muscles via the activation of cGMP (50,52–55). The mechanism by which the rise in cGMP results in smooth muscle relaxation is not clear. Many possibilities have been suggested including the inhibition of

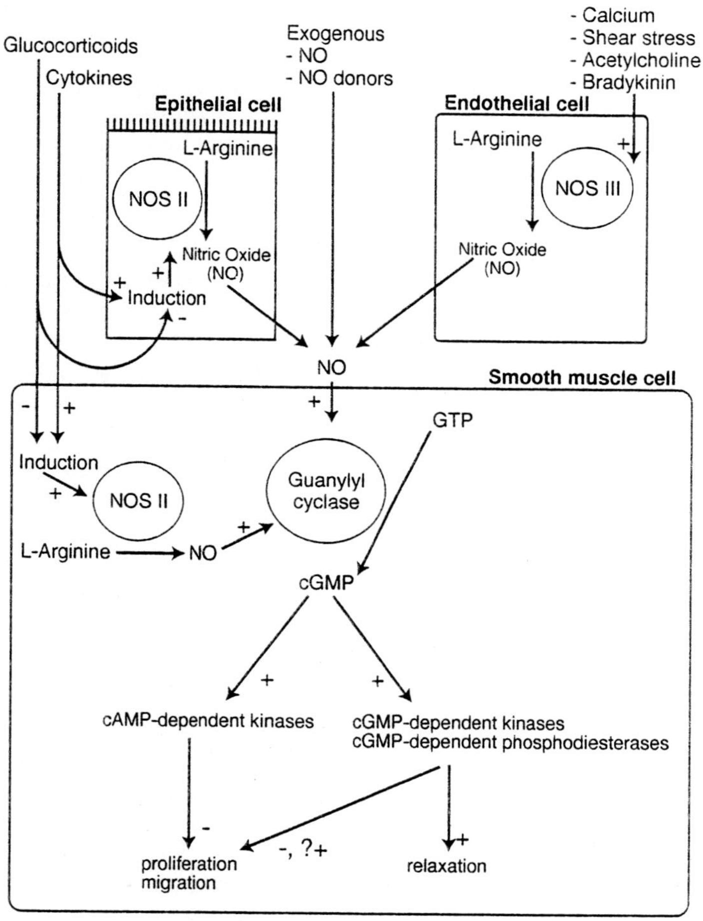

Figure 2 Nitric oxide induction of guanylyl cyclase and cGMP in smooth muscle leading to relaxation and inhibition of migration and proliferation. In normal blood vessels, NO is primarily produced by endothelial NOS (NOS III), which is constitutively expressed in these cells. The activation of endothelial cells by hormones, neurotransmitters, physical, and chemical stimuli triggers the production of NO, through the increase in intracellular concentration of calcium. The most important physiologic stimulus for release of NO is the increase in shear stress that can be produced by elevated flow velocity or viscosity of blood. NO then diffuses toward the lumen (not shown) and toward the underlying smooth muscle. In the smooth muscle, NO activates guanylyl cyclase, leading to an increase in intracellular cGMP concentration, which then inhibits smooth muscle tone and prevents proliferation of smooth muscle cells through its effects on cGMP-regulated phosphodiesterases, cGMP-dependent protein kinases, or cAMP-dependent kinases. Other endogenous sources of NO include smooth muscle cells, which when induced by cytokines or injury express NOS II. In the lung, epithelial cells also produce NO, which can affect vascular and airway smooth muscle cells. NO can also be administered exogenously as inhaled NO gas, or in the form of an NO generator, and can exert similar effects to endogenous NO.

inositol triphosphate, inhibition of a cAMP phosphodiesterase, dephosphorylation of the light chain of myosin, activation of protein kinases, stimulation of membrane Ca-ATPase, phosphorylation and opening of K-channels, increased sequestration of cytosolic calcium, and inhibition of calcium influx (46,47,49). Whatever the final mechanisms, NO has potent relaxant effects on vascular smooth muscle tone. Endogenous NO is especially important in the decrease in pulmonary artery resistance and increase in pulmonary blood flow at the time of birth and in maintaining the dilation of the pulmonary vascular bed in vivo (49,52,56). In this context, intravenous infusion of NOS inhibitor (L-NAME) in an intact-chest cat increased baseline pulmonary lobar arterial pressure, decreased responsiveness to endothelial dependent dilators, and increased the response to NO and NO generators (56). Similar effects were found in intact fetal pulmonary arteries in sheep (36). In human studies, exogenous NO administered as a gas is beneficial in pulmonary hypertension of the newborn of different etiologies (36,57–59).

In addition to its effects on vascular smooth muscle, NO also leads to relaxation of bronchial smooth muscle. Exogenous NO inhaled by mouth at 15 ppm decreased pulmonary airway resistance, which was additive to terbutaline in methacholine-pretreated pigs (3,60). S-nitrosothiols (NO generators) increased the levels of cGMP concentration and relaxed airway smooth muscle from guinea pig and human airways constricted with methacholine, histamine, or leukotriene D4 in vitro, while L-NAME markedly enhanced bronchoconstrictor effects of histamine in guinea pigs (3). These studies suggest a potential role for endogenous NO in modulating basal airway tone, in addition to pulmonary vascular tone (3).

B. Effects of NO on Cell Proliferation and Migration

NO inhibits vascular smooth muscle cell proliferation (62), DNA synthesis (50,55), and collagen production (63). NO also inhibits vascular smooth muscle cell migration independent of effects on proliferation (54). Similar to the effects on smooth muscle tone, the mechanisms of NO effects on vascular smooth muscle cell proliferation and migration are predominantly mediated through the activation of cGMP (50,54,55,62,63). For example, NO inhibition of DNA synthesis in vascular smooth muscle is associated with a concomitant rise in cGMP levels and can be reproduced by a cGMP analog (8-bromo-cGMP) (50,55). Further, NOS-mediated antiproliferative effects of IFN-γ on vascular smooth muscle cells are closely related to cGMP formation (62). However, experiments with smooth muscle cells demonstrate that higher levels of NO are required for inhibition of proliferation than are required to produce vasodilatation, suggesting that cGMP-dependent activation of the cAMP kinase may be responsible for the NO-dependent inhibition of proliferation in these cells (64). In support of this, complete relaxation of aortic strips/rings by NO generators occurs at low concentrations, which have no effect on smooth muscle cell proliferation, even though cGMP levels are elevated 10-fold (64). In contrast, concentrations of NO-generating compounds that inhibit proliferation also activate cGMP kinase, apparently through augmented cGMP elevation (64). Thus, although elevation of cGMP is as effective as or more effective than cAMP in relaxing smooth muscle from a variety of sources (21,65), higher levels of cGMP are necessary to inhibit proliferation (21).

NO generators can also inhibit proliferation in cells that lack soluble guanylate cyclase, suggesting that NO can inhibit smooth muscle cell proliferation through cGMP-independent mechanisms (21,66). In this context, endogeneous or exogeneous NO is able to upregulate Fas, a type 1 membrane protein belonging to the TNF receptor family, which mediates death signal in rat aorta smooth muscle cells and induces apoptosis (32). This effect is inhibited by L-NMMA (a NOS inhibitor) but is not affected by methylene blue (a cGMP inhibitor) and not reproduced by 8-Br-cGMP (a cGMP analog), suggesting that this effect of NO is independent of cGMP activation (32). Although the mechanism of NO-induced apoptosis remains unknown, there are reports implicating NO in deaminating purine and pyrimidine bases in DNA resulting in increased mutagenesis and DNA strand breaks (32,43). There is also evidence to suggest that NO may achieve its inhibitory effect on cell growth by exerting a feedback control on calcium responses to growth factors (67).

Inhibition of cell proliferation by NO has been demonstrated in other cell types including lymphocytes (68), cerebellar glial cells (69), endothelial cells (51), mesangial cells (70), chondrocytes (71), and bone marrow cells (72). NO also exerts antiproliferative effects on several tumor cell lines, an effect enhanced by glutathione (GSH) depletion in these cells, suggesting a possible protective effect for intracellular GSH against the antiproliferative effects of NO (73). On the other hand, exogeneous NO enhanced proliferation of endothelial cells cultured from bovine coronary postcapillary venules (74), and NO produced by NOS II in vascular smooth muscle cells had a stimulatory effect on adjacent endothelial cell proliferation and migration (33).

Thus, while most of the current evidence supports the notion that NO inihibits cell proliferation, there are reports that suggest that NO may stimulate cell proliferation. For example, NO has a biphasic effect on DNA synthesis in rat fetal pulmonary artery smooth muscle cells, with stimulation at micromolar concentrations and inhibition at higher levels (52). In addition, Hecker et al. demonstrated that in a model of carotid artery injury under conditions in which smooth muscle cell injury predominates, NO did not act as an antiproliferative agent (75). Finally, the effect of NO on cell proliferation is also dependent upon the passage number of cells in vitro, with potentiation of mitogenic effects by NO in primary and early subcultures of rat aortic smooth muscle cells and inhibition of DNA synthesis and cell proliferation by NO in more advanced subcultures (76).

VI. NO in the Lung

NO is produced endogenously in the human lung, evidenced by NO detectable in the exhaled air of humans (6–8 ppb) and NO as nitrosothiol and NO_2^- detectable in the airway aspirate and bronchoalveolar lavage fluid from human lungs (3). NO is recognized to play key roles in virtually all aspects of lung biology and has been implicated in the pathophysiology of lung and airway diseases (3). NO in the lung is involved in pulmonary neurotransmission (77), host defense and bacteriostasis, airway and vascular smooth muscle relaxation (i.e., V/Q matching), pulmonary capillary leak, inflammation, mucociliary clearance, airway mucus secretion, and cytotoxicity (3).

There is evidence that NO may be formed in high concentrations in the upper respiratory tract (nasopharynx and paranasal sinuses), but several studies have conclusively demonstrated that NO is also produced in the lower respiratory tract (78–80). Cellular sources of NO in the lung include epithelial cells, endothelial cells of pulmonary arteries and veins, inhibitory nonadrenergic noncholinergic neurons, smooth muscle cells, mast cells, mesothelial cells, fibroblasts, neutrophils, lymphocytes, and macrophages (3,11). Immunohistochemical studies have identified the presence of NOS I, II, and III in the human lung (3,77,81). Specifically, NOS I is located in inhibitory nonadrenergic noncholinergic neurons in the lung, while NOS III is found in endothelial cells and the brush border of ciliated epithelial cells (3,77,81). NOS II is found in the epithelial cells of the airway. Although NOS II may be induced in several types of cells in response to cytokines, endotoxin, or oxidants, NOS II is continuously expressed in normal human airway epithelium at basal airway conditions (82).

VII. NO in LAM

Alterations in NO levels have been found in pulmonary diseases such as asthma, pulmonary hypertension, immune complex–mediated lung injury, and the adult respiratory distress syndrome (3). Exhaled NO is increased in inflammatory airway diseases, such as asthma and upper respiratory tract infections/bronchiectasis, and likely reflects an increase in NOS II activity in epithelial cells of these patients (3,77). Exhaled NO levels are lower than normal in smoking individuals and the reduction is proportionate to the number of cigarettes currently smoked. Cigarette smoke contains high levels of NO (77), which may dysregulate NOS activity and contribute to the lung injury caused by smoking (83). There is also evidence that patients with primary pulmonary hypertension (PPH) have lower levels of expression of NOS III in pulmonary vascular endothelial cells and lower levels of exhaled NO (84,85).

No studies have directly addressed the role of NO or cGMP in smooth muscle proliferation in LAM. Most studies exploring a pathologic relationship between NO and smooth muscle have been in the context of vascular injury and atherosclerosis. However, since smooth muscle proliferation is the hallmark of LAM (86,87), data regarding smooth muscle proliferation in vascular injury or atherosclerosis can be used to gain insight into the potential role of NO in smooth muscle proliferation in general and LAM in particular. In this context, endogenous NO plays a role in limiting neointimal hyperplasia, while inhibitors of NOS have been shown to increase neointimal hyperplasia after balloon injury in animal models (88,89). NO generators inhibit smooth muscle cell proliferation following carotid angioplasty in pigs (88) and rats (89). L-Arginine (NO precursor) protects against atheroma formation in hypercholesterolemic rabbits and inhibits intimal hyperplasia following experimental aortic balloon injury, an effect that is blocked by L-NAME (NOS inhibitor) (88). Thus, NO inhibits smooth muscle cell proliferation under conditions of injury and inflammation.

LAM is a disease of women of childbearing age, and thus hormones (particularly estrogen) have been implicated in the pathogenesis of the disease (90). In support of this possibility, hormonal manipulation has been used with some success as treatment for LAM (91). Interestingly, NOS and NO production are affected by estrogen levels as shown by studies of women at different times during the menstrual cycle or during pregnancy. For example, exhaled NO levels are highest in women during the midcycle phase of the menstrual cycle corresponding to the midcycle peak of estrogen (92). Further, NOS I and III, traditionally considered "constitutive" NOSs, are induced in several tissues during pregnancy and in nonpregnant female and male animals by exogenous estradiol but not progesterone administration (93). Pregnancy or estradiol administration increased the activities of the calcium-dependent NOSs (I and III) in uterine artery, heart, kidney, skeletal muscle, esophagus, and cerebellum. Both pregnancy and estradiol have been shown to increase the mRNAs for NOS I and NOS III in skeletal muscle (93). Importantly, the hormonally induced increases in NOS activities are inhibited by treatment with the estrogen receptor antagonist, tamoxifen, an agent sometimes used in the treatment of LAM. Since both NOS I and III are subject to regulation by estrogen (93–95), hormonal therapy for LAM with antiestrogens, oophorectomy, or progesterone might lead to decreased NOS levels and NO production. Recently, we have measured exhaled NO in five women with LAM on medroxyprogesterone therapy, inhaled β-agonists, and inhaled corticosteroids. Despite these therapies, which might be expected to decrease NO levels, we found that exhaled NO levels in LAM individuals were higher than control women of childbearing age [LAM 15 ± 6.3 ppb (n = 5) vs. control 8.7 ± 1.8 ppb (n = 6); $p < 0.03$]. It is unclear from these preliminary findings if higher than normal levels of exhaled NO are involved in the pathogenesis of the disease, a response to the LAM, or an effect of medical therapy. Furthermore, it is unknown if the smooth muscle cells in LAM express NOS enzymes or if they have abnormalities in the response to NO, i.e., in guanylyl cyclase, cGMP, G-kinases, A-kinases, or phosphodiesterases, which might allow the smooth muscle cells to escape from growth-inhibitory effects of NO. Studies are needed to clarify the role that NO and cGMP play in the development of smooth muscle proliferation in LAM, how hormonal therapy affects NO production in these patients, and if exogeneous NO might be useful as a therapeutic modality for inhibition of smooth muscle proliferation.

References

1. Palmer RMJ, Gerrige AG, Moncada S. Nitric oxide release accounts for the biological activity of endothelium-derived relaxing factor. Nature 1987; 327:524–526.
2. Ignarro LJ, Buga GM, Wood KS, Byrnes RE, Chaudhuri G. Endothelium derived relaxing factor produced and released from artery and vein is nitric oxide. Proc Natl Acad of Sci USA 1987; 84:9265–9269.
3. Gaston B, Drazen JM, Loscalzo J, and Stamler JS. The biology of nitrogen oxides in the airways. Am J Respir Crit Care Med 1994; 149:538–551.
4. Schmidt HHH, Walter U. NO at work. Cell 1994; 78:919–925.
5. Nathan C. Nitric oxide as a secretory product of mammalian cells. FASEB J 1992; 6:3051–3064.
6. Garbers DL. Guanylyl cyclase receptors and their endocrine, paracrine, and autocrine ligands. Cell 1992; 71:1–4.
7. Schmidt HHH, Lohmann SM, Walter U. The nitric oxide cGMP signal transduction system: regulation and mechanism of action. Biochim Biophys Acta 1993; 1178:153–175.
8. Stuehr DJ, Griffith OW. Mammalian nitric oxide synthase. Adv Enzymol Relat Areas Mol Biol 1992; 65:287–346.
9. Nathan C, Xie Q. Nitric oxide synthases: roles, tolls, and controls. Cell 1994; 78:915–918.
10. Frandsen U, Lopez-Figueroa M, Hellsten Y. Localization of nitric oxide synthase in human skeletal muscle. Biochem Biophys Res Commun 1996; 227:88–93.
11. Gaston B, Stamler JS. Nitrogen oxides. In: Crystal RG, West JB, eds. The Lung: Scientific Foundations. 2d ed. Philadelphia: Lippincott-Raven, 1997:239–253.
12. Nathan C, Xie Q. Regulation of biosynthesis of nitric oxide. J Biol Chem 1994; 269:13725–13728.
13. Asano K, Chee CBE, Gaston B, Lilly CM, Gerard C, Drazen JM, Stamler JS. Constitutive and inducible nitric oxide synthase gene expression, regulation, and activity in human lung epithelial cells. Proc Natl Acad Sci USA 1994; 91:10089–10093.

14. Kim N, Vardi Y, Padma-Nathan H, Daley J, Goldstein I, Saenez de Tejeda I. Oxygen tension regulates the nitric oxide pathway. J Clin Invest 1993; 91:437–442.
15. Shaul PW, Wells LB. Oxygen modulates nitric oxide production selectively in fetal pulmonary endothelial cells. Am J Respir Cell Mol Biol 1994; 11:432–438.
16. Zehetgruber M, Conforto A, Bing RJ. Vascular smooth muscle and nitric oxide. Life Sci 1993; 52:1397–1406.
17. Durante W, Liao L, Iftikhar I, O'Brien WE, Schafer AI. Differential regulation of L-arginine transport and nitric oxide production by vascular smooth muscle and endothelium. Circ Res 1996; 78:1075–1082.
18. Schulz R, Triggle CR. Role of NO in vascular smooth muscle and cardiac muscle function. Trends Pharmacol Sci 1994; 15:255–259.
19. Nakayama DK, Geller DA, Lowenstein CJ, Davies P, Pitt BR, Simmons RL, Billiar TR. Cytokines and lipopolysaccharide induce nitric oxide synthase in cultured rat pulmonary artery smooth muscle. Am J Respir Cell Mol Biol 1992; 7:471–476.
20. Nunokawa Y, Ishida N, Tanaka S. Cloning of inducible nitric oxide synthase in rat vascular smooth muscle cells. Biochem Biophys Res Commun 1993; 191:89–94.
21. Newby AC, Southgate KM, Assender JW. Inhibition of vascular smooth muscle cell proliferation by endothelium-dependent vasodilators. Herz 1992; 17:291–299.
22. Nakayama DK, Geller DA, DiSilvio M, Bloomgarden G, Davies P, Pitt BR, Hatakeyama K, Kagamiyama H, Simmons RL, Billiar TR. Tetrahydrobiopterin synthesis and inducible nitric oxide production in pulmonary artery smooth muscle. Lung Cell Mol Physiol 1994; 10:L455–L460.
23. Hattori Y, Gross SS. Cycloheximide induces nitric oxide synthase mRNA in vascular smooth muscle cells by prolonging mRNA lifetime. Biochem Mol Biol 1995; 37:439–445.
24. Hattori Y, Campbell EB, Gross SS. Argininosuccinate synthase mRNA and activity are induced by immunostimulants in vascular smooth muscle. J Biol Chem 1994; 269:9405–9408.
25. Gross SS, Levi R. Tetrahydrobiopterin synthesis. J Biol Chem 1992; 267:25722–25729.
26. Moncada S, Higgs A. The L-arginine-nitric oxide pathway. N Engl J Med 1993; 2002–2012.
27. Hirokawa K, O'Shaughnessy KM, Ramrakha P, Wilkins MR. Inhibition of nitric oxide synthesis in vascular smooth muscle by retinoids. Br J Pharmacol 1994; 113:1448–1454.
28. Schini VB, Vanhoutte PM. Role of the L-arginine-nitric oxide pathway in vascular smooth muscle. Eur Heart J 1993; 14(suppl):16–21.
29. Geng Y, Hansson GK, Holme E. Interferon-γ and tumor necrosis factor synergize to induce nitric oxide production and inhibit mitochondrial respiration in vascular smooth muscle cells. Circ Res 1992; 71:1268–1276.
30. Stein CS, Fabry Z, Murphy S, Hart MN. Involvement of nitric oxide in IFN-γ-mediated reduction of microvessel smooth muscle cell proliferation. Mol Immunol 1995; 13:965–973.
31. Scott-Burden T, Schini VB, Elizondo E, Junquero DC, Vanhoutte PM. Platelet-derived growth factor suppresses and fibroblast growth factor enhances cytokine-in-

duced production of nitric oxide by cultured smooth muscles cells. Circ Res 1992; 71:1088–1100.
32. Fukuo K, Hata S, Suhara T, Nakahahi, T, Shinto Y, Tsujimoto Y, Morimoto S, Ogihara T. Nitric oxide induces upregulation of Fas and apoptosis in vascular smooth muscle. Hypertension 1996; 27(part 2):82–26.
33. Fukuo K, Inoue T, Morimoto S, Nakahashi T, Yasuda O, Shoichi K, Sasada R, Ogihara T. Nitric oxide mediates cytotoxicity and basic fibroblast growth factor release in cultured vascular smooth muscle cells. J Clin Invest 1995; 95:699–676.
34. Thomae KR, Joshi PC, Davies P, Pitt BR, Billiar TR, Simmons RL, Nakayama DK. Nitric oxide produced by cytokine-activated pulmonary artery smooth muscle cells is cytotoxic to cocultured endothelium. Surgery 1996; 119:61–66.
35. Geng Y, Hellstrand K, Wennmalm C, Hansson GK. Apoptotic death of human leukemic cells induced by vascular cells expressing nitric oxide synthase in response to γ-interferon and tumor necrosis factor-α. Cancer Res 1996; 56:866–874.
36. Zapol WM, Rimar S, Gillis N, Marletta M, Bosken CH. Nitric oxide and the lung. Am J Respir Crit Care Med 1994; 149:1375–1380.
37. Lipton SA, Choi YB, Pan ZH, Lei SZ, Chen HS, Sucher NJ, Loscalzo J, Singel DJ, Stamler JS. A redox-based mechanism for the neuroprotective and neurodestructive effects of nitric oxide and related nitroso-compounds. Nature 1993; 364:626–632.
38. Stamler JS, Single DJ, Loscalzo J. Biochemistry of nitric oxide and it redox-activated forms. Science 1992; 258:1898–1902.
39. Salvemini D, Misko TP, Masferrer JL, Seibert K, Currie MG, Needleman P. Nitric oxide activates cyclooxygenase enzymes. Proc Natl Acad Sci USA. 1993; 90:7240–7244.
40. Kwon NS, Stuehr DJ, Nathan CF. Inhibition of tumor cell ribonucleotide reductase by macrophage-derived nitric oxide. J Exp Med 1991; 174:761–767.
41. Garg UC, Hassid A. Mechanisms of nitrosothiol-induced antimitogenesis in aortic smooth muscle cells. Eur J Pharmacol 1993; 237:243–249.
42. Beinert H, Kennedy MC, Stout CD. Aconitase as iron-sulfur protein, enzyme, and iron-regulatory protein. Chem Rev 1996; 96:2335–2373.
43. Nguyen T, Brunson D, Crespi CL, Penman BW, Wishnok JS, Tannenbaum SR. DNA damage and mutation in human cells exposed to nitric oxide in vitro. Proc Natl Acad Sci USA 1992; 89:3030–3034.
44. Murad F. Regulation of cytosolic guanylyl cyclase by nitric oxide: the NO-cyclic GMP signal transduction system. Adv Pharmacol 1994; 26:19–33.
45. Wedel B, Humbert P, Harteneck C, Foerster J, Malkewitz J, Bohme E, Schultz G, Koesling D. Mutation of His-105 in the β_1 subunit yields a nitric oxide-insensitive form of soluble guanylyl cylcase. Proc Natl Acad Sci USA 1994; 91:2592–2596.
46. Lincoln TM, Cornwell TL. Intracellular cyclic GMP receptor proteins. FASEB J 1993; 7:328–338.
47. Lincoln TM. Cyclic GMP and mechanisms of vasodilation. Pharmacol Ther 1989; 41:479–502.
48. McDonald LJ, Murad F. Nitric oxide and cyclic GMP signaling. Proc Soc Exp Biol Med 1996; 211:1–6.
49. Archer SL, Huang JM, Hampl V, Nelson DP, Shultz PJ, Weir EK. Nitric oxide and

cGMP cause vasorelaxation by activation of a charybdotoxin-sensitive K channel by cGMP-dependent protein kinase. Proc Natl Acad Sci USA 1994; 91:7583–7587.
50. Garg UC, Hassid A. Nitric oxide-generating vasodilators and 8-bromo-cyclic guanosine monophosphate inhibit mitogenesis and proliferation of cultured rat vascular smooth muscle cells. J Clin Invest 1989; 83:1774–1777.
51. Yang W, Ando J, Korenaga R, Toyo-oka T, Kamiya A. Exogenous nitric oxide inhibits proliferation of cultured vascular endothelial cells. Biochem Biophys Res Commun 1994; 203; 1160–1167.
52. Thomae KR, Nakayama DK, Billiar TR, Simmons RL, Pitt BR, Davies P. The effect of nitric oxide on fetal pulmonary artery smooth muscle growth. J Surg Res 1995; 59:337–343.
53. Abman SH, Chatfield BA, Hall SL, McMurthry IF. Role of endothelium-derived relaxing factor during transition of pulmonary circulation at birth. Am J Physiol 1990; 259:H1921–H1927.
54. Sarkar R, Meinberg EG, Stanley JC, Gordon D, Webb RC. Nitric oxide reversibly inhibits the migration of cultured vascular smooth muscle cells. Circ Res 1996; 78:225–230.
55. Nakaki T, Nakayama M, Kato R. Inhibition by nitric oxide and nitric oxide-producing vasodilators of DNA synthesis in vascular smooth muscle cells. Eur J Pharmacol 1990; 189:347–353.
56. McMahon TJ, Ignarro LJ, Kadowitz PJ. Influence of Zaprinast on vascular tone and vasodilator responses in the cat pulmonary vascular bed. J Appl Physiol 1993; 74:1704–1711.
57. Roberts JD, Polaner DM, Lang P, Zapol WM. Inhaled nitric oxide in persistent pulmonary hypertension of the newborn. Lancet 1992; 340:818–819.
58. Roberts JD, Fineman JR, Morin FC, Shaul PW, Rimar S, Schreiber MD, Polin RA, Zwass MS, Zayek MM, Gross I, Heymann MA, Zapol WM. Inhaled nitric oxide and persitent pulmonary hypertension of the newborn. N Engl J Med 1997; 336:605–610.
59. The Neonatal Inhaled Nitric Oxide Study Group. Inhaled nitric oxide in full-term and nearly full-term infants with hypoxic respiratory failure. N Engl J Med 1997; 336:597–604.
60. Dupuy PM, Shore SA, Drazen JM, Frostell C, Hill WA, Zapol WM. Bronchodilator action of inhaled nitric oxide in guinea pigs. J Clin Invest 1992; 90:421–428.
61. Gaston B, Reilly J, Drazen JM, Feckler J, Ramdev P, Arnelle D, Mullins ME, Sugarbaker DJ, Chee C, Singel DJ, Loscalzo J, Stamler JS. Endogenous nitrogen oxides and bronchodilator S-nitrosothiols in human airways. Proc Natl Acad Sci USA 1993; 90:10957–10961.
62. Nunokawa Y, Tanaka S. Interferon-γ inhibits proliferation of rat vascular smooth muscle cells by nitric oxide generation. Biochem Biophys Res Commun 1992; 188:409–415.
63. Kolpakov V, Gordon D, Kulik TJ. Nitric oxide-generating compounds inhibit total protein and collagen synthesis in cultured vascular smooth muscle cells. Circ Res 1995; 76:305–309.
64. Cornwell TL, Arnold E, Boerth NJ, Lincoln TM. Inhibition of smooth muscle cell growth by nitric oxide and activation of cAMP-dependent protein kinase by cGMP. Am J Physiol 1994; 267:C1405–C1413.

65. Murray KJ. Cyclic AMP and mechanisms of vasodilation. Pharmacol Ther 1990; 47:329–345.
66. Garg UC, Hassid A. Nitric oxide-generating vasodilators inhibit mitogenesis and proliferation of BALB/C 3T3 fibroblasts by a cyclic GMP-independent mechanism. Biochem Biophys Res Commun 1990; 171:474–479.
67. Clementi E, Sciorati C, Nistico G. Growth factor-induced CA^{2+} responses are differentially modulated by nitric oxide via activation of a cyclic GMP-dependent pathway. Mol Pharmacol 1995; 48:1068–1077.
68. Albina JE, Abate JA, Henry WL. Nitric oxide production is required for murine resident peritoneal macrophages to suppress mitogen-stimulated T cell proliferation. J Immunol 1991; 147:144–148.
69. Garg UC, Lakshmi D, Turndorf H, Goldfrank LR, Bansinath M. Effect of nitric oxide on mitogenesis and proliferation of cerebellar glial cells. Brain Res 1992; 592:208–212.
70. Garg UC, Hassid A. Inhibition of rat mesangial cell mitogenesis by the nitric oxide-generating vasodilators. Am J Physiol 1989; 257:F60–F66.
71. Blanco FJ, Lotz M. IL-1 induced nitric oxide inhibits chondrocyte proliferation via PGE2. Exp Cell Res 1995; 218:319–325.
72. Punjabi CJ, Laskin DL, Heck DE, Laskin JD. Production of nitric oxide by murine bone marrow cells: Inverse correlation with cellular proliferation. J Immunol 1992; 149:2179–2184.
73. Petit JF, Nicaise M, Lepoivre M, Guissani A, Lemaire G. Protection by glutathione against the antiproliferative effects of nitric oxide. Biochem Pharmacol 1996; 52:205–212.
74. Ziche M, Morbidelli L, Masini E, Amerini S, Granger HJ, Maggi CA, Geppetti P, Ledda F. Nitric oxide mediates angiogenesis in vivo and endothelial cell growth and migration in vitro promoted by substance P. J Clin Invest 1994; 94:2036–2044.
75. Hecker G, Denzer D, Wohlfeil S. Elevation of circulating NO: its effects on hemodynamics and vascular smooth muscle cell proliferation in rats. Agents Actions Suppl 1995; 45:169–176.
76. Hassid A, Arabshahi H, Bourchier T, Dhaunsi GS, Matthews C. Nitric oxide selectively amplifies FGF-2 induced mitogenesis in primary rat aortic smooth muscle cells. Am J Physiol 1994; 267:H1040–H1048.
77. Barnes PJ, Belvisi MG. Nitric oxide and lung disease. Thorax 1993; 48:1034–1043.
78. Dweik RA, Laskowski D, Abu-Soud HM, Kaneko FT, Hutte R, Stuehr DJ, Erzurum SC. Nitric oxide synthesis in the lung: regulation by oxygen through a kinetic mechanism. J Clin Invest 1998; 101:660–666.
79. Tsujino I, Miyamoto K, Nishimura M, Shinano H, Makita H, Saito S, Nakano T, Kawakami Y. Production of nitric oxide (NO) in intrathoracic airways of normal humans. Am J Respir Crit Care Med 1996; 154:1370–1374.
80. Kharitonov SA, Chung KF, Evans D, O'Connor BJ, Barnes PJ. Increased exhaled nitric oxide in asthma is mainly derived from the lower respiratory tract. Am J Respir Crit Care Med 1996; 153:1773–1780.
81. Kobzik L, Bredt DS, Lowenstein CJ, Drazen J, Gaston B, Sugarbaker D, Stamler JS. Nitric oxide synthase in human and rat lung: immunocytochemical and histochemical localization. Am J Respir Cell Mol Biol 1993; 9:371–377.

82. Guo FH, De Raeve HR, Rice TW, Stuehr DJ, Thunnissen FB, Erzurum SC. Continuous nitric oxide synthesis by inducible nitric oxide synthase in normal human airway epithelium in vivo. Proc Natl Acad Sci USA 1995; 92:7809–7813.
83. Ischiropoulous H, Ignacio M, Fisher D, Fisher AB, Thom SR. Role of neutrophils and nitric oxide in lung alveolar injury from smoke inhalation. Am J Respir Crit Care Med 1994; 150:337–341.
84. Giaid A, Saleh D. Reduced expression of endothelial nitric oxide synthase in patients with pulmonary hypertension. N Engl J Med 1995; 333:214–221.
85. Cremona G, Higenbottam T, Borland C, Mist B. Mixed expired nitric oxide in primary pulmonary hypertension in relation to lung diffusing capacity. Q J Med 1994; 87:547–551.
86. Corrin B, Liebow AA, Friedman PJ. Pulmonary lymphangiomyomatosis: a review. Am J Pathol 1975; 79:347–382.
87. Carrington CB, Cugel DW, Gaensler EA, Merks A, Redding RA, Schaaf JT, Tomasian A. Lymphangioleiomyomatosis: physiologic-pathologic-radiologic correlations. Am Rev Respir Dis 1977; 116:977–995.
88. Groves PH, Banning AP, Penny WJ, Newby AC, Cheadle HA, Lewis MJ. The effects of exogenous nitric oxide on smooth muscle cell proliferation following porcine carotid angioplasty. Cardiovasc Res 1995; 30:87–96.
89. Seki J, Mishio M, Kato Y, Motoyama Y, Yoshida K. FK409, a new nitric-oxide donor, suppresses smooth muscle proliferation in the rat model of balloon angioplasty. Atherosclerosis 1995; 117:97–106.
90. Taylor JR, Ryu J, Colby TV, Raffin TA. Lymphangioleiomyomatosis: clinical course in 32 patients. N Engl J Med 1990; 323:1254–1260.
91. Eliasson AH, Phillips YY, Tenholder MF. Treatment of lymphangioleiomyomatosis: a meta-analysis. Chest 1989; 196:1352–1355.
92. Kharitonov SA, Logan-Sinclair RB, Busset CM, Shinebourne EA. Peak expiratory nitric oxide differences in men and women: relation to the menstrual cycle. Br Heart J 1994; 72:243–245.
93. Weiner CP, Lizasoain I, Baylis SA, Knowles RG, Charles IG, Moncada S. Induction of calcium-dependent nitric oxide synthases by sex hormones. Proc Natl Acad Sci USA 1994; 91:5212–5216.
94. Radomski MW. Nitric oxide: Biological mediator, modulator and effector. Ann Med 1995; 27:321–329.
95. Weiner CP, Knowles RG, Moncada S. Induction of nitric oxide synthases early in pregnancy. Am J Obstet Gynecol 1994; 171:838–843.

18

Role of Estrogen in Smooth Muscle Growth and Function

EDITH H. SPEIR and RICHARD O. CANNON, III

National Heart, Lung and Blood Institute
National Institutes of Health
Bethesda, Maryland

The near-exclusive diagnosis of lymphangioleiomyomatosis in reproductive-aged women, the identification of estrogen and progesterone receptors in smooth muscle cells from lung tissue of patients, and anecdotal responses in disease progression to estrogen-ablative or antagonist therapy have naturally led to consideration of the pathophysiological relevance of estrogen in this disease (1–3). Further, primary pulmonary hypertension, a disease characterized by plexiform vascular lesions associated with smooth muscle proliferation, is twice as common in women (usually of reproductive age) as in men (4–6). Accordingly, considerable interest has focused on the potential interaction between sex hormones and pulmonary smooth muscle proliferation in these diseases. In this chapter, genomic and nongenomic effects of estrogen on smooth muscle growth and function will be discussed, as will potential implications of these effects in the pathogenesis and treatment of these diseases.

I. Genomic Effects of Estrogen by Nuclear Receptor Activation

The cellular effects of steroid hormones, including the sex steroids estrogen and progesterone, have generally been thought to be mediated through interaction with specific intracellular receptors (7,8). Exposure of a cell to estrogen results in rapid diffusion of this lipophilic molecule across the cell membrane and binding to a specific hormone-binding domain of a 67 kDa receptor protein in the cytosol or in the nucleus (Fig. 1) (9–11). This binding is associated with phosphorylation of the receptor, resulting in a conformational change in the hormone-receptor complex with dissociation of inhibitory proteins, such as the 90 kDa heat-shock protein. The receptor-hormone unit then binds to another receptor-hormone unit to form a homodimer (12) or combines with other regulatory proteins to form a heterodimer. These complexes translocate into the nucleus and bind upstream to, or within, target genes at specific DNA segments that are arranged as two adjacent five to six base-pair units in mirror-imaged sequences (palindromes) or that exist as a single unit (half-palindrome) (13). The binding of each receptor-

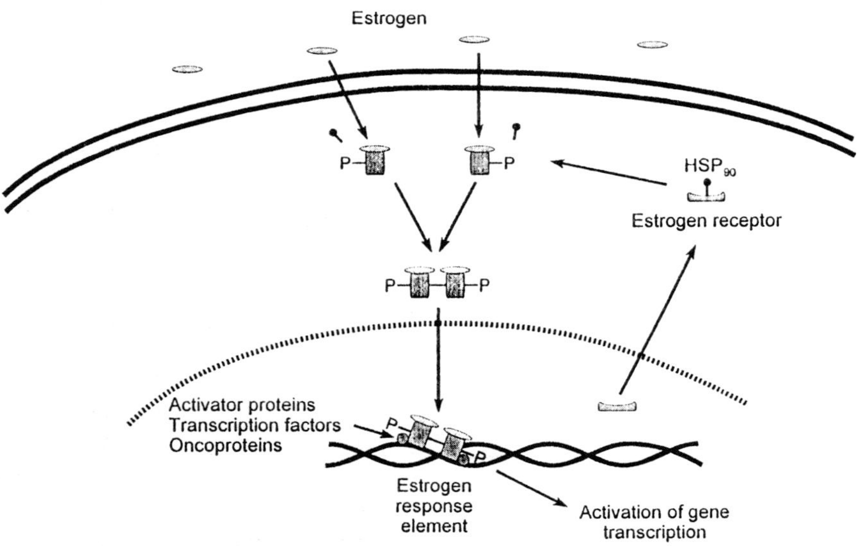

Figure 1 Estrogen rapidly crosses the cell membrane where it binds to the estrogen receptor in the nucleus or in the cytosol. Phosphorylation (P) of the receptor and dissociation of inhibitory proteins such as the 90 kDa heat-shock protein (HSP) results in a confirmational change in the receptor, dimerization with another estrogen-receptor complex, and translocation into the nucleus with binding to specific sites in the promoter region of target genes (estrogen response element). Activation of transcription of target genes is accomplished by the transcriptional activation domain of the estrogen receptor in concert with activator proteins, transcription factors, and oncoproteins.

hormone unit to these specific base-pair sequences, called estrogen response elements, is accomplished via two zinc-containing sites (zinc fingers) in the cysteine-rich DNA-binding domain of each receptor. Transcription of the target genes is then positively regulated by the transcriptional activation domain of the receptor with the participation of specific activator proteins, cAMP-responsive binding proteins, transcription factors, and nuclear oncoproteins (14–19). The estrogen receptor-ligand complex may also inhibit transcription of specific genes by antagonizing transcriptional factors or oncoproteins at their promoter region DNA-binding sites (20,21). The tissue, cell type, and target gene characteristics that determine transcriptional regulation by the estrogen receptor-ligand complex are unknown.

Estrogen and progesterone receptors are members of different subgroups of the steroid and thyroid hormone receptor superfamily (8). Because of a similarity in receptor structure and activity, liganded receptors from one member of the subgroup can act synergistically with the liganded receptor of another member, or can independently trigger transcription and expression of genes. For example, liganded thyroid receptor can bind to the estrogen response element of specific genes and cause expression of estrogen-dependent proteins (10). Further, steroid hormones of one receptor group may regulate the receptor concentration and binding activity of hormones of the other receptor group. Thus, estradiol treatment increases progesterone receptor content and binding in vascular tissue from ovariectomized dogs and rats (22,23). In the uterus and breast, estrogen upregulates progesterone receptors while progesterone downregulates its own receptor as well as the estrogen receptor (24–27). In the uterus and in endothelial cells in culture, estrogen upregulates its own receptor (28,29).

There is recent evidence for the existence of more than one nuclear estrogen receptor, with demonstration of a novel 54.2 kDa estrogen receptor in rat ovary and prostate (30). This receptor (ERβ) differs from the nuclear estrogen receptor (ERα) primarily in the N terminus, the site of transcriptional activation, but like the ERα receptor exhibits high-affinity binding of estrogen. The biological significance of multiple nuclear estrogen receptors remains to be defined.

II. Nonligand Activation of the Estrogen Receptor

Nuclear estrogen receptors may be activated independently of estrogen (Fig. 2). The catecholaminergic neurotransmitter dopamine and peptide growth factors have been shown to activate estrogen receptor-dependent transcription in the absence of estrogen (31,32). Further, because estrogen binding to its nuclear receptor activates genes that encode peptide growth factors and their receptors (33–35), continued estrogen receptor activation in the same cell or adjacent cells may be accomplished in the absence of additional estrogen through nuclear receptor

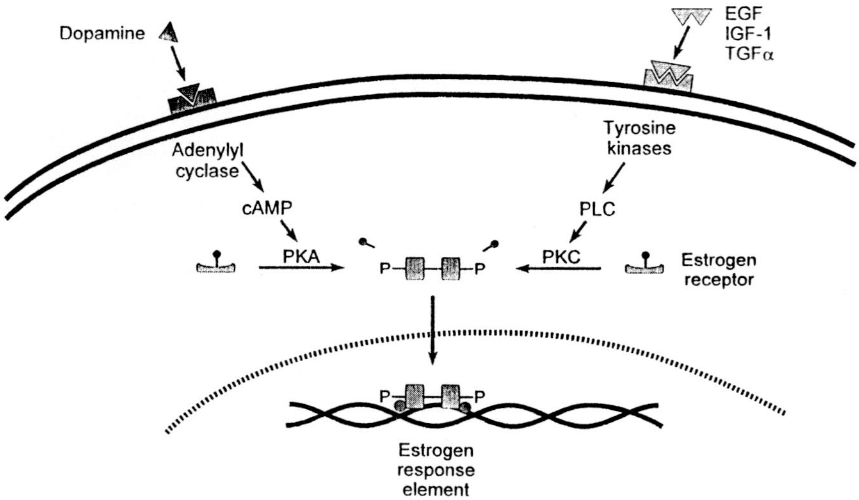

Figure 2 Proposed mechanism by which nuclear estrogen receptors may be activated in the absence of estrogen. Dopamine activation of protein kinase A (PKA) and cytokine growth factor [e.g., epidermal growth factor (EGF), insulin-like growth factor (IGF-1), transforming growth factor (TGF-α] activation of protein kinase C (PKC) may result in phosphorylation of the estrogen receptor, with translocation of the dimer to the nucleus where binding to estrogen response elements may occur.

activation by these growth factors (36). By this process, which may involve phosphorylation of the estrogen receptor as a consequence of growth factor–mediated kinase activation, genomic effects of small concentrations of estrogen may be amplified in an autocrine and paracrine manner (37–39).

III. Cell Membrane Receptor Activation by Estrogen

Steroid hormones may rapidly initiate intracellular events in the absence of genomic effects, possibly by activation of receptors on the cell membrane (Fig. 3) (40–44). Thus, estrogen promotes the release of prolactin within 5 minutes when added to rat pituitary tumor cells in culture (45). In this cell line, receptors structurally similar to the nuclear estrogen receptor were demonstrated on the cell membrane by the binding of monoclonal antibodies to multiple epitopes of the nuclear receptor using confocal scanning laser microscopy (44). Activation of membrane receptors by estrogen could account for the increase in intracellular cAMP levels within 5 minutes of incubation of rat vascular smooth muscle cells with supraphysiological concentrations of 17β-estradiol (46).

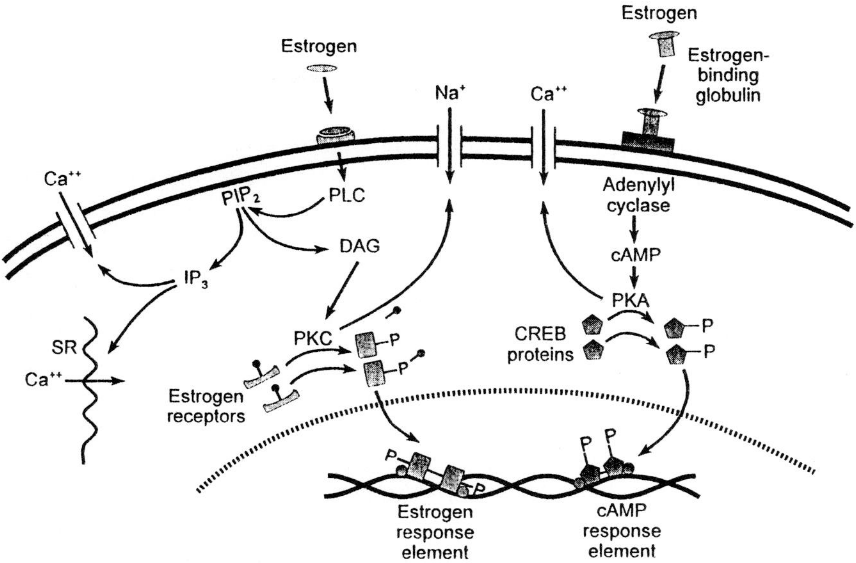

Figure 3 Proposed mechanism by which estrogen binding to estrogen receptors or estrogen-binding globulin receptors on the cell membrane may activate signal transduction pathways with subsequent activation of target gene transcription. The membrane estrogen receptor may activate membrane-bound phospholipase C (PLC), which converts phosphatidylinositol-4,5-biphosphate (PIP_2) to diacylglycerol (DAG) and inositol-1,4,5-triphosphate (IP_3). IP_3 stimulates the release of calcium from the sarcoplasmic reticulum (SR), increasing intracellular calcium content. Protein kinase C (PKC) is activated by DAG and may phosphorylate the estrogen receptor in the absence of estrogen, with subsequent binding to estrogen response elements of target genes. Estrogen-binding globulin receptor binding may activate adenylyl cyclase with increased cyclic AMP and activation of protein kinase A (PKA). PKA may phosphorylate cAMP response element–binding proteins (CREB), which form dimers and bind to cAMP-response elements of target genes. By either signal transduction pathway, genomic transcriptional activity may be accomplished in the absence of estrogen binding to a nuclear receptor. Activation of membrane receptors may also account for immediate, nongenomic actions of estrogen by activation of cAMP or by increases in intracellular sodium and calcium content.

Much of what is currently known regarding the acute cellular events following steroid hormone exposure has been learned from cell culture experiments with the mineralocorticoid aldosterone. In smooth muscle cells from rat aorta, physiological concentrations of aldosterone activate a sodium-proton exchanger in the cell membrane, raising intracellular sodium content within minutes of incubation (47,48). Inositol-1,4,5-triphosphate and diacylglycerol synthesis increases due to activation of phospholipase C followed by hydrolysis of membrane lipids. Inositol-1,4,5-triphosphate stimulates the release of calcium into the cytosol from intracellular stores in smooth muscle cells and from enhanced extracellular influx of calcium into endothelial cells within several minutes of incubation with aldosterone (49–51). Such a membrane receptor effect by estrogen that rapidly increases intracellular calcium, as has been demonstrated in chicken and pig ovarian granulosa cells (52), could activate the constitutively expressed, calcium-dependent enzyme nitric oxide synthase in endothelial cells (53), which enhanced synthesis and release of nitric oxide (54), and thus account for the acute vascular responses reported in humans (55,56).

Estrogen-mediated cell membrane activation may have genomic effects as well. In the aldosterone membrane receptor experiments discussed above, increased levels of diacylglycerol activate protein kinase C, which could ultimately have genomic effects, including activation of protooncogenes that lead to cell proliferation. In addition, estrogen bound to a 90 kDa sex hormone–binding globulin in a rat prostate cancer cell line was found to activate a membrane receptor, which in turn activated cAMP-dependent protein kinase A. This resulted in phosphorylation of a cAMP response element–binding protein and binding to a cAMP response element in the nucleus (57). Specific binding of this sex hormone–binding globulin has been identified thus far in breast, endometrium, testis, prostate, and liver. Further, estrogen-stimulated activation of a tyrosine kinase–dependent signal transduction pathway has been detected in cultured aortic endothelial cells (58). Thus, estrogen can activate multiple signal transduction pathways, which could play a role in regulating growth and proliferation of target cells.

IV. Estrogen Receptors and the Vasculature

Specific binding of estrogen to vascular cells was first demonstrated by injection of [^{3}H]estradiol to terminally ill men and women with accumulation of radioactivity in the intimal endothelium, and adventitia of normal and atheromatous arteries detected at necropsy (59). More recently, estrogen receptors were immunolocalized to coronary arteries from premenopausal and postmenopausal women, many of whom died with significant coronary artery disease (60). Using a radiolabeled RNA probe complementary to 123 base pairs of the estrogen receptor hormone–binding domain, estrogen receptor mRNA was demonstrated in human saphenous vein smooth muscle cells from men and women (61). These investigators further showed that in mammary artery smooth muscle cells, with use of a reporter gene, the ligand-bound estrogen receptor is capable of transcriptional activation. This group has recently screened and tested vascular smooth cell–derived mRNA for specific gene regulation by estrogen. Cells incubated for 48 hours with estradiol (10 nM) and stimulated for 6 hours with 10% fetal bovine serum expressed the mRNA and protein of nucleophosmin, a nucleolar phosphoprotein believed to contribute to cell growth (62).

Estrogen receptors have also been demonstrated in human umbilical vein, aortic, and coronary artery endothelial cells in culture (63,64). Nuclear extracts were found to contain proteins that were identical in size to the nuclear estrogen receptor, which reacted with three monoclonal antibodies to different epitopes of the estrogen receptor and bound specifically to estrogen response elements by electrophoretic mobility shift assay (63). mRNA for the estrogen receptor was also demonstrated by Northern blot analysis. Because these cells were not pretreated with estrogen, constitutive expression of the estrogen receptor by endothelial cells is suggested by the findings of this study. In another experiment, the addition of a near-physiological concentration of estradiol (3.7 nM) enhanced the proliferation of endothelial cells from human coronary arteries and umbilical veins, which incorporated more [^{3}H]thymidine than hormone-free cells (64). This effect of estrogen was blocked by the estrogen receptor antagonist ICI 182,780. mRNA for the estrogen receptor was detected by ribonuclease protection assay, as was binding of endothelial estrogen receptor protein to DNA estrogen response elements by use of an electrophoretic mobility shift assay. Radioligand studies showed similar kinetics of estrogen binding in cells from male donors as for cells from female donors, with receptor densities of approximately 6×10^4 receptors per cell.

V. Effects of Estrogen on Smooth Muscle Growth

The growth stimulatory effects of estrogen on hormonally sensitive tissues such as breast and uterus and the demonstration of estrogen receptors on vascular smooth muscle and endothelial cells make hormonal effects on cell growth within the vasculature likely. The dramatic smooth muscle cell growth that occurs in the uterine artery during pregnancy is associated with rising estrogen levels (65), suggesting that under some physiological settings estrogen may have a stimulatory effect on smooth muscle cell growth. In cultured rat aortic smooth muscle cells, a supraphysiological concentration of 17β-estradiol (10 nM) upregulated the expression of c-fos, a protooncogene expressed prior to cell growth and proliferation (66). This finding is consistent with growth stimulatory effects of estrogen observed in nonvascular cell lines (67–70).

In an experiment comparing growth characteristics of uterine and aortic smooth cells from pregnant versus nonpregnant guinea pigs, uterine cells from pregnant animals were found to have greater basal rates of DNA synthesis following serum withdrawal compared with uterine cells from nonpregnant animals or aortic cells from either group (71). Uterine and aortic smooth muscle cells from pregnant animals grew to a greater density with increased DNA synthesis in response to serum stimulation for 7 days and were more responsive to the addition of platelet-derived growth factor (PDGF) than smooth muscle cells from nonpregnant animals. Supraphysiological concentrations of estradiol (30–100 ng/ml) alone had minimal growth effects on serum-stimulated smooth muscle cells from nonpregnant animals. However, pretreatment of smooth muscle cells from nonpregnant animals with estradiol for as little as 1 hour increased the growth response to PDGF to levels observed in cells from pregnant animals. The synergistic effect of 17β-estradiol on the response of smooth muscle cells to PDGF was partially reproduced with 17α-estradiol, an isomer that does not bind the estrogen receptor and implies the contribution of a nonreceptor mechanism of estrogen. Further, the brief time course (1 hour) for estradiol enhancement of the PDGF effect on cell growth is consistent with a nongenomic effect of estrogen on PDGF-activated signal transduction. The synergy between estrogen and PDGF for stimulation of smooth muscle cell growth was dependent on activation of protein kinase C, perhaps as a final common pathway of membrane receptor activation and signal transduction for the two agonists.

Several experiments have shown inhibitory effects of estrogen on vascular smooth muscle cells from nonpregnant animals. A supraphysiological concentration of estradiol (20 ng/ml) inhibited the proliferative effect of hyperlipemic serum on stable cultures of rabbit aortic smooth muscle cells as measured by cell culture size and [^{3}H]thymidine uptake (72). Estradiol in supraphysiological concentrations ranging from 180 to 720 nM inhibited the uptake of [^{3}H]thymidine into vascular segments of porcine coronary artery, with thymidine uptake used as an index of smooth muscle cell proliferation (73). In this study, the estrogen receptor antagonist tamoxifen and its metabolite 4-hydroxytamoxifen also inhibited thymidine uptake, suggesting estrogenic effects of these compounds in vascular tissue. Incubation of rat aortic smooth muscle cells with a supraphysiological concentration of 17β-estradiol (10 μM) for 24 hours inhibited subsequent 1% fetal calf serum–stimulated [^{3}H]thymidine uptake over the next 24 hours by cells from female, but not male, animals, despite detection of estrogen receptors in cells from either gender (74). This effect of estradiol was blocked by coadministration of tamoxifen. This group recently reported inhibition of [^{3}H]thymidine uptake by estradiol (10 μM) in saphenous vein smooth muscle cells from men or postmenopausal women when cells were stimulated with either PDGF or with basic fibroblast growth factors (75).

In contrast to the findings in smooth muscle cells from the systemic vasculature, 17β-estradiol at concentrations extending into the supraphysiological range (3–300 nM) potentiated [^{3}H]thymidine uptake in cultures of rat pulmonary vascular smooth muscle cells in 10% fetal bovine serum following incubation for 24 hours in a concentration-dependent manner, an effect antagonized by prior administration of tamoxifen (76). This group also found that vascular strips from canine pulmonary artery showed increased DNA synthesis in the nuclei of the arterial media following incubation with estradiol, but only after removal of the endothelium.

The difference in the estrogenic response between pulmonary and systemic vessels may indicate the presence of two genomic pathways in smooth muscle cells: one for stimulation and one for inhibition (77). However, differences in responses may also relate to experimental design, differences in dosage of estradiol (usually supraphysiologic, even for pregnancy), and whether coadministration of growth factors or hyperlipemic serum (possibly enriched with growth factors) was required to show a hormone effect on smooth muscle cell growth.

VI. Inhibitory Effects of Estrogen on Vascular Response to Injury

In a necropsy study, the majority of normal arteries from premenopausal women expressed estrogen receptors, whereas only a minority of atherosclerotic vessels from premenopausal women were positive for estrogen receptors (60). This implies that the protective effect of estrogen is linked to an antiproliferative property, since smooth muscle cell proliferation and migration is an important feature of atherosclerosis (78). Such a possibility is supported by clinical observations that reproductive-aged women are particularly susceptible to atherosclerosis following bilateral oophorectomy unless treated with estrogen (79–81).

Several groups have looked at the effect of estrogen on the myointimal response to vascular injury in animal models. Estradiol was shown to decrease neointimal thickening following balloon injury of the common and external iliac arteries of male rabbits when administered one day prior to vascular injury and daily thereafter until sacrifice 3 weeks later (82). In this model, estradiol also inhibited thymidine uptake in major vessels following 3 days of treatment. A previous study had also shown inhibitory effects of estrogen on surgically induced vascular intimal hyperplasia in rabbits (83). Estrogen was also found to significantly decrease myointimal hyperplasia in both rabbit cardiac and aorta allografts (84,85).

Estradiol treatment was recently reported to significantly inhibit myointimal proliferation following carotid artery injury in a gonadectomized rat model of both sexes (86). In this study, gonadectomy of untreated female rats was associated with a greater increase in neointimal proliferation following balloon injury than observed in untreated, but gonadally intact females. Of note, carotid injury resulted in increases in vascular c-myc mRNA levels, with a greater increase in males compared with females. In the gonadally intact animals, balloon injury caused less neointimal formation in females compared with male animals. Estradiol administration to gonadally intact female rats did not affect the myointimal response to carotid injury.

The studies described above utilized supraphysiological doses of estrogen to inhibit the myointimal response to vascular injury. However, near-physiological doses of estrogen may also have smooth muscle inhibitory effects. Ovariectomized mice were treated for 7 days with 17β-estradiol, with continued daily treatment for 14 days (achieving plasma levels of approximately 2.4 nM) following wire injury to a carotid artery (87). The myointimal response noted in estrogen-deficient control animals was prevented with estrogen treatment and was associated with less histochemical evidence for cellular proliferation as assessed by bromodeoxyuridine labeling.

VII. Mechanism of Inhibitory Effects of Estrogen

The observation that presence of the endothelium prevented estrogen-stimulated smooth muscle cell growth in vascular strips from canine pulmonary artery (69) may provide insight into the mechanism of myointimal inhibitory effects of estrogen in animal models of vascular injury. As discussed previously in this chapter, endothelial cells express functional estrogen receptors (63,64), and in one study incubation of endothelial cells in a physiological concentration of estradiol augmented cell proliferation in culture (64). This same group had previously shown that near-physiological concentrations of 17β-estradiol (1–5 nM) increased adherence of endothelial cells to extracellular matrix proteins and augmented migration of cells into areas of the culture plate that were "wounded" by scraping when compared with untreated cells (88). These effects were blocked by the estrogen receptor antagonist ICI 182,780. Accordingly, the administration of estrogen to animals in vascular injury experiments may enhance the proliferation of endothelial cells into the traumatized vessel from the margins of injury, as was observed in a recent study (89). Endothelial cells may then secrete substances that inhibit smooth muscle cell proliferation.

In this regard, estrogen increases levels of mRNA for nitric oxide synthase in endothelial cells (54,90,91) likely due to transcriptional activation of the nitric oxide synthase gene via binding to associated estrogen response elements (92,93), with enhanced synthesis and release of nitric oxide. Increased production of nitric oxide by endothelial cells may diminish the proliferation of smooth muscle cells into the site of injury. This mechanism is supported by experiments utilizing chemical donors of nitric oxide showing inhibition of the migration and proliferation of smooth muscle cells in culture by blocking DNA synthesis (94–97). Nitric oxide may also diminish smooth muscle cell synthesis of extracellular matrix proteins considered important for cell migration into sites of vessel injury (98). Dietary supplementation with L-arginine, the precursor for nitric oxide, reduces the myointimal response to vascular injury (99,100), as does in vivo transfer of the endothelial nitric oxide synthase gene into the vessel wall

(101). Conversely, inhibitors of nitric oxide synthesis exacerbate the myointimal response to vascular injury (100).

Although smooth muscle cells do not express constitutive nitric oxide synthase, synthesis of the enzyme by vascular smooth muscle may be induced by cytokines (102–104). Nitric oxide released from vascular smooth muscle cells has been shown to inhibit proliferation of rat aorta smooth muscle cells in culture by means of a cytotoxic effect on cells (103,104), an effect that may prevent excessive proliferation of cells following injury. Whether estrogen augments inducible nitric oxide synthase levels or activity in smooth muscle cells is unknown.

VIII. Nitric Oxide and Pulmonary Vascular Function

Immunoreactive nitric oxide synthase has been demonstrated in the endothelium and epithelium of normal lung tissue (105). The physiologic relevance of nitric oxide in the regulation of pulmonary vascular tone is evidenced by increased pulmonary vascular resistance following infusion of an inhibitor of nitric oxide synthase into the pulmonary artery of healthy subjects (106). During acute hypoxemia in healthy volunteers, pulmonary vascular resistance increased by approximately 50%, with this pulmonary vasoconstrictor response exacerbated by simultaneous infusion of an inhibitor of nitric oxide synthase (107). Of interest, hypoxemia caused systemic vasodilation mediated by nitric oxide. Thus, despite evidence for hypoxemia-induced nitric oxide release in both the pulmonary and systemic circulations, release or activation of vasoconstrictor substances into the pulmonary circulation produced a net constrictor response in that vascular bed.

Nitric oxide may be of pathophysiological importance in patients with pulmonary hypertension. Diminished immunoreactive nitric oxide synthase and its mRNA (in situ hybridization) was detected in the pulmonary vascular endothelium of lung tissue from patients with primary pulmonary hypertension compared with normal lung tissue from transplantation donors, although epithelial nitric oxide synthase appeared to be preserved in the lung tissue from these patients (105). The etiologic significance of diminished nitric oxide is unclear in this study, because diminished nitric oxide synthase expression was evident in lung tissue from patients with either primary or secondary pulmonary hypertension. However, the inverse correlation between the magnitude of enzyme expression and severity of plexogenic pulmonary arteriopathy suggests that absence of nitric oxide may contribute to excessive vascular smooth muscle proliferation in this condition. In this regard, continuous administration of nitric oxide gas prevents the development of pulmonary hypertension in chronically hypoxic rats (108), and in animal models of pulmonary hypertension, administration of the nitric oxide substrate L-arginine improved endothelium-dependent pulmonary vascular responsiveness (109). Diminished nitric oxide in lung tissue of patients with pulmonary hypertension may account for increased plasma levels (110) and lung tissue expression (111) of endothelin-1 in these patients, due to its inhibitory effect on the synthesis of this potent vasoconstrictor and smooth muscle mitogen (112–115).

IX. Estrogen and Pulmonary Vascular Function

The discussion above would suggest that estrogen should have a vasodilator effect in the pulmonary circulation, given the evidence for estrogen-stimulated nitric oxide release from endothelial cells as well as clinical observations suggesting that estrogen may lower endothelin levels in plasma (116). However, estrogen has been reported to have pulmonary constrictor effects in experimental preparations. In the perfused rat lung, a supraphysiological concentration of 17β-estradiol (10 nM) or diethylstilbestrol (10 nM) increased the pulmonary perfusion pressure by approximately 60% in response to the thromboxane mimic U46619 (117). Diethylstilbestrol, but not estradiol, increased the pressure by approximately 70% in response to angiotensin II. Ovariectomy diminished the contribution of estradiol on the pressor effect of thromboxane in this series of experiments.

On the other hand, 17β-estradiol 0.001 mg/kg/day administered to female dogs for 2 weeks significantly reduced the elevation in pulmonary pressure and slightly increased the elevation in pulmonary vascular resistance during hypoxia compared with untreated dogs (118). Progesterone treatment did not affect the pulmonary vasoconstrictor response to hypoxia in this study. Other investigators found that estradiol (10–20 mg intramuscularly 2–5 days prior to study) attenuated the pulmonary vasoconstrictor response to hypoxia in the isolated perfused lung from juvenile female or male sheep (119). This effect of estrogen was prevented by pretreatment with indomethacin, suggesting estrogen-stimulated release of vasodilating prostaglandins (120).

X. Future Directions for Research

At the molecular level, further understanding of the control of smooth muscle gene transcription by the estrogen receptor complex, including variations in the transcriptional activation domains and the role of transcriptional activator proteins and nuclear oncoproteins, is required in order to understand regulation of transcription by estrogen and the tissue, cell type, and gene specificity of this activity. Mutations in any of these transcriptional regulatory components could result in inappropriate activation by estrogen of genes responsible for smooth muscle proliferation. Also of research interest would be determination of interactions between growth factor activation of signal transduction pathways and ligand or nonligand activation of the nuclear and membrane estrogen receptors. As progesterone downregulates estrogen receptors in uterine smooth muscle, effects of progesterone on estrogen receptor density and activity in smooth muscle from lung tissue should be determined, particularly given the anecdotal success of this hormone in some women with lymphangioleimyomatosis (2). Experiments should also be performed to determine the mechanism of the inhibitory effect of supraphysiological concentrations of estrogen on smooth muscle cell growth when stimulated by growth factors and cytokines in culture or following vascular injury in animal models.

Because of the inhibitory effects of nitric oxide on smooth muscle cell growth and proliferation, studies of nitric oxide synthetic capacity in various lung cell components (epithelium, smooth muscle, endothelium) and the inhibitory responsiveness of pulmonary smooth muscle to nitric oxide would be of considerable interest, as would determination of sex hormone effects on the pulmonary endothelial and epithelial synthesis of nitric oxide and endothelin-1. Therapies such as inhaled nitric oxide and L-arginine should be considered for clinical study if inhibitory effects of nitric oxide on smooth muscle proliferation can be demonstrated.

References

1. Kitaichi M, Nishimura K, Itoh H, Izumi T. Pulmonary lymphangioleiomyomatosis: a report of 46 patients including a clinicopathological study of prognostic factors. Am J Respir Crit Care Med 1995; 151:527–533.
2. Taylor JR, Ryu J, Colby TV, Raffin TA. Lymphangioleiomyomatosis. Clinical course in 32 patients. N Engl J Med 1990; 323:1254–1260.
3. Berger U, Khaghani A, Pomerance A, Yacoub MH, Coombes RC. Pulmonary lymphangioleiomyomatosis and steroid receptors. An immunocytochemical study. Am J Clin Pathol 1990; 93:609–614.
4. Wagenvoort CA, Waagenvoort N. Primary pulmonary hypertension. A pathological study of the lung vessels in 156 clinically diagnosed cases. Circulation 1970; 42:1163–1184.
5. Rich S, Dantzker DR, Ayres S, Bergofsky EH, Brundage BH, Detre KM, Fishman AP, Goldring RM, Groves RM, Groves BM, Koerner SK, Levy PC, Reid LM, Vreim CE, Williams GW. Primary pulmonary hypertension. A national prospective study. Ann Intern Med 1987; 107:216–223.
6. Tancredi RG. Pulmonary vascular disease: primary pulmonary hypertension. Cardiovasc Clin 1992; 22:113–124.
7. Evans RM. The steroid and thyroid hormone receptor superfamily. Science 1988; 240:889–895.
8. Beato M. Gene regulation by steroid hormones. Cell 1989; 56:335–344.

9. Kumar V, Green S, Stack G, Berry M, Jin J-R, Chambon P. Functional domains of the human estrogen receptor. Cell 1987; 51:941–951.
10. Tsai M-J, O'Malley BW. Molecular mechanisms of action of steroid/thyroid receptor superfamily members. Annu Rev Biochem 1994; 63:451–486.
11. Hard T, Gustafsson J-A. Structure and function of the DNA-binding domain of the glucocorticoid receptor and other members of the nuclear receptor supergene family. Acc Chem Res 1993; 26:644–650.
12. Chambraud B, Berry M, Redeuilh G, Chambon P, Baulieu E-E. Several regions of the human estrogen receptor are involved in the formation of receptor–heat shock protein 90 complexes. J Biol Chem 1990; 265:20686–20691.
13. Kumar V, Chambon P. The estrogen receptor binds tightly to its response element as a ligand-induced homodimer. Cell 1988; 55:145–156.
14. Onate SA, Tsai SY, Tsai M-J, O'Malley BW. Sequence and characterization of a coactivator for the steroid hormone receptor superfamily. Science 1995; 270:1354–1357.
15. Mclnerney EM, Tsai M-J, O'Malley BW, Katzenellenbogen BS. Analysis of estrogen receptor transcriptional enhancement by a nuclear hormone receptor coactivator. Proc Natl Acad Sci USA 1996; 93:10069–10073.
16. Smith CL, Onate SA, Tsai M-J, O'Malley BW. CREB binding protein acts synergistically with steroid receptor coactivator-1 to enhance steroid receptor-dependent transcription. Proc Natl Acad Sci USA 1996; 93:8884–8888.
17. Gaub M-P, Bellard M, Scheuer I, Chambon P, Sassone-Corsi P. Activation of the ovalbumin by the estrogen receptor involves the Fos-Jun complex. Cell 1990; 63:1267–1276.
18. Weisz A, Rosales R. Identification of an estrogen response element upstream of the human c-fos gene that binds the estrogen receptor and the AP-1 transcription factor. Nucl Acids Res 1990; 18:5097–5106.
19. Krishnan V, Wang X, Safe S. Estrogen receptor-Spl complexes mediate estrogen-induced cathepsin D gene expression in MCF-7 human breast cancer cells. J Biol Chem 1994; 269:15912–15917.
20. Yang-Yen H-F, Chambard J-C, Sun Y-L, Smeal T, Schmidt TJ, Drovin J, Karin M. Transcriptional interference between c-tun and the glucocorticold receptor: mutual inhibition of DNA binding due to direct protein-protein interactions. Cell 1990; 62:1205–1215.
21. Ray A, Prefontaine KE, Ray P. Down-modulation of interleukin-6 gene expression by 17β-estradiol in the absence of high affinity DNA binding by the estrogen receptor. J Biol Chem 1994; 269:12940-12946.
22. Horowitz KB, Horowitz LD. Canine vascular tissues are targets for androgens, estrogens, progestins, and glucocorticoids. J Clin Invest 1982; 69:750–758.
23. Chobanian AV. Effects of sex hormones on phospholipid, RNA and protein metabolism in the arterial intima. J Atheroscl Res 1968; 8:763–775.
24. Milgrom E, Thi L, Atger M, Baulieu E-E. Mechanisms regulating the concentration and the conformation of progesterone receptor(s) in the uterus. J Biol Chem 1973; 248:6366–6374.
25. Vu Hai MT, Logeat F, Warembourg M, Milgrom E. Hormonal control of progesterone receptors. Ann NY Acad Sci 1977; 286:199–209.

26. Bronson FH, Hamilton TH. A comparison of nucleic acid synthesis in the mouse oviduct and uterus: interactions between estradiol and progesterone. Biol Reprod 1972; 6:160–167.
27. Hsueh AJ, Peck EJ, Clark JH. Control of uterine estrogen receptor levels by progesterone. Endocrinology 1976; 98:438–444.
28. Bergman MD, Schachter BS, Karelus K, Combatsiaris EP, Garcia T, Nelson J-F. Upregulation of the uterine estrogen receptor and its messenger ribonucleic acid during the mouse estrus cycle: the role of estradiol. Endocrinology 1992; 130:1923–1930.
29. Caulin-Glaser T, Watson CA, Pardi R, Bender JR. Effects of 17β-estradiol on cytokine-induced endothelial cell adhesion molecule expression. J Clin Invest 1996 98:36–42.
30. Kuiper GGJM, Enmark E, Pelto-Huikko M, Nilsson S, Gustafssoll J-A. Cloning of a novel estrogen receptor expressed in rat prostate and ovary. Proc Natl Acad Sci USA 1996; 93:5925–5930.
31. Power RF, Mani SK, Codina J, Conneely OM, O'Malley BW. Dopaminergic and ligand-independent activation of steroid hormone receptors. Science 1991; 254:1636–1639.
32. Smith CL, Conneely OM, O'Malley BW. Modulation of the ligand-independent activation of the human estrogen receptor by hormone and antihormone. Proc Natl Acad Sci 1993; 90:6120–6124.
33. DiAugustine RP, Petrusz P, Bell GI, Brown CF, Korach KS, Melachlan JA, Teng CT. Influence of estrogens on mouse uterine epidermal growth factor precursor protein and messenger ribonucleic acid. Endocrinology 1988; 122:2355–2363.
34. Nelson KG, Takahashi T, Bossert NL, Walmer DK, McLachlan JA. Epidermal growth factor replaces estrogen in the stimulation of female genital-tract growth and differentiation. Proc Natl Acad Sci USA 1991; 88:21–25.
35. Nelson KG, Takahashi T, Lee DC, Luetteke NC, Bossert NL, Ross K, Eitzman BE, McLachlan JA. Transforming growth factor-α is a potential mediator of estrogen action in the mouse uterus. Endocrinology 1992; 131:1657–1664.
36. Smith CL, Conneely OM, O'Malley BW. Oestrogen receptor activation in the absence of ligand. Biochem Soc Trans 1995; 23:935–939.
37. Ignar-Trowbridge DM, Nelson KG, Bidwell MC, Curtis SW, Washburn TF, McLachlan JA, Korach KS. Coupling of dual signaling pathways: epidermal growth factor action involves the estrogen receptor. Proc Natl Acad Sci USA 1992; 89:4658–4662.
38. Cho H, Katzenellenbogen BS. Synergistic activation of estrogen receptor-mediated transcription by estradiol and protein kinase activators. Mol Endocrinol 1993; 7:441–452.
39. Ignar-Trowbridge DM, Pimentel M, Parker MG, McLachlan JA, Korach KS. Peptide growth factor cross-talk with the estrogen receptor requires the A/B domain and occurs independently of protein kinase C or estradiol. Endocrinology 1996; 137:1735–1744.
40. Dufy B, Vincent J-D, Fleury H, Du Pasquier P, Gourdji D, Tixier-Vidal A. Membrane effects of thyrotropin-releasing hormone and estrogen shown by intracellular recording from pituitary cells. Science 1979; 204:509–511.

41. Pietras RJ, Szego CM. Metabolic and proliferative responses to estrogen by hepatocytes selected for plasma membrane binding-sites for estradiol-17β. J Cell Physiol 1979; 98:145–160.
42. Nenci I, Marchetti E, Marzola A. Affinity cytochemistry visualizes specific estrogen binding sites on the plasma membrane of breast cancer cells. J Steroid Biochem 1981; 14:1139–1146.
43. Berthois Y, Pourreau-Schneider N, Gandilhon P, Mittre H, Tubiana N, Martin PM. Estradiol membrane binding sites on human breast cancer cell lines. Use of fluorescent estradiol conjugate to demonstrate plasma membrane binding systems. J Steroid Biochem 1981; 25:963–972.
44. Pappas TC, Gametchu B, Watson CS. Membrane estrogen receptors identified by multiple antibody labeling and impeded-ligand binding. FASEB J 1995; 9:404–410.
45. Pappas TC, Gametchu B, Yannariello-Brown J, Collins TJ, Watson CS. Membrane estrogen receptors in GH3/B6 cells are associated with rapid estrogen-induced release of prolactin. Endocrine 1994; 2:813–822.
46. Farhat MY, Abi-Younes S, Dingaan B, Vargas R, Ramwell PW. Estradiol increases cyclic adenosine monophosphate in rat pulmonary vascular smooth muscle cells by a nongenomic mechanism. J Pharmacol Exp Ther 1996; 276:652–657.
47. Wehling M, Christ M, Theisen K. Membrane receptors for aldosterone: a novel pathway for mineralocorticoid action. Am J Physiol 1992; 263:E974–E979.
48. Christ M, Douwes K, Eisen C, Bechtner G, Theisen K, Wehling M. Rapid effects of aldosterone on sodium transport in rat vascular smooth muscle cells. Hypertension 1995; 25:117–123.
49. Christ M, Meyer C, Sippel K, Wehling M. Rapid aldosterone signaling in vascular smooth muscle cells: involvement of phospholipase C, diacylglycerol and protein kinase Cα. Biochem Biophys Res Commun 1995; 213:123–129.
50. Wehling M, Ulsenheimer A, Schneider M, Neylon C, Christ M. Rapid effects of aldersterone on free intracellular calcium in vascular smooth muscle and endothelial cells: subcellular localization of calcium release by single cell imaging. Biochem Biophys Res Commun 1994; 204:475–481.
51. Wehling M, Neylon CB, Fullerton M, Bobik A, Funder JM. Nongenomic effects of aldosterone on intracellular calcium in vascular smooth muscle cells. Circ Res 1995; 76:973–979.
52. Morley P, Whitfield JF, Vanderhyden BC, Tsang BK, Schwartz J-L. A new, nongenomic estrogen action: The rapid release of intracellular calcium. Endocrinology 1992; 131:1305–1312.
53. Moncada S, Palmer RM, Higgs EA. Nitric oxide: physiology, pathophysiology, and pharmacology. Pharmacol Rev 1991; 43:109–142.
54. Caulin-Glaser TL, Sessa W, Sarrel P, Bender J. The effect of 17β-estradiol on human endothelial cell nitric oxide production (abstr). Circulation 1994; 90:I-30.
55. Gilligan DM, Quyyumi AA, Cannon RO. Effects of physiological levels of estrogen on coronary vasomotor function in postmenopausal women. Circulation 1994; 89:2545–2551.
56. Gilligan DM, Badar DM, Panza JA, Quyyumi AA, Cannon RO. Acute vascular effects of estrogen in postmenopausal women. Circulation 1994; 90:786–791.

57. Nakhla AM, Rosner W. Stimulation of prostate cancer growth by androgens and estrogens through the intermediacy of sex hormone-binding globulin. Endocrinology 1996; 137:4126–4129.
58. Gips SJ, Goldschmidt-Clermont PJ. Short term exposure to 17β-estradiol stimulates tyrosine phosphorylation of ppl25 focal adhesion kinase in cultured endothelial cells (abstr). Circulation 1994; 90:I–87.
59. Malinow MR, Moguilevsky JA, Lema B, Bur GE. Vascular and extravascular radioactivity after injection of estradiol 6,7[^{3}H] in the human being. J Clin Endocrinol Metab 1963; 23:306–310.
60. Losordo DW, Kearney BA, Kim EA, Jekanowski J, Isner JM. Variable expression of the estrogen receptor in normal and atherosclerotic coronary arteries of premenopausal women. Circulation 1994; 89:1501–1510.
61. Karas RH, Patterson BL, Mendelsohn ME. Human vascular smooth muscle cells contain functional estrogen receptor. Circulation 1994; 89:1943–1950.
62. Koike H, Karas RH, Baur WE, O'Donnell TF, Mendelsohn ME. Differential-display polymerase chain reaction identifies nucleophosmin as an estrogen-regulated gene in human vascular smooth muscle cells. J Vasc Surg 1996; 23:477–482.
63. Venkov CD, Rankin AB, Vaughan DE. Identification of authentic estrogen receptor in cultured endothelial cells. A potential mechanism for steroid hormone regulation of endothelial function. Circulation 1996; 94:727–733.
64. Kim-Schulze S, McGowan KA, Hubchak SC, Cid MC, Martin MB, Kleinman, HK, Greene GL, Schnaper HW. Expression of an estrogen receptor by human coronary artery and umbilical vein endothelial cells. Circulation 1996; 94:1402–1407.
65. Guenther AE, Conley AJ, Van Orden DE, Farley DB, Ford SP. Structural and mechanical changes of uterine arteries during pregnancy in the pig. J Anim Sci 1988; 66:3144–3152.
66. Orimo A, Inoue S, Ikegama A, Hosoi T, Akishita M, Ouchi Y, Maramatsu M, Orimo H. Vascular smooth muscle cells as a target for estrogen. Biochem Biophys Res Commun 1993; 195:730–736.
67. Lippman M, Bolan G, Huff K. The effects of estrogens and antiestrogens on hormone-responsive human breast cancer in long-term tissue culture. Cancer Res 1976; 36:4595–4601.
68. Chalbos D, Vignon F, Keydar I, Rochefort H. Estrogens stimulate cell proliferation and induce secretary proteins in a human breast cancer cell line ($T_{47}D$). J Clin Endocr Metab 1982; 55:276–283.
69. Nishizawa Y, Sato B, Miyashita Y, Tsukuda S, Hirose T, Kishimoto S, Matsumoto K. Autocrine regulation of cell proliferation by estradiol and hydroxytamoxifen of transformed mouse Leydig cells in serum-free culture. Endocrinology 1988; 122:227–235.
70. Francavilla A, Polimeno L, DiLeo A, Barone M, Ore P, Coetzee M, Eagon P, Makowka L, Ambrosino G, Mazzaferro V, Starzl TE. The effect of estrogen and tamoxifen on hepatocyte proliferation in vivo and in vitro. Hepatology 1989; 9:614–620.
71. Keyes LE, Moore LG, Walchak SJ, Dempsey EC. Pregnancy-stimulated growth of vascular smooth muscle cells: importance of protein kinase C-dependent synergy

between estrogen and platelet-derived growth factor. J Cell Physiol 1996; 166:22–32.
72. Fischer-Dzoga K, Wissler RW, Vesselinovitch D. The effect of estradiol on the proliferation of rabbit aortic medial tissue culture cells induced by hyperlipemic serum. Exp Mol Pathol 1983; 39:355–363.
73. Vargas R, Wroblewska B, Rego A, Hatch J, Ramwell PW. Oestradiol inhibits smooth muscle cell proliferation of pig coronary artery. Br J Pharmacol 1993; 109:612–617.
74. Espinoza E, Oemar BS, Luscher TF. 17β-Estradiol and smooth muscle cell proliferation in aortic cells of male and female rats. Biochem Biophys Res Commun 1996; 221:8–14.
75. Dai-Do D, Espinosa E, Liu G, Rabelink TJ, Julmy F, Yang Z, Mahler F, Luscher TF. 17β-estradiol inhibits proliferation and migration of human vascular smooth muscle cells: similar effects in cells from postmenopausal females and in males. Cardiovasc Res 1996; 32:980–985.
76. Farhat MY, Vargas R, Dingaan B, Ramwell PW. In vitro effect of oestradiol on thymidine uptake in pulmonary vascular smooth muscle cell: role of endothelium. Br J Pharmacol 1992; 107:679–683.
77. Sato B, Nishizawa Y, Maeda Y, Noma K, Kishimoto S, Matsumoto K. Stimulatory and inhibitory pathways for steroid receptor to regulate gene expression in hormone-responsive cells. In Sakamoto Y, Isohashi F, eds. Glucocorticoid Hormone: Mechanism of Action. Tokyo: Japan Scientific Society Press, 19XX:175–187.
78. Ross R. The pathogenesis of atherosclerosis: a perspective for the 1990s. Nature 1993; 362:801–809.
79. Wuest J, Day TJ, Edwards JE. The degree of coronary atherosclerosis in bilaterally oophorectomized women. Circulation 1953; 7:801–808.
80. Novac ER, Williams TJ. Autopsy comparison of cardiovascular changes in castrated and normal women. Am J Obstet Gynecol 1960; 80:863–872.
81. Colditz GA, Willett WC, Stampfer MJ, Rosner B, Speizer FE, Hennekens CH. Menopause and the risk of coronary heart disease in women. N Engl J Med 1987; 316:1105–1110.
82. Foegh MI, Asotra S, Howell NM, Ramwell PW. Estradiol inhibition of arterial neointimal hyperplasia after balloon injury. J Vasc Surg 1994; 19:722–726.
83. Rhee CY, Spaet TH, Stemerman MB, Lajam F, Shiang HH, Caruso E, Litwak RS. Estrogen supression of surgically induced vascular intimal hyperplasia in rabbits. J Lab Clin Med 1977; 90:77–84.
84. Foegh MEL, Khirabadi BS, Hakanishi T, Vargas R, Ramwell PW. Estradiol protects against experimental transplant atherosclerosis. Transplant Proc 1987; 19:90–95.
85. Cheng LP, Kuwahara M, Jacobsson J, Foegh ML. Inhibition of hyperplasia and macrophage infiltration by estradiol in aorta allografts. Transplantation 1991; 52:967–972.
86. Chen S-J, Li H, Durand J, Oparil S, Chen Y-F. Estrogen reduces myointimal proliferation after balloon injury of rat carotid artery. Circulation 1996; 93:577–584.
87. Sullivan TR, Karas RH, Aronovitz M, Faller GT, Ziar JP, Smith JJ, O'Donnell TF, Mendelsohn ME. Estrogen inhibits the response-to-injury in a mouse carotid artery model. J Clin Invest 1995; 96:2482–2488.

88. Morales DE, McGowan KA, Grant DS, Maheshwari S, Bhartiya D, Cid MC, Kleinman HK, Schnaper HW. Estrogen promotes angiogenic activity in human umbilical vein endothelial cells in vitro and in a murine model. Circulation 1995; 91:755–763.
89. Krasinski KL, Spyridopoulos I, Asahara T, vander Zee R, Isner JM, Losordo DW. Estradiol accelerates endothelial recovery after arterial injury. Circulation 1997; 95:1768–1772.
90. Hayashi T, Yamada K, Esaki T, Kuzuya M, Satake S, Ishikawa T, Hidaka H, Igushi A. Estrogen increases endothelial nitric oxide by a receptor-mediated system. Biochem Biophys Res Commun 1995; 214:847–855.
91. Hishikawa K, Nakaki T, Marumo T, Suzuki H, Kato R, Saruta T. Up-regulation of nitric oxide synthase by estradiol in human aortic endothelial cells. FEBS Lett 1995; 360:291–293.
92. Miyahara K, Kawamoto T, Sase K, Yui Y, Toda K, Yang L-X, Hattori R, Aoyama T, Yamamoto Y, Doi Y, Ogoshi S, Hashimoto K, Kawal C, Sasayama S, Shizuta Y. Cloning and structural characterization of the human endothelial nitric-oxide-synthase gene. Eur J Biochem 1994; 223:719–726.
93. Venema RC, Nishida K, Alexander RW, Harrison DG, Murphy TJ, Organization of the bovine gene encoding the endothelial nitric oxide synthase. Biochim Biophys Acta 1994; 218:413–420.
94. Garg UC, Hassid A. Nitric oxide-generating vasodilators and 8-bromo-cyclic guanosine monophosphate inhibit mitogenesis and proliferation of cultured rat vascular smooth muscle cells. J Clin Invest 1989; 83:1774–1777.
95. Nakaki T, Nakayama M, Kato R. Inhibition by nitric oxide and nitric oxide-producing vasodilators of DNA synthesis in vascular smooth muscle cells. Eur J Pharmacol 1990; 189:347–353.
96. Cornwell TL, Arnold E, Boerth NJ, Lincoln TM. Inhibition of smooth muscle cell growth by nitric oxide and activation of cAMP-dependent protein kinase by cGMP. Am J Physiol 1994; 267:C1405–C1413.
97. Sarkar R, Meinberg EG, Stanley JC, Gordon D, Webb RC. Nitric oxide reversibly inhibits the migration of cultured vascular smooth muscle cells. Circ Res 1996; 78:225–230.
98. Kolpakov V, Gordon D, Kulik TJ. Nitric oxide-generating compounds inhibit total protein and collagen synthesis in cultured vascular smooth muscle cells. Circ Res 1995; 76:305–309.
99. Tarry WC, Makhoul RG. L-arginine improves endothelium-dependent vasorelaxation and reduces intimal hyperplasia after balloon angioplasty. Arterioscler Throm 1994; 14:938–943.
100. McNamara DB, Bedi B, Aurora H, Tena L, Ignarro LJ, Kadowitz PJ, Akers DL. L-arginine inhibits balloon catheter-induced intimal hyperplasia. Biochem Biophys Res Commun 1993; 193:291–296.
101. von der Leyen HE, Gibbons GH, Morishita R, Lewis NP, Zwang L, Nakajima M, Kaneda Y, Cooke JP, Dzau VJ. Gene therapy inhibiting neointimal vascular lesion: in vivo transfer of endothelial cell nitric oxide synthase gene. Proc Natl Acad Sci USA 1995; 92:1137–1141.
102. Busse R, Muisch A. Induction of nitric oxide synthase by cytokines in vascular smooth muscle cells. FEBS Lett 1990; 275:87–90.

103. Scott-Burden T, Schini VB, Elizondo E, Junquero DC, Vanhoutte PM. Platelet-derived growth factor supresses and fibroblast growth factor enhances cytokine-induced production of nitric oxide by cultured smooth muscle cells. Effects on cell proliferation. Circ Res 1992; 71:1088–1100.
104. Fukuo K, Inoue T, Morimoto S, Nakahashi T, Yasuda O, Kitano S, Sasada R, Ogihara T. Nitric oxide mediates cytotoxicity and basic fibroblast growth factor release in cultured vascular smooth muscle cells. A possible mechanism of neovascularization in atherosclerotic plaques. J Clin Invest 1995; 95:669–676.
105. Giaid A, Saleh D. Reduced expression of endothelial nitric oxide synthase in the lungs of patients with pulmonary hypertension. N Engl J Med 1995; 333:214–221.
106. Cooper CJ, Landzberg MJ, Anderson TJ, Charbonneau F, Creager MH, Ganz P, Selwyn AP. Role of nitric oxide in the local regulation of pulmonary vascular resistance in humans. Circulation 1996; 93:266–271.
107. Blitzer ML, Loh E, Roddy M-A, Stamler JS, Creager MA. Endothelium-derived nitric oxide regulates systemic and pulmonary vascular resistance during acute hypoxia in humans. J Am Coll Cardiol 1996; 28:591–596.
108 Kouyoumdjian C, Adnot S, Levame M, Eddahibi S, Bousbaa H, Ratrestin B. Continuous inhalation of nitric oxide protects against development of pulmonary hypertension in chronically hypoxic rats. J Clin Invest 1994; 94:578–584.
109. Eddahibi S, Adnot S, Carville C, Blouquit Y, Raffestin B. L-arginine restores endothelium-dependent relaxation in pulmonary circulation of chronically hypoxic rats. Am J Physiol 1992; 263:L194–L200.
110. Stewart DJ, Levy RD, Cernacek P, Langleben D. Increased plasma endothelin-1 in pulmonary hypertension: marker or mediator of disease? Ann Intern Med 1991; 114:464–469.
111. Giaid A, Yanagisawa M, Langleben D, Michael RP, Levy R, Shennib H, Kimura S, Masaki T, Duguid WP, Steward DJ. Expression of endothelin-1 in the lungs of patients with pulmonary hypertension. N Engl J Med 1993; 328:1732–1739.
112. Boulanger C, Luscher TF. Release of endothelin from the porcine aorta. Inhibition by endothelium-derived nitric oxide. J Clin Invest 1990; 85:587–590.
113. Yanagisawa M, Kurihara H, Kimura S, Tomobe Y, Kobayashi M, Mitsui Y, Yazaki Y, Goto K, Masaki T. A novel potent vasoconstrictor peptide produced by vascular endothelial cells. Nature 1988; 332:411–415.
114. Dubin D, Pratt RE, Cooke JP, Dzau VJ. Endothelin, a potent vasoconstrictor, is a vascular smooth muscle mitogen. J Vasc Med Biol 1989; 1:150–154.
115. Hirata Y, Takagi Y, Fukuda Y, Marumo F. Endothelin is a potent mitogen for rat vascular smooth muscle cells. Atherosclerosis 1989; 78:225–228.
116. Polderman KH, Stehouwer CD, van Kamp GJ, Dekker GA, Verheugt FW, Gooren LJ. Influence of sex hormones on plasma endothelin levels. Ann Intern Med 1993; 118:429–432.
117. Farhat MY, Ramwell PW. Estradiol potentiates the vasopressor response of the perfused rat lung to the thromboxane mimic U-46619. J Pharmacol Exp Ther 1992; 261:686–691.
118. Moore LG, Reeves JT. Pregnancy blunts pulmonary vascular reactivity in dogs. Am J Physiol 1980; 239:H297–H301.

119. Wetzel RC, Zacur HA, Sylvester JT. Effect of puberty and estradiol on hypoxic vasomotor response in isolated sheep lungs. J Appl Physiol 1984; 56:1199–1203.
120. Sylvester JT, Gordon JB, Malamet RL, Wetzel RC. Prostaglandins and estradiol-induced attenuation of hypoxic pulmonary vasoconstriction. Chest 1995; 88(suppl):252S–254S.

19

Lymphangioleiomyomatosis and Leiomyoma

Possibility of Shared Genetic Origins?

FRANCIS X. McCORMACK, TERESA A. SMOLAREK, and ANIL G. MENON

University of Cincinnati Medical Center
Cincinnati, Ohio

I. Background

A. Lymphangioleiomyomatosis

Lymphangioleiomyomatosis (LAM) is a rare interstitial lung disease that predominantly affects young women of childbearing age (1). The prevalence of the disease is not accurately known, but fewer than 150 cases had been reported prior to 1993 (2). The mean survival time following diagnosis has been estimated at less than 10 years (2), but recent reports have been somewhat more optimistic (3).

The most common symptom of LAM is dyspnea upon exertion, which is frequently accompanied by the development of spontaneous pneumothorax, chylothorax, or hemoptysis. The chest x-ray is often normal or may show cystic changes or reticular densities, but the most definitive changes are typically found on high-resolution chest computed tomography (CT) scans where multiple thin-walled cysts are seen throughout the lung parenchyma. Over half of LAM patients also have renal and retroperitoneal angiomyolipomas (4,5).

The diagnosis of LAM is established by thoracoscopic or open lung biopsy, or occasionally by transbronchial biopsy (1). Histologic examination of lung tissue shows extensive proliferation of smooth muscle–like cells of uncertain origin along bronchovascular axes. The infiltrating cells expand alveolar septa and line the walls of cystic spaces. In other areas, more nodular lesions are formed from fascicles of interdigitating smooth muscle cells (6). Obstruction of lymphatic channels, blood vessels, and airways is readily demonstrated, and these pathological findings correlate with the clinical manifestations of chylous effusions, hemoptysis, and airflow obstruction (7). Immunohistochemistry has shown that the cells from the LAM lesion stain positively for α-smooth muscle actin (α-SMA) (Fig. 1a), and less frequently desmin antibodies, markers consistent with myoid lineage (1,8–10) (Fig. 1a). We have determined that these cells are positive for the antibody HUC-1 (Fig. 1b), which recognizes an epitope common to all muscle actins (11). Electron microscopy also demonstrates features that are consistent with smooth muscle cells, but in addition reveals abundant endoplastic reticulum, which is more characteristic of fibroblasts (12). The smooth muscle cells of the LAM lesion stain strongly with an antibody to the intracellular transforming growth factor-β1 (TGF-β1) (13), and there is preliminary evidence that the platelet-derived growth factor receptor (PDGF-R) is abundantly expressed in LAM cells (14). One of the most unusual but consistent findings in LAM is that the lung and kidney lesions are positively stained using the monoclonal antibody HMB-45 (1,10,15–18) (Fig. 1c). HMB-45, used in the diagnosis of melanoma, has been shown to react with immature melanosome (19,20). In both normal and diseased lung, HMB-45 is very specific for the LAM lesion (16). The antigen recognized by HMB-45 is a protein called gp100, which, like its nearly identical counterpart pMel 17, was identified by screening a melanoma library (21).

Although there is no clear evidence for a hormonal abnormality, therapy for LAM has focused on estrogen reduction because of the demographics of the population affected and anecdotal reports of response to antiestrogen therapies (2,22). Standard treatment includes oophorectomy and/or progesterone therapy. Single lung transplantation has become an established therapeutic option in patients with advanced disease (23). Recurrence of LAM has been reported in the transplanted lung of at least two patients, suggesting that a systemic component may be involved in the pathogenesis of LAM (24,25).

B. Uterine Leiomyomata and LAM

The clinical presentation and cellular biology of uterine leiomyomata (UL), the most common benign neoplasm of smooth muscle origin, have interesting parallels to LAM. The UL are often multiple, vary considerably in size, and occur in approximately 20–30% of women over the age of 30 years (26,27). The tumors affect all races and do not to appear to be familial, although this has not yet been conclusively determined. In the United States alone, approximately 175,000

(27%) of the 650,000 hysterectomies performed annually are for the removal of uterine myomas.

The common symptoms of these tumors include pelvic pain and abnormal bleeding. Polycythemia, due to high levels of erythropoeitin resulting from arterial backpressure on renal parenchyma and an increased frequency of spontaneous abortion, are frequently reported sequela.

Leiomyomas are thought to be of mesenchymal origin, and although they are seen most often in the uterus, they also arise in the alimentary tract, the kidney, the skin, and the soft tissues of the oral cavity (26). The characteristic cellular pathology of leiomyoma involves the presence of interlacing fascicles of spindle-shaped or fusiform cells, indistinct cell borders, and an abundant eosinophilic cytoplasm. Because they are usually benign in nature, rapidly dividing cells and mitotic figures are rarely seen in these tumors. Based on histopathological features, leiomyoma are divided into three major categories: The first category comprises "typical" leiomyoma, which show a pattern of uniform smooth muscle cells containing elongated nuclei and small nucleoli arranged in whirled fascicles. Regions of fibrosis, cystic degeneration, and calcification are sometimes seen, though mitoses are rarely observed. The second category consists of "cellular" leiomyoma, which show dense, cellular fascicles, few cellular aberrations, and less than five mitoses per 10 high-powered fields. The third category consists of "atypical" leiomyoma (sometimes also called bizarre or symplastic leiomyoma). These tumors are characterized by large, hyperchromatic nuclei sometimes present in multiple copies in giant cells. Generally, five or fewer mitoses per 10 high-powered fields are seen on microscopic examination of these tumors. The distinction of an atypical, cellular or mitotically active leiomyoma from a leiomyosarcoma remains a difficult problem. Initially, a count of 10 mitotic figures in 10 high-powered fields was considered diagnostic for sarcoma. Subsequently, it was shown that a count of five tumors with atypical nuclei was diagnostic of sarcoma, and even later mitotic activity up to 15 per 10 high-power fields was consistent with a diagnosis of leiomyoma if nuclear atypicality was lacing (28). Occasionally even tumors that are "benign" by any of these criteria can metastasize, typically 5–10 years after a hysterectomy, to secondary sites in the lung or pelvic lymph nodes (29). The clinical presentation of benign metastasizing leiomyoma in the lung is occasionally confused with LAM.

Western blot and immunohistochemical analyses have been used to show that uterine leiomyomas, as well as the adjacent normal myometrium, are positive for smooth muscle differentiation markers, such as vinculin, desmin, α-smooth muscle actin, caldesmon, and calponin (30). Although some smooth muscle neoplasms, such as renal leiomyomas and leiomyosarcomas, have been shown to be positive for HMB-45 (31), UL are reportedly negative for this antibody (10).

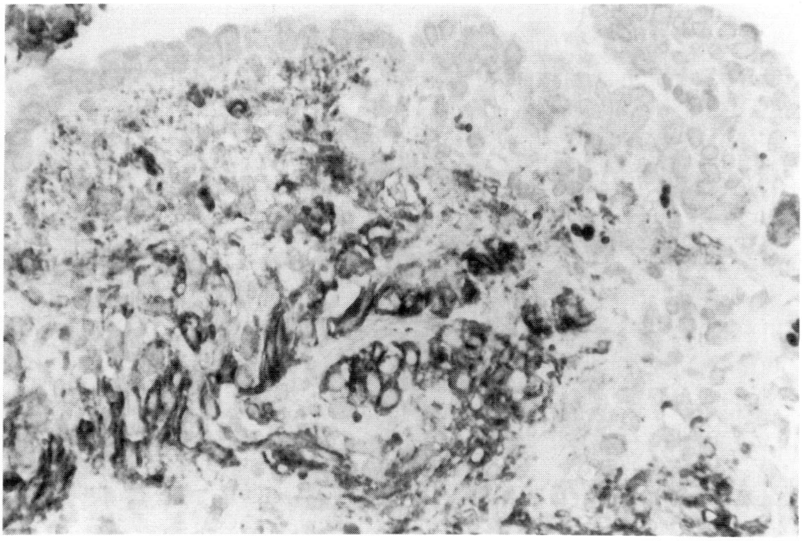

A

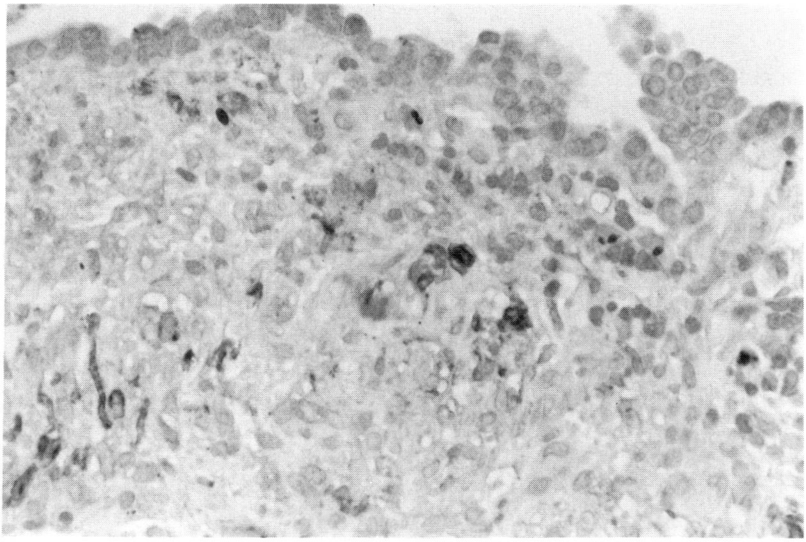

B

Figure 1 Cells from lymphangioleiomyomatosis stained with (A) α-smooth muscle actin antibody (Sigma), (B) HUC 1-1 (kindly provided by J. Lessard), (C) HMB-45 (Dako Corporation).

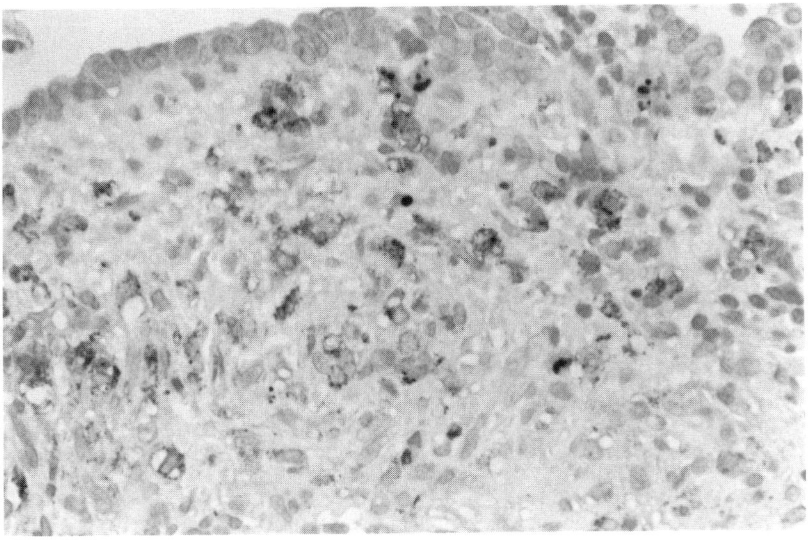

C

Figure 1 Continued.

Growth factors that have been implicated in the formation of UL include insulin-like growth factor (IGF), epidermal growth factor (EGF), PDGF, TGF-β, and basic fibroblast growth factor (bFGF) (32–36). Most recently, a major mitogen for human smooth muscle–like cells called leiomyoma-derived growth factor (LDGF) was identified in uterine smooth muscle extracts (37).

Hormonal factors play an important role in both LAM and UL. The occurrence of UL and LAM is largely restricted to the years between menarche and menopause. It has been reported that contraceptive use (38) and pregnancy (39) exacerbate UL in some cases, as is true for LAM. Conversely, antiestrogen therapies such as oophorectomy and progesterone administration have been reported to decrease the size of the lesions in both diseases (22,40). In some but not all of UL and LAM lesions, estrogen and progesterone receptors have been demonstrated by immunohistochemical analysis (8,41–43). It is not clear whether patients with LAM have an increased incidence of UL when compared to normal controls, although attempts to define such correlations have been reported (44).

C. Tuberous Sclerosis, UL, and LAM

There are several interesting phenotypic similarities between LAM and tuberous sclerosis (TSC). About 2.5% of patients with TSC present with a lung lesion that is indistinguishable from that which occurs in LAM (43). The cystic lung disease occurs almost exclusively in females after menarche (45), with an average age of onset of 33–35 years in both disease (2,22). Like LAM, common complications of TSC lung disease include pneumothorax and chylous effusions, and most patients with TSC have angiomyolipomas. The abnormal proliferating cells in the lungs and kidneys of patients with TSC also stain with the HMB-45 antibody (46). Thus, although patients with pulmonary TSC almost invariably also have skin, eye, and brain involvement that do not occur in LAM patients, the shared clinical features have led many to speculate that LAM is the forme fruste of TSC (4,17,45). Rarely, women who present with LAM and no peripheral manifestation of TSC are found to have calcified cerebral lesions suggestive of TSC on head CT (F. McCormack, unpublished observation). These patients almost certainly represent incomplete penetration of TSC. Two genes have been implicated in TSC (47), both of which act as tumor growth suppressors (48,49). The gene for the first is located on chromosome 9 at 9q34 (TSC1) and has not been identified. The second gene is on chromosome 16, located at 16p 13.3 (TSC2). TSC2 encodes the protein tuberin (50), which may play a role in control of cell growth and/or endocytic processes (51). Genotyping of patients with familial TSC affected by lung disease will be an important advance in the understanding of TSC lung disease. We have received verbal reports of mutations in TSC2 in two patients with pulmonary TSC (Dr. V. Whittemore, National Tuberous Sclerosis Association, personal communication). Although UL are not a prominent feature of TSC, the Eker rat, which has a germline insertion in the TSC2 locus (52), develops spontaneous UL (33). The growth of smooth muscle cells derived from Eker rat UL is stimulated by estrogen and inhibited by tamoxifen (53). These observations provide evidence that hormonally responsive smooth muscle proliferation can result from mutations in a tumor suppressor gene.

D. Cytogenetics of UL and LAM

The genetics of UL is an active area of investigation that may ultimately yield insights into the mechanisms underlying unregulated growth of smooth muscle cells (54). Analyses of nonrandom inactivation of the X chromosome have shown that each UL within the uterus is a distinct clone (55,56). About 40–50% of all UL have structural chromosome rearrangements (57), which presumably arise by spontaneous somatic mutation. Six major cytogenetic groups have been identified, including deletion of 7q, trisomy 12, rearrangements involving 6q, l0q22, and 13q, and translocations between 12q and 14q [t(12;14)(q13-15;q24)] (58). A few of these genetic abnormalities may have relevance to LAM. A chromosomal deletion of 14q24 has been reported in the only karyotypic analysis of cells from a LAM lesion (59). This region is of particular interest, since it is the same locus involved in the t(12;14)(ql3-15;q24) reported in UL (58). In addition, the gene that encodes the HMB-45 epitope gp100 localizes to a region near chromosome 12ql3-14 (60). This region of chromosome 12 is also frequently rearranged in other benign mesenchymal tumors, and alterations in the level of expression of the high mobility group protein gene (HMGI-C) in this region have been identified in UL, pulmonary hamartoma, and lipoma (61). A second candidate locus is on chromosome 13. Deletions of chromosome 13 that would include the retinoblastoma gene locus (Rb) at 13ql4 have been previously reported in UL (62). Rb is an important tumor suppressor gene involved in cell cycle regulation. Mutations in Rb have been reported as early events in the development of a wide variety of tumors, such as osteosarcoma and bladder and lung carcinomas (reviewed in Ref. 63). Preliminary studies in our laboratory showed loss of heterozygosity at the Rb locus in two of five informative LJL cases tested, suggesting that Rb also may have a role in the etiology of UL (T. Smolarek, unpublished data).

II. Cytogenetic Analysis of LAM Cells

A. Hypothesis

Our hypothesis is that the genetic lesion causing LAM may be the same as that causing smooth muscle proliferation in leiomyoma. Several lines of evidence have been considered in formulating this hypothesis:

1. There is an abnormal proliferation of smooth muscle–like cells in both disorders.
2. Both disorders appear to be largely limited to females of reproductive age.
3. The LAM lesion and the leiomyoma lesion both show increased growth in response to estrogen and related hormones, indicating possible hormonal involvement in both disorders.
4. Aberrations in the same chromosomal regions (13q14 and 14q24) have been identified in both disorders. A marker for LAM (HMB-45) is located in 12ql3-15, a region frequently rearranged in UL.

In order to test this hypothesis, we are attempting to develop an in vitro system for the study of LAM. Dispersed cells from the LAM lungs removed at transplant have been grown in culture and clonally expanded. We report here the initial characterization and genetic analysis of LAM cell lines.

B. LAM Cell Lines

Lung tissues from seven patients with LAM were disaggregated using a collagenase/dispase solution and plated in RPMI with 16% FBS, MGM3 (a melanocyte growth media from Clonetics), or RPMI 1640 supplemented with SmGM3 (smooth muscle growth medium supplements from Clonetics). The heterogeneous

Table 1 Karyotype of Lymphangioleiomyomatosis Samples

Patient	Karyotype (passage number)
UCLAM2	46,XX (P1)
	46,XX,del(13)(q?14-21)[25]/
	46,XX[18](P13 and P14)
	46,XX (P13, flask 2-1)
UCLAM3	46,XX
UCLAM4	LAM4A: 46,XX
	LAM4B: 46,XX
UCLAM5	LAM5A: 45,XX,-22[3]/46,XX
	LAM5B: 46,XX
UCLAM6	46,XX
UCLAM7	46,XX
UCLAM22	46,XX

cell populations obtained, comprised of both normal and abnormal cells, were named UCLAM2, UCLAM3, UCLAM4, UCLAM5, UCLAM6, UCLAM7, and UCLAM22 (Table 1). In some cases, multiple tissues from a single patient were received and processed. The percentage of cells that stained positively for HMB-45 at the earliest culture passages was consistently very low and not enriched by clonal isolation and expansion of the HMB-45–positive cells. However, HMB-45–positive cells were detected as far out as passage 11, indicating that these cells can survive in culture. Cells from the LAM lesion may require special matrix or alternative cell culture conditions, as has been shown to be the case for other types of cells, such as lung epithelial cells (64). Metaphase cells from the mixed populations were analyzed at different cell passages. UCLAM3, UCLAM4A, UCLAM4B, UCLAM5B, UCLAM6, UCLAM7, and UCLAM 22 were karyotypically normal at early passage. In the case of UCLAM2, the cells were karyotypically normal at passage 1, but at passages 13 and 14 approximately 50% of the cells were identified with a partially deleted chromosome 13. A second flask, also at passage 13, was harvested and the cells were found to be karyotypically normal. Studies are underway to determine whether cells with the deleted chromosome 13 were present initially in the lesion or whether this abnormality was an artifact that arose in culture. Monosomy 22 was found in a small population of cells from UCLAM5A, and the relevance of this abnormality is under investigation. It is likely that the majority of the cells that were karyotyped were representative of normal cells within the lung and not cells from the lesion, based on the low percentage of HMB-45–positive cells identified in culture. The conclusions that can be drawn from these efforts to determine karyotypes are: (1) no recurrent constitutional karyotypic rearrangements were evident in the metaphase spreads from the seven individuals that we have examined to date; (2) unlike UL, which are well-circumscribed smooth muscle proliferative lesions, and which show recurrent karyotypic abnormalities at detectable frequencies, LAM lesions are generally disseminated and therefore less easily karyotyped. Therefore, disaggregation of the cells from LAM lung is not the method of choice when processing these tissues for karyotypic analysis, and alternative approaches should be considered.

To date there have been no reports of a consistent karyotypic abnormality in LAM cells and we have not detected, in any of the UCLAM cell lines, any deletions of chromosome 14 as reported in one LAM patient by Popper et al. (59). It is possible that the lack of chromosomal abnormalities may be due to the mixed population of cells being examined, or that the karyotypically normal cells have a growth advantage and are therefore overrepresented in the genetic analysis. The significance of the terminal deletion of chromosome 13 in UCLAM2, with a breakpoint estimated between 13q14-21, is not clear. This deletion may involve the Rb locus but does not appear to interrupt the BRCA2 gene locus at 13q12-13, which is involved in breast cancer susceptibility (65) and tumors of the prostate, ovary, cervix, colon, and ureter (66). Deletions of chromosome 13 that would include the Rb gene locus at 13ql4 have been described in UL (54). If this deletion in UCLAM2 is not an artifact of cell culture, then it is possible that Rb may have a role in the development of LAM. Certainly, the karyotypic analysis of cells from LAM lesions is a subject for much more detailed analysis.

III. Summary

The investigation of the pathogenesis of LAM has been hindered by the absence of representative cell lines or an appropriate animal model. Because of the rarity of the illness, obtaining clinical specimens for research purposes is logistically difficult. Until these reagents have been collected and characterized, utilizing related model systems may provide the most practical means of obtaining useful information. Uterine leiomyomas, in rodents and in humans, provide an attractive model of hormonally dependent smooth muscle proliferation that may have relevance to LAM.

IV. Future Directions

Our primary objective is to develop an in vitro model that will be useful for the study of LAM. We will continue our attempts to isolate cell lines from LAM tissue obtained at transplant and to maintain the expression of the LAM cell phenotype using a variety of matrix and soluble factors. Karyotypic analysis of clonally derived LAM cell lines promises to yield more definitive results than we have been able to achieve to date. If cell lines can be established, the effects of hormonal manipulation on cell growth in culture and on the development and progression of LAM cell tumors in xenografted nude mice will be determined.

References

1. Guinee D, Jr., Feuerstein I, Koss MN, Travis WD. Pulmonary lymphangioleiomyomatosis. Diagnosis based on results of transbronchial biopsy and immunohistochemical studies and correlation with high-resolution computed tomography findings. Arch Pathol Lab Med 1994; 118:846–849.
2. Kitiachi M, Nishmura K, Izumi T. Pulmonary lymphangioleiomyomatosis: a report of 46 patients including a clinicopathologic study of prognostic factors. Am J Respir Crit Care Med 1995; 151(2 Pt 1):527–533.
3. Johnson SR, Tattersfield AE. Treatment and outcome of lymphangioleiomyomatosis in the UK. Am J Respir Crit Care Med 1997; 155:A327.
4. Kerr LA, Blute ML, Ryu JH, Swensen SJ, Malek RS. Renal angiomyolipoma in association with pulmonary lymphangioleiomyomatosis: forme fruste of tuberous sclerosis? Urology 1993; 41:440–444.
5. Bernstein SM, Newell J, Jr., Adamczyk D, Mortenson RL, King T, Jr., Lynch DA. How common are renal angiomyolipomas in patients with pulmonary lymphangiomyomatosis? Am J Respir Crit Care Med 1995; 152:2138–2143.
6. Peyrol S, Gindre D, Cordier JF, Loire R, Grimaud JA. Characterization of the smooth muscle cell infiltrate and associated connective tissue matrix of lymphangiomyomatosis. Immunohistochemical and ultrastructural study of two cases. J Pathol 1992; 168:387–395.
7. Carrington CB, Cugell DW, Gaensler EA, et al. Lymphangioleiomyomatosis. Physiologic-pathologic-radiologic correlations. Am Rev Respir Dis 1977; 116:977–995.
8. Johnson SF, Davey DD, Cibull ML, Schwartz RW, Strodel WE. Lymphangioleiomyomatosis. Am Surg 1993; 59:395-399.
9. Matthews TJ, Hornall D, Sheppard MN. Comparison of the use of antibodies to alpha smooth muscle actin and desmin in pulmonary lymphangioleiomyomatosis. J Clin Pathol 1993; 46:479–480.
10. Chan JKC, Tsang WYW, Pau MY, Tang MC, Pang SW. Lymphangiomyomatosis and angiomyolipoma: closely related entities characterized by hamatomatous proliferation of HMB-45 positive smooth muscle. Histopathology 1993; 22:445–455.
11. Sawtell NM, Lessard JL. Cellular distribution of smooth muscle actins during myogenesis: expression of the a-vascular but not the g-enteric isoform in differentiating striated myocytes. J Cell Biol 1989; 109:2929–2937.
12. Basset F, Soler P, Marsac J, Corrin B. Pulmonary lymphangiomyomatosis. Three new cases studied with electron microscopy. Cancer 1976; 38:2357–2366.

13. Corrin B, Butcher D, McAnulty BJ, et al. Immunohistochemical localization of transforming growth factor-b1 in the lungs of patients with systemic sclerosis, cryptogenic fibrosing alveolitis, and other lung diseases. Histopathology 1994; 24:145–150.
14. Glassberg MK, Alexis J, Krieger BP, Stylbo JL. Platelet-derived growth factor b receptor and B chain are more abundant in LAM. Am J Respir Crit Care Med 1997; 155:A327.
15. Koutsilieris M. Pathophysiology of uterine leiomyomas. Biochem Cell Biol 1992; 70:273–278.
16. Bonetti F, Pea M, Martignoni G, Zamboni G, Iuzzolino P. Cellular heterogeneity in lymphangiomyomatosis of the lung. Human Pathol 1991; 22:727–728.
17. Bonetti F, Chiodera PL, Pea M, et al. Transbronchial biopsy in lymphangiomyomatosis of the lung: HMB-45 for diagnosis. Am J Surg Pathol 1993; 17:1092–1102.
18. Hoon V, Thung SN, Kaneko M, Unger PD. HMB-45 reactivity in renal angiomyolipoma and lymphangioleiomyomatosis. Arch Pathol Lab Med 1994; 118:732–4.
19. Gown AM, Vogel AM, Hoak D, Gough F, McNutt MA. Monoclonal antibodies specific for melanocytic tumors distinguish subpopulations of melanocytes. Am J Pathol 1986; 123:195–203.
20. Kapur RP, Bigler SA, Skelly M, Gown AM. Anti-melanoma monoclonal antibody identifies an oncofetal glycoconjugate associated with immature melanosomes. J Histochem Cytochem 1992; 40:207–212.
21. Adema GJ, de Boer AJ, Vogel AM, Loenen WAM, Figdor CG. Molecular characterization of the melanocyte specific antigen gp 100. J Biol Chem 1994; 269:20126–20133.
22. Taylor JR, Ryu J, Colby TV, Raffin TA. Lymphangioleiomyomatosis. Clinical course in 32 patients. N Engl J Med 1990; 323:1254–1260.
23. Boehler A, Speich R, Russi EW, Weder W. Lung transplantation for lymphangioleiomyomatosis. N Engl J Med 1996; 335:1275–1280.
24. O'Brien JD, Lium JH, Parosa JF, DeYound BR, Wick MR, Trulock EP. Lymphangiomyomatosis recurrence in the allograft after single-lung transplantation. Am J Respir Crit Care Med 1995; 151:2033–2036.
25. Nine JS, Yousem SA, Paradis IL, Keenan R, Griffith BP. Lymphangioleiomyomatosis: recurrence after lung transplantation. J Heart Lung Transplant 1994; 13:714–719.
26. Kraus F. Pathology of female genitalia. In: Kissane J, ed. Anderson's Pathology. 1990:1620–1725.
27. Zaloudek C, Norris H. Mesenchymal tumors of the uterus. In: Blaustein A, ed. Pathology of the Female Genital Tract. Berlin: Springer-Verlag, 1982:352.
28. Norris H, Zaloudek C. Mesenchymal tumors of the uterus. In: Blaustein A, ed. Pathology of the Female Genital Tract. Berlin: Springer-Verlag, 1982.
29. Bell SW, Kempson RL, Hendirckson MR. Problematic uterine smooth muscle neoplasms. A clinicopathologic study of 213 cases. Am J Surg Pathol 1994; 18:535–558.

30. Draeger A, Graf A-H, Staudach A, North AJ, Small JV. Smooth muscle differentiation in human myometrium and uterine leiomyoma. Virch Arch B Cell Pathol 1993; 64:21–27.
31. Bonsib SM. HMB-45 reactivity in renal leiomyomas and leiomyosarcomas. Mod Path 1996; 9:664–669.
32. Fayed YM, Tsibris JC, Langenberg PW, Robertson ALJ. Human uterine leiomyoma cells: binding and growth responses to epidermal growth factor, platelet-derived growth factor and insulin. Lab Invest 1989; 60:30–37.
33. Howe SR, Gottardis MM, Everitt JI, Goldsworthy TL, Wolf DC, Walker C. Rodent model of reproductive tract leiomyomata. Establishment and characterization of tumor-derived cell lines. Am J Pathol 1995; 146:1568–1579.
34. Mangrulkar RS, Ono M, Ishikawa M, Takashima S, Klagsbrun M, Nowak RA. Isolation and characterization of heparin-binding growth factors in human leiomyomas and normal myometrium. Biol Reprod 1995; 53:636–646.
35. Rauk PN, Surti U, Roberts JM, Michalopolus G. Mitogenic effect of basic fibroblast growth factor and estradiol on cultured human myometrial and leiomyoma cells. Am J Obstet Gynecol 1995; 173:571–577.
36. Strawn EY, Novy MJ, Burry KA, Bethea CL. Insulin-like growth factor 1 promotes leiomyoma cell growth in vitro. Am J Obstet Gynecol 1995; 172:1837–1843.
37. Souria A, Koutsilieris M. Purification and partial sequencing of the major mitogen for human uterine smooth muscle like cells in leiomyoma extracts. J Clin Invest 1995; 96:751–758.
38. Shen A, Iseman MD, Waldron JA, King TE. Exacerbation of pulmonary lymphangioleiomyomatosis by exogenous estrogens. Chest 1987; 91:782–785.
39. Brunelli A, Catalini G, Fianchini A. Pregnancy exacerbating unsuspected mediastinal lymphangioleiomyomatosis and chylothorax. Internat J Gynecol Obstet 1996; 52:289–290.
40. Jourdain O, Descamps P, Abusada N, et al. Treatment of fibromas. Eur J Obstet Gyn Reprod Biol 1996; 66:99–107.
41. Berger U, Khaghani A, Pomerance A, Yacoub MH, Coombes RC. Pulmonary lymphangioleiomyomatosis and steroid receptors. An immunocytochemical study. Am J Clin Pathol 1990; 93:609–614.
42. Ohori NP, Yousem SA, Sonmez-Alpan E, Colby TV. Estrogen and progesterone receptors in lymphangioleiomyomatosis, epithelioid hemangioendothelioma, and sclerosing hemangioma of the lung. Am J Clin Pathol 1991; 96:529–535.
43. Uzzo RG, Libby DM, Vaughan E, Jr., Levey SH. Coexisting lymphangioleiomyomatosis and bilateral angiomyolipomas in a patient with tuberous sclerosis. J Urol 1994; 151:1612–1615.
44. Wahenda I, Cooper S, Williams J, Paterson IC, Britton JR, Tattersfield AE. Relation of pulmonary lymphangioleiomyomatosis to use of the oral contraceptive pill and fertility in the U.K.: a national case control study. Thorax 1994; 49:910-914.
45. Bonetti F, Chiodera P. Lymphangioleiomyomatosis and tuberous sclerosis: Where is the border? Eur Respir J 1996; 9:399–401.
46. Gyure KA, Hart WR, Kennedy AW. Lymphangiomyomatosis of the uterus associated with tuberous sclerosis and malignant neoplasia of the female genital tract: a report of two cases. Int J Gynecol Pathol 1995; 14:344–351.

47. Povey S, Burley MW, Attwood J, et al. Two loci for tuberous sclerosis: one on 9q34 and one on 16p13. Ann Hum Genet 1994; 58:107–127.
48. Green AJ, Johnson PH, Yates JRW. The tuberous sclerosis gene on chromosome 9q34 acts as a growth suppressor. Hum Mol Gen 1994; 3:1833–1834.
49. Green A, Smith M, Yates JRW. Loss of heterozygosity on chromosome 16pl3.3 in hamartomas from tuberous sclerosis patients. Nature Genetics 1994; 6:193–196.
50. Wienecke R, Konig A, DeClue JE. Identification of tuberin, the tuberous sclerosis-2 gene product. J Biol Chem 1995; 270:16409–16414.
51. Xiao G-H, Shoarinejad F, Jin F, Golemis EA, Yeung RS. The tuberous sclerosis 2 gene product, tuberin, functions as a rab5 GTPase activating protein (GAP) in modulating endocytosis. J Biol Chem 1997; 272:6097–6100.
52. Kobayashi T, Hirayama Y, Kobayashi E, Kubo Y, Hino O. A germ-line insertion in the tuberous sclerosis (TSC2) gene gives rise to the Eker rat model of dominantly inherited cancer. Nat Genet 1995; 9:70–74.
53. Howe SR, Gottardis MM, Everitt JI, Walker C. Estrogen stimulation and tamoxifen inhibition of leiomyoma cell growth in vitro and in vivo. Endocrinology 1995; 136:4996–5003.
54. Quade BJ. Pathology, cytogenetics, and molecular biology of uterine leiomyomas and other smooth muscle lesions. Curr Opin Obstet Gynecol 1995; 7:35–42.
55. Nilbert M, Heim S, Mandahl N, Floderus U-M, Willen H, Mitelman F. Independent origin of uterine leiomyomas with karyotypically identical alterations. Gynecol Obstet Invest 1988; 33:300–304.
56. Mashal RD, Schoenberg, Fejzo ML, et al. Analysis of androgen receptor DNA reveals the independent clonal origins of uterine leiomyomata and the secondary nature of cytogenetic aberration in the development of leiomyomata. Cancer 1994; 7:1–6.
57. Rein MS, Friedman AJ, Barbieri RL, Pavelka K, Fletcher JA, Morton CC. Cytogenetic abnormalities in uterine leiomyomata. Obstet Gynecol 1991; 77:923–926.
58. Heim S, Nilbert M, Vanni R, et al. A specific translocation, t(12;14)(ql4-15;q23-24), characterizes a subgroup of uterine leiomyomas. Cancer Genet Cytogenet 1988; 32:13–17.
59. Popper HH, Gamperl R, Pongratz MG, Kullnig P, Juttner-Smolle FM, Pfragner R. Chromosome typing in lymphangioleiomyomatosis of the lung with and without tuberous sclerosis. Eur Respir J 1993; 6:753–759.
60. Kubota R, Wang Y, Minoshima S, et al. Mapping of the human gene for a melanocyte protein Pmel 17 (Dl2S53E) to chromosome 12ql3-14. Genomics 1995; 26:430–431.
61. Schoenmakers EF, Wanschura S, Mols R, Bullerdiek J, Van den Berghe H, Van de Ven WJ. Recurrent rearrangements in the high mobility group protein gene, HMG-IC, in benign mesenchymal tumors. Nat Genet 1995; 10:436–444.
62. Meloni AM, Surti U, Sandberg AA. Deletion of chromosome 13 in leiomyomas of the uterus. Cancer Genet Cytogenet 1991; 53:199–203.
63. Cordon-Carlo C. Mutation of cell cycle regulators. Biological and clinical implications from human neoplasia. Am J Pathol 1995; 147:545–560.
64. Shannon JM, Mason RJ, Jennings SD. Functional differentiation of alveolar type II

epithelial cells in vitro: effects of cell shape, cell-matrix interactions, and cell-cell interactions. Biochim Biophys Acta 1987; 931:143–156.
65. Greene MH. Genetics of breast cancer. Mayo Clin Proc 1997; 72:54–65.
66. Gudmundsson J, Johannesdottir G, Bergthorsson JT, et al. Different tumor types from BRCA2 carriers show wild type chromosome deletions on 13ql2-ql3. Cancer Res 1995; 55:4830–4832.

20

Clinical and Genetic Aspects of Tuberous Sclerosis Complex I and II

M. PRISCILLA SHORT

University of Chicago
Chicago, Illinois

DAVID J. KWIATKOWSKI

Brigham and Women's Hospital
Boston, Massachusetts

I. Introduction

Tuberous sclerosis complex (TSC) is an autosomal dominant, neurocutaneous disorder characterized by benign tumors (harmartomas and harmatias) which derived from all three primary germ layers. It is the second most common neurocutaneous syndrome after neurofibromatosis, type I, with an incidence of 1 in 10,000–15,000 (1). The two disease-causing genes (TSC2 and TSC1) were isolated by efforts of international consortia in 1993 and 1997, respectively (2,3). TSC demonstrates genetic heterogeneity, with the two disease genes accounting for nearly 100% of the cases.

The name tuberous sclerosis was coined by Bourneville in 1880 on the basis of the gross neuropathological findings: areas of the cerebral cortex that are firmer and paler than normal brain tissue, reminiscent of tubers. Sclerosis was added to reflect the firmness of the tuberous protuberances (4). The clinical spectrum of tuberous sclerosis complex was further expanded by Vogt's observation of the clinical triad of mental retardation, seizures, and adenoma sebaceum (a misnomer) (5). Unlike other neurocutaneous disorders, TSC is unique in its involvement of all three primary germ layers. The neurofibromatoses types I and II preferentially involve tissues derived from the ectoderm.

II. Clinical Features

The diagnosis of TSC is made on the basis of the presence of the multiple tumors that characterize this disorder. By consensus the features have been grouped into primary features, secondary features, and tertiary features after extensive review of the literature and ongoing genetic linkage studies (see Table 1). To make a definite diagnosis of TSC, the presence of one primary feature, two secondary features, or one secondary feature and two tertiary features is required. A probable diagnosis of TSC requires the presence of either one secondary plus one tertiary feature or three tertiary features. A diagnosis of suspected TSC requires one secondary feature or two tertiary features. These categories will need to be revisited now that both genes have been isolated. It would not be surprising that, like NF1, the clinical diagnostic features will remain important due to the difficulty of finding disease mutations in the genes. The validity of these clinical features in making a diagnosis of TSC must take into account the temporal sequences in which the features appear in affected individuals (7). Cardiac rhabdomyomas are present prenatally, whereas renal angiomyolipomas occur gradually over time, usually after the second decade. With further genotype-phenotype correlations possible, it may be that the timelines for specific features will have to be shifted further to the right with earlier onsets than previously appreciated.

A. Dermatological Features

Cutaneous involvement in TSC includes hypomelanotic macules, confetti-sized hypomelanotic macules, ungual fibromas, Shagreen patch, and fibrous forehead plaque. The first lesion, the hypomelanotic "ashleaf spot," is frequently the earliest sign of TSC. However, the frequency of hypomelanotic macules in the general population diminishes its diagnostic specificity. The last four findings are robust clinical features of TSC consisting of benign proliferation of fibrous and vascular elements of the dermal layer of the skin. Angiofibromas (also erroneously known as adenoma sebaceum) have a characteristic malar distribution on the face and can develop as early as the first decade. With the onset of puberty, there can be a phase of exuberant growth of angiofibromas which persists. Cosmesis using various forms of laser therapy has been effective in decreasing the cosmetic effect of these lesions due to their vascular nature. Ungual fibroma involving both the fingers and toes usually develops in the second decade and can continue to appear throughout life. Despite surgical excision, these lesions can recur. The Shagreen patch is usually a cluster of hamartoma typically located on the lower back and, together with hypomelanotic macules, is frequently the

Table 1 Diagnostic Features of Tuberous Sclerosis Complex

Primary features
Multiple facial angiomas[a]
Multiple ungual fibromas[a]
Cortical tuber (histologically confirmed)
Subependymal nodule or giant cell tumor (histologically confirmed)
Multiple calcified periventricular subependymal nodules (radiographically demonstrated)
Multiple retinal astrocytomas (phakomas)
Secondary features
Affected first-degree relative
Cardiac rhabdomyomas (histologic or echocardiographic confirmation)
Other retinal hamartoma or achromic patch
Cerebral tubers (radiographic confirmation)
Noncalcified subependymal nodeules (radiographic confirmation)
Shagreen patch[a]
Forehead plaque[a]
Pulmonary lymphangiomyomatosis (histologic confirmation)
Renal angiomyoliomas (radiographic or histologic confirmation)
Renal cysts (histologic confirmation)
Tertiary features
Hypomelanotic macules ("ashleaf spots")[a]
"Confetti" skin lesions[a]
Cerebral white matter "migration tracts" or heterotopias (radiographic evidence)
Infantile spasms (hypsarrhythmia on EEG)
Gingival fibroma[a]
Enamel pits in deciduous and/or permanent teeth
Renal cysts (radiographic evidence)
Hamartomatous rectal polyps (histologic confirmation)
Bone cysts (radiographic evidence)
Pulmonary lymphangiomyomatosis (radiographic evidence)
Hamartomas of other organs (histologic confirmation)

[a]No histological confirmation necessary if clinically obvious.
Source: Adapted from Ref. 6.

earliest feature of TSC. Fibrous plaques on the forehead are fleshy plaquelike lesions which lack the vascularity of angiofibromas. Both Shagreen and fibrous plaques demonstrate proliferation of collagen and elastic tissue within the dermis.

B. Neurological/Psychiatric Features

The neurological signs of TSC are common. The extent to which one patient with TSC is neurologically symptomatic varies from 30% to 90% with wide variation between and within affected families (8,9). Severe involvement may cause intractable seizures, severe mental retardation, or progressive hydrocephalus due to the growth of a subependymal giant cell tumor. More mild involvement could involve a readily controlled seizure disorder. In the absence of seizures, the incidence of mental retardation is low; conversely, most affected TSC patients with mental retardation do have seizures. Vogt's triad of mental retardation, seizures, and angiofibromas refers to a minority of patients with TSC (10).

Seizures are the most frequent symptom to initiate an evaluation for TSC in both inherited and sporadic cases. Of seizures that begin within the first year of life, infantile spasms, a form of generalized seizure activity, is a very common type and has a typical EEG signature. Seizure types with later onset are usually focal in onset.

Neuroimaging is frequently abnormal in patients with TSC. Magnetic resonance imaging is very sensitive to demonstrating cortical tubers, which are best seen as circumscribed areas on T_2-weighted images versus subependymal nodules, which are better seen on T_1-weighted images. Contrast enhancement has been seen in subependymal nodules which have shown growth. Obstructive hydrocephalus can occur with growth of nodules located at the foramen of Monro, obstructing the outflow of cerebrospinal fluid from the lateral ventricles into the third ventricle.

The incidence of mental retardation varies from 30% to 46% depending on the series. Such figures represent a bias of ascertainment which has been recognized as more families have been recognized in the course of genetic linkage studies (8,9).

Other neuropsychiatric features of TSC include autism, behavioral disturbances, sleep disorders, and frank psychiatric disturbances such as depression with and without psychotic features (11).

C. Renal Features

Renal angiomyolipomas and cysts are relatively common in patients with TSC. Angiomyolipomas are more common in affected adults. Compared to the incidence of these tumors in the general population, where they are preferentially seen in older woman as unilateral tumors, in affected TSC patients the tumors are multiple, bilateral, and with earlier onset of symptoms. They are vascular tumors consisting of smooth muscle, adipose tissue, and fibrous tissue. Renal angiomyolipomas can be a source of morbidity due to unexpected hemorrhage. Renal transplantation has been done successfully in TSC-associated end-stage renal disease (12).

Renal cysts are more common in affected TSC children (13). Renal cystic disease in children can be asymptomatic or present with hypertension and mild renal failure. Analysis of patients linked to TSC2 on chromosome 16 has shown that in some cases in which affected children present with early, severe cystic disease, the mutation has deleted parts of both TSC2 and the contiguous gene for polycystic kidney disease (14). However, renal cysts do occur on the basis of TSC1 and 2 alone without involvement of the polycystic kidney disease genes.

There is a slightly increased risk of malignant transformation of renal angiomyolipomas. Bjornsson et al. reported six TSC-associated renal cell carcinomas, four of which demonstrated positive immunoreactivity for the melanocyte-associated marker HMB-45. positive immunoreactivity for HMB-45 has been reported in TSC-associated renal angiomyolipomas and pulmonary lymphangiomyomatosis (15).

D. Cardiac Features

Rhabdomyomas are very common in children with TSC. They can be detected as early as 20 weeks on fetal echocardiography. Usually they are multiple and clinically silent. The association with tuberous sclerosis is strong; nearly 50%–80% of children presenting with cardiac rhabdomyomas will be found to have other signs of tuberous sclerosis (16). When the tumors are clinically symptomatic, producing outflow obstruction or arrhythmias, experience has shown that observation and medical therapy is the preferred treatment. Over time on serial echocardiography, rhabdomyomas have decreased in size without surgical intervention (17).

Pathologically the rhabdomyomas are circumscribed, white-yellow tumors consisting of enlarged, glycogen-filled myocytes which on electron microscopy more closely represent myoblasts than mature myocytes (17).

E. Other Clinical Features

Ophthalmological findings of TSC, retinal hamartomas (phakomas), are very common in patients with TSC, presenting as either a noncalcified hamartoma, a calcified mulberrylike lesion, or a transitional form (18). Pathologically the tumors are an extension of hamartomas of the central nervous system, representing a proliferation of astroglial cells involving the superficial layers of the retin or optic nerve head.

Pulmonary involvement in TSC is relatively rare, occurring exclusively in women. It was not recognized as a feature of TSC until the 1940s, when Berg et al. described changes consistent with pulmonary lymphangiomyomatosis (LAM) in patients with TSC (19). In various series of clinical features in TSC, it has been reported in less than 1% of all cases. In a Mayo series of patients with LAM, 80% had angiofibroma, 60% had angiomyolipoma, and 25% had retinal phakomas (20).

Clinically patients present with symptoms of recurrent pulmonary pneumothoraces with eventual pulmonary hypertension and cor pulmonale. Pathologically there is a histological difference between TSC-associated pulmonary LAM and that occurring sporadically. Whether or not sporadic pulmonary LAM represents a form fruste of TSC, a segmental variant of TSC, awaits further investigation. Involvement of regional lymph nodes has been reported more frequently in non–TSC-associated pulmonary LAM.

Recently, Boehler et al. reported results of lung transplantation patients in those patients who have pulmonary lymphangiomyomatosis (21). Traditional treatment has symptomatic therapy for acute pneumothoraces with additional evidence supporting the use of progesterone therapy or oophorectomy with stabilization and/or improvement of disease.

Other organ involvement has included reports of microhamartomatous polyps in the rectum and hepatic hamartomas. The latter in some cases have proven to be angiomyolipomas of the liver.

III. Clinical Genetics

Tuberous sclerosis is an autosomal dominant genetic disorder in which about two-thirds of patients present with no family history and detailed clinical investigation of the parents are negative (1,22,23). The birth incidence worldwide appears to be about 1 in 10,000, with one estimate as high as 1 in 5800 considering cases with a mild presentation (1). Families in which TSC is seen to be segregating are generally small, likely due to the negative survival effects of the condition, particularly in those severely affected and in past times. Although clinical expression of tuberous sclerosis varies greatly, with thorough physical examination and imaging studies of the brain, heart, and kidneys, there are rare instances of skipped generations within a family that would be consistent with a complete lack of expression (24,25).

A single family has been described that appears exceptional with respect to penetrance (26). Smalley et al. have described an extended Utah kindred in which a generally mild form of tuberous sclerosis appears to be inherited, with the dominant features being psychiatric in nature. Six members of this extended 74-member kindred meet formal criteria for a diagnosis of tuberous sclerosis. An additional 13 individuals in the family have possible or suspected TSC by formal diagnostic criteria. Among these 19 individuals, 13 had psychiatric disorders, including 6 with mood disorder and 10 with anxiety disorder. Considering all 19 of these individuals as affected during linkage analysis gives a lod score of over 6 for TSC2 region markers, with segregation of a common D16S85-D16S291 haplotype among all "affected" family members. To determine whether or not a family is truly segregating a mild mutation within TSC2, explaining the clinical syndromes seen in family members will require demonstration of such a pathogenic mutation. Although inferences derived from analysis of this family must be considered tentative until such evidence is obtained, the family suggests the possibility that tuberous sclerosis may occur in a milder low-penetration form in some families. This observation also suggests that the TSC genes may have an important role in psychiatric disorders.

Tuberous sclerosis is one of a few human genetic diseases for which genetic mosaicism has been demonstrated (27). When parents of a sporadic case of tuberous sclerosis have a second child, the risk of tuberous sclerosis is much higher than for a child born to someone in the general population and is conventionally estimated at about a 2% risk. Verhoef and colleagues (27) have demonstrated the occurrence of germline mosaicisim in a parent of a sporadic tuberous sclerosis patient. The parent had no major clinical manifestations of TSC. The same group has also demonstrated the occurrence of a TSC2 point mutation in a family with some features of TSC but not meeting formal diagnostic criteria (28). As mutational analysis of the TSC2 gene continues, we can anticipate identification of additional individuals with mutations and subclinical disease.

A. Linkage Analysis in Tuberous Sclerosis

Genetic linkage studies in tuberous sclerosis were first initiated over 10 years ago and initially resulted in the identification of a probable locus (TSC1) in the 9q34 region (29). Subsequent studies indicated that there were clearly families without linkage to this region of the genome (30–32). This confusion was resolved when several TSC families without linkage to chromosome 9q34 were studied in 1992, resulting in the identification of linkage to the 16p13 region (33). Subsequent studies led to identification of the TSC2, as described below. Other follow-up studies, however, have indicated that the proportion of 9q34-linked to 16pl3-linked families is approximately equal (34). This is consistent with each gene accounting for about half of all cases of tuberous sclerosis. Since family studies are based upon a small fraction of the overall TSC population, it is possible that in the larger sporadic population one or the other of these two genes accounts for a larger fraction of cases. At present, linkage analyses suggest that the two genes TSC1 and TSC2 account for all cases of TSC; that is, there is no evidence for an additional third locus (34; Haines and Pericak-Vance, personal communication).

B. TSC2: Identification, Gene Structure, and Mutations

The TSC2 gene was identified from the chromosome 16pl3.3 region in 1993 by a positional cloning strategy that relied upon the careful evaluation of two critical individuals (2). One individual had undergone a deletion of the terminal portion of 16pl3 and had a number of developmental defects related to that loss. However, the individual had none of the stigmata of tuberous sclerosis. Second, there was a family that was segregating polycystic kidney disease (PKD) in whom a child was recognized to have both renal disease and features of tuberous sclerosis. A chromosomal translocation was found to be segregating in the family which interrupted the PKD1 gene, causing PKD in members of the family with a balanced translocation. In the child affected with TSC as well as PKD1, the translocation was unbalanced due to loss of the region of 16pl3 telomeric to PKD1. Comparison of the genomic regions lost in the two individuals restricted the search for TSC2 to a 100 kb region, facilitating its identification. TSC2 and PKD1 lie adjacent to each other in the genome, with transcriptional orientations aimed toward each other.

The TSC2 gene is composed of 45 kb of genomic DNA, contains 41 coding exons, and encodes a message of size 6 kb and protein of 1741–1807 amino acids (35). Alternative splicing occurs within the gene, affecting exons 25, 31 and the splice acceptor site for exon 26, creating the possibility of a total of 8 different tuberin isoforms (35–38). The size of the TSC2 locus has complicated efforts at mutation detection. Preliminary reports utilizing a variety of mutation detection methods have appeared (14,27,28,39–42). Large deletions within the TSC2 gene (>5 kb) occur in 1–5% of unselected TSC patients (14). Fourteen distinct small mutations have been described, including five missense, two nonsense, five small deletion, one duplication, and one splice site mutation. A single mutation has been seen in two different patients (27), and the remainder are unique. The small number of mutations described thus far and their diversity has made it impossible to derive any meaningful correlation between mutation type and clinical signs. This is likely to be difficult in any case, since the expression of TSC varies widely among members of a family in which the same mutation is segregating. Preliminary results from centers where comprehensive efforts at mutation detection are being made show that about a third of unselected patients are found to have TSC2 mutations (Haines et al., personal communication). Given the inherent limitations of current mutation-detection methods, this fraction must be considered a lower limit on the proportion of TSC cases due to mutations in TSC2.

The single clinical correlation that has derived from these studies is that TSC patients with severe renal cystic disease that presents before age 20 are likely to have large deletions involving both the TSC2 and the adjacent PKD1 gene (14). In one series carefully analyzed for such deletions, nearly all patients who presented with early onset renal cystic disease, 10% of a series of 90 unselected sporadic cases, had significant genomic deletions involving both genes (J. Sampson, personal communication).

Apart from this single distinction, there is little or no evidence that the clinical manifestations of TSC due to mutations in TSC2 are different from those seen in patients with TSCl disease (30,32,34). In adding, the wide variability in the manifestations of TSC in families with mutations in each gene suggests that such gene-specific clinical manifestations are likely to be subtle.

C. TSC1: Identification, Gene Structure, and Mutations

The TSC1 gene was identified from the chromosome 9q34 region surrounding the ABO blood group locus (3,25) by the use of positional cloning. Polymerase chain reaction (PCR) was used to amplify putative and confirmed exons from a 208 kb sequence from unrelated familial TSC cases with linkage to 9q34 and 40 sporadic TSC cases. Amplification products that produced heteroduplex formation on weak, denaturing polyacrylamide gels were subsequently sequenced. Seven small frame-shifting deletions, one nonsense mutation, and one missense mutation were found. Eight of the nine mutations were from the 20 familial cases tested. Analysis of other family members confirmed the segregation of the mutation with the disease phenotype. On full gene sequence analysis, the TSC1 gene consists of 23 exons of which the last 21 contain coding sequence. The predicted TSC1 protein, hamartin, consists of 1164 amino acids of a mass of 130 kDa. There were no strong matches to other known vertebrate proteins. A possible yeast homolog of TSC1 was identified.

Mutations in 40% of the familial cases and 5% of the sporadic cases were identified by screening of all coding exons in 20 familial cases and 152 sporadic patients. Of the 32 distinct mutations found, 30 predicted a truncated protein (3).

Analysis from a renal cell carcinoma from a patient with a germline TSC1 mutation revealed an additional mutation in the wild type allele. Similar to the earlier findings in TSC2, TSC1 appears to function as a tumor suppressor gene.

D. Allelic Loss Studies in TSC

Allelic loss or loss of heterozygosity (LOH) is the phenomenon in which DNA derived from a TSC lesion, or more generally any tumor, demonstrates loss of one allele for a DNA marker in comparison with analysis of DNA from some unaffected tissue from the same individual. LOH has been observed in numerous tumors at many genomic sites and often reflects loss of one copy of a gene crucial for suppression of tumor development. In these cases, the other copy of the gene may be nonfunctional due to a germline mutation, as in the case of TSC and other hereditary tumor suppressor gene syndromes, or due to a smaller inactivating mutation affecting the other allele of the critical locus. LOH can also occur nonspecifically, due to global and nonspecific genomic instability, particularly in advanced carcinomas. When it occurs in a specific region, it can be used as a guide to identify the gene that is being lost, through comparison of the minimal region of overlap of the "lost" genomic regions.

In TSC, LOH studies were first reported in 1994 for the chromosome 16pl3.3 region where TSC2 is found (44). These observations provided some of the first support for the hypothesis that the TSC genes acted as tumor suppressor genes, in that loss of the second, normal germline allele occurred in TSC lesions. The observations also helped to confirm the localization of the TSC2 gene by linkage studies, accelerating the positional cloning efforts going on at that time to identify TSC2 (44).

LOH in the TSC2 region has now been reported for over 50 different TSC lesions from over 40 different TSC patients (45–47). In addition, similar LOH for the TSC2 region has been found in sporadic renal angiomyolipomas (non-TSC patients) in 3 cases out of 30 examined (48). This suggests that inactivation of the TSC2 gene occurs in sporadic angiomyolipomas as well as in TSC-related angiomyolipomas.

On the other hand, LOH for the TSC1 region has been seen much less (45–57). Seven patients with 10 different lesions have been reported to have 9q34 LOH, using markers that span the critical region for TSC1 and beyond. Four of the six cases of LOH were seen in lesions collected from a single patient, in whom four of six angiomyolipomas collected at autopsy demonstrated LOH (46). Why there is such a great disparity in the frequency of observed LOH for the TSC2 versus TSC1 genomic regions is not clear. It is possible that the LOH phenomenon occurs much less in the 9q34 region because of genomic structure there, i.e., point mutations or other mechanisms to inactivate the normal TSC1 allele may occur much more frequently than large genomic deletions. However, this is exceptional in comparison with other tumor suppressor genes and the abundance of LOH observations throughout the genome. A second possibility is that in the sporadic TSC population in whom most of the observations regarding LOH have been made, TSC1 disease is much less frequent that TSC2 disease, in contrast to familial linkage studies (34). This seems unlikely to explain such a wide disparity in the frequency of LOH, as observed by three different groups in different patient populations. A third possibility is that lesions that come to medical attention and are resected from TSC patients, or are found at autopsy, typically occur in patients with TSC2 disease and not TSC1 disease. This is possible, but so far familial studies have shown no evidence of a difference in the clinical-pathological phenotype for TSC1 versus TSC2 disease (30,32,34).

A final and most interesting possibility is that the TSC1 gene is subjected to a restricted set of inactivating or even activating mutations, so that LOH occurs much less commonly. Activating mutations with TSC1 seem unlikely since the lesions that occur in TSC1 patients, as in TSC2 patients, are focal hamartomas/hamartias rather than global organ hyperplasia, suggesting that a second hit of some sort is required. The identification of TSC1 and further analysis of mutations within the second allele of the gene within TSC lesions from TSC1 patients should indicate which possibility is correct.

E. The Eker Rat

The Eker rat was recognized as a unique animal model of malignancy by Eker in 1954 (49) due to a spontaneous germline mutation in the Wistar rat; heterozygous carriers develop multiple and often bilateral renal carcinoma which often prove fatal. Animals with this mutation were maintained and bred for 40 years, and it was not until the TSC2 gene was identified that it was recognized that the molecular defect in the Eker rat is due to a mutation within the rat TSC2 homolog (50,51). The renal cell lesions of the Eker rat develop through a series of defined stages, beginning as atypical tubules, progressing to adenomatous lesions, and finally to invasive carcinomas (52). All heterozygotes have at least one renal adenoma by age 1 year. Past the age of 1 year, Eker rats also develop pituitary adenomas, splenic hemangiosarcomas, and uterine leiomyosarcomas at lower frequency. Mixed cell tumors or tumors with prominent Smc involvement are not seen in the Eker rat.

The germline genetic lesion in the Eker rat is the insertion of a 6.3 kb retroviral-like sequence into an intron in the 3′ region of the rat TSC2 (rTSC2) locus (50,53). This results in the generation of an altered mRNA transcript from the rTSC2 locus, which does not contain the normal 3′ 30% of the mRNA. Tissues and cells isolated from renal and other lesions which develop in the Eker rat have undergone a second event eliminating transcription from the remaining normal TSC2 locus. In most cases, this second hit can be detected through loss of heterozygosity analysis of the lesions (54–56) as in TSC.

IV. Pathogenesis

The variety of benign proliferative lesions associated with tuberous sclerosis define it as a tumor suppressor gene syndrome. In addition, mutational analyses of the germline TSC2 allele and allelic loss studies performed in TSC lesions (45–57) demonstrate that for TSC2 patients many TSC lesions have lost both alleles of the TSC2 gene, also consistent with a growth suppressor function for the TSC genes, and TSC2 in particular. However, TSC is only rarely a cancer suppressor gene syndrome. That is, malignant progression of TSC lesions rarely occurs. Some lesions do give rise to devastating complications, e.g., giant cell astrocytomas that cause obstructive hydrocephalus. The sole organ where malignant transformation of TSC lesions occurs is in the kidney, where an association between malignant renal tumors occurring at a young age and TSC have been seen (15,57), albeit at low frequency (1–2% of TSC patients, without regard to age; compares with lifetime risk of renal cancer of 1% in United States).

These observations contrast with most other tumor suppressor gene syndromes (58). The Li-Fraumeni syndrome, due to mutations in p53, and the retinoblastoma gene syndrome, due to mutations in the retinoblastoma gene, are characterized by development of frankly malignant tumors at an early age and in multiple organ systems. Neurofibromatosis type 1, a “nearest neighbor” of TSC, is characterized by development of numerous benign neurofibromas, which progress to malignant sarcoma in about 3% of lesions (59). Many other malignant tumors occur at increased frequency in neurofibromatosis type 1 patients. In keeping with the benign nature of TSC tumors is the observation that cells from such lesions are difficult to culture and passage (D.J. Kwiatkowski, unpublished observations).

Accepting TSC as a tumor suppressor gene syndrome, several questions regarding its pathogenesis then follow, many of which are difficult to answer at this time. They include: Are all lesions that occur in TSC due to allelic loss of the second wild-type allele, or are some TSC lesions due to haplo-insufficiency? What explains the tissue distribution of lesions seen in TSC? Why is it that nearly all TSC lesions undergo growth during a defined developmental interval and then become stable in size or actually recede (the cardiac rhabdomyomas are most notable in this regard)? Why are the tumors associated with TSC so rare in the general population (among TSC lesions, only renal angiomyolipomas are seen in the sporadic non-TSC population at any appreciable frequency)? Are additional genetic hits (e.g., ras mutations) required for development of TSC lesions, or is loss of the remaining wild-type TSC2 or TSC1 allele sufficient? What is the biochemical function of the TSC genes, by which they serve a growth regulatory function? None of these questions can be answered fully at this time.

Haplo-insufficiency may explain some TSC lesions, particularly given the wide range of clinical manifestations in TSC patients. However, all of the pathological manifestations of TSC are focal in nature and never occupy the entire organ of involvement, Nonetheless, possibility deserves consideration, particularly in the brain, where brain tubers might occur by this mechanism. In contrast to renal angiomyolipomas and cardiac rhabdomyomas, in which LOH for the TSC2 or TSC1 region was seen in over 60% of cases, we saw no LOH for these genomic regions in 14 carefully dissected cortical tubers (46). In addition, LOH was seen in only 1 of 11 subependymal giant cell astrocytomas. Similar but more limited results have been obtained by others (45,47). Two groups have reported preliminary analyses of tuberin expression in brain sections from TSC patients (60,61). In both of these reports, neither linkage or mutational analysis was available to indicate whether the disease was due to TSC1 or TSC2. In one study looking at six brains from TSC patients, the tuberin staining pattern of normal neurons was on different from controls (60). Cytomegalic dysmorphic neurons (CDNs) in tubers showed enhanced tuberin staining compared with adjacent normal brain. Early subependymal lesions from these patients also expressed tuberin at levels comparable to that of normal adjacent ependyma. In the second study five TSC patient brains were analyzed for expression of tuberin mRNA and other mRNAs using an elegant single cell mRNA amplification approach (61). CDNs from three of the five patients contained tuberin mRNA, while similar cells from the other two patients did not. This study also demonstrated by antibody staining that most CDNs were positive for expression of nestin, Ki-67, and PCNA. Nestin is an intermediate filament protein which is usually expressed during brain embryogenesis, but not in the adult. Ki-67 and PCNA are both markers of cell proliferation, which again are not normally present in the post-mitotic neurons of the postnatal brain.

Analysis of LOH and clonality of tubers certainly may be compromised by admixture of normal and reactive cells. In addition, tuberin would likely be expressed in the tuber CDNs that were derived from TSC1 patients, and TSC2 expression might occur in some CDNs when the protein is expressed but nonfunctional due to missense mutation. Thus, at this point, the evidence is not clear. The focal nature of tubers within the TSC brain would certainly argue that some type of second hit is required to lead to their generation.

Tuberin expression has been analyzed in a variety of tissues, cells, and organs by several research groups using both antibody and RNA expression methods in an effort to correlate sites of expression with the lesions seen in TSC (60,62–66). In general, tuberin expression occurs at a low level, probably much less than 0.01% of total cell protein (D.J. Kwiatkowski, unpublished observations).

There is generally good concordance between antibody staining analysis of tuberin expression and analysis of tuberin RNA expression (in situ hybridization, ISH). Tuberin is expressed in a variety of cell types and organs, although smooth muscle cells (SMCs) in many tissues and certain brain cell types have the highest levels of expression (60,64,65). Multiple cell types, including keratinocytes, melanocytes, fibroblasts, and SMCs, express tuberin in the skin, and eccrine sweat gland cells have particularly high-level expression. Expression, as assessed by antibody studies, in several other adult human organs (kidney, adrenal gland, kidneys, pancreas) appears minimal, apart from SMCs associated with the vasculature. In mouse and rat, and in human fetal tissues, tuberin expression is more widespread and abundant. Within the brain, multiple neuronal cell types express tuberin at appreciable levels: cortical pyramidal neurons, the molecular and granular cell layers of the cerebellum, cerebellar Purkinje cells, and motor neuron cells of the brainstem and spinal cord (60,62). Ependymal cells and choroid plexus cells also express tuberin. In contrast, astrocytes and other nonneuronal brain cell types contain very little tuberin. Heart has also been observed to contain tuberin (64).

Thus, there is a reasonable correlation between tuberin expression and sites where lesions develop in TSC patients. As smooth muscle proliferation is a prominent component of many TSC lesions, the observation of relatively high-level tuberin expression in SMCs does fit well.

In general TSC lesions are rare in patients who do not have TSC. Sporadic renal angiomyolipomas and ungual and other fibromas do occur at a very low rate in the general population, and it is possible that other sporadic TSC lesions often go unrecognized in patients without a formal diagnosis of TSC. Methods for precise and comprehensive assessment of TSC1 and TSC2 mutations will prove valuable for analysis of TSC-like lesions in non-TSC patients both to determine if there is a larger pool of subclinical TSC patients and whether other sporadic lesions occurring in non-TSC patients are due to mutation of the TSC1 or TSC2 genes.

At the time of its identification, TSC2 was seen to contain a 39-amino-acid region near its C-terminus with homology to the protein rap1GAP (2,67,68). Subsequent in vitro studies have demonstrated that tuberin when immunoprecipitated from cultured cells has a modest degree of GTPase-activating protein (GAP) activity for rap1 as well (69). Although for GAP activity that has been shown is modest, it also appears to be specific for rap1 and not other ras family members, suggesting it is physiologically relevant. In addition, rap1 and tuberin have both been localized to the Golgi/late endosome compartment of the cell, consistent with an interaction between these proteins (63,70). However, the original rap1GAP appears to be a more abundant and biochemically dominant GAP for rap1 based upon brain extract analysis (68).

To understand the implications of this finding for the pathogenesis of tuberous sclerosis, it is necessary to understand the ras family of small GTPases and current models of how they function to regulate cell growth (71,72). The ras superfamily of GTPases consist of over 40 proteins and genes that have roles in transduction of external cytokine signs for cell physiology (73). The ras subfamily of the ras superfamily consists of 10 family members: H-ras, Ki-ras, N-ras, ralA and B, raplA and B, rap2, R-ras, and TC21. H-ras, Ki-ras, and N-ras all function similarly. They bind guanine nucleotide as either GDP or GTP and have an intrinsic GTPase that leads to conversion of bound GTP to GDP. When GDP is bound by these proteins, they are in an inactive state for signaling. When GTP is bound, they are active for signaling. The three ras proteins translocate to the cell member when they bid GTP, and there they serve to dock or coordinate a complex of proteins which transmit signals to the cell interior. Arguably most important among these proteins downstream of ras in signaling is the raf kinase. Raf is activated by binding to ras, and a kinase cascade is initiated leading to activation and phosphorylation of MAP kinase, which translocates to the cell nucleus and phosphorylates transcription factors leading to initiation of DNA synthesis and eventually cell division (71).

Much less is known about the functions of the other members of the ras subfamily, including rapl (74–76). Rap1 is expressed in many cell types, including neurons and SMCs. It is capable of reverting v-K-ras transformation of NIH 3T3 cells (77), suggesting that it may act to inhibit ras-related signaling. However, microinjection of rap1 into Swiss 3T3 cells leads to DNA synthesis (78), indicating that it can also stimulate cell growth in some circumstances. Rapl binds relatively poorly to raf, but binds to and activates a brain isoform of raf, B-raf (79). It also binds tightly to a potential effector protein, ralGDS, whose gene happens to map to the TSC1 critical region (80).

All ras subfamily GTPases (71,72) are regulated by a large group of proteins with the ability to (1) enhance or retard nucleotide exchange (leading to larger or smaller amounts of protein in the GTP-bound, activated state) and (2) enhance the hydrolysis of GTP, so-called GTPase-activating protein (GAP) activity, leading to larger amounts of protein in the inactive GDP-bound state.

Thus, the finding of modest GAP activity of tuberin for rap1 is consistent with a model for the pathogenesis of TSC in which in certain cell types lack of tuberin leads to a higher level of rap1 GTP, leading to inappropriate cell growth or survival and TSC lesion development. The lack of strong growth-promoting activity by rap1 in cell culture systems is also consistent with the benign character of most TSC lesions and the poor in vitro growth qualities of cells derived from such lesions. However, this model must be considered an hypothesis at present, and many details remain to filled in. For example, if this model is correct then one would predict a high level of rap1 GTP in TSC lesions compared with normal tissues. Second, one must explain why the other rapl GAP, which has dominant rapl GAP activity in organ extracts, appears to be ineffective in curbing rapl activity in TSC lesions. Third, why TSC lesions occur at certain developmental stages and not others remains a mystery. Presumably, tuberin (and therefore rapl) has a critical role in growth control in different cells/organs at different times. The actual function of hamartin awaits similar studies that have been conducted looking at tuberin. Further, presumably changes in the importance of tuberin and hamartin for cell growth control occur as a function of development. Further understanding of this phenomenon will likely require a better understanding of tuberin and hamartin's biochemical function in cellular physiology.

References

1. Osborne JP, Fryer A, Webb D. Epidemiology of tuberous sclerosis. Ann NY Acad Sci 1991; 615:125–127.
2. European Chromosome 16 Tuberous Sclerosis Consortium. Identification and characterization of the tuberous sclerosis gene on chromosome 16. Cell 1993; 75:1305–1315.
3. van Slegtenhorst M, de Hoogt R, Hermans C, Nellist M, Janssen B, Verhoef S, Lindhout D, van den Ouweland A, Halley D, Young J, Burley M, Jeremiah S, Woodward K, Nahmias J, Fox M, Ekong R, Osborne J, Wolfe J, Povey S, Snell RG, Cheadle JP, Jones AC, Tachataki M, Ravine D, Sampson JR, Reeve MP, Richardson P, Wilmer F, Munro C, Hawkins TL, Sepp T, Ali JBM, Ward S, Green AJ, Yates JRW, Kwiatkowska J, Henske DP, Short MP, Haines JH, Jozwiak S, Kwiatkowski

DJ. Identification of the tuberous sclerosis gene TSC1 on chromosome 9q34. Science 1997; 277:805–808.
4. Bournville DM. Sclerose tebereuse des circonvolutions cerebrales: Idiotie et epilepsie hemiplegique. Arch Neurol (Paris) 1880; 1:81–91
5. Vogt H. Zue Diagnostik der terosen Sklerose. Z Erforsch Behandl Jegendl Schwachsinns 1903; 2:1–12.
6. Roach E, Smith M, Huttenlocher P, Bhat M, Alcorn D, Hawley L. Diagnostic criteria: tuberous sclerosis complex. J Child Neurol 1991; 7:221–224.
7. Short MP, Richardson, Jr EP, Haines JL, Kwiatkowski DJ. Clinical, neuropathological and genetic aspects of the tuberous sclerosis complex. Brain Pathol 1995; 5:173–179.
8. Gomez MR. Neurologic and psychiatric features in tuberous sclerosis. In: Gomez MR, ed. Tuberous Sclerosis, 2nd ed. New York: Raven Press, 1988:21–36.
9. Short MP, Haines J, Jewell A, Beijani B, Yang CH, Wyandt H, MacFarlane H, Andermann E, Kwiatkowski DJ, Amos J. Clinical Findings and linkage studies in familial tuberous sclerosis. Ann NY Acad Sci 615:382–383.
10. Gomez MR. Criteria for diagnosis in tuberous sclerosis. In: Gomez MR, ed. Tuberous Sclerosis, 2nd ed. New York: Raven Press, 1988:14.
11. Hunt A. Development, Behavior and siezures in 300 cases of tuberous sclerosis. J Intell Disabil Res 1993; 37:47–51.
12. Cohnen M, Weber F, Wagner K, Philipp T. Tuberous sclerosis: typical complications of a hereditary disesase and therapeutic opitons. Med Klin 1995; 90:506–512.
13. Bernstein J Robbins TO. Renal involvement in tuberous sclerosis. Ann NY Acad Sci 1991; 615:36–49.
14. Brook-Carter PT, Peral B, Ward CJ, Thompson P, Hughes J, Maheshwar MM, Nellist M, Gamble V, Harris PC, Sampson JR. Deletion of the TSC2 and PKD1 genes associated with severe infantile polycystic kidney disease—a contiguous gene syndrome. Nat Genet 1994; 8:328–332.
15. Bjornsson J, Short MP, Kwiatkowski DJ, Henske EP. Tuberous sclerosis-associated renal cell carcinoma. Am J Pathol 1996; 149:1201–1208.
16. Webb D, Thomas RD, Osborne J. Cardiac rhabdomyomas and their association with tuberous sclerosis. Arch Dis Child 1993; 63:367–370.
17. Watson GH. Cardiac rhadbomyomas in tuberous sclerosis. Ann NY Acad Sci 1991; 615:50–57.
18. Robertson DM. Ophthalmic manifestations of tuberous sclerosis. Ann NY Acad Sci 1991; 615:17–25.
19. Berg G, Zacharissoon CG. Cystic lungs of rare origin: tuberous sclerosis. Acta Radiol (Stockh) 1939; 22:16–30.
20. Lie JT. Cardiac, pulmonary, and vascular involvements in tuberous sclerosis. Ann NY Acad Sci 1991; 615:58–70.
21. Boehler A, speich R, Russi EW, Weder W. Lung transplantation for lymphangioleiomyomatosis. NEJM 1996; 335:1275–1280.
22. Sampson JR, Scahill JS, Stephenson JB, Mann L, Connor JM. Genetic aspects of tuberous sclerosis in the west of Scotland. J Med Genet 1989; 26:28–31.
23. Hunt A. Prevalence of Autism in TS. TSA of Great Britain meeting abstracts. A26, 1991.

24. XX al GL, Arthur RJ, Lamb JT, Hammer HM, Coker TP, Hirschmann PN, Gibbs J, Mueller RF. Diagnostic and counselling difficulties using a fully comprehensive screening protocol for families at risk for tuberous sclerosis. J Med Genet 1989; 26:694–703.
25. Webb DW, Osborne JP. Non-penetrance in tuberous sclerosis. J Med Genet 1991; 28:417–419.
26. Smalley SL, Burger F, Smith M. Phenotypic variation of tuberous sclerosis in a single extended kindred. J Med Genet 1994; 31:761–765.
27. Verhoef S, Vrtel R, van ET, Bakker L, Sikkens E, Halley D, Lindhout D van den, Ouweland, A. Somatic mosaicism and clinical variation in tuberous sclerosis complex [letter]. Lancet 1995; 345:202.
28. Vrtel R, Verhoef S, Bouman K, Maheshwar MM, Nellist M, van Essen AJ, Bakker PLG, Hermans CJ, Bink-Boelkens MTE, van Elburg RM, Hoff M, Lindhout D, Sampson J, Halley DJJ, van den Ouweland AMW. Identification of a nonsense mutation at the 5′ end of the TSC2 gene ina family with a resumptive diagnosis of tuberous sclerosis complex. J Med Genet 1996; 33:47–51.
29. Fryer AE, Connor JM, Povey S, Yates JRW, Chalmers A, Fraser I, Yates AD, Osborne JP. Evidence that the gene for tuberous sclerosis is on chromosome 9. Lancet 1987; i:659–661.
30. Haines JL, Short MP, Kwiatkowski DJ, Jewell A, Andermann E, Bejjani B, Yang CH, Gusella JF, Amos JA. Localization of one gene for tuberous sclerosis within 9q32-9q34, and further evidence for heterogeneity. Am J Hum Genet 1991; 49:764–72.
31. Kandt R, Pericak-Vance M, Hung W-Y, Gardner R, Nellist M, Phillips K, Warner K, Speer M, Crossen P, Laing N, Roses A. Absence of linkage of ABO blood group locus to familial tuberous sclerosis. Exp Neurol 1989; 104:223–228.
32. Northrup H, Kwiatkowski D, Roach E, Dobyns W, Lewis R, Herman G, Rodriguez E, Daiger S, Blanton S. Evidence for genetic heterogeneity in tuberous sclerosis: one locus on chromosome 9 and at least one locus elsewhere. Am J Hum Genet 1992; 51:709–720.
33. Kandt R, Haines J, Smith M, Northrup H, Gardner R, Short M, Dumars K, Roach E, Steingold S, Wall S, Blanton S, Flodman P, Kwiatkowski D, Jewell A, Weber J, Roses A, Pericak-Vance M. Linkage of a major gene locus for tuberous sclerosis to a chromosome-16 marker for polycystic kidney disease. Nature Genet 1992; 2:37–41.
34. Povey S, Burley MW, Attwood J, Benham F, Hunt D, Jeremiah SJ, Franklin D, Gillett G, Malas S, Robson EB, et al. Two loci for tuberous sclerosis: one on 9q34 and one on 16p13. Ann Hum Genet 1994; 107–127.
35. Maheshwar MM, Sandford R, Nellist M, cheadle JP, Sgotto B, Vaudin M, Sampson JR. Comparative analysis and genomic structure of the tuberous sclerosis 2 (TSC2) gene in human and pufferfish. Hum Mol Genet 1996; 5:131–137.
36. Kobayashi T, Nishizawa M, Hirayama Y, Kobayashi E, Hino O. cDNA structure, alternative splicing and exon-intron organization of the predisposing tuberous sclerosis (Tsc2) gene of the Eker rat model. Nucleic Acids Res 1995; 23:2608–2613.
37. Xiao GH, Jin F, Yeung RS. Identification of tuberous sclerosis 2 messenger RNA

splice variants that are conserved and differentially expressed in rat and human tissues. Cell Growth Differ 1995; 6:1185–1191.
38. Xu L, Sterner C, Maheshwa MM, Wilson PH, Nellist M, Short PM, Haines JL, Sampson JR, Ramesh V. Alternative splicing of the tuberous sclerosis 2 (TSC2) gene in human and mouse tissues. Genomics 1995; 27:475–480.
39. Kumar A, Kandt RS, Wolpert C, Roses AD, Pericak-Vance MA, Gilbert JR. Mutation analysis of the TSC2 gene in an African-American family. Human Mol Genet 1995; 4:2295–2298.
40. Wilson PJ, Ramesh V, Kristiansen A, Bove C, Jozwiak S, Kwiatkowski DJ, Short MP, Haines JL. Novel mutations detected in the TSC2 gene from both sporadic and familial TSC patients. Hum Mol Genet 1996; 5:249–256.
41 Verhoef S, Vrtel R, Bakker L, Stolte-Dijkstra I, Nellist M, Begeer JH, Zaremba J, Jozwiak S, Tempelaars AMP, Lindhout D, Halley DJJ, van den Ouweland AMW. Recurrent mutation 4882delTT in the GAP-related domain of the tuberous sclerosis TSC2 gene. Human Mutation. 1996; 8:XX
42. Kumar A, WOlpert C, Kandt RS, Segal J, Pufky J, Roses AD, Pericak VM, Gilbert JR. A de novo frame-shift mutation inthe tuberin gene. Hum Mol Genet 1995; 4:1471–1472.
43. Au KS, Murrell J, Buckler A, Blanton SH, Northrup H. Recombination further narrowing the TSC1 region. J med Genet 1996; 33:559–561.
44. Green AJ, Smith M, Yates JR. Loss of heeterozygosity on chromosome 16p13.3 in hamartomas from tuberous sclerosis patients. Nat Genet 1994; 6:193–196.
45. Carbonara C, Longa L, Grosso E, Mazzucco G, Borrone C, Garre ML, Brisigotti M, Filippi G, Scabar A, Giannotti A, Falzoni P, Monga G, Garini G, Gabrielli M, Riegler P, Danesino C, Ruggieri M, Magro G, Migone N. Apparent preferential loss of heterozygosity at TSC2 over TSC1 chromosomal region in tuberous sclerosis hamartomas. Genes Chrom Cancer 1996; 15:18–25.
46. Henske EP, Scheithauer BW, Short MP, Wollmann R, Nahmias J, Hornigold N, van SM, Welsh CT, Kwiatkowski DJ. Allelic loss is frequent in tuberous sclerosis kidney lesions but rare in brain lesions. Am J Hum Genet 1996; 59:400–406.
47. Sepp T, Yates JRW, Green AJ. Loss of heterozygosity in tuberous sclerosis hamartomas. J Med Genet 1996; 33:962–964.
48. Henske EP, Neumann HP, Scheithauer BW, herbst EW, Short MP, Kwiatkowski DJ. Loss of heterozygosity in the tuberous sclerosis (TSC2) region of chromosome band 16p13 occurs in sporadic as well as TSC-associated renal angiomyolipomas. Genes Chrom Cancer 1995; 13:295–298.
49. Eker R, Mossige J, Johannessen JV, Aars H. Hereditary renal adenomas and adenocarcinomas in rats. Diagn Histopathol 1981; 4:99–110.
50. Kobayashi T, Hirayama Y, Kobayashi E, Kubo Y, Hino O. A germline insertion in the tuberous sclerosis (Tsc2) gene gives rise to the Eker rat model of dominantly inherited cancer [published erratum appears in Nat Genet 1995; 9(2):218)]. Nat Genet 1995; 9:70–74.
51. Yueng RS, Xiao GH, Jin F, Lee WC, Testa JR, Knudson AG. Predisposition to renal carcinoma in the Eker rat is determined by germ-line mutation of the tuberous sclerosis 2 (TSC2) gene. Proc Natl Acad Sci USA 1994; 91:11413–6.

52. Hino O, Klein-Szanto AJP, Freed JJ, Testa JR, Brown DQ, Vilensky M, Yeung RS, Tartof KD, Knudson AG. Spontaneous and radiation-induced renal tumors in the Eker rat model of dominantly inherited cancer. Proc Natl Acad Sci USA 1993; 90:327–331.
53. Xiao GH, Jin F, Yeung RS. Germ-line Tsc2 mutation in a dominantly inherited cancer model defines a novel family of rat intracisternal-A particle elements. Oncogene 1995; 11:81–87.
54. Kubo Y, Klimek F, Kikuchi Y, Bannasch P, Hino O. Early detection of Knudson's two-hits in preneoplastic renal cells fo the Eker rat model by the laser microdissection procedure. Cancer Res 1995; 55:989–990.
55. Yeung RS, Ziao GH, Everitt JI, Jin F, Walker CL. Allelic loss at the tuberous sclerosis 2 locus in spontaneous tumors in the Eker rat. Mol Carcinogen 1995; 14:28–36.
56. Kubo Y, Kikuchi Y, Mitani H, Kobayashi E, Kobayashi T, Hino O. Allelic loss at the tuberous sclerosis (Tsc2) gene locus in spontaneous uterine leiomyosarcomas and pituitary adenomas in the Eker rat model. Jpn J Cancer Res. 1995; 86:828–832.
57. Cook JA, Oliver K, Mueller RF, Sampson J. A cross-sectional study of renal involvement in tuberous sclerosis. J Med Genet 1996; 33:480–484.
58. Hodgson SV, Maher ER. A Practical Guide to Human Cancer Genetics. Cambridge: Cambridge University, 1993.
59. Huson SM, Compston DAs, Harper PS. A genetic study of von Recklinghausen neurofibromatosis in southeast Wales. II Guidelines for genetic counseling. J Med Genet 1989; 26:712–721.
60. Kerfoot C, Wienecke R, Menchine M, Emelin J, Maize JC, Welsh CT, Norman MG, DeClue JE, Vinters HV. Localization of tuberous sclerosis 2 mRNA and its protein product tuberin in normal human brain and in cerebral lesions of patients with tuberous sclerosis. Brain Pathol 1996; 6:367–377.
61. Crino PB, Trojanowski JW, Dichter MA, Eberwine J. Embryonic neuronal markers in tuberous sclerosis; single-cell molecular pathology. Proc Natl Acad Sci USA 1996; 93:14152–14157.
62. Geist RT, Reddy AJ, Zhang J, Gutmann DH. Expression of the tuberous sclerosis 2 gene product, tuberin, in adult and developing nervous system tissues. Neurobiol Dis 1996; 3:111–120.
63. Wienecke R, Maize JC, Shoarinejad F, Vass WC, Reed J, Bonifacino JS, Resau JH, de Gunzberg J, Yeung RS, deClue JE. Co-localization of the TSC2 product tuberin with its target rap1 in the Golgi apparatus. Oncogene 1996; 13:913–923.
64. Menchine M, Emelin JK, Mischel PS, Haag TA, Norman MG, Pepkowitz SH, Welsh CT, Townsend JJ, Vinters HV. Tissue and cell-type specific expression of the tuberous sclerosis gene, TSC2, in human tissues. Mod Pathol 1996; 9:1071–1080.
65. Wienecke R, Maize JC, Reed J, de Gunzberg J, Yeung RS, DeClue JE. Expression of the TSC2 product tuberin and its target rap1 in normal human tissues. Am J Pathol 1997; 150:1–8.
66. Geist RT, Gutmann DH. The tuberous sclerosis 2 gene is expressed at high levels in the cerebellum and developing spinal cord. Cell Growth Differ 1995; 6:1477–1483.

67. Kikuchi A, Saski T, Araki S, Hata Y, Takai Y. Purification and characterization from bovine brain cytosol of two GTPase-activating proteins specific for smg p21, a GTP-binding protein having the same effector domain as c-ras p21s. J Biol Chem 1989; 264:9133–9136.
68. Rubinfeld B, Munemitsu S, Clark R, Conroy L, Watt K, Crosier WJ, McCormick F, Polakis P. Molecular cloning of a GTPase activing protein specific for the Krev-1 protein p21rap1. Cell 1991; 65:1033–1042.
69. Wienecke R, Konig A, DeClue JE. Identification of tuberin, the tuberous sclerosis-2 product. Tuberin possesses specific Rap1GAP activity. J Biol Chem 1995; 270:16409–16414.
70. Pizon V, Desjardins M, Bucci C, Parton RG, Zerial M. Association of Rap1a and Rap1b proteins with late endocytic/phagocytic compartments and Rap2a with the Golgi complex. J Cell Sci 1994; 1661–1670.
71. McCormick F, Wittinghofer A. Interactions between Ras proteins and their effectors. Curr Opin Biotechnol 1996; 7:449–456.
72. Boguski M, McCormick F. Proteins regulating Ras and its relatives. Nature 1993; 366:643–654.
73. Hall A. The cellular functions of small GTP-binding proteins. Science 1990; 249:635–640.
74. Pizon V, Chardin P, Lerosey I, Olofsson B, Tavitian A. Human cDNAs rap1 and rap2 homologous to the Drosophila gene Dras2 encode proteins closely related to ras the "effector" region. Oncogene 1988; 3:201–204.

21

Tuberous Sclerosis Complex and LAM

JAY H. RYU

Mayo Clinic
Mayo Medical School
Rochester, Minnesota

I. Introduction

Tuberous sclerosis complex (TSC) is a congenital hamartomatosis of autosomal dominant inheritance with high penetrance and variable expressivity (1). However, approximately 60% of all TSC patients appear to represent sporadic cases with no prior family history of the disease (2). Clinical manifestations of this disorder are extremely variable from patient to patient, even within the same family, and are age-dependent. TSC is a hamartomatosis of multifocal origin and is diagnosed by the presence of specific lesions in certain organs. Most commonly, the pathognomonic lesions are detected on the skin, brain, or retina. Other abnormalities involve the kidneys, endocrine glands, heart, gastrointestinal tract, lungs, and other organs. Classical clinical triad of Vogt (adenoma sebaceum, epileptic seizures, and mental retardation) is present in only 29% of TSC patients (1). To date, two mutations have been identified which appear to lead to the TSC phenotype. These loci have been named TSC1 and TSC2 genes located at chromosome 9q34 and chromosome 16pl3.3 regions, respectively (2). These genes appear to behave as tumor suppressor genes (3).

Lung involvement in tuberous sclerosis complex (pulmonary tuberous sclerosis) was initially described by Lutembacher in 1918 (4), who reported a 36-

year-old woman with bilateral pneumothoraces. She was found to have cystic changes in the lungs at autopsy. In 1939, Berg and Vejlens (5) gave an account of another young woman who suffered recurrent pneumothoraces and progressive respiratory insufficiency. This report included a description of interstitial infiltrates and cystic changes on the chest radiograph as well as diffuse cystic changes and smooth muscle proliferation seen in the lungs on postmortem examination. In 1971, Dwyer et al. reviewed 28 cases in the literature and added three additional cases of their own (6). Since the initial description by Berg and Vejlens, there have been about 60 cases reported (7–31). Most of these papers are single case reports. A recent report by Castro and associates (31) summarizing nine pulmonary tuberous sclerosis (PTS) patients seen at the Mayo Clinic represents the largest series of original cases.

Over the past 30 years, several authors have debated the relationship between pulmonary lymphangioleiomyomatosis (LAM) and PTS (17,20,31–37). These two entities share striking similarities in their epidemiological, clinical, radiographic, and histopathological features. In addition, both entities are associated with chylothorax, extrapulmonary lymphangiomyomas, and renal angiomyolipomas (6,8,9,12,15,17,18,20,27,31,32,34–36,39–45). The question of whether pulmonary lymphangioleiomyomatosis is a form fruste of TSC will be discussed later in this chapter.

II. Lung Involvement in Tuberous Sclerosis Complex

A. Epidemiology

Lung involvement in TSC is uncommon. It has previously been reported to occur in less than 1% of the cases (6). A more recent report suggests a prevalence of 2.3% in a series of 388 patients with TSC (31). However, even this figure may be an underestimate since lung involvement in TSC may be clinically and radiographically silent in earlier stages.

Although TSC affects both males and females with no sex predilection, pulmonary involvement occurs almost exclusively in women (6,8,12,15, 17,20,31,34,36,39,46–48). In contrast to epileptic seizures, the lung disease usually develops during adult life. Detection of the lung involvement is usually made during the childbearing ages of third through fifth decades of life (8,12,15,20,31). The mean age at the onset of respiratory symptoms is 33–34 years (8,31). In approximately one-third of these patients, respiratory problems may be the initial clue that leads to the diagnosis of TSC (31).

B. Histopathology

Most authors believe the histopathological features of PTS to be identical to LAM (15,20,21,34,35,50). Both conditions are characterized by diffuse cystic changes and proliferation of immature-appearing smooth muscle cells in the lung parenchyma. Smooth muscle elements can be seen in the walls of the cysts (12,49,50). Although the microscopic picture is unique, macroscopically, the cystic change may be confused for honeycombing seen in idiopathic pulmonary fibrosis. On the pleural surface of the lungs, cystic changes are manifest as numerous subpleural blebs. Lung parenchyma between the cysts appear normal. As in LAM, hemosiderin-laden macrophages may be seen in the alveolar spaces as well as the interstitial compartment. Even at the ultrastructural level, the features are similar to those reported for LAM (20). Estrogen receptors have been demonstrated in patients with PTS (23). Torres and associates (5) reported the presence of estrogen and progesterone receptors in extrapulmonary lymphangiomyomatous tissue obtained from TSC patients. In addition, cells cultured from one of these patients exhibited a mitogenic response to estradiol. Another recent report describes positive staining with HMB45 monoclonal antibody of the proliferating smooth muscle cells in a lung biopsy specimen from a woman with TSC (52).

Histopathological differences that have been noted by some authors have been relatively minor. Stovin and associates (17) described differences in the distribution of the lesion with the tendency of smooth muscle to involve the blood vessels in PTS compared to LAM. Lie and associates (18) noted proliferation of smooth muscle involving lymph nodes and lymphatics to be more widespread in LAM compared to PTS. Recently, an atypical case of lung involvement in TSC was described consisting of micronodular hyperplasia of type II pneumocytes (28).

C. Clinical Manifestations

Similar to LAM, the clinical manifestations in PTS relate to the proliferation of immature smooth muscle around the airways, blood vessels, and lymphatics in the lungs. The most common symptom in PTS is dypnea, which is usually progressive over several years. The next most common manifestation is pneumothorax, which may occasionally be bilateral. Pneumothorax is frequently recurrent unless treated with pleurodesis. Other symptoms include hemoptysis, cough, chest pain, and chyloptysis. Since the respiratory manifestations usually occur during adult life, the majority of patients have a known history of TSC. Occasionally, lung involvement in TSC may be detected in an asymptomatic stage by an abnormal chest radiograph or computed tomography (CT) of the thorax. In addition, we have seen several asymptomatic patients whose lung involvement was diagnosed by CT of the abdomen which happened to include views of the lower thorax.

Physical signs that relate to PTS include tachypnea, signs of hyperinflation, and expiratory slowing. Lung auscultation usually reveals distant breath sounds without adventitial noises. Occasionally, crackles or wheezes may be heard. Clubbing of the digits has been reported but is not a characteristic feature of PTS (6). Cyanosis and signs of cor pulmonale are present in advanced cases. Most patients with PTS have obvious cutaneous signs of TSC, which may at times be recognized only in retrospect (31). When present, pleural effusion is detected by the presence of dullness and decreased breath sounds over the lower part of the involved hemithorax. Pleural effusion is not seen in PTS as commonly as in LAM but does occur and is usually chylous.

TSC patients with pulmonary involvement have been noted to have less mental retardation than the general TSC population (6,8). This may be due to premature deaths of those patients with more severe forms of TSC at an early age since pulmonary disease develops during adult life.

D. Laboratory Findings

Chest Radiography

Chest radiograph in patients with PTS usually shows diffuse interstitial infiltrates with reticular or reticulonodular character (Fig. 1). These infiltrates may be accompanied by signs of hyperinflation, pneumothorax, or chylothorax. In advanced cases cystic or bullous changes are seen. However, serial chest radiographs may not correlate well with changes occurring in symptoms or pulmonary function results (31).

Computed Tomography of the Chest

For optimal visualization of the changes in the lung parenchyma, high-resolution (HRCT) technique is employed in computed tomography of the thorax. Characteristic findings include numerous well-defined cysts with thin walls that are distributed diffusely throughout all lobes of the lungs with no predominance or sparing of any particular regions (Fig. 2) (30,31,53–56). Cysts vary in size from a few millimeters to several centimeters in diameter. They are usually round but may assume irregular and bizarre shapes as they enlarge and coalesce. These features are indistinguishable from LAM (47,53).

As with the chest radiograph, one may also see evidence of pneumothorax, chylothorax, and hyperinflation. Pneumothorax may be loculated and not apparent by conventional chest radiography. HRCT of the chest is clearly more sensitive than chest radiography in detecting pulmonary involvement in TSC. Diffuse cystic changes in the lung parenchyma can be seen in the presence of normal chest radiograph and pulmonary function (31). On the other hand, Müller and associates (57) have reported a case of biopsy-proven LAM with a normal CT of the chest.

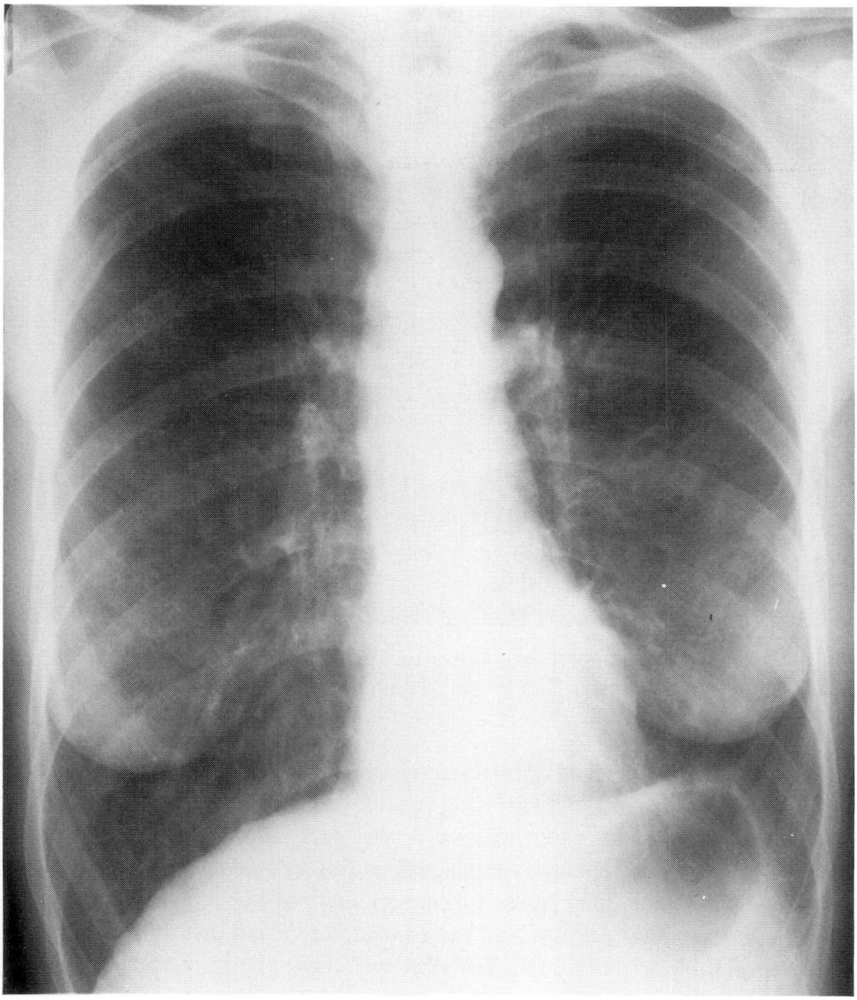

Figure 1 Posteroanterior chest radiograph in a 37-year-old woman with advanced PTS demonstrating diffuse reticular infiltrates, cystic changes, and hyperinflation. Her pulmonary function testing showed very severe obstructive changes with an FEV_1 of 19% predicted normal.

Pulmonary Function Tests

Pulmonary function testing is useful in assessing the degree of pulmonary impairment. Most patients show an obstructive pattern. In a recent report, an average value of forced expiratory volume in one second (FEV_1) was 43%, which represents obstructive airways disease of moderate to severe degree (31). Some

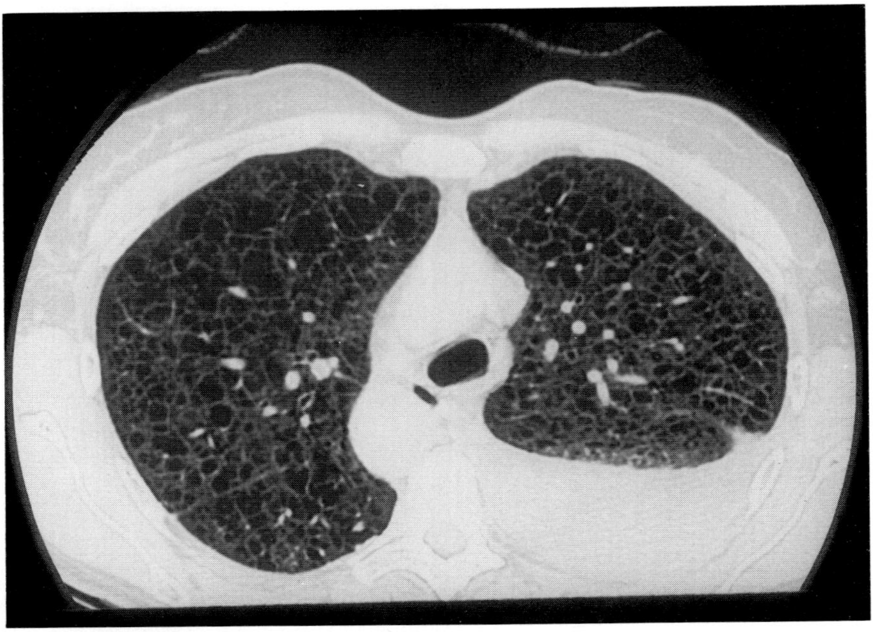

Figure 2 High resolution CT of the chest on a 42-year-old woman with PTS demonstrating diffuse cystic changes and a right chylothorax.

patients may show evidence of hyperreactive airways with a significant response to an inhaled bronchodilator. Diffusing capacity is usually low, reflecting diffuse cystic changes in the lung parenchyma. Signs of air trapping and hyperinflation are seen in increased residual volume and total lung capacity. A superimposed restrictive component may be seen in the presence of a pleural effusion or previous lung resection, resulting in a mixed obstructive and restrictive defect.

Arterial blood gas study reveals hypoxemia at rest in the majority of patients with further oxygen desaturation on exercise. However, in the early asymptomatic stage arterial oxygen levels may be normal at rest as well as with exercise.

E. Diagnosis

In patients with confirmed diagnosis of TSC, lung involvement is usually suspected on the basis of an abnormal chest radiograph. Presumptive diagnosis of pulmonary tuberous sclerosis can be made in the presence of diffuse interstitial infiltrates combined with signs of hyperinflation. Unilateral or bilateral chylothorax may also be present. In addition, a history or the presence of pneumothorax is also suspicious for lung involvement in TSC. HRCT of the chest demonstrating typical cystic changes throughout both lungs provides adequate confirmation of PTS in patients with pathognomonic features of TSC. Lung biopsy is usually not necessary unless there are atypical features on thoracic imaging or the underlying diagnosis of TSC is in question. If histological confirmation is needed, brochoscopic biopsy may provide enough tissue to demonstrate typical histological findings (31,47). If not, thoracoscopic or open lung biopsy can be pursued.

F. Treatment

There are a limited amount of data regarding treatment of PTS. In 1983, Capron and associates (20) initially raised the question of whether hormonal therapy used in treating LAM should also be tried in PTS, given the similarities in these two conditions. In 1985, Luna and associates (23) reported a case of a 44-year-old woman who was treated with tamoxifen and showed improvement in her clinical status and pulmonary function. Few years later, Murray and associates (25) described a 35-year-old woman treated with progesterone who experienced a reduction in her chylous pleural effusion and no further worsening in her lung infiltrates. However, there have also been reports of treatment failure to tamoxifen and progesterone (24). The most commonly used medication has been progesterone, usually given by the intramuscular route. Other agents used have included gonadotrophin-releasing hormone analogs as well as oophorectomy (31).

Recently, Castro and associates (31) described nine PTS patients, five of whom were treated with hormonal manipulation including progesterone, leuprolide, and oophorectomy. Three of these patients appeared to benefit with either improvement or stabilization of their lung disease. Two of these nine patients subsequently underwent lung transplantation (one single lung transplant, one double lung transplant).

G. Prognosis

In Dwyer's series (6), 60% of the PTS patients were dead with an average time interval of 4 years and 6 months between the onset of respiratory symptoms and death. Eighty-six percent of these deaths were due to the progressive lung disease leading to recurrent pneumothoraces, cor pulmonale, and respiratory failure. However, in a recent report by Castro, seven of nine (78%) patients were alive after an average follow-up of 17 years since the diagnosis of TSC. Two patients had died of respiratory failure at ages 46 and 53 years, respectively. Both of these patients had severe obstructive lung disease at presentation and were never treated with hormonal therapy Thus, survival in PTS patients appeared to be more favorable than previously described and not significantly different from that of TSC patients without lung involvement (Fig. 3). It is also similar to the prognosis re-

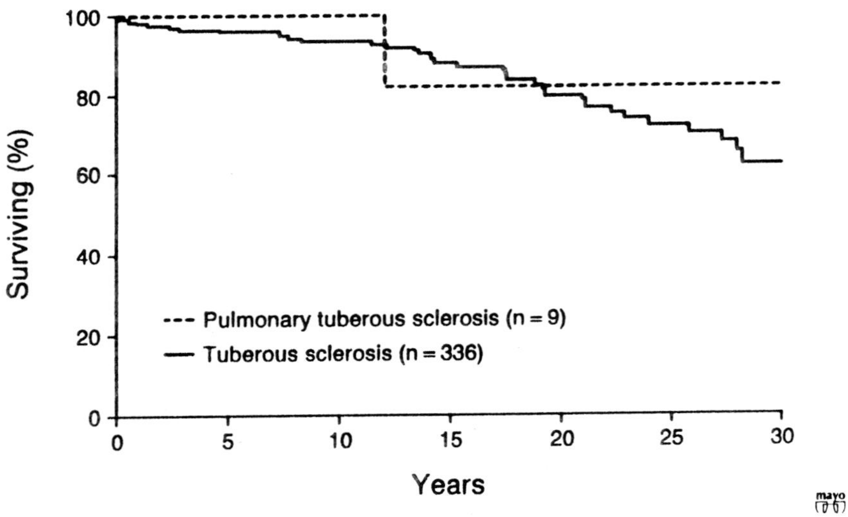

Figure 3 Kaplan-Meier survival curve of PTS patients compared with survival of TSC patients without lung involvement demonstrating no significant difference. Seven of nine PTS patients are alive after a mean follow-up of 17 years since the TSC diagnosis. (From Ref. 31.)

ported by Taylor and associates (47) for patients with LAM. Clinical course for individual PTS patients is variable, and stability over a number of years has been observed in some patients, even without hormonal therapy (13,31).

III. Relationship to LAM

In 1966, Cornog and Enterline (32) reported six cases of lymphangiomyoma and noted similarities to lesions associated with TSC. In 1972, Jao and associates (15) described a 41-year-old woman with TSC who had diffuse interstitial lung infiltrates and chylothorax. Needle biopsy of the lung showed features consistent with LAM. On the basis of similarities in epidemiological (nearly all women), clinical, radiographic, and histopathological features, PTS and LAM were felt to be either identical or variable expressions of the same disorder. Valensi (33) also considered LAM to be in the spectrum of presentations of TSC. He argued that the absence of family history does not exclude LAM as a form of TSC, since most cases of TSC are sporadic. Wolff (34) described LAM as a forme fruste or incomplete expression of TSC with both conditions presenting as multifocal hamartomatosis. On the other hand, Stovin and associates (I 7) concluded these disorders to be distinct in their report of two patients with LAM and one patient with PTS, along with review of the literature. Their argument was based on differences in the incidence of chylothorax and the distribution of lesions histologically, as well as the absence of family history in LAM.

Gomez (1) has stated that the presence of LAM or renal angiomyolipomas represents a "presumptive" diagnosis of TSC. Similarly, according to the diagnostic criteria proposed by the National Tuberous Sclerosis Association (59), the presence of LAM (histologically confirmed) is considered as "probable" TSC, and the combined presence of LAM and renal angiomyolipomas represents "definite" TSC.

As already described, PTS and LAM are indeed nearly identical in their epidemiological, histopathological, clinical, and radiographic features. Similarities in their natural history have also been observed. In addition, both lung diseases can be associated with chylothorax, extrapulmonary lymphangiomyomas, and renal angiomyolipomas. However, there has never been a familial case of LAM described even in those LAM patients with associated extrapulmonary lymphangiomyomas and renal angiomyolipomas. In contrast, PTS has been seen in first-degree relatives as expected for an autosomal dominant syndrome (60).

TSC is a disorder with protean clinical manifestations. The boundaries of TSC are not clearly defined, and its diagnosis remains a clinical judgment. Recent studies have demonstrated genetic heterogeneity with two TSC loci identified to date. The question of whether LAM is an expression of TSC will remain unresolved until a reliable molecular marker for TSC is available. In the absence of demonstrated TSC markers in LAM patients, TSC and LAM may be considered separate entities since TSC has never been reported in the offspring of LAM patients.

References

1. Gomez MR. Tuberous Sclerosis, 2nd ed. New York: Raven Press, 1988.
2. Sampson JR, Harris PC. The molecular genetics of tuberous sclerosis. Hum Mol Genet 1994; 3:1477–1480.
3. Webb DW, Osborne JP. Tuberous sclerosis. Arch Dis Child 1995; 72:471–474.
4. Lutembacher R. Dysembryomes metatypiques des reins: carcinose submiliaire aigue du poumon avec emphyseme generalise et double pneumothorax. Ann Med 1918; 5:435–450.
5. Berg G, Vejlens G. Maladie kystique du poumon et sclerose tubereuse du cerveau. Acta Paediatr Uppsala 1939; 26:16–30.
6. Dwyer JM, Hickie JB, Garvan J. Pulmonary tuberous sclerosis: report of three patients and a review of the literature. Q J Med 1971; 40:115–125.
7. Boberg A. Clinical and genetic investigations into tuberous sclerosis and Recklinghausen's neurofibromatosis. Acta Phys Neurol Paediatr Scand 1951; 71(suppl):11–239.

8. Dawson J. Pulonary tuberous sclerosis and its relationship to other forms of the disease. Q J Med 1954; 23:113–146.
9. Wilson GC. Tuberous sclerosis: a case with pulmonary and lymph node involvement. Med J Austral 1964; 2:795–796.
10. Rumberg J, Herzog I. Tuberous sclerosis. NY State J Med 1966; 66:642–648.
11. Milledge RD, Gerald BE, Carter WJ. Pulmonary manifestations of tuberous sclerosis. Am J Roentgenol Rad Ther Nucl Med 1966; 98:734–743.
12. Harris JO, Waltuck BL, Swenson EW. The pathophysiology of the lungs in tuberous sclerosis: a case report and literature review. Am Rev Respir Dis 1969; 100:379–387.
13. Malik SK, Pardee N, Martin CJ. Involvement of the lungs in tuberous sclerosis. Chest 1970; 58:538–540.
14. Broughton RBK. Pulmonary tuberous sclerosis presenting with pleural effusion. BMJ 1970; 1:477–478.
15. Jao J, Gilbert S, Messer R. Lymphangiomyoma and tuberous sclerosis. Cancer 1972; 29:1188–1192.
16. Master K, Ting EY, Katz M. Pathophysiology in pulmonary tuberous sclerosis. NY State J Med 1974; 74:2000–2003.
17. Stovin PGI, Lum C, Flower CDR, Drake CS, Becley M. The lungs in lymphangiomyomatosis and in tuberous sclerosis. Thorax 1975; 30:497–509.
18. Lie JT, Miller RD, Williams DE. Cystic disease of the lungs in tuberous sclerosis: clinicopathologic correlation, including body plethysmographic lung function tests. Mayo Clin Proc 1980; 55:547–553.
19. Babcock TL, Snyder BA. Spontaneous pneumothorax associated with tuberous sclerosis. J Thorac CV Surg 1982; 83:100–104.
20. Capron F, Ameille J, Lecelrc P, Mornet P, Barbagellata M, Reynes M, Rochemaure J. Pulmonary lymphangioleiomyomatosis and Bourneville's tuberous sclerosis with pulmonary involvement: the same disease? Cancer 1983; 52:851–855.
21. Kaku T, Toyoshima S, Enjoji M. Tuberous sclerosis with pulmonary and lymph node involvement: relationship to lymphangiomyomatosis. Acta Pathol Jpn 1983; 33:395–401.
22. Lieberman BA, Chamberlain DW, Goldstein RS. Tuberous sclerosis with pulmonary involvement. Can Med Assoc J 1984; 130:287–289.
23. Luna CM, Gene R, Jolly EC, Nahmod N, Defranchi HA, Patino G, Elsner B. Pulmonary lymphangiomyomatosis associated with tuberous sclerosis: treatment with tamoxifen and tetracycline pleurodesis. Chest 1985; 88:473–475.
24. Westermann CJJ, Oostveen ACM, Wagenaar SS, Hilvering C, Overbeek SE, Verheijen-Breemhaar D, Corrin B. Pulmonary tuberous sclerosis treated with tamoxifen and progesterone. Thorax 1986; 41:892–893.
25. Murray DP, O'Sullivan DJ. Pulmonary tuberous sclerosis responds to progesterone treatmetn. Ir J Med Sci 1988; 157:196–197.
26. Slingerland JM, Grossman RF, Chamberlain D, Trembley CE. Pulmonary manifestations of tuberous sclerosis in first degree relatives. Thorax 1989; 44:212–214.
27. Hauck RW, Konig G, Permanetter W, Weiss M. Wockel W, Iruhmann G. Tuberous sclerosis with pulmonary involvement. Respiration 1990; 57:289–292.

28. Popper HH, Gamperl R, Pongratz MG, Kullnig P, Juttner-Smolle FM, Pfragner R. Chromosome tying in lymphangioleiomyomatosis of the lung with and without tuberous sclerosis. Eur Respir J 1993; 6:753–759.
29. Uzzo RG, Libby DM, Vaughan ED Jr, Levey SH. Coexisting lymphangioleiomyomatosis and bilateral angiomyolipomas in a patient with tuberous sclerosis. J Urol 1994; 151:1612–1615.
30. Meysman M., Noppen M, Herregodts P, Vincken W. A patient with seizures, haemoptysis and dyspnoea. Eur Respir J 1995; 8:1433–1434.
31. Castro M, Shepherd CW, Gomez MR, Lie JT, Ryu JH. Pulmonary tuberous sclerosis. Chest 1995; 107:189–195
32. Cornog JL, Enterline HT. Lymphangiomyoma, a benign lesion of chyliferous lymphatics synonymous with lymphangiopericytoma. Cancer 1966; 19:1909–1930.
33. Valensi QJ. Pulmonary lymphangiomyoma, a probable forme fruste of tuberous sclerosis; a case report and survey of the literature. Am Rev Respir Dis 1973; 108:1411–1415.
34. Wolff M. Lymphangiomyoma: clinicopathologic study and ultrastructural confirmation of its histogenesis. Cancer 1973; 31:988–1007.
35. Monteforte WJ Jr, Kohnen PW. Angiomyolipomas in a case of lymphangiomyomatosis syndrome: relationships to tuberous sclerosis. Cancer 1974; 34:317–321.
36. Corrin B, Liebow AA, Friedman PJ. Pulmonary lymphangiomyomatosis: a review. Am J Pathol 1975; 79:348–367.
37. Bonetti F, Chiodera P. Lymphangiomyomatosis and tuberous sclerosis: Where is the border? Eur Respir J 1966; 9:399–401.
38. Vadas G, Pare JAP, Thurlbeck WM. Pulmonary and lymph node myomatosis: review of the literature and report of a case. Can Med Assoc J 1967; 96:420–424.
39. Frack MD, Simon L, Dawson BH. The lymphangiomyomatosis syndrome. Cancer 1968; 22:428–437.
40. Farrow GM, Harrison EG Jr, Utz DC, Jones DR. Renal angiomyolipoma: a clinicopathologic study of 32 cases. Cancer 1968; 22:564–570.
41. Bush JK, Mclean RL, Seeker HO. Diffuse lung disease due to lymphangiomyoma. Am J Med 1969; 46:645–654.
42. Lack EE, Dolan MF, Finisio J, Grover G, Singh M, Triche TJ. Pulmonary and extrapulmonary lymphangioleiomyomatosis: report of a case with bilateral renal angiomyolipomas, multifocal lymphangioleiomyomatosis, and a glial polyp of the endocervix. Am J Surg Pathol 1986; 10:650–657.
43. Kerr LA, Blute ML, Ryu JH, Swensen SJ, Malek RS, Renal angiomyolipoma in association with pulmonary lymphangioleiomyomatosis: forme fruste of tuberous sclerosis? Urology 1993; 41:440–444.
44. Bernstein SM, Newell JD Jr, Adamczyk D, Mortenson RL, King TE Jr, Lynch DA. How common are renal angiomyolipomas in patients with pulmonary lymphangiomyomatosis. Am J Respir Crit Care Med 1995; 152:2138–2143.
45. Maziak DE, Kesten S, Rappaport DC, Maurer J. Extrathoracic angiomyolipomas in lymphangioleiomyomatosis. Eur Respir J 1996; 9:402–405.
46. Carrington CB, Cugell DW, Gaensler EA, Marks A, Redding RA, Schaff JT,

Tomasian A. Lymphangioleiomyomatosis: physiologic-pathologic-radiologic correlation. Am Rev Respir Dis 1977; 116:977–995.

47. Taylor JR, Ryu J, Colby TV, Raffin TA. Lymphangioleiomyomatosis: clinical course in 32 patients. N Engl J Med 1990; 323:1254–1260.
48. Kitaichi M, Nishimura K, Itoh H, Izumi T. Pulmonary lymphangioleiomyomatosis: a report of 46 patients including a clinicopathologic study of prognostic factors. Am J Respir Crit Care Med 1995; 151:527–33.
49. Sobonya RE, Quan SF, Fleishman JS. Pulmonary lymphangioleiomyomatosis: quantitative analysis of lesions producing airflow limitation. Hum Pathol 1985; 16:1122–1128.
50. Colby TV, Carrington CB. Interstitial lung disease. In: Thurlbeck WM, Churg AM, eds. Pathology of the Lung. New York: Thieme Medical Publishers, 1995:675–732.
51. Torres VC, Bjomsson J, King B, Kumar R, Zincke H, Edell ES, Wilson TO, Hattery RR, Gomez MR. Extrapulmonary lymphangioleiomyomatosis and lymphangiomatous cysts in tuberous sclerosis complex. Mayo Clin Proc 1995; 70:641–648.
52. Nakajima J, Kotsuka Y, Yagyuu K, Takeshita M, Furuse A, Osa T. Pulmonary hamartoangiomyomatosis (lymphangiomyomatosis) in tuberous sclerosis–a case in which clinical course had been modified by previous surgical intervention. Nippon Kyobu Shikkan Gakkai Zasshi 1995; 33:80–84.
53. Lenoir A, Grenier P, Brauner MW, Frija J, Remy-Jardin M, Revel D, Cordier J. Pulmonary Lymphangiomyomatosis and tuberous sclerosis: comparison of radiographic and thin-section CT findings. Radiology 1990; 175:329–334.
54. Stem EJ, Webb WR, Golden JA, Gamsu G. Cystic lung disease associated with eosinophilic granuloma and tuberous sclerosis: air trapping at dynamic ultrafast high-resolution CT. Radiology 1992; 182:325–329.
55. Perez VL, Shimkin PM. Computed tomography in pulmonary tuberous sclerosis. Connect Med 1993; 57:13–14.
56. Williams DE, Rosenow EC. Exertional dyspnea, hemoptysis, and skin lesions in a 34-year-old woman. Chest 1993; 104:587–588.
57. Müller NL, Chiles , Kullnig P. Pulmonary lymphangiomyomatosis: correlation of CT with radiographic and functional findings. Radiology 1990; 175:335–339.
58. Aberle DR, Hansell DM, Brown K, Tashkin DP. Lymphangiomyomatosis: CT, chest radiographic, and functional correlations. Radiology 1990; 176:381–387.
59. Roach ES, Smith M, Huttenlocher P, Bhat M, Alcorn D, Hawley L. Diagnostic criteria: tuberous sclerosis complex. Report of the Diagnostic Criteria Committee of the National Tuberous Sclerosis Association. J Child Neurol 1992; 7:221–224.
60. Slingerland JM, Grossman RF, Chamberlain D, Trembly CE. Pulmonary manifestations of tuberous sclerosis in first degree relatives. Thorax 1989; 44:212–214.

22

Tuberin

JEFFREY E. DECLUE

National Cancer Institute
National Institutes of Health
Bethesda, Maryland

I. Introduction

The identification of the *TSC2* gene in 1993 represented the culmination of a long, determined effort by scores of investigators (1). This discovery was not only a breakthrough in its own right, but it also allowed for the beginning of an investigation into the properties of the *TSC2* product, tuberin. In turn, it is the hope of tuberous sclerosis (TSC) patients and investigators alike that a better understanding of the normal cellular role of this protein will allow for the development of specific therapies to both prevent and treat the manifestations of TSC. The investigations described here, including the identification and characterization of the protein, were begun with an eye toward these goals.

II. From Gene to Protein

The human *TSC2* gene spans approximately 43 kb in the region of 16p13.3 and lies adjacent to the polycystic kidney disease gene (*PKD1*) (2). In fact, large deletions affecting both of these genes have been reported in some patients with severe infantile kidney disease (3). The *TSC2* transcript is encoded by 41 exons and is approximately 5.5 kb in length. *TSC2* is widely conserved between vertebrate species, including rat, where *TSC2* functions as a tumor suppressor gene in the Eker rat strain (4,5). This strain of rats develops bilateral renal cell carcinomas as a result of a heterozygous germline mutation in the rat homolog of *TSC2*, and the tumors display frequent loss of heterozygosity (LOH) at the normal *TSC2* allele, consistent with a "two-hit" mechanism of carcinogenesis (6). *TSC2* has also been found to be conserved in the pufferfish *Fugu rubipes*, with four regions of the predicted protein products displaying greater than 80% similarity between human and pufferfish (7). Moreover, the intron/exon structure of the *F. rubipes* and Homo sapiens genes are nearly identical (7). Based on these results, it is likely that *TSC2* plays a role in the growth or development of a wide variety of vertebrate species.

The *TSC2* transcript has been found to be expressed in many different tissues in human, mouse, and rat (1,4,8–10). In general, these studies are consistent with the wide spectrum of organs affected in TSC patients (11). Affected tissues that show significant expression of the *TSC2* mRNA include brain, heart, lung, and kidney. More detailed studies have examined the expression of *TSC2* mRNA in the nervous system during development and in adults (12,13). Abundant *TSC2* mRNA was detected in the cerebellum, the choroid plexus epithelium, neurons of the cerebral cortex, and the spinal cord.

The predicted product of the human *TSC2* gene, designated tuberin (1), comprises 1784 amino acids (excluding the alternately spliced exon 31; see below) (Fig. 1). The predicted sequence contains several areas of significant interest. These include a potential leucine-zipper motif in the amino-terminal region. As these motifs have been shown to be involved in protein-protein interactions (14), this region of tuberin may also serve such a role. The middle portion of tuberin includes two short proline-rich regions (the regions surrounding amino acids 670 and 1265). The more N-terminal of these regions is found within a portion of *TSC2* that is highly conserved between human and pufferfish (7). These proline-rich regions may also represent potential sites of protein-protein interaction, as they have been shown to serve as binding sites for the SH3 domains found in many structural and regulatory proteins (15).

Most interestingly, a 58-amino-acid region near the C-terminus has been found that displays limited homology (19 identical amino acids) with a portion of the catalytic domain of Rap1GAP (16). Further examination of this region of tuberin has revealed that the homology between tuberin and GAP extends to a larger region than the 58 amino acids originally described (R. Wienecke and J. DeClue, unpublished data). Rap1GAP acts as a negative regulator of the Rap1a and Rap1b GTPases, which share greater than 50% amino acid identity with Ras

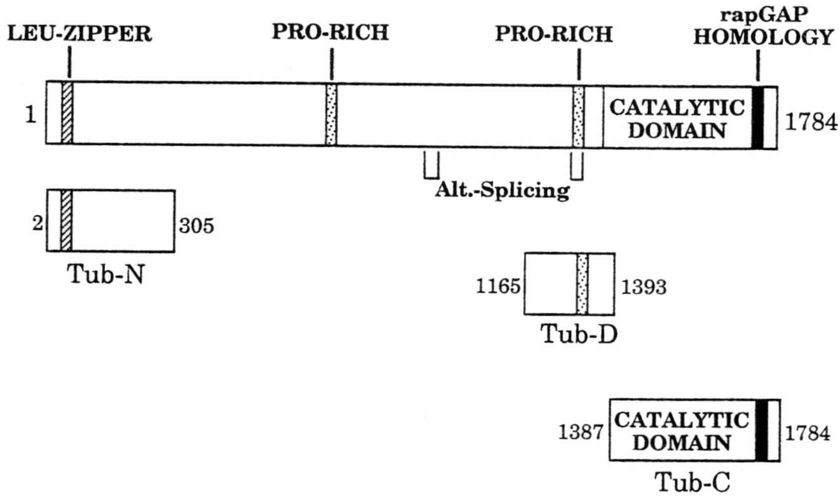

Figure 1 Structure of tuberin and bacterial fusion proteins. Tuberin contains a potential leucine zipper domain (LZ), two proline-rich regions, and a region of homology to the catalytic domain of Rap1GAP, in which 19 of 58 amino acid residues are identical. The locations of the two alternately spliced exons, exon 25 (amino acids 947–989) and exon 31 (amino acids 1272–1294), are noted (see text for details). The numbering shown does not include exon 31, which was absent from the original cDNA clone and also from the clones used to generate recombinant GST-fusion constructs and raise antibodies. If exon 31 is included, the length of human tuberin is 1807 amino acids. The recombinant GST-fusion constructs (GST-Tub-N, GST-Tub-D, and GST-Tub-C) encode different portions of human tuberin, as shown. GST-Tub-C, representing the C-terminus, includes the putative catalytic (GAP) domain of tuberin, based on sequence alignment with Rap1GAP.

(17). The homology between tuberin and Rap1GAP suggested that tuberin might also function as a GAP protein for Rap1 (see below).

Analyses of the expression of *TSC2* in mouse, human, and rat tissues have revealed that the gene undergoes alternative splicing (9,18). Exon 25, encoding a 43-amino-acid segment corresponding to amino acids 947–989 of human tuberin, and exon 31, which encodes a 23-amino-acid segment (1272–1294) were found to be variably expressed. All four isoforms were found to be expressed in both newborn and adult tissues. The existence of exon 31, which was absent from the sequence originally published for the human gene, was also identified through the analysis of the pufferfish *TSC2* gene (7). The functional consequences of these splicing events, and their effects on the properties of tuberin, remain to be identified.

III. Identification of Tuberin

To initiate studies of tuberin, antisera were raised against bacterial fusion proteins encoding different regions of the human *TSC2* product (19). Different cDNA fragments encoding regions of the human *TSC2* gene were obtained by polymerase chain reaction (PCR) amplification from a human fetal brain cDNA library. The sequences of the DNA fragments were verified, and they were then transferred to a plasmid vector for expression as glutathione-S-transferase (GST) fusion proteins. The fusion proteins were then purified and used as antigens to raise polyclonal antisera in rabbits. Three different fusion proteins were utilized for these studies (Fig. 1). These were designated Tub-N (amino acids 2–305), Tub-D (1165–1393), and Tub-C (1387–1784). Each of the fusion proteins, and the antisera generated against them, possess distinct properties. The antisera against Tub-N proved useful in immunoprecipitation assays, but failed to recognize tuberin in immunoblots. The Tub-D protein, which is the smallest of the three, is soluble when expressed as a GST-fusion. This allowed for the Tub-D protein to be coupled to a column and used to affinity-purify antibodies from the rabbit serum raised against it. These affinity-purified sera were subsequently used in many of the studies described below. The Tub-C protein encompasses the C-terminal 398 amino acids of tuberin, including the entire region of homology with Rap1GAP. Purified preparations of this protein were therefore used to test the potential GAP activity of tuberin. In addition, certain preparations of antisera against the Tub-C peptide were species cross-reactive, allowing these sera to be utilized for analyses of the rat and murine *TSC2* products.

To allow for the specific detection of tuberin, combined immunoprecipitation/immunoblotting was carried out, using combinations of the antisera raised against different regions of tuberin (19). Extracts of the human K-562 erythroleukemia cell line, previously shown to express *TSC2* mRNA (1), were subjected to immunoprecipitation with either anti-Tub-N, unrelated, or preimmune sera. After SDS-PAGE analysis, immunoprecipitates were transferred to a filter, and the filter was incubated with anti-Tub-C serum (Fig. 2). A specific band of 180 kDa was present in the anti-Tub-N immunoprecipitates (Fig. 2, lane 3); this band was absent in the immunoprecipitates prepared using preimmune (lane 1) or unrelated (lane 2) antisera. The identity of this band as the authentic product of *TSC2* was further confirmed by analyses using extracts prepared from other cell lines, and also in experiments in which immunoprecipitation of the 180 kDa protein was blocked by preincubation with the cognate GST-fusion protein used to generate the antiserum. Additional confirmation of the 180 kDa band as the *TCS2* product came from analyses of cells derived from tumors of the Eker rat strain. Using species cross-reactive sera, it was found that the 180 kDa band, which is present in normal rat cell lines, is absent from tumor cell lines derived from Eker

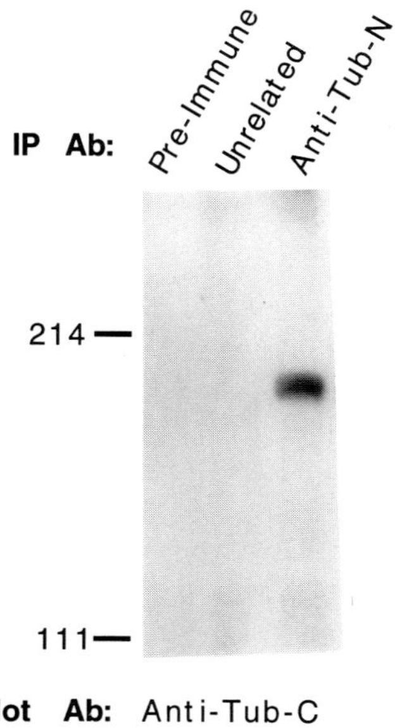

Figure 2 Identification of tuberin by combined immunoprecipitation/Western blot analysis. Protein extracts were prepared from K-562 cells and subjected to immunoprecipitation (IP) with preimmune, unrelated, or anti-Tub-N serum. Immunoprecipitates were washed, separated by SDS-PAGE, and transferred to PVDF membranes, and immunoblotting was carried out with anti-Tub-C serum. A specific band of 180 kDa corresponding to tuberin was observed (arrowhead).

rat tumors lacking an intact copy of *TSC2*. On the basis of these different analyses, it is possible to conclude that the 180 kDa band detected in these experiments represents the authentic *TSC2* product.

IV. Biochemical (GAP) Activity of Tuberin

The region of tuberin originally identified as homologous to Rap1GAP (58 amino acids) is substantially shorter than the Rap1GAP catalytic domain (331 residues) and is also shorter than the homology typically observed among different Ras-specific GAP proteins (ca. 350 residues) (20,21). Nevertheless, to determine if tuberin functions as a GAP for Rap1, immunoprecipitates of tuberin were prepared from K-562 cell lysates, and the immunoprecipitates were incubated with [γ-^{32}P]GTP-bound Rap1a to assay potential GAP activity (19). Significant levels of GAP activity toward Rap1a were observed in the tuberin immunoprecipitates, but not in immunoprecipitates in which a control (unrelated) antiserum was used (Fig. 3, top three panels). As a positive control, the GAP activity toward Rap1a present in nonimmunoprecipitated lysates of K-562 cells was assayed. It was found that the K-562 lysate contained GAP activity toward Rap1a well in excess of that found int he tuberin immunoprecipitates, implying that K-562 cells may express other sources of Rap1-specific GAP activity, such as one of the previously characterized Rap1GAP activities (16,22). The results described above strongly suggest that tuberin itself possesses GAP activity for Rap1, although the possibility that this activity was due to a coimmunoprecipitating Rap1GAP could not be excluded. To distinguish between these possibilities, the ability of the GST-Tub-C fusion protein to stimulate the GTPase activity of Rap1a was assayed. GST-Tub-C purified from either *Escherichia coli* or Sf9 insect cells was found to possess GAP activity toward Rap1, verifying that the Rap1GAP activity is an intrinsic property of tuberin (19).

To determine the specificity of tuberin GAP activity, immunoprecipitates of native tuberin were incubated with [γ-^{32}P]GTP-bound recombinant Rap2, Ha-Ras, or Rho proteins (Fig. 3, bottom three panels). The GAP activity of tuberin toward these other GTPase proteins was measured together with Rap1a in the same experiment. In contrast to the results with Rap1, the intrinsic GTPase activity of Rap2, Ras, and Rho was not stimulated by incubation with the anti-turberin immunoprecipitates. In additional experiments, the GTPase activity of Rac and Ran were not enhanced by tuberin (not shown). These results describe a high degree of specificity for the GAP activity of tuberin, as Rap2 is greater than 60% identical to Rap1, while Ras is approximately 50% identical. However, the possibility that other small GTPase proteins, either known or as yet unidentified, do interact with tuberin and are subject to its GAP activity, cannot be excluded.

V. Subcellular Localization of Tuberin

To investigate the subcellular localization of tuberin, K-562 cells were lysed by Dounce homogenization in the absence of detergent. The postnuclear supernatant was centrifuged at 100,000 xg to yield membrane/particulate (P100) and nonparticulate (S100) fractions, each of which were then analyzed by immunoprecipitation/immunoblotting. A substantial majority of the tuberin was recovered in the P100 fraction, raising the possibility that tuberin may associate with the cell plasma membrane or with intracellular membranes or organelles (19).

To explore further the subcellular localization of tuberin, indirect immunofluorescence was carried out, using the affinity-purified antibodies prepared against the GST-fusion peptide Tub-D (23). First, the pattern of tuberin immunofluorescence was analyzed in cultured cells, including tumor cell lines derived from human kidney, adrenal gland, and brain. While preimmune IgG or anti-Tub-

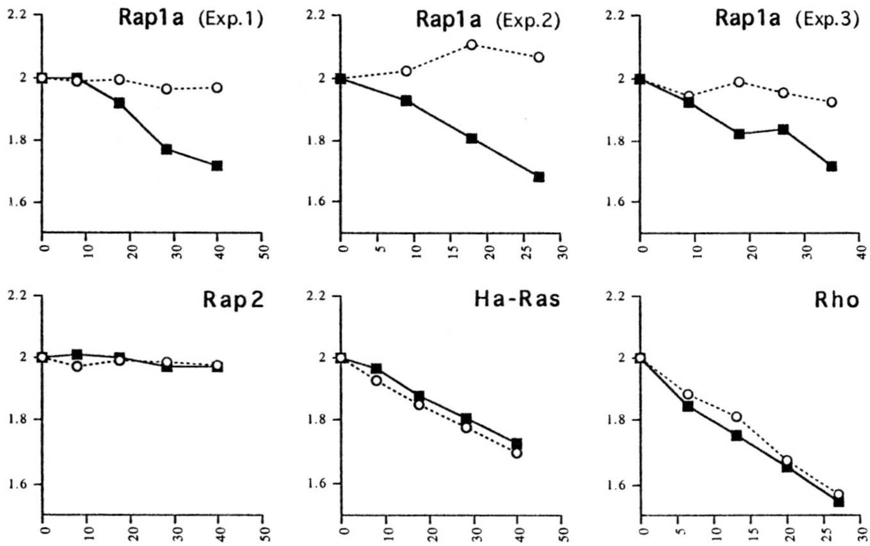

Figure 3 Tuberin possesses specific GAP activity toward Rap1a. Immunoprecipitates of K-562 cells obtained by anti-Tub-C (■) or control antibody (○) were used to test sensitivity of different Ras-like proteins toward GAP activity of native tuberin. (Top three panels) GTP remaining bound to Rap1a was determined following binding of [γ-^{32}P]GTP to Rap1a, using a nitrocellulose filter assay. The plots represent Log_{10}(Rap1a•GTP$\{t_n\}$/Rap1a•GTP$\{t_0\}$ [as %]) versus time. Immunoprecipitation of K-562 lysates (120 ml per GAP reaction) was performed using either anti-Tub-C or control antibody. Immune complexes were collected using protein A-Sepharose and washed, then incubated with [γ-^{32}P]GTP•Rap1a. An equal amount of protein A-Sepharose beads with anti-Tub-C or control antibody was used. Similar assays were also conducted using other small GTPases, including (bottom row, left) Rap2; (bottom row, center) Ha-Ras; and (bottom row, right) Rho. The different slopes of the curves reflect the different intrinsic GTPase activities of these proteins. Two or three independent experiments were performed for Rap2, Ras, and Rho; the data shown are representative of the results obtained in each trial.

D serum that was preabsorbed against GST-Tub-D protein yielded no detectable signal, anti-Tub-D serum that was preabsorbed against GST alone yielded a strong, specific pattern of fluorescence. Most of the fluorescence was localized to the perinuclear region, either as a ring or as a distinct perinuclear cluster (23). The staining pattern observed in these cells suggested that tuberin might be localized to the Golgi complex.

To verify that tuberin was localized to the Golgi apparatus, we compared the fluorescent staining pattern of tuberin with that of two different known Golgi marker proteins, nontagged mouse mannosidase-II and hemagglutinin (HA)-

tagged furin (24,25). Because antibodies against the endogenous human marker proteins were not available, HeLa cervical carcinoma cells were transfected with plasmids encoding either of the markers, and double-indirect immunofluorescence was carried out to detect tuberin (using anti-Tub-D followed by fluorescein) and either mouse mannosidase-II (Fig. 4A–C) or HA-tagged furin (Fig. 4D–F) (both stained with rhodamine). The staining pattern of tuberin was nearly identical to that of mannosidase-II, a protein that localizes to the *cis*/medial-Golgi compartment of the Golgi stacks (24). In contrast, the staining of tuberin only partially overlapped with that of furin, which is localized to the *trans*-Golgi network in the periphery of the cell (24,26). The partial overlap of the furin and tuberin signals was seen near the nucleus, but not in the periphery of the cell. Taken together, these studies show that most of the immunoreactive tuberin resides in the Golgi stacks. The localization of tuberin to the Golgi apparatus was confirmed by treatment of HeLa cells with brefeldin A, an agent that specifically disrupts the Golgi apparatus (27). A 30-minute incubation with brefeldin A abolished the normal perinuclear tuberin fluorescence seen with these cells (23). From these findings, it is apparent that the majority of cellular tuberin is localized in the Golgi stacks.

The observation that tuberin is capable of stimulating the GTPase activity of Rap1 in vitro (19) suggested that these proteins might also interact and co-localize in vivo. To test this possibility, double-indirect immunofluorescence and confocal microscopy immunofluorescence were carried out, using affinity-purified antibodies against tuberin and Rap1 (Fig. 5). In this technique, a single plane of focus is analyzed, eliminating the possibility that an apparent co-localization is due to overlapping staining patterns in different focal planes. The staining patterns of tuberin (visualized with rhodamine; Fig. 5A) and Rap1 (visualized with fluorescein; Fig. 5B) were found to overlap significantly (Fig. 5C). Again, the staining was perinuclear, as determined by comparison with a Nomarski image of the same cell (Fig. 5D), consistent with localization to the Golgi apparatus. Previous studies of the intracellular localization of Rap1 have indicated that this protein is localized to the Golgi apparatus (28) as well as in the late endocytic/phagocytic compartment of some cells (29).

VI. Expression Pattern of Tuberin

The wide variety of organ systems affected in TSC patients suggests that the *TSC2* product is expressed in many different cell types. To verify this, the expression of tuberin in a panel of 13 different human cell lines was analyzed (Fig. 6). These lines represent a variety of cell types (see Fig. 6). Cells were lysed and subjected to combined immunoprecipitation/immunoblot analysis. With the exception of HL-60 and U-937 cells, tuberin was abundantly expressed in all of the cell lines tested. Interestingly, each of the tuberin-negative cell lines represents a different maturation level of the myelocytic/monocytic lineage; abnormalities in this lin-

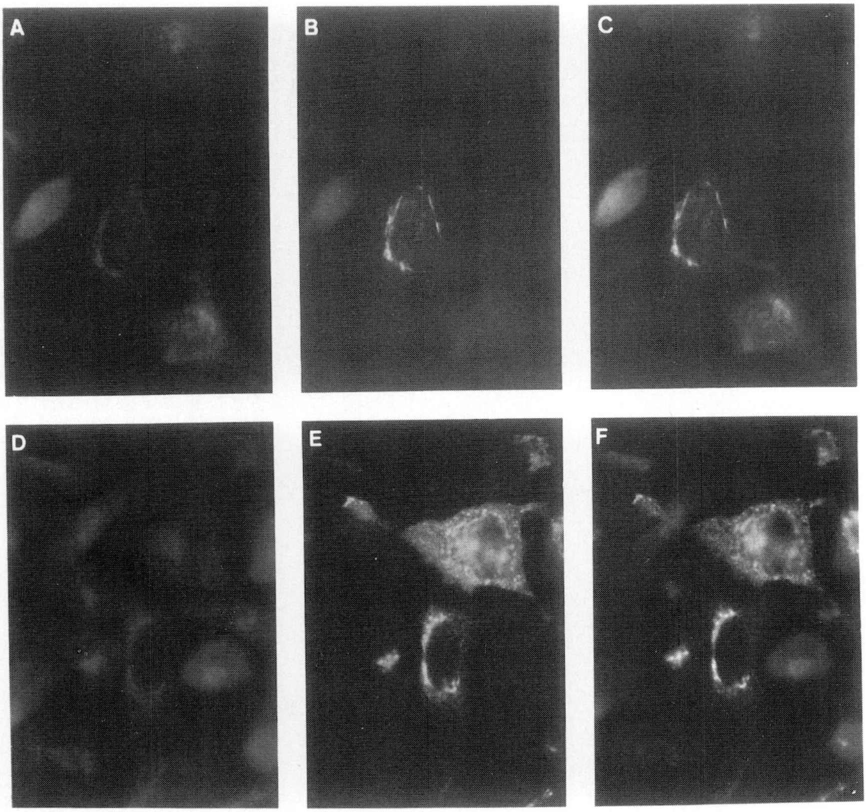

Figure 4 Co-localization of endogenous tuberin (with fluorescein) (A,D) and Golgi marker proteins (with rhodamine) (B,E) by double-indirect immunofluorescence. Expression plasmids encoding nontagged mannosidase-II (B), which is located in the *cis*/medial-Golgi compartment of the Golgi stacks, or hemagglutinin (HA)-tagged furin (E), which localizes to the *trans*-Golgi compartment of the Golgi stacks as well as the *trans*-Golgi network in the periphery of the cell, were transiently transfected into HeLa cells. The transfection efficiency was approximately 10%, leaving most cells untransfected. (C) Double exposure of (A) and (B), showing overlap of mannosidase II and tuberin in the Golgi stacks. (F) Double exposure of (D) and (E), demonstrating partial co-localization of HA-furin and tuberin near the nucleus, but not in the periphery of the cell. Staining of tuberin and marker proteins was detected as described in Ref. 23. Original magnification was 250×; size marker represents 10 μM.

eage have not been linked to TSC patients (30,31). The small differences in the migration rate of tuberin observed in some of the cell lines may reflect posttranslational modification of tuberin or the products of alternatively-spliced variants of the *TSC2* mRNA (see above).

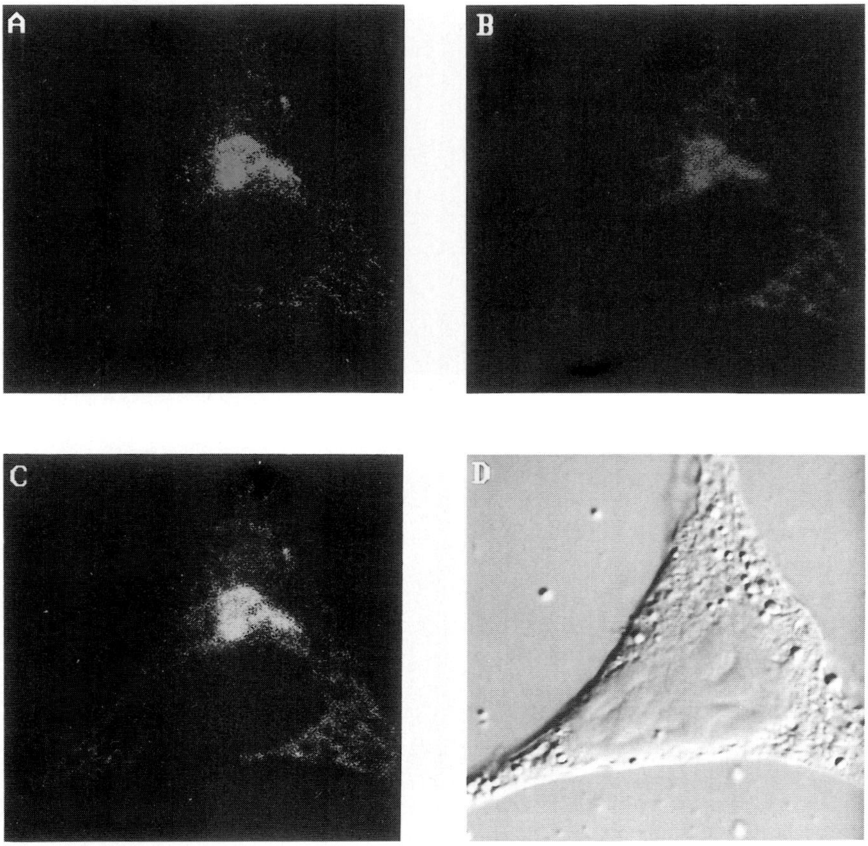

Figure 5 Confocal microscopic analysis of G-402 cells stained with anti-Tub-D1 (detected by rhodamine) (A) and anti-Rap1 (detected by fluorescein) (B). (C) represents an overlay of (A) and (B). (D) Nomarski optics image of the same cell. The staining patterns of tuberin and Rap1 in a single plane of focus revealed significant overlap. Original magnification was 250×; size marker represents 10 μM.

In addition to testing the expression in cultured cells, the levels of tuberin present in various adult human and rat tissues were analyzed by immunoblot analysis (Table 1). In humans the highest levels of tuberin were found in brain, heart, and kidney, while lower amounts were detected in lung, skeletal muscle, and liver. In general, there was a good correlation between the tissues with the highest tuberin expression and the primary organs affected in patients with TSC. A similar, but somewhat distinct, pattern of tuberin expression was observed in tissues of the adult rat. Tuberin was detected in many different rat tissues, with the highest levels observed in liver, testis, and brain.

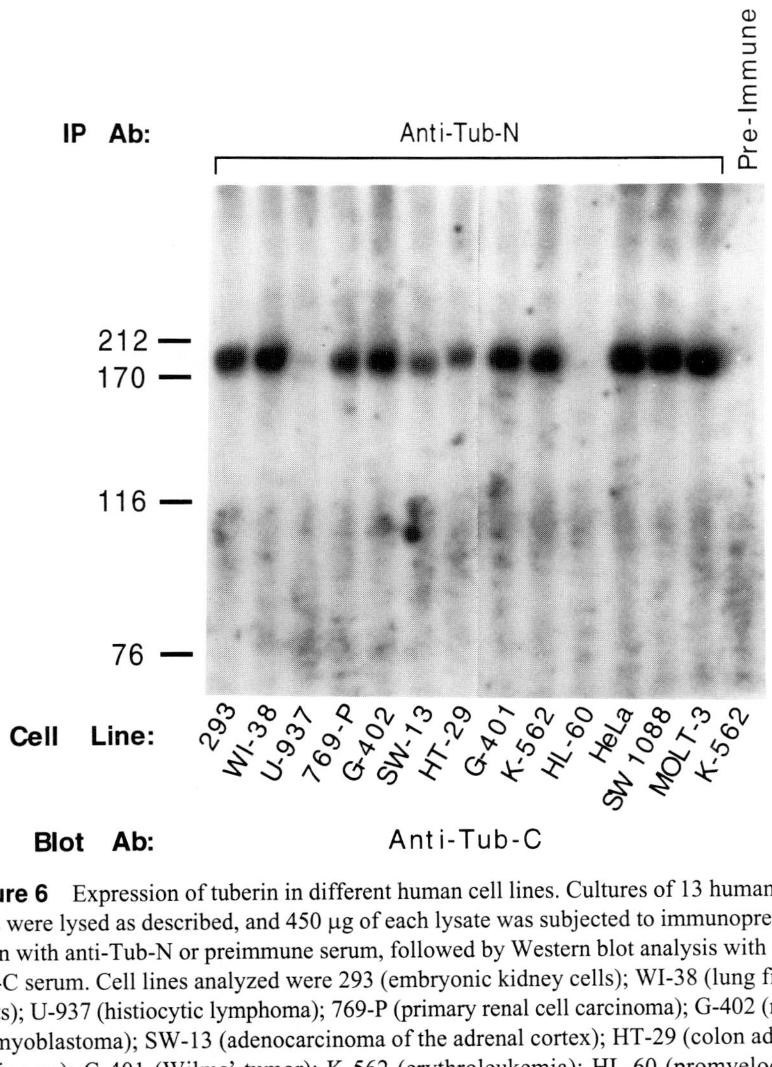

Figure 6 Expression of tuberin in different human cell lines. Cultures of 13 human cell lines were lysed as described, and 450 μg of each lysate was subjected to immunoprecipitation with anti-Tub-N or preimmune serum, followed by Western blot analysis with anti-Tub-C serum. Cell lines analyzed were 293 (embryonic kidney cells); WI-38 (lung fibroblasts); U-937 (histiocytic lymphoma); 769-P (primary renal cell carcinoma); G-402 (renal leiomyoblastoma); SW-13 (adenocarcinoma of the adrenal cortex); HT-29 (colon adenocarcinoma); G-401 (Wilms' tumor); K-562 (erythroleukemia); HL-60 (promyelocytic leukemia); HeLa (cervical carcinoma); SW 1088 (astrocytoma); and MOLT-3 (T-cell lymphoblastic leukemia). Arrowhead denotes the position of the 180 kDa tuberin band.

To better define the expression of tuberin within specific tissues, the staining pattern of tuberin was analyzed by immunohistochemistry (32). Again, the affinity-purified antibodies prepared against the Tub-D peptide were used for these assays. The analyses included both cryosections and paraffin sections, while

Table 1 Expression of Tuberin in Adult Human and Rat Tissues[a]

Tissue	Human[b]	Rat[c]
Brain	++++	+++
Kidney	+++	+
Heart	++++	+
Lung	+	+
Liver	+	+++
Skeletal muscle	++	+
Testis	ND	++++
Spleen	ND	++
Small intestine	ND	+/–

[a]Based on immunoblot analysis with either anti-Tub-D serum (for human tissues) or species cross-reactive anti-Tub-C serum (for rat).
[b]Commercially prepared filter with lysates of adult human male tissues.
[c]Tissues obtained from adult rat were lysed and electro-blotted onto filter.
ND, not determined.

focusing on the organs which are most commonly involved in the phenotype of TSC patients. For example, as patients are often afflicted with skin lesions, such as angiofibromas, subungual fibromas, and hypomelanotic macules (33), the expression of tuberin in normal human skin was analyzed. Tuberin staining was observed in many different cell types including keratinocytes, melanocytes, fibroblasts, and smooth muscle cells of dermal small blood vessels, with especially high levels in vascular cells and cells of the eccrine sweat glands (32). Additional analyses revealed strong staining of tuberin in the arterioles of the adrenal gland, in the cells in the islets of Langerhans in the pancreas, at the nuclear poles of cardiac myocytes, and in the cells of arterioles within the heart.

Given the in vitro interaction between tuberin and Rap1, as well as their colocalization in cultured cells, the staining patterns of these proteins within certain tissues were compared by immunohistochemistry. The kidneys are frequently affected in TSC patients (34). Staining of the renal cortex using anti-Tub-D revealed weak staining of cells, mainly in the distal tubules (Fig. 7A). A significantly higher level of tuberin expression was found in the small blood vessels of the kidney. In striking parallel to the expression of tuberin, Rap1 was also found to be expressed at high levels in the small blood vessels, and to a lesser extent in the distal tubules (Fig. 7B). Although patients with TSC do not show clinical signs of cerebellar dysfunction, focal atrophy of the cerebellar cortex and a paucity of Purkinje cells have been documented in these patients (11,35). Staining of tuberin was observed in the molecular layer (Mo.L.), which contains neuronal processes, and in cells of the granular cell layer (Gr.L.), while the Purkinje cells exhibited striking immunoreactivity in their perikaryons and dendritic processes (Fig. 7C). Again, the pattern of staining for Rap1 was quite similar to that of tuberin, both within the molecular and granular cell layers and in the Purkinje cells (Fig. 7D). The similar staining of tuberin and Rap1 suggests a functional interaction between these proteins in organs commonly affected in TSC patients.

A more detailed analysis of the expression of tuberin throughout the central nervous system was conducted in order to compare the expression of *TSC2* mRNA (by in situ hybridization) and tuberin (by immunohistochemistry) (12). These studies revealed a generally widespread expression of tuberin, including neurons of the neocortex, the hippocampus, the choroid plexus epithelium, ependymal cells, neurons of the brainstem, and spinal cord motor neurons (Table 2). Rap1 was also detected in the neurons and in the gray matter of the neocortex (32). When examined at higher magnification, the tuberin immunoreactivity within cortical tissue was most prominent in the perikaryons and processes of

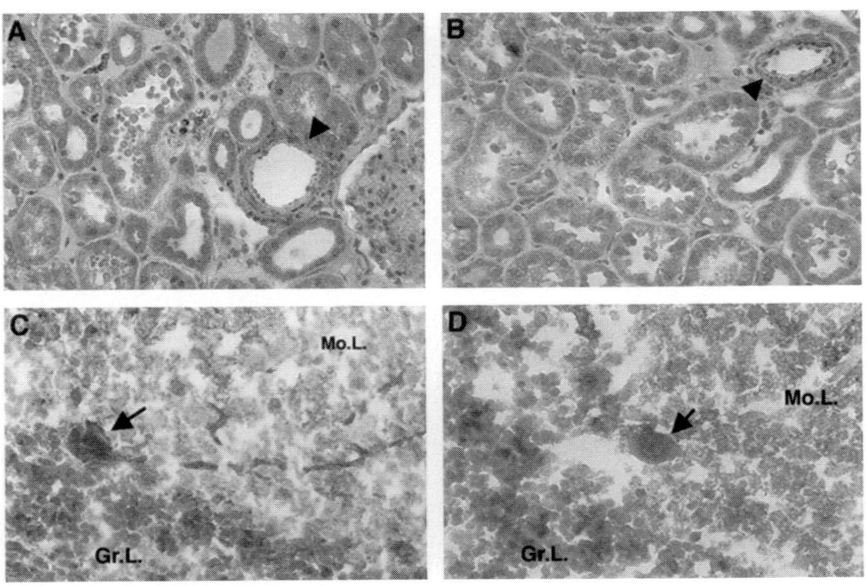

Figure 7 Immunohistochemical analyses of human kidney (A, B) and human cerebellum (C,D) for the expression of tuberin (A, C) and Rap1 (B, D). High levels of expression of tuberin and Rap1 are visible in the small blood vessels (arrowhead) of the kidney, and in the cerebellar Purkinje cells (arrow). Weak expression of tuberin was found in the renal tubules and in the granular (Gr.L.) and molecular layers (Mo.L.) of the cerebellum. All panels were hematoxylin-counterstained. (200×)

neurons, whereas other cell types such as astrocytes contained much lower levels. The sole area where virtually no tuberin was found was in the subcortical white matter of the neocortex (Table 2). Loss of tuberin in the precursors of the cortical neurons might lead to defects in differentiation and/or migration, thereby contributing to the formation of the characteristic cortical tubers that occur in TSC patients.

VII. Growth-Inhibitory Properties of Tuberin

Several lines of evidence suggest that *TSC2* functions as a tumor suppressor gene. Many of the clinical features of TSC resemble those of other disorders involving tumor suppressor genes, such as neurofibromatosis type 1 and 2 (NF1 and NF2) and von Hippel-Lindau disease. The tumor suppressor genes underlying

Table 2 Distribution of *TSC2* mRNA and Tuberin in Normal Human Brain

Cell type	mRNA[a]	Antibody 1[b]	Antibody 2[c]
Neocortex			
Pyramidal neurons	+++	++	+++
Subcortical white matter	–	–	–
Cerebellum			
External granule cell layer	+++	+++	ND
Molecular layer	++	++	++
Purkinje cells	+++	++	+++
Internal granule cell layer	+++	+	++
Hippocampus			
Dentate gyrus (granule cell layer)	+++	+	ND
Pyramidal cell layer	+++	+	ND
Choroid plexus:			
Epithelium	+++	+++	ND
Ependyma			
Ependymal cells	+++	+++	ND
Astrocytes			
Astrocytes	+	ND	+
Brain stem			
Motor neurons	+++	++	ND
Spinal cord			
Motor neurons, Clarke's column	+++	++	ND

[a]In situ hybridization of paraffin sections with 3′ probe (nt 5101–5371).
[b]Immunohistochemistry of paraffin sections with anti-TubD2 (aa 1165–1393).
[c]Immunohistochemistry of cryosections with anti-TubD1 (aa 1165–1393).
ND, Not determined.

these disorders are representative of a class of genes that are mutationally inactivated in a wide variety of human cancers (36).

In addition to the loss of heterozygosity (LOH) of *TSC2* seen in tumors of the Eker rat strain (see above), LOH has also been reported for lesions of human TSC patients and in sporadic lesions of non-TSC patients (37,38). LOH is especially prevalent for alterations involving the kidney (39). These data are consistent with a tumor suppressor function for *TSC2*.

One common measure of the function of tumor suppressor genes is their ability, when reintroduced or overexpressed in cells, to inhibit cell proliferation or tumorigenicity (40,41). To address this aspect of the tumor suppressor activity of *TSC2*, the effects of overexpression of tuberin were analyzed using a conditional expression system (42). The full-length rat *TSC2* gene was placed under the control of a regulatable tetracycline promoter and introduced into a strain of Rat1 fibroblasts (R12) stably expressing the tetracycline repressor/VP16 transactivator fusion protein (43). This line was designated Tub6. After removal of tetracycline from Tub6 cells for 4–6 days, a 2- to 5-fold elevation in the level of tuberin over the basal expression level was observed (Fig. 8A). In contrast, the control R12 cell line lacking the *TSC2* plasmid showed no difference in tuberin expression in the presence or absence of tetracycline. Removal of tetracycline also caused specific inhibition of the growth of Tub6 cells over the same time course as that in which tuberin expression was elevated (Fig.8B). Orimoto et al. also reported suppression of the growth of cells following the induction of tuberin expression (44). In that report, a cell line derived from a tumor of the Eker rat strain was used. As a direct measure of the tumor suppressor function of *TSC2*, it was found that reintroduction of the rat *TSC2* into an Eker rat-derived line abolished the tumorigenicity of these cells in SCID mice (42). These results provide direct evidence for the tumor suppressor function of *TSC2* and may also provide a useful bioassay for evaluating the relevant contribution of different features of tuberin with respect to this tumor suppressor function.

VIII. Tuberin: Other Potential Functions

The large size of the *TSC2* product, as well as the pleiotropic effect of *TSC2* mutations in TSC patients, suggest that tuberin may have multiple, diverse functions. As discussed in the preceding sections, several regions within the primary sequence of tuberin may serve as sites of protein-protein interactions. These interactions may serve to ensure the proper localization of tuberin within the cell, to specify the cellular proteins that are regulated by tuberin, or to define interactions through which tuberin may mediate one or more intracellular signaling pathways.

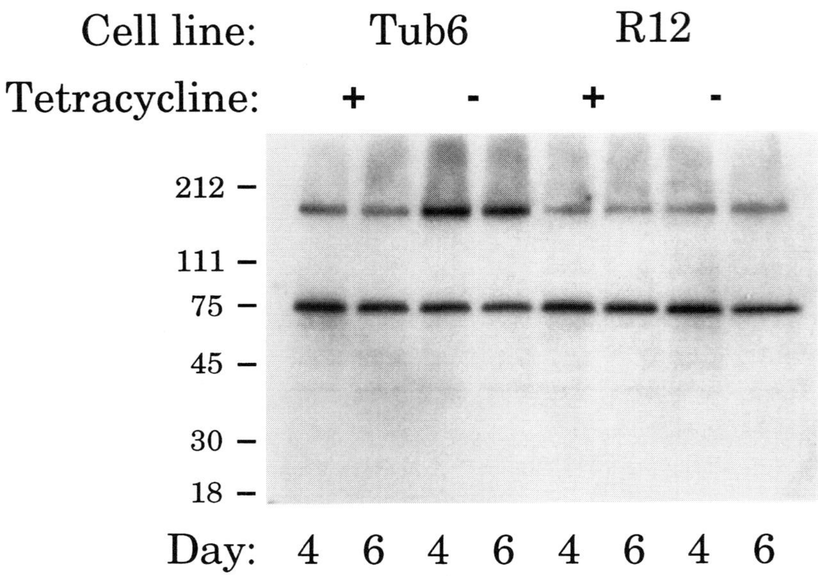

A

Figure 8 Overexpression of tuberin inhibits cell growth. (A) Conditional overexpression of tuberin in R12 and derivatives. Tub6 and R12 cells contain the tetracycline repressor/VP16 transactivator construct. Tub6 cells were transfected with full-length *TSC2* under the control of a tetracycline-repressible promoter. Tuberin protein (arrow) was assayed by immunoblot after cells were grown in the presence (+) or absence (–) of tetracycline for 4 or 6 days. The reactivity of the nonspecific band at ~75 kDa indicates equal loading of protein. (B) Inhibition of growth upon conditional overexpression of tuberin by the removal of tetracycline. Tub6 cells were grown in the presence (+) or absence (–) of tetracycline. Slower growth of Tub6 cells in the absence of tetracycline mirrors the increased tuberin expression shown in (A).

One recent report described a completely novel potential function for tuberin (45). In this report, it was found that certain portions of tuberin, particularly the C-terminus, could induce a potent transactivation of transcription when expressed as GAL4-fusion proteins in yeast. However, no activity was detected when similar constructs were tested in mammalian cells, and the reason(s) for this discrepancy are unknown. Furthermore, while overexpression of full-length tuberin resulted in a protein that was localized to the perinuclear region, a smaller, C-terminal fragment (amino acids 1006–1743 of the rat protein) displayed partial nuclear fluorescence (45). While it is not known if such a smaller protein is expressed in cells in a natural setting (e.g., in TSC patients), the results do suggest that tuberin may have a potential role as a transcriptional regulator.

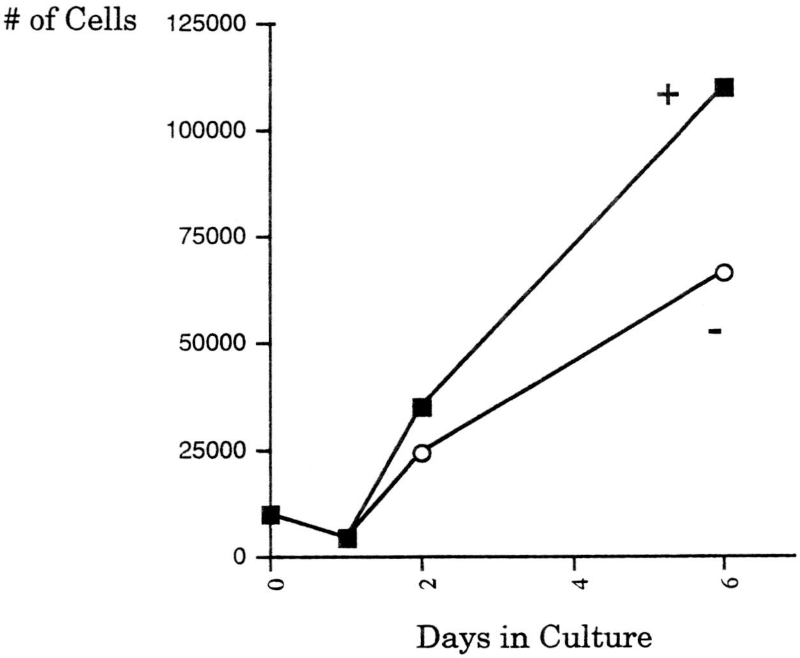

B

Figure 8 Continued.

The concentration of tuberin in many different regions of organs that are typically involved in secretion points to another potential function of this protein. Tuberin was found to be expressed at high levels in the eccrine sweat glands of the skin, the islets of Langerhans of the pancreas, the steroid hormone–secreting cells of the adrenal cortex, and epithelial cells of the choroid plexus (32). These results echo the conclusions from an analysis of the expression of *TSC2* mRNA in adult human tissues (10). Together with the demonstration of a Golgi localization for tuberin, these findings suggest that tuberin may play a role in the processing, secretion, or trafficking of growth factors, growth factor receptors, or cell-surface molecules involved in cell adhesion and cell-cell interactions. Such a role is consistent with the aberrant migration, differentiation, and growth of the cells that give rise to lesions in TSC patients (11).

With respect to the Rap1GAP activity of tuberin, it remains to be seen whether Rap1 is the sole, or even the primary, target for this activity. The level of activity detected in tuberin immunoprecipitates was low (19), and there are other known sources of Rap1GAP activity within cells (16,22). While the high degree of specificity seen for GAP proteins in general (20), and tuberin in particular (19), support Rap1 as a primary target for tuberin, other small molecular weight GTPases remain to be directly tested in these assays.

IX. Summary

The studies described here represent, on the one hand, the culmination of a long search for the molecular determinants of the pathology of TSC and, on the other hand, the mere beginning of an investigation of the properties of the *TSC2* product tuberin. Many aspects of the studies of tuberin described here relate to its interaction with the small GTPase Rap1. These studies represent a direct outgrowth of the suggestion of sequence homology between tuberin and Rap1GAP, which followed from the identification of *TSC2* (1). Not only do tuberin and Rap1 interact in vitro, but tuberin is capable of stimulating the intrinsic GTPase activity of Rap1, thereby inactivating it. Furthermore, these proteins shows a similar in-

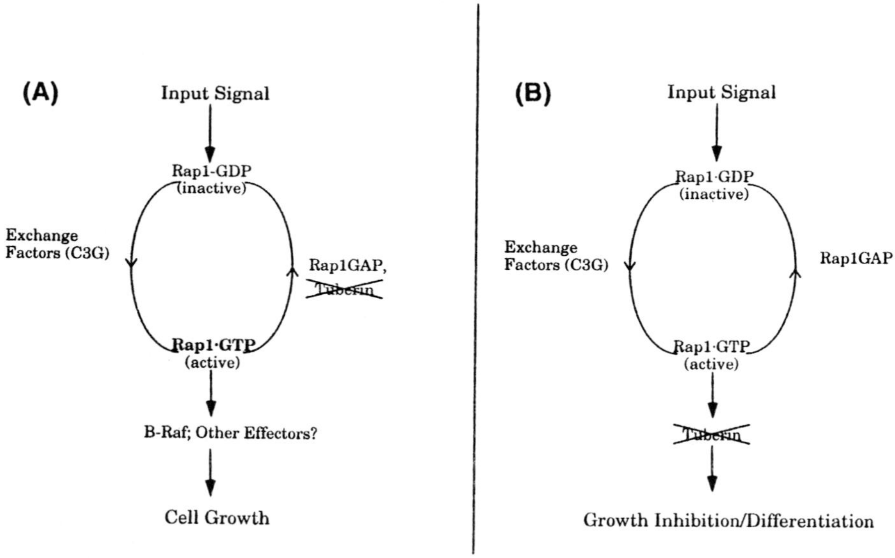

Figure 9 Models for the function of tuberin and Rap1 in regulating cell growth. The interaction of these proteins in vitro and their co-localization in vivo and in tissues suggests that the growth-suppressive function of tuberin is manifested, at least partly, through the interaction with Rap1. (A) Tuberin functions to negatively regulate Rap1-GTP levels. Loss of tuberin expression leads to increased Rap1 activity, which in turn stimulates cell growth. (B) Tuberin functions together with Rap1 to transmit antiproliferative/differentiation signals, and the loss of tuberin expression terminates the transmission of these signals. See text for further explanation.

tracellular localization and are found within the same cells of many different tissues. These findings suggest several potential models for the role of tuberin and Rap1 in growth regulation and tumorigenesis, two of which are described in Figure 9. In the first of these models (Fig. 9A), the negative regulation of Rap1-GTP levels by tuberin represents its primary function, and the consequence of the loss of tuberin expression is an overactive Rap1 protein, leading to activation of effector proteins such as B-Raf (46) and increased mitogenesis. Consistent with this model, Rap1 has been shown to induce DNA synthesis and morphological changes when microinjected into cultured cells (47). In this model, the molecular pathology of TSC presents striking parallels to that of neurofibromatosis type 1, where loss of expression of the *NF1* product neurofibromin (a specific Ras-GAP) leads to the constitutive activation of Ras within the tumor cells of NF1 patients (48,49). An alternative model, which is also consistent with certain experimental properties of Rap1 (50,51), is shown in Figure 9B. Here, Rap1 transmits a signal that leads to growth inhibition or differentiation of the cells, and tuberin is a critical mediator of these antiproliferative signals. In this case, the loss of tuberin expression would leave the cells in a cycling, undifferentiated state. It is important to note that these models are not necessarily mutually exclusive, particularly as the true biological role of Rap1 is not yet completely clear. Furthermore, different models may apply in different cell types, and many different cells are affected in TSC patients. Future studies of tuberin will no doubt lead to a better understanding of the role of this protein in normal cell growth and in the development of lesions in TSC patients.

References

1. The Europeean Chromosome 16 Tuberous Sclerosis Consortium. Identification and characterization of the tuberous sclerosis gene on chromosome 16. Cell 1993; 75:1305-1313.
2. The European Polycystic Kidney Disease Consortium. The polycystic kidney disease 1 gene encodes a 14kb transcript and lies within a duplicated region on chromosome 16. Cell 1994; 77:881–894.
3. Brook-Carter PT, Peral B, Ward CJ, Thompson P, Hughes J, Maheshwar MM, Nellist M, Gamble V, Harris PC, Sampsom JR. Deletion of the *TSC2* and *PKD1* genes associated with severe infantile polycystic kidney disease—a contiguous gene syndrome. Nature Genet 1994; 8:328-332.
4. Yeung RS, Xiao G-H, Jin F, Lee W-C, Testa JR, Knudson AG. Predisposition to renal cell carcinoma in the Eker rat is determined by germ-line mutation of the tuberous sclerosis 2 (TSC2) gene. Proc Natl Acad Sci USA 1994; 91:11413-11416.
5. Kobayashi T, Hirayama Y, Kobayashi E, Kubo Y, Hino O. A germline insertion in the tuberous sclerosis (Tsc2) gene gives rise to the Eker rat model of dominantly inherited cancer. Nature Genet 1995; 9:70–74.

6. Knudson AG. Mutation and cancer: statistical study of retinoblastoma. Proc Natl Acad Sci USA 1971; 68:802–823.
7. Maheshwar MM, Sandford R, Nellist M, Cheadle JP, Sgotto B, Vaudin M, Sampson JR. Comparative analysis and genomic structure of the tuberous sclerosis 2 (TSC2) gene in human and pufferfish. Hum Mol Genet 1996; 5:131–137.
8. Geist RT, Gutmann DH. The tuberous sclerosis 2 gene is expressed at high levels in the cerebellum and developing spinal cord. Cell Growth Diff 1995; 6:1477–1483.
9. Xiao G-H, Jin F, Yeung R. Identification of tuberous sclerosis 2 messenger RNA splice variants that are conserved and differentially expressed in rat and human tissues. Cell Growth Diff 1995; 6:1185–1191.
10. Menchine M, Emelin JK, Mischel PS, Haag TA, Norman MG, Pepkowitz SH, Welsh CT, Townsend JJ, Vinters, HV. Tissue and cell-type specific expression of the tuberous sclerosis gene, *TSC2*, in human tissues. Modern Pathol 1996; 9:1071–1080.
11. Short MP, Richardson EP jr., Haines JL, Kwiatkowski DJ. Clinical, neuropathological and genetic aspects of the tuberous sclerosis complex. Brain Pathol 1995; 5:173–179.
12. Kerfoot C, Wienecke R, Menchine M, Emelin J, Maize JC, Welsh CT, Norman MG, DeClue JE, Vinters HV. Localization of tuberous sclerosis-2 mRNA and its protein product tuberin in normal human brain and in cerebral lesions of patients with tuberous sclerosis. Brain Pathol 1996; 6:367–377.
13. Geist RT, Reddy AJ, Zhang J, Gutmann DH. Expression of the tuberous sclerosis 2 gene product, tuberin, in adult and developing nervous system tissues. Neurobiol Dis 1996; 34:111–120.
14. Landschulz WH, Johnson PF, McKnight SL. The leucin zipper: a hypothetical structure common to a new class of DNA binding proteins. Science 1988; 240:1759–1764.
15. Morton CJ, Campbell ID. SH3 Domains: Molecular 'velcro.' Curr Biol 1994; 4:615–617.
16. Polakis PG, Rubinfeld B, Evans T, McCormick F. Purification of a plasma membrane-associated GTPase-activating protein specific for *rap*1/*Krev*-1 from HL60 cells. Proc Natl Acad Sci USA 1991; 88:239–243.
17. Pizon V, Lerosey I, Chardin P, Tavitian A. Nucleotide sequence of a human cDNA encoding a *ras*-related protein (*rap*1B). Nucl Acid Res 1988; 16:7719–7719.
18. Xu L, Sterner C, Maheshwar MM, Wilson PJ, Nellist M, Short PM, Haines JL, Sampson JR, Ramesh V. Alternative splicing of the tuberous sclerosis 2 (TSC2) gene in human and mouse tissues. Genomics 1995; 27:475–480.
19. Wienecke R, König A, DeClue J. Identification of tuberin, the tuberous sclerosis-2 product. J Biol Chem 1995; 270:16409–16414.
20. Boguski MS, McCormick F. Proteins regulating Ras and its relatives. Nature 1993; 366:643–654.
21. Rubinfeld B, Crosier WJ, Albert I, Conroy L, Clark R, McCormick F, Polakis P. Localization of the rap1GAP catalytic domain and sites of phosphorylation by mutational analysis. Mol Cell Biol 1992; 12:4634–4642.
22. Zhang K, Papageorge AP, Martin P, Vass WC, Olah Z, Polakis P, McCormick F, Lowy DR. Heterogeneous amino acids in Ras and Rap1A specifying sensitivity to GAP proteins. Science 1991; 254:1630–1634.

23. Wienecke R, Maize JC, Shoarinejad F, Vass WC, Reed J, Bonifacino JS, Resau JH, de Gunzburg J, Yeung RS, DeClue JE. Co-localization of the TSC2 product tuberin with its target Rap1 in the Golgi apparatus. Oncogene 1996; 13:913–923.
24. Novikoff PM, Tulsiani DR, Touster O, Yam A, Novikoff AB. Immunohistochemical localization of a-D-mannosidase II in the Golgi apparatus of rat liver. Proc Natl Acad Sci USA 1983; 80:4364–4368.
25. Bosshart H, Humphrey J, Deignan E, Davidson J, Drazba J, Yuan L, Oorschot V, Peters PJ, Bonifacino JS. The cytoplasmic domain mediates localization of furin to the trans-Golgi network en route to the endosomal/lysosomal system. J Cell Biol 1994; 126:1157–1172.
26. Molloy SS, Thomas L, VanSlyke JK, Stenberg PE, Thomas G. Intracellular trafficking and activation of the furin proprotein convertase: localization to the TGN and recycling from the cell surface. EMBO J 1994; 13:18–33.
27. Donaldson JG, Lippincott-Schwartz J, Bloom GS, Kreis TE, Klausner RD. Dissociation of a 100-kD peripheral membrane protein from the Golgi apparatus is an early event in brefeldin A action. J Cell Biol 1990; 111:2295–2306.
28. Béranger F. Goud B, Tavitian A, de Gunzburg J. Association of the Ras-antagonistic Rap1/Krev-1 proteins with the Golgi complex. Proc Natl Acad Sci USA 1991; 88:1606–1610.
29. Pizon V, Desjardins M, Bucci C, Parton RG, Zerial M. Association of Rap1a and Rap1b proteins with late endocytic/phagocytic compartments and Rap2a with the Golgi complex. J Cell Sci 1994; 107:1661–1670.
30. Gomez MR. Tuberous Sclerosis. New York: Raven Press, 1988.
31. Lübbert M, Herrmann F, Koeffler HP. Expression and regulation of myeloid-specific genes in normal and leukemic myeloid cells. Blood 1991; 77:909–924.
32. Wienecke R, Maize JC, Reed J, de Gunzburg J, Yeung RS, DeClue JE. Expression of the *TSC2* product tuberin and its target Rap1 in normal human tissues. Am J Pathol 1997; 150:43–50.
33. Zvulunov A, Esterly NB. Neurocutaneous syndromes associated with pigmentary skin lesions. J Am Acad Dermatol 1995; 32:915–935.
34. Bernstein J, Robbins TO. Renal involvement in tuberous sclerosis. In: Johnson WG, Gomez, MR, eds. Tuberous Sclerosis and Allied Disorders: Clinical, Cellular, and Molecular Studies, 2d ed. New York: New York Academy of Sciences. 1991:36–49.
35. Richardson EP Jr. Pathology of tuberous sclerosis: neuropathologic aspects. In: Johnson WG, Gomez MR, eds. Tuberous Sclerosis and Allied Disorders: Clinical, Cellular, and Molecular Studies. 2d ed. New York: New York Academy of Sciences, 1991:128–139.
36. Levine AJ. The tumor suppressor genes. Ann Rev Biochem 1993; 62:623–651.
37. Green AJ, Smith M, Yates JRW. Loss of heterozygosity on chromosome 16p13.3 in hamartomas from tuberous sclerosis patients. Nature Genet 1994; 6:193–196.
38. Henske EP, Neumann HPH, Scheithauer BW, Herbst EW, Short MP, Kwiatkowski DJ. Loss of heterozygosity in the tuberous sclerosis (TSC2) region of chromosome band 16p13 occurs in sporadic as well as TSC-associated renal angiomyolipomas. Genes Chrom Cancer 1995; 13:295–298.

39. Henske EP, Scheithauer BW, Short MP, Wollmann R, Nahmias J, Hornigold N, van Slegtenhorst M, Welsh CT, Kwiatkowski DJ. Allelic loss is frequent in tuberous sclerosis kidney lesions but rare in brain lesions. Am J Hum Gen 1996; 59:400–406.
40. Huang H-JS, Yee J-K, Shew J-H, Chen P-L, Bookstein R, Friedman T, Lee EY-HP, Lee W-H. Suppression of the neoplastic phenotype by replacement of the RB gene in human cancer cells. Science 1988; 242:1563–1566.
41. Johnson MR, DeClue JE, Felzmann S, Vass WC, Xu G, White R, Lowy DR. Neurofibromin can inhibit Ras-dependent growth by a mechanism independent of its GTPase-accelerating function. Mol Cell Biol 1994; 14:641–645.
42. Jin F, Wienecke R, Xiao G-H, Maize JC Jr., DeClue JE, Yeung RS. Suppression of tumorigenicity by the wild-type tuberous sclerosis 2 (Tsc2) gene and its C-terminal region. Proc Natl Acad Sci USA 1996; 93:9154–9159.
43. Resnitzky D, Gossen M, Bujard H, Reed SI. Acceleration of the G1/S phase transition by expression of cyclins D1 and E with an inducible system. Mol Cell Biol 1994; 14:1669–1679.
44. Orimoto K, Tsuchiya H, Kobayashi T, Matsuda T, Hino O. Suppression of the neoplastic phenotype by replacement of the *TSC2* gene in Eker rat renal carcinoma cells. Biochem Biophys Res Commun 1996; 219:70–75.
45. Tsuchiya H, Orimoto K, Kobayashi T, Hino O. Presence of potent transcriptional activation domains in the predisposing tuberous sclerosis (Tsc2) gene product of the Eker rat model. Cancer Res 1996; 56:429–433.
46. Ohtsuka T, Shimizu K, Yamamori B, Kuroda S, Takai Y. Activation of brain B-raf protein kinase by Rap1B small GTP-binding protein. J Biol Chem 1996; 271:1258–1261.
47. Yoshida Y, Kawata M, Miura Y, Musha T, Sasaki T, Kikuchi A, Takai Y. Microinjection of *smg/rap1/Krev*-1 p21 into swiss 3T3-Cells induces DNA synthesis and morphological changes. Mol Cell Biol 1992; 12:3407–3414.
48. DeClue JE, Papageorge AG, Fletcher JA, Diehl SR, Ratner N, Vass WC, Lowy DR. Abnormal regulation of mammalian $p21^{ras}$ contributes to malignant tumor growth in Vonrecklinghausen (Type-1) neurofibromatosis. Cell 1992; 69:265–273.
49. Basu TN, Gutmann DH, Fletcher JA, Glover TW, Collins FS, Downward J. Aberrant regulation of ras proteins in malignant tumour cells from type-1 neurofibromatosis patients. Nature 1992; 356:713–715.
50. Kitayama H, Sugimoto Y, Matsuzaki T, Ikawa Y, Noda M. A *ras*-related gene with transformation suppressor activity. Cell 1989; 56:77–84.
51. Hariharan IK, Carthew RW, Rubin GW. The Drosophila roughened mutation: activation of a rap homolog disrupts eye development and interferes with cell discrimination. Cell 1991; 67:717–722.

23

Structure and Function of Ras Superfamily Small GTPases

JONATHAN MOORMAN and DAVID A. BOBAK

University of Virginia School of Medicine
Charlottesville, Virginia

WALTER A. PATTON and JOEL MOSS

National Heart, Lung and Blood Institute
National Institutes of Health
Bethesda, Maryland

I. Introduction

Pulmonary lymphangioleiomyomatosis (LAM) is characterized by an abnormal proliferation of smooth muscle throughout the lung (24,241) and occurs exclusively in women, usually of reproductive age. Tuberous sclerosis (TS) is a neurocutaneous hereditary disorder in which the lung may exhibit smooth muscle proliferation indistinguishable from LAM (37,245), leading some investigators to believe that LAM is in fact a forme fruste of TS (150). While other disease manifestations differ, the striking similarities in terms of pulmonary disease suggest that the underlying mechanisms of disease may be similar as well. TS is a dominantly transmitted disorder with protean and variable clinical manifestations, including skin lesions, cystic kidney, liver and spleen lesions, angiofibromas, rhabdomyomas, and angiomyolipomas (122). Certain aspects of pulmonary pathology are identical to those seen in patients with LAM (37). Genetic linkage studies have demonstrated that deletions in two chromosomal loci (TSC1 on chromosome 9 and TSC2 on chromosome 16) are responsible for TS (122). Notably, TSC2 has been cloned (10) and the gene has been found to encode a

Table 1 Subfamilies and Selected Members of the Ras GTPase Superfamily

Ras-like	Rho-like	Rab-like	ARF-like	Miscellaneous
H-Ras	RhoA-C	Rab1-24	ARF 1-6	Ran
N-Ras	Rac1,2	Ypt1	ARL 1-5	Rad
K-RasA, B	Cdc42	Sec4		Gem/Kir
R-Ras1	TC10			
R-Ras2/TC21	RhoD			
RalA, B	RhoE			
	RhoG			

GTPase-activating protein (GAP3 or rap1GAP) associated with the Rap1 oncogene. In another neurocutaneous syndrome, neurofibromatosis, investigators have demonstrated that neurofibromin, the product of the neurofibromatosis gene (NF1), shares homology with another GAP, rasGAP (270), and regulates the activity of the GTPase Ras (146). LAM as a distinct disease or as a manifestation of TS will likely be the result of dysregulated GTPase activity, and thus an understanding of the superfamily of GTPases is necessary.

The Ras superfamily of monomeric GTPases is a heterogeneous group of proteins that function as molecular switches to coordinate a remarkable variety of cellular processes. The group includes more than 50 known members and has been divided into four major subfamilies based on structural and functional similarities: Ras-like proteins, Rho-like proteins, Rab-like proteins, and ARF-like proteins (20) (Table 1). Behaving as binary switches, these GTPases cycle between an active (GTP-bound) conformation and an inactive (GDP-bound) conformation. A series of guanine nucleotide-exchange factors (GEFs), guanine nucleotide-dissociation inhibitors (GDIs), and GTPase-activating proteins (GAPs) regulate nucleotide exchange and GTP hydrolysis, thereby controlling the activation/inactivation cycle of each GTPase (Fig. 1).

The Ras proteins were initially discovered as the translation products of mutant ras genes that were capable of disrupting normal cell proliferation and differentiation (139). Between 10 and 30% of human cancers have transforming ras mutations (112). Ras proteins regulate the flow of signals from receptor tyrosine kinases via a complex cascade of protein kinases to the nucleus and thereby regulate cell proliferation and differentiation (140).

The Rho-like [subfamily of] GTPases coordinate a diverse array of cytoskeleton-dependent events (201). Microinjection of Rho induces stress fiber formation and adhesion plaques; Rac induces lamellipodia formation, and Cdc42 promotes filopodia formation (168). Rho family proteins play important roles in protein kinase cascades, cell morphogenesis, phospholipid metabolism, neutro-

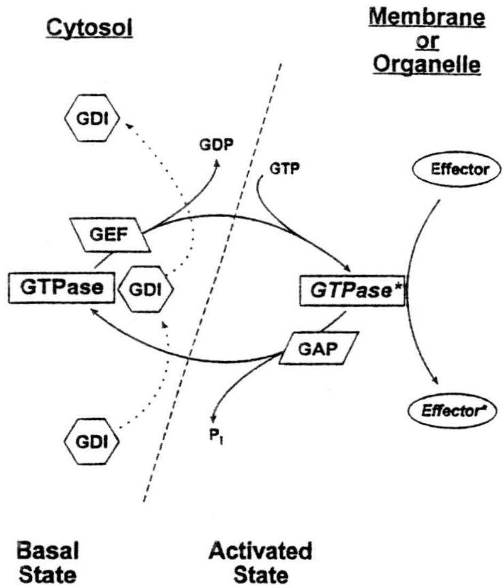

Figure 1 Regulation of the guanine nucleotide–dependent activation and inactivation of Ras superfamily GTPases. See text for details.

phil activation, and nuclear transcription regulation (51,95,127,201). Cross-talk between Rho and Ras subfamilies likely occurs via a variety of exchange factors, effector proteins, and upstream regulatory proteins (20).

The ARF-like and Rab-like GTPases appear to be involved in most types of intracellular vesicle assembly, loading, and targeting (218). ARFs are cytosolic proteins that, after activation by GTP, recruit other proteins to membranes to initiate the formation of transport vesicles (59). In addition, ARFs can activate specific isoforms of phospholipase D (31,48), possibly to facilitate the formation of vesicles or their fusion with target membranes. Rab proteins are believed to function by recruiting and targeting proteins required for the vectoral movement of vesicles between intracellular compartments, thus coordinating vesicle docking and fusion (29,72,182).

The recently described small GTPase Ran or TC4 is thought to regulate nuclear import and export (160). Ran has been implicated in numerous nuclear functions, most notably cell cycle progression, RNA processing, and DNA replication; Ran may work by coordinating nuclear import and export of mRNA and/or other macromolecules (155,160,272).

Activity of the Ras superfamily of GTPases is regulated by at least three classes of proteins: GAPs, GEFs, and GDIs (Fig. 1) (20). GAPs accelerate the intrinsic GTPase activity of the Ras superfamily members, and thereby promote formation of the GDP-bound, inactive conformation (22). The exchange of GDP for GTP is necessary for activation of the small GTPase; it is regulated by GEFs, which facilitate the exchange, and GDIs, which inhibit this exchange (20,69). These proteins integrate information from a range of intracellular signalling pathways to control GTPase function.

The Ras superfamily members thus coordinate an incredibly diverse array of intracellular functions, including cytoskeletal organization, vesicular trafficking, nuclear transport, and cellular proliferation and differentiation. Their ability to behave as molecular switches, to control protein kinase cascades, and to interact with critical effectors serves as a model for understanding fundamental intracellular signal transduction. Determining the specific functions of these proteins has been facilitated by understanding their structures.

II. Structure of Ras Superfamily Members

Although members of the Ras superfamily have quite divergent sequences, their overall structures are quite similar (268). The most highly conserved residues are those responsible for GTP binding and hydrolysis, including the sequences GXXXXGKS/T, DXXGQ, NKXD, and (S/C)A(K/L/T) (Fig. 2). Several core residues that provide a hydrophobic interior in the folded molecule appear also to be quite conserved (e.g., F156 in Ras) (267,268). The so-called effector domain differs in sequence among family members, although its position relative to the N-terminus is retained (27). A threonine within this region (e.g., T35 in Ras), as well as a glycine within the conserved DXXGQ sequence (e.g., G60 in Ras), is known to be critical for binding the γ-phosphate of GTP.

The N- and C-termini vary greatly among the small GTPases, being divergent both in size and sequence. For the majority of small GTPases, the C-termi-

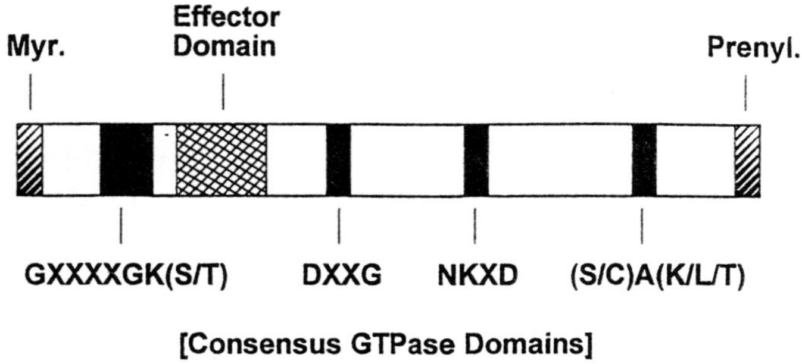

Figure 2 Schematic of key sequence motifs in small GTPases. Key motifs implicated in GTP-binding and GTPase activity, prenylation, myristoylation, and effector specificity are indicated in this representation of small GTPase protein structure.

nus serves as the site of crucial posttranslational modifications necessary for subcellular localization. Members of the Ras and Rho subfamilies contain a C-terminal CAAX sequence motif, whereas Rab proteins have a C-terminal CXC or CC motif. These motifs serve as signals for proteolytic cleavage, carboxymethylation, and prenylation. ARF proteins differ from other small GTPases in that their amino terminus is myristoylated. The amino-terminal myristate appears to function as a GTP-dependent switch to facilitate membrane localization and nucleotide exchange (74,75).

The three-dimensional structures of several small GTPases have been solved (268). The structure of Ras is most clearly understood and provides a model for other small GTP-binding proteins. The site for nucleotide binding and hydrolysis is a pocket formed by the highly conserved sequence motifs outlined in Figure 2. The GXXXXGKS/T sequence forms a loop (the P-loop) that is responsible for binding charged phosphate groups. The NKXD motif links regions of the nucleotide-binding site and provides the high specificity for the purine base. The Ras crystal structure has been used to elucidate the mechanism of GTP hydrolysis (211,214). The interaction between RasGDP and one of its GTPase-activating proteins, p120GAP, has been studied in the presence of aluminum fluoride, which binds to the active site of RasGDP and mimics a γ-phosphate group (211). These studies indicate that a critical arginine residue (termed an arginine finger) in GAP extends into the active site of Ras, perhaps stabilizing the transition state induced by aluminum fluoride binding.

Mutations that alter the position of the arginine residue in the active site, (e.g., Gln62 or Glyl2 in Ras), impair intrinsic and GAP-enhanced GTP hydrolysis, allowing Ras-GTP to accumulate; high levels of Ras-GTP appear to have oncogenic potential (27,112,268). Similarly, three-dimensional structures of the cdc42/RhoGAP complex demonstrate a crucial arginine in RhoGAP that directly interacts with the P-loop of Cdc42 and is thought to stabilize the transition state in the GTP hydrolysis reaction (97).

III. Regulation of Small GTPases

To function, members of the Ras superfamily must cycle between inactive and active conformations. Multiple proteins [e.g., guanine nucleotide-exchange factors (GEFs), GTPase-activating proteins (GAPs), guanine nucleotide-dissociation inhibitors (GDIs)] can alter the intrinsic GTPase activity, nucleotide-exchange rate, and membrane localization (20). In addition, prosttranslational modifications, which involve peptidases, carboxymethyltransferases, and prenyltransferases, may serve a regulatory function. A general schematic for the role of several of these factors during nucleotide cycling is shown in Figure 1.

A. Guanine Nucleotide-Exchange Factors

Guanine nucleotide-exchange factors catalyze the replacement of GDP by GTP and thus the formation of active GTPase (69). Interactions between several of the small GTPases and their exchange factors (GEFs) appear to occur via two specific domains that correspond to Ras residues 62–78 and 100–108 (152). GEFs first associate with the inactive, GDP-bound form of the small GTPase, thereby accelerating GDP dissociation, leading to an "empty," GEF-bound GTPase. Binding of GTP causes dissociation of GEF, leaving an active, GTP-bound GTPase (20). For Ras, the first GEF to be identified was CDC25 from *Saccharomyces cerevisiae* (107,112). A mammalian analog of CDC25, mSOS1, was later identified as an H-ras specific GEF that increased GDP dissociation and GTP association (25). mSOS1 is primarily cytosolic and appears to target Ras to the plasma membrane via an adaptor protein, GRB2, which contains SH3 domains that bind mSOS1 (42,66).

An individual GEF can catalyze nucleotide exchange for all members of a given subfamily. Rho- and Rac-specific GEFs, including Dbl, Vav, Ost, and Lbc, have been described that contain conserved domains with putative exchange properties (20). Mss4, a Rab family GEF, stimulates GDP release from rab3A, Ypt1, and Sec4 (35). The RCC1 gene encodes a 46 kDa GEF that catalyzes nucleotide exchange on Ran in vitro (19). It is likely that GEFs are essential for normal regulation of small GTPase function; in the Ras model, for example, genetic loss of GEF function has effects similar to those resulting from the loss of Ras proteins themselves.

B. GTPase-Activating Proteins

GTPase-activating proteins stimulate the low intrinsic GTPase activity of the GTP-binding proteins in vivo; GAP activity appears to be required for recycling the GTPase back to its inactive state (22). Oncogenic Ras mutants, for example, are constitutively locked in an active, GTP-bound state because they are resistant to GAP enhancement of GTP hydrolysis (84).

p120GAP (rasGAP) contains an ~250-residue domain at the C-terminus that specifically recognizes GTP-bound Ras and stimulates GTPase activity (78). The full-length protein differs in kinetic behavior from the isolated GAP domain and thus may contain sequences that modulate its GAP activity. Given that Ras interacts directly with Raf-1 (260), it seems likely that other proteins interacting with domains (such as SH2/SH3 and PH) found in p120GAP influence its ability to stimulate GTPase activity.

Neurofibromin (NF1) contains a catalytic domain similar to that of p120GAP (112,270). NF1 has Ras-GAP activity (146) and is a major regulator of Ras in neural crest cells. Defective alleles of NF1 are responsible for von Recklinghausen's disease (neurofibromatosis) (270), suggesting that loss of NF1 leads to accumulation of active Ras in neural crest cells (269). Alternatively, neurofibromin may control cell differentiation and proliferation in a manner unrelated to Ras function.

Interactions among the small GTPases may be coordinated by a different GAP, known as p190 (219). This protein has multiple domains, including a 145-residue domain near its C-terminus with GAP activity toward members of the Rho subfamily. Interestingly, this protein also binds p120GAP via its SH2 domain and appears to regulate p120GAP activity. The postulate of both parallel and interdependent GTPase signal transduction pathways is supported by the presence of these multifunctional GAPs.

C. Guanine Nucleotide-Dissociation Inhibitors

Guanine nucleotide-dissociation inhibitors are regulatory proteins that bind to the GTPase and inhibit the exchange of GDP for GTP; by interacting with the prenylated C-terminus, they maintain the GTPase as a soluble, inactive cytoplasmic complex. Described primarily for the Rho and Rab subfamilies, GDIs are believed to regulate the pool of plasma membrane–associated active GTPases. Rho undergoes posttranslational modification by geranlgeranylation near the C-terminus, which facilitates membrane localization (173). RhoGDI is able to extract Rho from cellular membranes in cell-free systems (22) and inhibits dissociation of GDP from prenylated Rho (173). Most types of cells contain RhoGDI in the cytoplasm, where it forms heterodimers with RhoA, CDC42, or Rac (8,89,173). Similarly, RabGDI forms a complex with prenylated Rab3A GTPases (22), inhibiting the exchange of GDP for GTP and the interaction of Rab3A-GDP with membranes.

D. Prenyltransferases

Prenyltransferases catalyze the posttranslational addition of farnesyl or geranylgeranyl groups to cysteine residues near the C-termini of Ras superfamily GTPases, a modification necessary for targeting of the GTPase to membranes (20,31,86). Mutations that prevent posttranslational modifications lead to inactive proteins (90). Three types of prenyltransferases catalyze the reactions that utilize different substrates: CAAX farnesyltransferases, CAAX geranylgeranyltransferases, and Rab geranylgeranyltransferases. These enzymes contain α and β subunits with repetitive sequence motifs that are responsible for their catalytic function and Zn^{2+}-binding capability (20,217).

Farnesyltransferases modify one cysteine in Ras proteins that contain a CAAX, in which A is an aliphatic amino acid and X is a serine or methionine residue (20,215). In contrast, members of the Rho family and Rap are substrates of CAAX-specific geranylgeranyltransferases (Type I GGTases) (216), where X is a leucine rather than a serine or methionine. The Rab-specific geranylgeranyltransferases (Type II GGTases) recognize the carboxy-terminal motifs CXXC or CC (20,216).

Newly synthesized small GTPases are first modified by either farnesylation or geranylgeranylation while in the cytosolic compartment. The prenylated protein then undergoes proteolytic removal of the three C-terminal amino acid residues (86,210). Finally, the carbon of the resulting terminal cysteine is methylated (88). These modifications are essential for GTPase membrane binding and cellular localization and do not affect intrinsic GTPase activity per se: they are, however, important for interaction of the GTPases with their GEFs and GDIs.

Ras proteins, with the exception of K-Ras, undergo palmitoylation of a cysteine relatively near the CAAX sequence (86,90). Certain other Ras and Rho proteins contain a series of polybasic amino acids in that region; both the palmitoylation and basic amino acids help to localize these proteins correctly (91). For the Rab proteins, a pair of escort proteins (REP1 and REP2) are required to present the unprenylated Rab protein to the Rab GGTase and to direct the prenylated form to the membrane (5,9). Notably, ARF proteins do not contain isoprenoid modification motifs, and instead are cotranslationally myristoylated at an N-terminal glycine residue (125). No lipid modification of Ran protein has been reported (86).

IV. Subfamilies

A. Ras Subfamily

Ras Proteins

The *ras* oncogene was discovered in 1981 and soon thereafter was determined to be a key regulator of both mitogenesis and oncogenesis (17,112). Expression of constitutively active Ras mutants induces specific cellular phenotypic changes typical of malignant transformation. Oncogenic mutants of Ras are found in up to 30% of all malignancies; those of epithelial origin (e.g., pancreatic adenocarcinoma) have an even higher incidence (17,112). Ras regulates signal transduction from the plasma membrane to the nucleus via several complex signaling pathways (112,139,140).

Ras proteins mediate signals transmitted from both receptor and nonreceptor tyrosine kinases as well as from heterotrimeric G protein-coupled receptors (140,151). A recently described adaptor molecule, Grb2, appears to associate with both receptor tyrosine kinases (e.g., EGF or PDGF) and with a guanine nucleotide-exchange factor known as SOS (42,256). Activation of growth factor receptors induces receptor autophosphorylation and subsequent association of a Grb2/SOS complex. Activated SOS then interacts with Ras to catalyze the exchange of GDP for GTP, resulting in activated Ras (33,77,135,209). A second protein, Shc, also can associate with the Grb2/SOS complex and is phosphorylated during activation of both receptor and nonreceptor tyrosine kinases (66,153,178,209).

Activated GTP-bound Ras likely interacts with multiple downstream effectors, including Raf1 kinase (260), and promotes localization of Raf to membranes. Raf activates a complex serine/threonine kinase cascade known as the mitogen-activated protein kinase or MAPK signaling pathway (42,140,259). This cascade, some form of which is found in all eukaryotes, stimulates both nuclear transcriptional factors (e.g., c-Myc, c-Jun) and key kinases involved in transcriptional activation (111,247). The importance of the pathway is demonstrated by the observation that upon transformation, some Ras mutants persistently interact with Raf1.

The Ras-Raf signaling pathway appears to be more complex than initially thought. For example, Ras-transformed cells do not always demonstrate activation of the MAPK cascade; in addition, heterotrimeric G proteins, and constituents of the MAPK cascade itself, can activate the pathway independent of Ras and Raf1. It seems clear that alternative effectors for Ras exist, and it is likely that Ras transformation requires the coordination of multiple downstream effectors. Potential downstream Ras effectors include phosphatidylinositol 3-kinase (PI3-kinase) (206), Rin1 (87), and RalGDS (114), a Ral GEF.

The Ras subfamily consists of numerous GTPases that share a high degree of similarity. H-, N-, and K-RasA/B are closely related proteins involved in signaling events described above (112,139). R-Ras1, while sharing significant structural similarity with these Ras molecules and interacting with Raf1, does not transform rat fibroblasts in its constitutively active form (138). Instead, R-Ras may interact with the apoptosis suppressor proto-oncogene Bcl-2 to control programmed cell death (71). R-Ras also binds to RalGDS in a GTP-dependent manner and may use this as its effector (4,231). Mutant R-Ras2 is transforming (80), but its effectors remain unknown.

Rap and Ral proteins

Rap proteins are closely related to Ras GTPases. Rap1A and Rap1B are Ras-related proteins that appear to be localized to the endoplasmic reticulum, late endosomes, and lysosomes (185). Expression of Rap1a protein antagonizes Ras transformation, perhaps by interfering with MAP kinases or by competing for Raf1 (50,118,185). Rap1A has also been shown to regulate the highly specialized phagocyte NADPH oxidase system (1,119,192). Rap2A appears to be localized to the ER and may have a role in vesicular trafficking, acting in a Ras-independent manner (18,105). Rap2B is involved in platelet aggregation, at the level of cytoskeletal reorganization (246).

Ras subfamily proteins RalA and RalB are ~50% identical to Ras in amino acid sequence, but diverge notably from Ras within the Ral-effector domains

(39,40). The Rap proteins are themselves very similar and differ primarily in their C-terminal sequences. RalGDS catalyzes nucleotide exchange on these and other Ras subfamily proteins (98,231). The functions of RalA and RalB are unknown, although they may play a role in early endocytosis/receptor internalization and likely are involved in Ras-dependent signaling as well (70).

B. Rho Subfamily

Rho and Rho-Related Proteins

The Rho subfamily consists of the primary Rho proteins (RhoA, B, C) and Rho-like proteins (Rac1, 2; Cdc42; TC10; Rho D, E, G). The *rho* gene was initially identified in *Aplysia* in 1985; since then, Rho proteins have been found to be highly conserved among nearly all eukaryotic organisms (13,201,239). Rho GTPases share ~30% overall amino acid sequence similarity with Ras and were originally described as key regulators of the actin cytoskeleton. More recently, these proteins have been implicated in a diverse array of cellular functions, including cellular transformation, cell cycle progression, and transcriptional regulation (51,95,201).

Rho Family and the Cytoskeleton

Many aspects of cytoskeletal organization are regulated by Rho family GTPases (201,239). Microinjection of constitutively active RhoA caused stress fiber formation and promoted the development of focal adhesions (204). In cells, stress fiber formation was inhibited by treatment with *Clostridium botulinum* exoenzyme C3, a bacterial ADP-ribosyltransferase that selectively ADP-ribosylates (and inactivates) RhoA, B, and C. Rac1 has been implicated as a regulator of lamellipodia formation and membrane ruffling (203), and Cdc42 in filopodia formation (168). Hall and colleagues suggested that a hierarchy of Rho-modulated pathways acts to control microfilament organization (123,129,168). Rho subfamily members appear also to play important roles in other types of cytoskeletal-dependent functions, including cell-cell adhesion, cell motility, and cytokinesis.

Rho A, B, and C Proteins

Rho A, B, and C are very similar proteins that induce actin stress fiber formation via protein kinases (201). The newly identified Rho-associated kinases, such as Rho kinase (ROK) (103,116,133,134,149) and protein kinase N (PKN) (6), appear to be molecular links between RhoA and the myosin-binding subunit (MBS) of myosin light-chain phosphatase (MLC), which controls the binding of myosin to actin filaments. MBS is phosphorylated by Rho-kinase in a Rho-dependent manner (116). One model proposes that activation of Rho proteins leads to binding of Rho kinase and/or PKN, which can phosphorylate MBS. In this hypothesis, Rho could stimulate the phosphorylation of MBS, thus inhibiting MLC activity. The accumulation of phosphorylated MLC could then increase myosin-actin filament binding and the formation of actin stress fibers.

RhoB and C are less well studied than RhoA. Microinjection of either protein into Swiss 3T3 fibroblasts induced actin stress fiber formation and focal adhesion assembly (204). Like RhoA, both RhoB and C are ADP-ribosylated by exoenzyme C3 (41). RhoA and RhoB are nearly identical in amino acid sequence and appear to function similarly. RhoA and RhoC are both geranylgeranylated, whereas RhoB is palmitoylated and either farnesylated or geranylgeranylated (2). In addition, RhoB is associated with early endosomes and prelysosomes in Rat-2 and MDCK cells (3), whereas RhoA and C are primarily cytosolic. The *rhoB* gene appears to be an immediate-early gene inducible by activation of protein tyrosine kinases (104). Recently, Zalcman and colleagues found that EGF-induced RhoB expression is regulated during the cell cycle in HeLa cells, with peak expression during S phase (274). RhoB was perinuclear and localized to vesicles, suggesting that RhoB may be involved in regulating assembly/translocation of cytoskeletal elements necessary for mitosis.

Rac proteins

Rac1 and 2 are also involved in cytoskeletal organization and actin polymerization. Rac proteins, which share ~92% identity at the amino acid level, are widely expressed in many types of cells and tissues, although in neutrophils, Rac2 appears to predominate (1,53,55). Microinjection of Rac proteins induces lamellipodia formation and membrane ruffling, effects similar to those of PDGF, EGF, or insulin (168,169,204); subsequent formation of actin stress fibers requires Rho. Rac proteins are essential to the phagocyte NADPH oxidase system, along with p47-phox, p67-phox, and cytochrome b 558 (1,62,119,120). In cell-free systems, both Rac1 and 2 activate the oxidase system (8,94) efficiently. Rac2-dependent activation of NADPH oxidase is, in turn, regulated by a series of Rac-specific GEFs, GAPs, and GDIs (94,159).

Cdc42

Cdc42 regulates cytoskeletal events in concert with Rac and Rho (85). The cognate protein in yeast appears to coordinate certain changes in cell polarity required during growth. Initially, microinjection of activated forms of Cdc42 demonstrated a role of this protein in regulating the formation of bradykinin-induced filopodia (123,169) and the assembly of intracellular integrin-actin complexes (100,167,169). A hierarchical relationship in which Rac and Rho function downstream from Cdc42 has been postulated (169,205). Subsequent studies suggested that this interaction is not sequential, but rather occurs by means of GTPase crosstalk (130,282). In helper T cells, Cdc42 has also been implicated in the control of cell polarity during T-cell interactions with antigen-presenting cells (130).

Cdc42 has been linked to the Wiskott-Aldrich syndrome (WAS), a condition associated with an abnormal WAS gene product (WASP) (202,238). WASP appears to modulate the function of Cdc42 and, possibly, Rac (12,82), to induce pathological actin reorganization. Although it did not affect filopodia formation, WASP overexpression in Jurkat cells induced clusters of polymerized actin. WASP appeared to co-localize with these clusters; its localization was inhibited by the expression of a dominant negative form of Cdc42, but not Rac or Rho (238). A sequence of 16 amino acids (referred to as the CRIB motif) (12,238) in WASP is thought to be necessary for Cdc42 or Rac binding.

Rho Subfamily and Cellular Growth

Members of the Rho subfamily coordinate cytoskeletal events, but appear also to regulate aspects of cellular growth, development, and transformation. Both Rho and Rac were necessary for Ras-induced fibroblast transformation (82,113, 179,191); activated mutants of both transformed NIH3T3 fibroblasts (179,190,191). The recent recognition that several oncogenes (e.g., Dbl and Ost) (92,99) are Rho GEFs led to intense investigation of Rho control of cellular growth pathways. Rho proteins have important functions in several aspects of nuclear signaling, including growth factor–mediated activation of the serum response factor (SRF). SRF binds to the serum response element (SRE) in the promoter of many genes that are upregulated in response to certain serum growth factors, e.g., lysophosphatidic acid (LPA). Rho, Rac, and Cdc42 each can stimulate SRF activity; however, only Rho is required for serum- and LPA-induced activation of SRF (95,201). The roles of Rho in the transcriptional events and in the well-described cytoskeletal events may be distinct.

Recently pathways by which Rac and Cdc42 potentially regulate cellular growth responses include several elements that are quite similar to the Ras-Raf-MAPK paradigm of cellular activation and nuclear signaling. Both Rac1 and Cdc42 specifically associated with and activated the p21-activated kinase (PAK) family of serine/threonine kinases (145). Similar to WASP, PAKs contain CRIB motifs. Expression of a constitutively active PAK stimulated the activity of a novel family of kinases that are structurally related to MAPK, the so-called stress-activated protein kinases (SAPKs) or jun N-terminal kinases (JNKs) (14). JNK and the p38 kinase, but not MAPK, were stimulated by expression of activated forms of Rac and Cdc42 (51,82,128). Similarly, inhibition of growth factor–stimulated JNK activity was achieved using dominant negative Rac or Cdc42 mutants (51,157,175). How stimulation of these pathways leads to mitogenic responses is unclear, although it is presumed that kinase-dependent activation of transcription factors is involved.

Rho Effectors and Modulators

As described for Ras proteins, many potential regulators and effectors have been identified for Rho family GTPases. Numerous GAPs, GEFs, GDIs, kinases, and effectors have been identified using a variety of screening techniques, including the yeast two-hybrid system, affinity chromatography, and overlay assays. Several of these Rho family–associated proteins and their potential roles are outlined in Table 2.

C. ADP-Ribosylation Factors

Identification and Initial Characterization of ARF

Initial studies revealed that guanine nucleoside triphosphates (68,137,162,163, 166,264) and tissue factors (67,68,163,184,213) were required for cholera toxin–catalyzed ADP-ribosylation of G_{sa} (79,106,110,170). A major tissue factor turned out to be a family of 20 kDa GTP-binding proteins termed ADP-ribosylation factors (ARFs), which was found in both membrane (253) and cytosolic (252) forms and was especially abundant in brain. Myristoylation of ARF at its amino terminus (125) and GTP binding facilitate its membrane localization (93). ARFs have been found in species from *Giardia* to humans, and they appear to be ubiquitous in eukaryotes.

Nucleotide Exchange and Hydrolysis by ARF

Upon activation, ARF moves from the soluble/cytosolic fraction to the particulate/membrane fraction (74,108,197,261), where it exerts its action; unlike heterotrimeric GTP-binding proteins, it is not activated by GDP-AIF_4^- (108). In vitro, lipids and detergents facilitate nucleotide exchange (195,243) by decreasing the apparent K_a for GTP (165). The fungal fatty acid metabolite brefeldin A (BFA) can block ARF activation (60) and the association of ARF with Golgi membranes (61,249). In some instances, BFA is believed to block ARF activation by directly inhibiting guanine nucleotide-exchange factor(s) (161). BFA-insensitive exchange factors have also been identified (154,250,251).

Several ARF guanine nucleotide exchange proteins (GEPs) have been identified in different tissues. A BFA-insensitive ARF-GEP of ~55 kDa was found in bovine brain and rat spleen cytosol (250,251); like the protein studied by Franco et al. (75), it activated only myristoylated ARF (251). Several characteristics of this family of ARF exchange proteins are emerging. They appear to fall into two categories: higher molecular weight, BFA-sensitive molecules and smaller molecular weight, BFA-insensitive molecules. Most of the ARG GEPs

Table 2 Rho Subfamily Proteins and Putative Modulators

Modulator	Action	Subfamily specificity	Ref.
Dbl	GEF	Rho, Cdc42	92
			38
Ost	GEF	RhoA, Cdc42	99
Lbc	GEF	RhoA	279
Cdc24 (yeast)	GEF(?)	Cdc42	63
smgGDS	GEF	RhoA, Rac1	96
Tiam-1	GEF	Rac1,Cdc42>RhoA	156
			83
RhoGDI	GDI	Rho, Rac	96
			173
Ly-GDI	GDI	RhoA	212
Bcr	GAP	Rac, Cdc42	57
			47
Abr	GAP	Rac, Cdc42	47
n-, -chimaerin	GAP	Rac	123
p190 RhoGAP	GAP	Rho>Rac, Cdc42	220
			129
Myr-5	GAP	Rho, Cdc42>Rac1	199
ROK	Kinase	RhoA	133, 134
			149
$P160^{ROCK}$	Kinase	RhoA	103
Rho kinase	Kinase	Rho	149
PAK	Kinase	Cdc42, Rac	263
			143
$p120^{ACK}$	Kinase	Cdc42	6
			144
$p70^{S6K}$	Kinase	Cdc42, Rac	46
	PKN	Kinase	RhoA
263			
			6
Rhophilin	?	RhoA	263
Rhotekin	?	RhoA	198
MBS (MLCP)	Phosphatase	RhoA	116
$p67^{phox}$	Rac		189
			56
WASP	Cdc42		238
			12
PIP 5-kinase	Kinase	Rho, Rac	45
PI 3-kinase	Kinase	Rac, Cdc42	237
			278
			21

contain sequences similar to a *Saccharomyces cerevisiae* protein Sec7 and may reflect the existence of a distinct class of ARF GEPs.

The first identified larger Sec7 domain GEP, p200, is a protein of ~200 kDa, which contains sequences that are 47% identical to Sec7 and retained its BFA sensitivity after purification by gel electrophoresis (161). A second larger Sec7 domain GEP of 500–600 kDa, Gea1, was identified in *S. cerevisiae* as a critical component of ER-Golgi transport and shown to be BFA sensitive (181). A slightly larger Golgi-localized, BFA-sensitive protein, p619, in which a Sec7 domain has not been identified, was found in human breast carcinoma cells (207). p619 contains two domains with sequences similar to RCC1, an exchange factor for the Ran GTPase, and a C-terminus that interacts specifically with myristoylated ARF1 and an N-terminus that catalyzes nucleotide exchange on ARF1 and Rab-related proteins, but not Ran or R-Ras2/TC21 (207).

Two smaller, BFA-insensitive GEPs—cytohesin-1 (154), a ~46 kDa protein product of the B2-1 gene that may regulate α1β2 integrin function (121), and cytohesin-2 or ARNO (ARF nucleotide binding site opener) (43), a protein that appears to exchange the nucleotide only of myristoylated ARF—contain Sec7 domains. These appear to be the minimal catalytically active segments of the proteins, which also contain pleckstrin homology (PH) domains for lipid interaction.

Unlike other Ras superfamily members, ARF has no detectable intrinsic GTPase activity (266) and requires a GAP for conversion to the inactive (GDP-bound) state. Several partially pure ARF GAPs have been reported (58,141,194); a hallmark of this family of proteins appears to be a critical amino-terminal zinc finger motif. The ARF-GAP described by Makler et al. (141) was identified as a 45 kDa protein whose Golgi localization was BFA sensitive (52). An additional zinc finger–containing ARF GAP is the 39 kDa protein from *Saccharomyces* termed GSC1 (187), originally described as mediating the transition from stationary to proliferation (102), now known to be required for efficient secretion of invertase in yeast (187).

Role of ARF in Vesicle Traffic

Yeast and bovine ARF sequences were the first to be determined (188,221), and it was work on *S. cerevisiae* ARFs that yielded the first clues to their intracellular function. Deletion of yeast ARF 1 (yARF1), which was localized to the Golgi, resulted in defects in the secretory pathway; specifically, invertase was shown to accumulate intracellularly and that which was secreted was only partially glycosylated (233). Thereafter, deletion of yARFs 1 and 2 was reported to be lethal (234). ARFs were found to be associated with coat proteins or COPs that form the coatomer complex on the surface of non–clathrin-coated, Golgi-derived vesicles (218); activation of ARF by GTP and its association with Golgi was required for the recruitment of βCOP, a coatomer component, to Golgi (59,176). The model for ARF action in vesicular trafficking in the Golgi, originally proposed by Serafini et al. (218), suggested that after its formation, ARF-GTP binds to a membrane and initiates COP recruitment and membrane budding. Following vesicle formation and release, ARF remains associated with the vesicle until acted upon by an ARF-GAP, which triggers GTP hydrolysis and release of ARF and COP from the membrane, which then fuses with the acceptor membrane. Besides regulating membrane traffic in the ER and Golgi, ARFs appear to function in nuclear membrane dynamics (23) and endocytosis (132).

An additional level of control of ARF-initiated vesicular trafficking might be exerted by one of several proteins that fall into the diverse category of signaling proteins and include an isoform of phospholipase D (PLD) as well as heterotrimeric G protein subunits. An ARF-activated isoform of phosphatidylcholine-specific PLD (the products of which are phosphatidic acid and choline) was dependent on divalent cations and phosphatidylinositol 4,5-bisphosphate (PIP_2) (31,48,148). With an ARF-GAP activity that was inhibited by phosphatidylcholine and stimulated by phosphatidic acid (194), the possibility exists of both negative and positive modification of ARF function and half-life in vesicle production, but no direct evidence has been presented. Rho A (28,142), protein kinase C (174,227), cdc42 (225,226), and unidentified proteins of 50 (26,126,131) and 36 kDa (222) have also been shown to activate or synergize with ARF in the activation of ARF-dependent PLD. They demonstrated that the production of phosphatidic acid (PA) by bacterial PLD (an enzyme that does not require ARF) resulted in the recruitment of coatomer (124) is consistent with either additional levels of control in the regulation of ARF-stimulatable PLD activity or the existence of several distinct PLD isoforms.

Possible involvement of the heterotrimeric G proteins in the control of ARF-mediated vesicular transport was suggested when a bovine brain G_α protein was shown to inhibit the binding of ARF and βCOP to Golgi membranes (61). Later, ARF was shown to interact with both G_α (49) and $G_{\beta\gamma}$ (49,76) subunits. The $G_{\beta\gamma}$ interaction had been shown also to be important for the inhibition of endosome fusion (49,132,232).

ARF Sequence and Structure

To date, six mammalian ARFs have been identified by cDNA cloning (ARF2 has been identified only in bovine tissues and has not been detected in primates). Multiple ADP-ribosylation factor–like proteins (ARLs) have also been identified by cDNA cloning including five from humans ARLs and numerous others (e.g., rat, *S. cerevisiae*), but their function remains elusive. Numerous ARF family members are still being added to sequence databases, but these by definition can be designated as ARFs only if the ability of the protein to rescue the *Saccharo-*

myces arf1⁻, arf2⁻ double mutant and/or stimulate the ADP-ribosyltransferase activity of cholera toxin A subunit is demonstrated. If a protein does not meet these requirements, it is designated an ARL. Thus, many new ARF family members cannot be correctly named until their activities have been defined. Activation of a specific PLD is an ARF characteristic, but it is not established that all ARFs activate PLD and all ARLs do not.

Mammalian ARFs have been grouped, based on protein and DNA sequence homology as well as gene structure, into three classes (254), which now appear also to correlate with subcellular localization and function. Class I ARFs include ARFs 1, 2, and 3, class II, ARFs 4 and 5, and class III, ARF 6. Utilizing sequence alignment or dendritic tree analysis, ARFs from other species can also be assigned to these classes. Hallmarks of ARF structure include (1) a glycine at position two, which is the site of co-translational acylation, usually with myristic acid, and (2) consensus GXXXXGK, DXXG (commonly DVGG) and NKQD sequences of the putative GTP-hydrolysis/phosphate-binding, Mg^{2+}/guanine nucleotide phosphate-binding, and guanine nucleotide purine ring interaction sites, respectively.

Before determination of the crystal structure of ARF (7,81), Ras was considered the best available model for ARF structure; with the putative GTP-binding and hydrolysis regions of the two sequences aligned, ARF has an N-terminal extension that is absent in Ras, and it was postulated that this could explain the lack of intrinsic GTP hydrolysis by ARF. Structural analysis of ARF crystallized as a monomer (81) and a dimer (7,81) revealed that ARF differs from Ras not only by the amphipathic α-helix and loop at the N-terminus, but by an additional β-sheet, in the Ras effector region, through which the two molecules in the dimer appeared to interact. Other important features in the crystal structure include a positively charged area on the surface of the molecule that may be important for its interaction with membrane lipids and the location of Gln71, which is important for GTP hydrolysis by ARF (109,240,242,277). Gln71 was approximately 5 Å farther away from the putative γ-phosphate binding site than is the corresponding Gln in Ras, which was mentioned as possibly accounting for the higher GTPase activity of Ras.

Intracellular Localization of ARF

It is becoming increasingly apparent that ARF class is related to specific intracellular localization and presumably function. Yeast ARF1 was the first to be localized to the Golgi (233); based on studies with recombinant wild-type and mutant human and native bovine ARFs, this localization appears to be a characteristic of all ARFs that have been grouped as members of class I (109,240, 242,248,277). Data on a class II ARF (ARF5) are also consistent with their binding and interaction with Golgi (93,248,249) and perhaps other compartments.

Most distinct in its localization is the class III ARF, human ARF6, which is localized and appears to function at the plasma membrane (64,180,193).

D. Rab Proteins

The Rab subfamily of small GTPases consists of more than 30 proteins that help to regulate intracellular vesicular trafficking. This diverse group of GTPases is the largest of the Ras subfamilies, and its members are localized to distinct subsets of intracellular organelles involved in exocytic, transcytotic, and endocytic pathways (275). It was originally proposed that Rabs act as molecular "tags" to direct vesicles to particular intracellular targets (72). Later investigation indicated that, more likely, Rab proteins function as molecular switches to regulate vesicle docking and fusion, playing roles that are much more complex than initially envisioned (29,65).

Rab Distribution and Function

In general, Rab proteins are localized to specific intracellular compartments and transport pathways. Rab1, for example, is localized to the endoplasmic reticulum (ER), pre-Golgi, and Golgi and regulates transport of vesicles from the ER to the Golgi (16,186,244). Overexpression of the GDP-bound form of Rab1 inhibited both ER to Golgi and intra-Golgi transport (172,244) apparently by reducing the rate of vesicle formation from the ER (172). A GTP-bound active mutant of Rab1, which has a high rate of GTP exchange, inhibited vesicle transport (172,183,244). Therefore, whereas vesicle formation may require recruitment of Rab1 in its GDP-bound form, vesicle fusion per se may additionally require a conformational change induced by GTP hydrolysis (16). Some evidence, however, suggests that it is the presence of Rab-GTP and not the process of GTP hydrolysis or the presence of Rab-GDP that is necessary for vesicle fusion (29,235,262,276).

In some systems, multiple Rabs have been localized to the same specific compartment, yet each appears to have different functions. Rab4a and 5a, for example, are both found in early endocytic compartments. Whereas Rab4a regulates recycling of early endosomes, Rab5a regulates endocytosis from coated pits to the early endosomes (32,257,275). Even closely related Rabs (e.g., Rab3a,3b,3c, and 3d) appear to differ somewhat in their intracellular distribution and functions (275).

Conversely, membrane compartments may contain several different Rab proteins with similar functions. For example, the trafficking between ER and Golgi apparatus requires not only isoforms of Rab1, but also Rab2 (183,244). This redundancy is not found in yeast and may be a reflection of vesicle regulation in both directions (147). Cells that have specialized functions may contain Rab proteins with apparently redundant functions as well as those with unique roles, as is evidenced in polarized epithelial cells with Rabs 3b, 8, and 13 (101,265,273).

The Rab Model and the SNARE Hypothesis

In one model for Rab regulation of docking and fusion of vesicles with target membrane compartments (72,171), inactive Rab-GDP is believed to exist associated with RabGDI in the cytosol (11,171,196,229,255). This complex is then incorporated into the transport vesicle either just before or after its formation at the donor membrane. At the acceptor membrane, RabGDI dissociates, Rab-bound GDP is replaced by GTP, and the ensuing conformational change in Rab-GTP allows the vesicle to dock (171). The specific role of Rab proteins in vesicle docking and fusion may involve interaction with and/or regulation of putative vesicle and target membrane receptors (72,182), which have not been identified. They may be analogous to the v-SNARE protein and t-SNARE receptor described for synaptic vesicle fusion at nerve terminals (72,230). The SNARE hypothesis of neuronal membrane fusion provides a useful paradigm for vesicle docking and fusion events. Several proteins, such as soluble *N*-ethylmaleimide-sensitive factor (NSF) and soluble NSF-attachment proteins (SNAPs), are required for intracellular membrane fusion (230). Rothman et al. (208) proposed that a membrane protein present on transport vesicles, v-SNARE, binds to a receptor on the target membrane, t-SNARE, that is itself complexed with a SNAP. The specificities of a given v-SNARE and t-SNARE would ensure correct targeting of vesicle to membrane, and the interaction of NSF with SNAP would initiate fusion (208). In nerve terminals, synaptobrevin appears to function as a v-SNARE, syntaxin as a t-SNARE, and SNAP-25 as the SNAP associated with the t-SNARE.

Recent data suggest that Rab proteins may directly or indirectly regulate SNARE function (30,136,228). Rab3a is highly expressed in secretory cells, such as neurons and endocrine cells, and is concentrated at neuronal synaptic vesicles (115,158). One potential effector for Rab3a, Rabphilin-3a, provides a link to vesicle fusion. Rabphilin 3a appears to interact with GTP-bound Rab3a (223,224), perhaps stabilizing it in the active conformation (117). In addition, Rabphilin contains a region of similarity to synaptotagmin and protein kinase C, both of which bind phospholipid in a calcium-dependent manner (271). Rabphilin-3a may thus serve as a calcium-sensitive barrier to the SNARE pathway of vesicle fusion (54), thereby permitting fusion of synaptic vesicles upon Ca^{2+} influx during synaptic transmission. Rabaptin-5 has recently been described as an effector for Rab5 (236), which is required for membrane docking and fusion (140,236). Rab5 recruits this effector to early endosomes in a GTP-dependent manner. Although its exact role is unclear, Rabaptin-5 does not appear to have a role in membrane recycling or regulated membrane trafficking in the early steps of endocytosis.

Regulation of Rab Function

As is typical for most GTPases of the Ras superfamily, Rab proteins undergo C-terminal modifications, which are likely to be particularly important for these small proteins because each must move between specific membrane sites and the cytosol. Rab GTPases are geranylgeranylated at cysteines located near the C-termini (275). Geranylgeranylation allows membrane association, but does not confer specificity of localization, which appears to be determined by domains upstream of the prenylation site (29,44,275). The geranylgeranylation requires escort proteins (5,9), designated REP-1 and REP-2, to present the Rab protein to the transferase. These proteins then deliver the geranylgeranylated Rab to the target membrane (5,9,86). Certain Rab proteins, notably Rab1a and Rab4a, may also undergo phosphorylation as a means of regulating membrane association (15,257). Given the importance of guanine nucleotide exchange in Rab function, the existence of Rab GEFs and GAPs seems likely. Mss4p, a mammalian counterpart of DSS4p (a yeast GEF for Ypt1 and Sec4), was identified as a GEF for Rab3a (35). Similarly, GAP activity for this Rab has been detected (34).

E. Miscellaneous Small GTPases

The Ran/TC4 GTPase was identified as an essential component of the nuclear protein transport mechanism (155,160). Ran GTPases are involved in mRNA processing and export, DNA replication, and cell cycle progression, possibly as a consequence of Ran-mediated control of nuclear import and export (155). Factors transported into the nucleus generally contain short stretches of amino acids designated as nuclear-localizing sequences (NLS). NLS act to facilitate import of molecules through the nuclear pore complex (NPC). In this multistep process, several cytosolic factors, including Ran, appear to be required.

There is evidence that the NLS receptor importin (NLS-R) binds the NLS-containing ligand on the cytosolic side of the NPC (272). A stabilizing component of the NPC-docking complex, p97, or karyopherin, may promote ligand binding at the NPC. Ran-GTP localizes to the cytoplasmic region of the NPC, possibly by binding to RanBP2, a nuclear pore complex protein found at the cytoplasmic surface (272). Ran-GTP interacts with the NLS-R/ligand complex and GTP is hydrolyzed, an event that appears to be necessary for commitment of the NLS-R/ligand to distal transport (155). A Ran-binding domain, present on RanBP2 and other putative Ran-binding partners (272), can activate RNA1p, a RanGAP, to facilitate this GTP hydrolysis. Subsequent steps in the import pathways are still unclear. Other putative targets of Ran include RCC1, which functions as an exchange factor for Ran and is involved in cell entry into and exit from mitosis.

The Rad GTPase was initially found to be overexpressed in the skeletal muscle of type II diabetics (36,200,280,281). Immunolocalization studies suggest that Rad is localized to thin filaments in muscle (177). It also appeared to interact with skeletal muscle β-tropomyosin in a guanine nucleotide–dependent manner (280). Rad and its related proteins, Gem and Kir, are unique among the Ras-related GTPases in that they lack prenylation motifs and contain significant N- and C-terminal extensions (164,258). They also contain several nonconservative changes within the GTP-binding domain which are not present in other Ras-related GTPases (73,164). The C-terminus extension of ~30 amino acids exhibits features of a calmodulin-binding domain (73), and these GTPases have been shown to bind to calmodulin in a calcium-dependent manner (73,164). Phosphorylation of Rad by protein kinase A (PKA) may occur (281). These data suggest a role for Rad in integrating Ca^{2+}/calmodulin-dependent phosphorylation pathways and growth factor signal transduction pathways.

References

1. Abo A, Pick E, Hall A, Totty N, Teahan CG, Segal AW. Activation of the NADPH oxidase involves the small GTP-binding protein p21rac1. Nature, 1991; 353:668–670.
2. Adamson P, Marshall CJ, Hall A, Tilbrook PA. Post-translational modifications of p21rho proteins. J Biol Chem, 1992; 267:20033–20038.
3. Adamson P, Paterson HF, Hall A. Intracellular localization of the p21rho proteins. J Cell Biol 1992; 119:617–627.
4. Albright CF, Giddings, BW, Liu J, Vito M, Weinberg RA. Characterization of a guanine nucleotide dissociation stimulator for a ras-related GTPase. EMBO J 1993; 12:339–347.
5. Alexandrov K, Horiuchi H, Steel-Mortimer O, Seabra M, Zerial M. Rab escort protein-1 is a multifunctional protein that accompanies newly prenylated Rab proteins to their target membranes. EMBO J 1994; 13:5262–5273.
6. Amano M, Mukai H, Ono Y, Chihara K, Matsui T, Hamajima Y, Okawa K, Iwamatsu A, Kaibuchi K. Identification of a putative target for Rho as the serine-threonine protein kinase N. Science 1996; 271:648–650.
7. Amor J, Harrison D, Kahn R, Ringe D. Structure of the human ADP-ribosylation factor 1 complexed with GDP. Nature 1994; 372:704–708.
8. Ando S, Kaibuchi K, Sasaki T, Hiraoka K, Nishiyama T, Mizuno T, Asada M, Nunoi N, Matsuda I, Matsuura Y, et al. Post-translational processing of rac p21s is important both for their interaction with the GDP/GTP exchange proteins and for their activation of NADPH oxidase. J Biol Chem 1992; 267:25709–25713.
9. Andres DA, Seabra MC, Brown MS, Armstrong SA, Smeland TE, Cremers FPM, Goldstein JL. cDNA cloning of component A of Rab geranylgeranyl transferase and demonstration of its role as a rab escort protein. Cell 1993; 73:1091–1099.
10. Anonymous. Identification and characterization of the tuberous sclerosis gene on chromosome 16. The European Chromosome 16 Tuberous Sclerosis Consortium. Cell 1993; 75:1305–1315.
11. Araki S, Kikuchi A, Hata Y, Isomura M, Takai Y. Regulation and reversible binding of smg p25a, a ras p21-like GTP-binding protein, to synaptic plasma membranes and vesicles by its specific regulatory protein, GDP dissociation inhibitor. J Biol Chem 1990; 265:13007–13015.

12. Aspenstrom P, Lindberg U, Hall A. Two GTPases, Cdc42 and Rac, bind directly to a protein implicated in the immunodeficiency disorder Wiskott-Aldrich syndrome. Curr Biol 1996; 6:70–75.
13. Avraham H, Weinberg RA. Characterization and expression of the human *rhoH12* gene product. Mol Cell Biol 1989; 9:2058–2066.
14. Bagrodia S, Derijard B, Davis RJ, Cerione RA. Cdc42 and PAK-mediated signaling leads to Jun kinase and p38 mitogen-activated protein kinase activation. J Biol Chem 1995; 270:27995–27998.
15. Bailly E, McCaffrey M, Touchot N, Zahraoui A, Goud B, Bornens M. Phosphorylation of two small GTP-binding proteins of the Rab family by p34cdc2. Nature 1991; 350.
16. Balch WE. Rab1a,b. In: Zerial M, Huber LA, eds. Guidebook to the Small GTPases. New York: Oxford University Press Inc., 1995:307–310.
17. Barbacid M. ras genes. Ann Rev Biochem 1987; 56:779–827.
18. Beranger F, Tavitian A, deGunzburg J. Post-translational processing and subcellular localization of the ras-related rap2 protein. Oncogene 1991; 6:1835–1842.
19. Bischoff RF, Ponstingl H. Mitotic regulator protein RCC1 is complexed with a nuclear ras-related polypeptide. Proc Natl Acad Sci USA 1991; 88:10830–10834.
20. Boguski MS, McCormick F. Proteins regulating Ras and its relatives. Nature 1993; 366:643–654.
21. Bokoch GM, Vlahos CJ, Wang Y, Knaus UG, Traynor-Kaplan AE. Rac GTPase interacts specifically with phosphatidylinositol 3-kinase. Biochem J 1996; 315:775–779.
22. Bollag G, McCormick FA. Regulators and effectors of Ras proteins. Annu Rev Cell Biol 1991; 7:601–632.
23. Boman AL, Taylor TC, Melancon P, Wilson KL. A role for ADP-ribosylation factor in nuclear vesicle dynamics. Nature 1992; 358:512–514.
24. Bonetti F, Chiodera P. Lymphangioleiomyomatosis and tuberous sclerosis: Where is the border? [editorial]. Eur Respir J 1996; 9:399–401.
25. Botwell, D, Fu P, Simon M, Senior P. Identification of murine homologues of the Drosophila son of sevenless gene: potential activators of ras. Proc Natl Acad Sci 1992; 89:6511–6515.
26. Bourgoin S, Harbour D, Desmarais Y, Takai Y, Beaulieu A. Low molecular weight GTP-binding proteins in HL-60 granulocytes. Assessment of the role of ARF and of a 50-kDa cytosolic protein in phospholipase D activation. J Biol Chem 1995; 270:3172–3178.
27. Bourne HR, Sanders DA, McCormick F. The GTPase superfamily: conserved structure and molecular mechanism. Nature 1991; 349:117–126.
28. Bowman EP, Uhlinger DJ, Lambeth JD. Neutrophil phospholipase D is activated by a membrane-associated Rho family small molecular weight GTP-binding protein. J Biol Chem 1993; 268:21509–21512.
29. Brennwald P, Novick P. Interactions of three domains distinguishing the Ras-related GTP-binding proteins Ypt1 and Sec4. Nature 1993; 362:560–563.
30. Brennwald PB, Kearns K, Champion S, Keranen S, Bankaitis V, Novick P. Sec9 is a SNAP-25-like component of a yeast SNARE complex that may be the effector of Sec4 function in exocytosis. Cell 1994; 79:245–258.

31. Brown HA, Gutowski S, Moomaw CR, Slaughter C, Sternweis PC. ADP-ribosylation factor, a small GTP-dependent regulatory protein, stimulates phospholipase D activity. Cell 1993; 75:1137–1144.
32. Bucci C, Parton RG, Mather IM, Stunnenberg H, Simons K, Hoflack B, Zerial M. The small GTPase rab5 functions as a negative regulatory factor in the early endocytic pathway. Cell 1992; 70:715–728.
33. Buday L, Downward J. Epidermal growth factor regulates p21ras through the formation of a complex of receptor, Grb2 adaptor protein, and SOS nucleotide exchange factor. Cell 1993; 73:611–620.
34. Burstein E, Macara IG. Characterization of a guanine nucleotide-releasing factor and a GTPase-activating protein that are specific for the ras-related protein p25rab3a. Proc Natl Acad Sci USA 1992; 89:1154–1158.
35. Burton J, Roberts D, Montaldi M, Novick P, De CP. A mammalian guanin-nucleotide-releasing protein enhances function of yeast secretory protein Sec4. Nature 1993; 361:464–467.
36. Caldwell JS, Moyers JS, Doria A, Reynet C, Kahn RC. Molecular cloning of the human rad gene: gene structure and complete nucleotide sequence. Biochim Biophys Acta 1996; 1316:145–148
37. Capron F, Ameille J, Leclerc P, Mornet P, Barbagellata M, Reynes M, and Rochemaure J. Pulmonary lymphangioleiomyomatosis and Bourneville's tuberous sclerosis with pulmonary involvement: the same disease? Cancer 1983; 52:851–855.
38. Cerione RA, Zheng Y. The Dbl family of oncogenes. Curr Opin Cell Biol 1996; 8:216–222.
39. Chardin P. RalA. In: Zerial M, Huber LA, eds. Guidebook to the Small GTPases. New York: Oxford University Press Inc., 1995:83–85.
40. Chardin P. RalB. In: Zerial M, Huber LA, eds. Guidebook to the Small GTPases. New York: Oxford University Press Inc., 1995:85–86.
41. Chardin P, Boquet P, Madaule P, Popoff MR, Rubin EJ, Gill DM. The mammalian G proton *rhoC* is ADP-ribosylated by *Clostridium botulinum* exoenzyme C3 and affects actin microfilaments in Vero cells. EMBO J 1989; 8:1087–1092.
42. Chardin P, Camonis JH, Gale NW, Van Aelst L, Schlessinger J, Wigler M, Bar-Sagi D. Human Sos1: a guanine nucleotide exchange factor for Ras that binds to Grb2. Science 1993; 260:1338–1343.
43. Chardin P, Paris S, Antonny B, Robineau S, Beraud-Dufor S, Jackson CL, Chabre M. A human exchange factor for ARF contains Sec-7 and pleckstrin-homology domains. Nature 1996; 384:481–484.
44. Chavrier, P, Gorvel JP, Simons K, Gruenberg J, Zerial M. The hypervariable C-terminal domain of rab proteins acts as a targeting signal. Nature 1991; 353:769–772.
45. Chong LD, Traynor-Kaplan A, Bokoch GM, Schwartz MA. The small GTP-binding protein Rho regulates a phosphatidylinositol 4-phosphate 5-kinase in mammalian cells. Cell 1994; 79:507–513.
46. Chou MM, Blenis J. The 70 kDa S6 kinase complexes with and is activated by the Rho family G proteins Cdc42 and Rac1. Cell 1996; 85:573–583.

47. Chuang TH, Xu X, Kaartinen V, Heisterkamp N, Groffen J, Bokoch GM. Abr and Bcr are multifunctional regulators of the Rho GTP-binding protein family. Proc Natl Acad Sci USA 1995; 92:10282–10286.
48. Cockcroft S, Thomas GMH, Gensome A, Geny B, Cunningham E, Gout I, Hiles I, Totty NF, Truong I, Hsuan JJ. A downstream effector of ARF in granulocytes. Science 1994; 263:523–526.
49. Colombo MI, Inglese J, D'Souza-Schorey C, Beron W, Stahl PD. Heterotrimeric G proteins interact with the small GTPase ARF: possibilities for the regulation of vesicular traffic. J Biol Chem 1995; 270:24564–24571.
50. Cook J, Rubinfeld B, Albert I, McCormick F. RapV12 antagonizes Ras-dependent activation of ERK1 and ERK2 by LPA and EGF in Rat1 fibroblasts. EMBO J 1993; 12:3475–3485.
51. Coso OA, Chiariello M, Yu JC, Teramoto H, Crespo P, Xu N, Miki T, Gutkind JS. The small GTP-binding proteins Rac1 and Cdc42 regulate the activity of the JNK/SAPK signaling pathway. Cell 1995; 81:1137–1146.
52. Cukierman E, Huber I, Rotman M, Cassel D. The ARF1 GTPase activating protein: zinc finger motif and Golgi localization. Science 1995; 270:1999–2002.
53. Dagher MC, Fuchs A, Bourmeyster N, Jouan A, Vignais PV. Small G proteins and the neutrophil NADPH oxidase. Biochimie 1995; 77:651–660.
54. DeBello WE, Betz H, Augustine GJ. Synaptotagmin and neurotransmitter release. Cell 1993; 74:947–950.
55. Didsbury J, Weber RF, Bokoch GM, Evans T, Snyderman R. Rac, a novel ras-related family of proteins that are botulinum toxin substrates. J Biol Chem 1989; 264:16378–16381.
56. Diekmann D, Abo A, Johnston C, Segal AW, Hall A. Interaction of Rac with p67phox and regulation of phagocytic NADPH oxodase activity. Science 1994; 265:531–533.
57. Diekmann D, Brill S, Garrett MD, Totty N, Hsuan J, Monfries C, Hall C, Lim L, Hall A. Bcr encodes a GTPase-activating protein for p21rac. Nature 1991; 351:400–402.
58. Ding M, Vitale N, Tsai S-C, Adamik R, Moss J, Vaughan M. Characterization of a GTPase-activating protein that stimulates GTP hydrolysis by both ADP-ribosylation factor (ARF) and ARF-like proteins. J Biol Chem 1996; 271:24005–24009.
59. Donaldson JG, Cassel D, Kahn RA, Klausner RD. ADP-ribolyation factor, a small GTP-binding protein, is required for binding of the coatomer protein beta-COP to Golgi membranes. Proc Natl Acad Sci USA 1992; 89:6408–6412.
60. Donaldson JG, Finazzi D, Klausner RD. Brefeldin A inhibits Golgi-membrane catalysed exchange of guanine nucleotide onto ARF protein. Nature 1992; 360:350–352.
61. Donaldson JG, Kahn RA, Lippincott-Schwartz J, Klausner RD. Binding of ARF and β-COP to Golgi membranes: possible regulation by a trimeric G protein. Science 1991; 254:1197–1199.
62. Dorseuil O, Vazquez A, Lang P, Bertoglio J, Gacon G, Leca G. Inhibition of superoxide production in B lymphocytes by rac antisense oligonucleotides. J Biol Chem 1992; 267:20540–20542.

63. Drubin DG. Development of cell polarity in budding yeast. Cell 1991; 65:1093–1096.
64. D'Souza-Schorey C, Li G, Colombo MI, Stahl PD. A regulatory role for ARF6 in receptor-mediated endocytosis. Science 1995; 267:1175–1178.
65. Dunn B, Stearns T, Botstein D. Specificity domains distinguish the Ras-related GTPases Ypt1 and Sec4. Nature 1993; 362:563–565.
66. Egan SE, Giddings BW, Brooks MW, Buday L, Sizeland AM, Weinberg RA. Association of sos ras exchange protein with Grb2 is implicated in tyrosine kinase signal transduction and transformation. Nature 1993; 363:45–51.
67. Enomoto K, Gill DM. Cholera toxin activation of adenylate cyclase. J Biol Chem 1980; 255:1252–1258.
68. Enomoto K, Gill DM. Requirement for guanosine triphosphate in the activation of adenylate cyclase by cholera toxin. J Supramol Struct 1979; 10:51–60.
69. Feig L. Guanine nucleotide-exchange factors: a family of positive regulators of Ras and related GTPases. Curr Opin Cell Biol 1994; 6:204–211.
70. Feig L, Urano T, Cantor S. Evidence for a Ras/Ral signaling cascade. Trends Biol Sci 1996; 21:438–441.
71. Fernandez-Sarabia MJ, Bischoff JR. Bcl-2 associates with the ras-related protein R-ras p23. Nature 1993; 366:274–275.
72. Ferro-Novick S, Reinhard J. Vesicle fusion from yeast to man. Nature 1994; 370:191–193.
73. Fischer R, Wei Y, Anagli J, Berchtold MW. Calmodulin binds to and inhibits GTP binding of the ras-like GTPase Kir/Gem. J Biol Chem 1996; 271:25067–25070.
74. Franco M, Chardin P, Chabre M, Paris S. Myristoylation of ADP-ribosylation factor 1 facilitates nucleotide exchange at physiological Mg+2 levels. J Biol Chem 1995; 270:1337–1341.
75. Franco M, Chardin P, Chabre M, Paris S. Myristoylation-facilitated binding of the G protein ARF1GDP to membrane phospholipids is required for its activation by a soluble nucleotide exchange factor. J Biol Chem 1996; 271:1573–1578.
76. Franco M, Paris S, Chabre M. The small G-protein ARF1GDP binds to the Gt subunit of transducin, but not to Gt GDP-Gt. FEBS Lett 1995; 362:286–290.
77. Gale NW, Kaplan S, Lowenstein EJ, Schlessinger J, Bar-Sagi D. Grb2 mediates the EGF-dependent activation of guanine nucleotide exchange on Ras. Nature 1993; 363:88–92.
78. Gibbs JB, Schaber MD, Allard WJ, Sigal IS, Scolnick EM. Purification of ras GTPase activating protein from bovine brain. Proc Natl Acad Sci USA 1988; 85:5026–5030.
79. Gill DM, Meren R. ADP-ribosylation of membrane proteins catalyzed by cholera toxin: Basis of the activation of adenylate cyclase. Proc Natl Acad Sci USA 1978; 75:3050–3054.
80. Graham SM, Cox AD, Drivas G, Rush MR, D'Eustachio P, Der CJ. Aberrant function of the Ras-related TC21/R-Ras2 protein triggers malignant transformation. Mol Cell Biol 1994; 14:4108–4115.
81. Greasley SE, Jhoti H, Teahan C, Solari R, Fensome A, Thomas GMH, Cockcroft S, Bax B. The structure of rat ADP-ribosylation factor-1 (ARF-1) complexed to GDP determined from two different crystal forms. Nat Struct Biol 1995; 2:797–806.

82. Gutkind JS, Vitale-Cross L. The pathway linking small GTP-binding proteins of the Rho family to cytoskeletal components and novel signaling kinase cascades. Cell Dev Biol 1996; 7:683–690.
83. Habets GG, Scholtes EH, Zuydgeest D, van der Kammen RA, Stam JC, Berns A, Collard JG. Identification of an invasion-inducing gene, Tiam-1, that encodes a protein with homology to GDP-GTP exchangers for Rho-like proteins. Cell 1994; 77:537–549.
84. Hall A. Ras and GAP—Who's controlling whom? Cell 1990; 61:921–923.
85. Hall A. Small GTP-binding proteins and the regulation of the actin cytoskeleton. Annu Rev Cell Biol 1994; 10:31–54.
86. Hall A, Zerial M. General introduction. In: Zerial M, Huber LA, eds. Guidebook to the Small GTPases. New York: Oxford University Press Inc., 1995:3–11.
87. Han L, Colicelli J. A human protein selected for interference with Ras function interacts directly with Ras and competes with Raf1. Mol Cell Biol 1995; 15:1318–1323.
88. Hancock JF, Cadwallader K, Marshall CJ. Methylation and proteolysis are essential for efficient membrane binding of prenylated p21K-ras(B). EMBO J 1991; 10:641–646.
89. Hancock JF, Hall A. A novel role for RhoGDI as an inhibitor of GAP proteins. Embo J 1993; 12:1915–1921.
90. Hancock JF, Magee AI, Childs JE, Marshall CJ. All ras proteins are polyisoprenylated but only some are palmitoylated. Cell 1989; 57:1167–1177.
91. Hancock JF, Paterson H, Marshall CJ. A polybasic domain or palmitoylation is required in addition to the CAAX motif to localize p21ras to the plasma membrane. Cell 1990; 63:133–139.
92. Hart MJ, Eva A, Zangrilli D, Aaronson SA, Evans T, Cerione RA, Zheng Y. Cellular transformation and guanine nucleotide exchange activity are catalyzed by a common domain on the dbl oncogene product. J Biol Chem 1994; 269:62–65.
93. Haun R, Tsai S-C, Adamik R, Moss J, Vaughan M. Effect of myristoylation on GTP-dependent binding of ADP-ribosylation factor to Golgi. J Biol Chem 1993; 268:7064–7068.
94. Heyworth PG, Knaus UG, Settleman J, Curnutte JT, Bokoch GM. Regulation of NADPH oxidase activity by Rac GTPase activating protein(s). Mol Biol Cell 1993; 4:1217–1223.
95. Hill CS, Wynne J, Treisman R. The Rho family GTPases RhoA, Rac1, and CDC42Hs regulate transcriptional activation by SRF. Cell 1995; 81:1159–1170.
96. Hiraoka K, Kaibuchi K, Ando S, Musha T, Takaishi K, Mizuno T, Asada M, Menard L, Tomhave E, Disbury J, et al. Both stimulatory and inhibitory GDP/GTP exchange proteins, smg GDS and rho GDI, are active on multiple small GTP-binding proteins. Biochem Biophys Res Commun 1992; 182:921–930.
97. Hirshberg M, Stockley RW, Dodson G, Webb MR. The crystal structure of human Rac1, a member of the Rho-family complexed with GTP analogue. Nature Struct Biol 1997; 4:147–152.
98. Hofer F, Fields S, Schneider C, Martin GS. Activated Ras interacts with the Ral guanine nucleotide dissociation stimulator. Proc Natl Acad Sci USA 1994; 91:11089–11093.

99. Horri Y, Beeler JF, Sakaguchi K, Tachibana M, Miki T. A novel oncogene, ost, encodes a guanine nucleotide exchange factor that potentially links Rho and Rac signaling pathways. EMBO J 1994; 13:4776–4786.
100. Hotchin NA, Hall A. The assembly of integrin adhesion complexes requires both extracellular matrix and intracellular RHO/RAC GTPases. J Cell Biol 1995; 131:1857–1865.
101. Huber LA, Pimplikar S, Parton RG, Virta H, Zerial M, Simons K. Rab8, a small GTPase involved in vesicular traffic between the TGN and the basolateral membrane. J Cell Biol 1993; 123:35–45.
102. Ireland LS, Johnston GC, Drebot MA, Dhillon N, DeMaggio N, Hoekstra MF, Singer RA. A member of a novel family of yeast "Zn-finger" proteins mediates the transition from stationary phase to cell proliferation. EMBO J 1994; 13:3812–3821.
103. Ishizaki T, Maekawa M, Fujisawa K, Okawa K, Iwamatsu A, Fujita A, et al. The small GTP-binding protein Rho binds to and activates a 160 kDa Ser/Thr protein kinase homologous to myotonic dystrophy kinase. EMBO J 1996; 8:1885–1893.
104. Jahner D, Hunter T. The ras-related gene rhoB is an immediate-early gene inducible by v-src, epidermal growth factor, and platelet-derived growth factor in rat fibroblasts. Mol Cell Biol 1991; 11:3682–3690.
105. Jimenez B, Pizon V, Lerosey I, Beranger F, Tavitian A, deGunzburg J. Effects of the ras-related rap2 protein on cellular proliferation. Int J Cancer 1991; 49:471–479.
106. Johnson GL, Kaslow HR, Bourne HR. Genetic evidence that cholera toxin substrates are regulatory components of adenylate cyclase. J Biol Chem 1978; 253:7120–7123.
107. Jones S, Vignais M-L, Broach JR. The CDC25 protein of Saccharomyces cerevisiae promotes exchange of guanine nucleotides bound to ras. Mol Cell Biol 1991; 11:2641–2646.
108. Kahn RA. Fluoride is not an activator of the smaller (20-25 kDa) GTP-binding proteins. J Biol Chem 1991; 266:15595–15597.
109. Kahn RA, Clark J, Rulka C, Stearns T, Zhang C-J, Randazzo PA, Terui T, Cavenagh M. Mutational analysis of *Saccharomyces cerevisiae* ARF1. J Biol Chem 1995; 270:143–150.
110. Kaslow HR, Johnson GL, Brothers VM, Bourne HR. A regulatory component of adenylate cyclase from human erythrocyte membranes. J Biol Chem 1980; 255:3736–3741.
111. Khosravi-Far R, Chrzanowska-Wodnicka M, Solski PA, Eva A, Burridge K, Der CJ. Dbl and Vav mediate transformation via mitogen-activated protein kinase pathways that are distinct from those activated by oncogenic Ras. Mol Cell Biol 1994; 14:6848–6857.
112. Khosravi-Far R, Der CJ. The Ras signal transduction pathway. Center Metastasis Rev 1994; 13:67–89.
113. Khosravi-Far R, Solski PA, Clark GJ, Kinch MS, Der CJ. Activation of Rac1, RhoA, and mitogen-activated protein kinases is required for Ras transformation. Mol Cell Biol 1995; 15:6443–6453.
114. Kikuchi A, Demo SD, Ye ZH, Chen YW, Williams LT. RalGDS family members interact with the effector loop of ras p21. Mol Cell Biol 1994; 14:7483–7491.

115. Kikuchi A, Takai Y. Rab3a. In: Zerial M, Huber LA, eds. Guidebook to the Small GTPases. New York: Oxford University Press Inc., 1995:312–316.
116. Kimura K, Ito M, Amano M, et al. Regulation of myosin phosphatase by rho and rho-associated kinase (Rho-kinase). Science 1996; 273:245–248.
117. Kishida S, Shiritaki H, Sasaki T, Dato M, Kaibuchi K, Takai Y. Rab3a GTPase-activating protein-inhibiting activity of Rabphilin-3a, a putative Rab3a target protein. J Biol Chem 1993; 268:
118. Kitayama H, Sugimoto Y, Matsuzaki T, Ikawa Y, Noda M. A ras-related gene with transformation suppressor activity. Cell 189; 56:77–84.
119. Knaus UG, Heyworth PG, Evans T, Curnutte JT, Bokoch GM. Regulation of phagocyte oxygen radical production by the GTP-binding protein Rac 2. Science 1991; 254:1512–1515.
120. Knaus UG, Heyworth PG, Kinsella BT, Curnutte JT, Bokoch GM. Purification and characterization of Rac 2. A cytosolic GTP-binding protein that regulates human neutrophil NADPH oxidase. J Biol Chem 1992; 267:23575–23582.
121. Kolanus W, Nagel W, Schiller B, Zeitlmann L, Godar S, Stockinger H, Seed B. L 2 integrin/LFA-1 binding to ICAM-1 induced by cytohesin-1, a cytoplasmic regulatory molecule. Cell 1996; 86:233–242.
122. Korf BR. Neurocutaneous syndromes: neurofibromatosis 1, neurofibromatosis 2, and tuberous sclerosis. Curr Opin Neurol 1997; 10:131–136.
123. Kozman R, Ahmed S, Best A, Lim L. The Ras-related protein Cdc42Hs and bradykinin promote formation of peripheral actin microspikes and filopodia in Swiss 3T3 fibroblasts. Mol Cell Biol 1995; 15:1942–1952.
124. Ktistakis NT, Brown HA, Waters MG, Sternweis PC, Roth MG. Evidence that phospholipase D mediates ADP ribosylation factor-dependent formation of Golgi coated vesicles. J Biol Chem 1996; 134:295–306.
125. Kunz BC, Muczynski KA, Welsh CF, Stanley SJ, Tsai S-C, Adamik R, Chang PP, Moss J, Vaughan M. Characterization of recombinant and endogenous ADP-ribosylation factors synthesized in Sf9 insect cells. Biochemistry 1993; 32:6643–6648.
126. Kwak J-Y, Lopez I, Uhlinger DJ, Ryu SH, Lambeth DJ. RhoA and a cytosolic 50-kDa factor reconstitute GTP S-dependent phospholipase D activity in human neutrophil subcellular fractions. J Biol Chem 1995; 270:2431–2434.
127. Kwong CH, Malech HL, Rotrosen D, Leto TL. Regulation of the human neutrophil NADPH oxidase by rho-related G-proteins. Biochemistry 1993; 32:5711–5717.
128. Kyriakis JM, Avurch J. Protein kinase cascades activated by stress and inflammatory cytokines. BioEssays 1996; 18:567–577.
129. Lamarche N, Hall A. GAPs for rho-related GTPases. Trends Genet 1994; 10:436–440.
130. Lamarche N, Tapon N, Stowers L, Burbelo PD, Aspenstrom P, Bridges T, Chant J, Hall A. Rac and Cdc42 induce actin polymerization and G1 cell cycle progression independently of p65 PAK and the JNK/SAPK MAP kinase cascade. Cell 1996; 87:519–529.
131. Lambeth JD, Kwak JY, Bowman EP, Perry D, Uhlinger DJ, Lopez I. ADP-ribosylation factor functions synergistically with a 50-kDa cytosolic factor in cell-

free activation of human neutrophil phospholipase D. J Biol Chem 1995; 270:2431–2434.

132. Lenhard JL, Kahn RA, Stahl PD. Evidence for ADP-ribosylation factor (ARF) as a regulator of in vitro endosome-endosome fusion. J Biol Chem 1992; 267:13047–13052.

133. Leung T, Chen X-Q, Manser E, Lim L. The p160 RhoA-binding kinase ROKA is a member of a kinase family and is involved in the reorganization of the cytoskeleton. Mol Cell Biol 1996;

134. Leung T, Manser E, Tan L, Lim L. A novel serine/threonine kinase binding the Ras-related RhoA GTPase which translocates the kinase to peripheral membranes. J Biol Chem 1995; 270:29051–29054.

135. Li N, Batzer A, Daly R, Yajnik V, Skolnik E, Chardin P, Bar-Sagi D, Margolis B, Schlessinger J. Guanine-nucleotide-releasing factor hSos1 binds to Grb2 and links receptor tyrosine kinases to Ras signaling. Nature 1993; 363:85–88.

136. Lian JP, Stone S, Jiang Y, Lyons P, Ferro-Novick S. Ypt1 implicated in v-SNARE activation. Nature 1994; 372:698–701.

137. Lin MC, Welton AF, Berman MF. Essential role of GTP in the expression of adenylate cyclase activity after cholera toxin treatment. J Cycl Nuc Res 1978; 4:159–168.

138. Lowe DG, Goeddel DV. Heterologous expression and characterization of the human R-ras gene product. Mol Cell Biol 1987; 7:

139. Lowy DR, Willumsen BM. Function and regulation of ras. Ann Rev Biochem 1993; 62:851–891.

140. Macara IG, Lounsbury KM, Richards SA, McKiernan C, Bar-sagi D. The Ras superfamily of GTPases. FASEB J 1996; 10:625–630.

141. Makler V, Cukierman E, Rotman M, Admon A, Cassel D. ADP-ribosylation factor-directed GTPase-activating protein: purification and partial characterization. J Biol Chem 1995; 270:5232–5237.

142. Malcolm KC, Ross AH, Qiu RG, Symons M, Exton JH. Activation of rat liver phospholipase D by the small GTP-binding protein RhoA. J Biol Chem 1994; 269:25951–25954.

143. Manser E, Chong C, Zhao ZS, Leung T, Michael G, Hall C, Lim L. Molecular cloning of a new member of the p21-Cdc42/Rac-activated kinase (PAK) family. J Biol Chem 1995; 270:25070–25078.

144. Manser, E, Leung T, Salihuddin H, Zhao S, Lim L. A brain serine/threonine protein kinase activated by Cdc42 and Rac1. Nature 1994; 367:40–46.

145. Manser, E, Leung T, Salihuddin H, Zhao S, Lim L. A brain serine/threonine protein kinase activated by Cdc42 and Rac1. Nature 1994; 367:40–46.

146. Martin GA, Viskochil D, Bollag G, McCabe PC, Crosier WJ, Haubruck H, Conroy L, Clark R, P OC, Cawthon M, et al. The GAP-related domain of the neurofibromatosis type 1 gene product interacts with ras p21. Cell 1990; 63:843–849.

147. Martinez, O, Schmidt A, Salamero J, Hoflack B, Roa M, Goud B. The small GTP-binding protein rab6 functions in intra-Golgi transport. J Cell Biol 1994; 127:1575–1588.

148. Massenburg D, J-S Han, Liyanage M, Patton WA, Rhee SG, Moss J, Vaughan M. Activation of rat brain phospholipase D by ADP-ribosylation factors 1, 5, and 6:

separation of ADP-ribosylation factor-dependent and oleate-dependent enzymes. Proc Natl Acad Sci USA 1994; 91:11718–11722.

149. Matsui T, Amano M, Yamamoto T, Chihara K, Nakafuku M, Ito M, Nakano T, Okawa K, Iwamatsu A, Kaibuchi K. Rho-associated kinase, a novel serine/threonine kinase, as a putative target for the small GTP-binding protein Rho. EMBO J 1996; 15:2208–2216.
150. Maziak DE, Kesten S, Rappaport DC, Maurer J. Extrathoracic angiomyolipoma in lymphangioleiomyomatosis. Eur Respir J 1996; 9:402–405.
151. McCormick F. How receptors turn Ras on. Nature 1993; 363:15–16.
152. McCormick F, Wittinghofer A. Interactions between Ras proteins and their effectors. Curr Opin Biotech 1996; 7:449–456.
153. McGlade J, Cheng A, Pelicci G, Pelicci PG, Pawson T. Shc proteins are phosphorylated and regulated by the v-SRC and v-Fps protein-tyrosine kinases. Proc Natl Acad Sci USA 1992; 89:8869–8873.
154. Meacci E, Tsai S-C, Adamik R, Moss J, Vaughan M. Cytohesin-1, a cytosolic guanine nucleotide-exchange protein for ADP-ribosylation factor (ARF). Proc Natl Acad Sci USA. 1997;
155. Melchior F, Gerace L. Mechanisms of nuclear protein import. Curr Opin Biol 1995; 7:310–318.
156. Michiels F, Habets GG, Stam JC, van der Kammen RA, Collard JG. A role for Rac in Tiam1-induced membrane ruffling and invasion. Nature 1995; 375:338–340.
157. Minden A, Lin A, Claret FX, Abo A, Karin M. Selective activation of the JNK signaling cascade and c-Jun transcriptional activity by the small GTPases Rac and Cdc42Hs. Cell 1995; 81:1147–1157.
158. Mizoguchi A, Kim S, Ueda T, Takai Y. Tissue distribution of smgp25a, a ras p21-like GTP-binding protein, studied by use of a specific monoclonal antibody. Biochem Biophys Res Commun 1989; 162:1438–1445.
159. Mizuno T, Kaibuchi K, Ando S, Musha T, Hiraoka K, Takaishi K, Asada M, Nunoi H. Matsuda I, Takai Y. Regulation of the superoxide-generating NADPH oxidase by a small GTP-binding protein and its stimulatory and inhibitory GDP/GTP exchange proteins. J Biol Chem 1992; 267:10215–10218.
160. Moore MS, Blobel G. The GTP-binding protein Ran/TC4 is required for protein import into the nucleus. Nature 1993; 365:661–663.
161. Morinaga N, Tsai S-C, Moss J, Vaughan M. Isolation of a brefeldin A-inhibited guanine nucleotide-exchange protein for ADP-ribosylation factor (ARF) 1 and ARF3 that contains a Sec7-like domain. Proc Natl Acad Sci USA 1996; 93:12856–12860.
162. Moss J, Vaughan M. Choleragen activation of solubilized adenylate cyclase: Requirement for GTP and protein activator for demonstration of enzymatic activity. Proc Natl Acad Sci USA 1977; 74:4396–4400.
163. Moss J, Vaughan M. Mechanism of action of choleragen: evidence for ADP-ribosyltransferase activity with arginine as an acceptor. J Biol Chem 1977; 252:2455–2457.
164. Moyers JS, Bilan PJ, Zhu J, Kahn CR. Rad and Rad-related GTPases interact with calmodulin and calmodulin-dependent protein kinase II. J Biol Chem 1997; 272:11832–11839.

165. Murayama T, Tsai S-C, Adamik R, Moss J, Vaughan M. Effects of temperature on ADP-ribosylation factor stimulation of cholera toxin activity. Biochemistry 1993; 32:561–566.
166. Nakaya S, Moss J, Vaughan M. Effects of nucleoside triphosphates on choleragen-activated brain adenylate cyclase. Biochemistry 1980; 19:4871–4874.
167. Nobes C, Hall A. Regulation and function of the Rho subfamily of small GTPases. Curr Opin Genet Dev 1994; 4:77–81.
168. Nobes CD, Hall A. Rho, rac, and cdc42 GTPases regulate the assembly of multimolecular focal complexes associated with actin stress fibers, lamellipodia, and filopodia. Cell 1995; 81:53–62.
169. Nobes CD, Hawkins P, Stephens L, Hall A. Activation of the small GTP-binding proteins rho and rac by growth factor receptors. J Cell Sci 1995; 108:225–233.
170. Northup JK, Sternweis PC, Smigel MD, Schleifer LS, Ross EM and Gilman AG. Purification of the regulatory component of adenylate cyclase. Proc Natl Acad Sci USA 1980; 77:6516–6520.
171. Novick P, Brennwald P. Friends and family: the role of the rab GTPases in vesicular traffic. Cell 1993; 75:597–601.
172. Nuoffer C, Davidson HW, Matteson J, Meinkoth J, Balch WE. A GDP-bound form of Rab1 inhibits protein export from the endoplasmic reticulum and transport between Golgi compartments. J Cell Biol 1994; 125:225–237.
173. Ohga N, Kikuchi A, Ueda T, Yamamoto J, Takai Y. Rabbit intestine contains a protein that inhibits the dissociation of GDP from and the subsequent binding of GTP to rhoB p20, a ras p21-like GTP-binding protein. Biochem Biophys Res Commun 1989; 163:1523–1533.
174. Ohguchi K, Banno Y, Nakashima S, Nozawa Y. Activation of membrane-bound phospholipase D by protein kinase C in HL60 cells: synergistic action of a small GTP-binding protein RhoA. Biochem Biophys Res Commun 1995; 211:306–311.
175. Olsen MF, Ashworh A, Hall A. An essential role for Rho, Rac, and Cdc42 GTPases in cell cycle progression through G_1. Nature 1995; 269:1270–1272.
176. Palmer DJ, Helms JB, Beckers CJM, Orci L, Rothman JE. Binding of coatomer to Golgi membranes requires ADP-ribosylation factor. J Biol Chem 1993; 268:12083–12089.
177. Paulik MA, Hamacher LL, Yarnall DP, Simmons CJ, Maianu L, Pratley RE, Garvey WT, Burns DK, Lenhard JM. Identification of Rad's effector-binding domain, intracellular localization, and analysis of expression in Pima Indians. J Cell Biochem 1997; 65:527–541.
178. Pelicci G, Lanfrancone L, Grignani F, McGlade J, Cavallo F, Forni G, Nicoletti I, Pawson T, Pelicci PG. A novel transforming protein (SHC) with an SH2 domain is implicated in mitogenic signal transduction. Cell 1992; 70:93–104.
179. Perona R, Esteve P, Jimenez B, Ballestero RP, Ramon y Cajal S, Lacal JC. Tumorigenic activity of *rho* genes from *Aplysia californica*. Oncogene 1993; 8:1285–1292.
180. Peters PJ, Hsu VW, Ooi CE, Finazzi D, Teal SB, Oorschot V, Donaldson JG, Klausner RD. Overexpression of wild-type and mutant ARF1 and ARF6: distinct perturbations of nonoverlapping membrane compartments. J Biol Chem 1995; 128:1003–1017.

181. Peyroche A, Paris S, Jackson CL. Nucleotide exchange on ARF mediated by yeast Gel protein. Nature 1996; 384:479–481.
182. Pfeffer SR. Rab GTPases: master regulators of membrane trafficking. Curr Opin Cell Biol 1994; 6:522–526.
183. Pind SN, Nuoffer C, McCaffery JM, Plutner H, Davidson HW, Farquhar MG, Balch WE. Rabl and Ca2+ are required for fusion of carrier vesicles mediating endoplasmic reticulum to Golgi transport. J Cell Biol 1994; 125:239–252.
184. Pinkett MO, Anderson WB. Plasma membrane-associated component(s) that confer(s) cholera toxin sensitivity to adenylate cyclase. Biochim Biophys Acta 1982; 714:337–343.
185. Pizon V. Rap1a and Rap1b. In. Zerial M, Huber LA, eds. Guidebook to the Small GTPases. New York: Oxford University Press Inc., 1995:87–89.
186. Plutner H, Cox, AD, Pind S, Khosravi-Far R, Bourne JR, Schwaninger R, Der CJ, Balch WE. Rab1b regulates vesicular transport between the endoplasmic reticulum and successive Golgi compartments. J Cell Biol 1994; 115:
187. Poon PP, Wang X, Rotman M, Huber I, Cukierman E, Cassel D, Singer RA, Johnston GC. *Saccharomyces cerevisiae* Gcs1 is an ADP-ribosylation factor GTPase-activating protein. Proc Natl Acad Sci USA 1996; 93:10074–10077.
188. Price SR, Nightingale M, Tsai S-C, Williamson KC, Adamik R, Chen H-C, Moss J, Vaughan M. Guanine nucleotide-binding proteins that enhance choleragen ADP-ribosyltransferase activity: nucleotide and deduced amino acid sequence of an ADP-ribosylation factor cDNA. Proc Natl Acad Sci USA 1988; 85:5488–5491.
189. Prigmore E, Ahmed S, Best A, Kozma R, Manser E, Segal AW, Lim L. A 68-kDa kinase and NADPH oxidase component p67phox are targets for Cdc42Hs and Rac1 in neutrophils. J Biol Chem 1995; 270:10717–10722.
190. Qiu R, Chen J, McCormick F, Symons M. A role for rho in ras transformation. Proc Natl Acad Sci 1995; 92:11781–11785.
191. Qiu RG, Chen J, Kirn D, McCormick F, Symons M. An essential role for Rac in Ras transformation. Nature 1995; 374:457–459.
192. Quinn M, Mullen M, Jesaitis A, Linner J. Subcellular distribution of the Rap1A protein in human neutrophils: colocalization and cotranslocation with cytochrome b559. Blood 1992; 79:1563–1573.
193. Radhakrishna H, Klausner RD, Donaldson JG. Aluminum fluoride stimulates surface protrusions in cells overexpressing the ARF6 GTPase. J Cell Biol 1996; 134:935–947.
194. Randazzo PA, Kahn RA. GTP hydrolysis by ADP-ribosylation factor is dependent on both an ADP-ribosylation factor GTPase-activating protein and acid phospholipids. J Biol Chem 1994; 269:10758–10763.
195. Randazzo PA, Yang YC, Rulka C, Kahn RA. Activation of ADP-ribosylation factor by Golgi membranes. J Biol Chem 1993; 268:9555–9563.
196. Regazzi R, Kikuchi A, Takai Y, Wollheim CB. The small GTP-binding proteins in the cytosol of insulin-secreting cells are complexed to GDP dissociation inhibitor proteins. J Biol Chem 1992; 267:17512–17519.
197. Regazzi R, Ullrich S, Kahn RA, Wollheim CB. Redistribution of ADP-ribosylation factor during stimulation of permeabilized cells with GTP analogues. Biochem J 1991; 275:639–644.

198. Reid T, Furuyashiki T, Ishizaki T, et al. Rhotekin, a new putative target for Rho bearing homology to a serine/threonine kinase, PKN, and Rhophilin in the Rho-binding domain. J Biol Chem 1996; 271:13556–13560.
199. Rienhard J, Scheel AA, Diekmann D, Hall A, Ruppert C, Bahler M. A novel type of myosin implicated in signalling by rho family GTPases. EMBO J 1995; 14:697–704.
200. Reynet C, Kahn CR. Rad: a member of the Ras family overexpressed in muscle of type II diabetic humans. Science 1993; 262:1441–1444.
201. Ridley A. Rho: theme and variations. Curr Biol 1996; 6:1256–1264.
202. Ridley AJ. Rho-related proteins: actin cytoskeleton and cell cycle. Curr Opin Genet Dev 1995; 5:24–30.
203. Ridley AJ, Hall A. Distinct patterns of actin organization regulated by the small GTP-binding proteins Rac and Rho. Cold Spring Harb Symp Quant Biol 1992; 57:661–671.
204. Ridley AJ, Hall A. The small GTP-binding protein rho regulates the assembly of focal adhesions and actin stress fibers in response to growth factors. Cell 1992;70:389–399.
205. Ridley AJ, Paterson HF, Johnston CL, Diekmann D, Hall A. The small GTP-binding protein rac regulates growth factor-induced membrane ruffling. Cell 1992; 70:401–410.
206. Rodriguez-Viciana P, Warne PH, Dhand R, Vanhaesebroeck B, Gout I, Fry MJ, Waterfield MD, Downward J. Phosphatidylinositol-3-OH kinase as a direct target of Ras. Nature 1994; 370:527–532.
207. Rosa JL, Casaroli-Marano RP, Buckler AJ, Vilaró S, Barbacid M. p619, a giant protein related to the chromosome condensation regulator RCC1, stimulates guanine nucleotide exchange on ARF1 and Rab proteins. EMBO J 1996; 15:4262–4273.
208. Rothman JE. Mechanisms of intracellular protein transport. Nature 1994; 372:55–63.
209. Rozakis-Adcock M, McGlade J, Mbanalu G, Pelicci G, Daly R, Li W, Batzer A, Thomas S, Brugge J, Pelicci PG, Schlessinger J, Pawson T. Association of the Sch and Grb-2/Sem-5 SH2-containing proteins is implicated in activation of the Ras pathway by tyrosine kinases. Nature 1992; 360:689–692.
210. Schafer WR, Rine J. Protein prenylation: genes, enzymes, targets, and functions. Ann Rev Genet 1992; 30:209–237.
211. Scheffzek K, Ahmadian MR, Mittal R, Kabsch W, Wittinghofer A. The mechanism of GAP-mediated GTP Hydrolysis. FASEB Summer Research Conference, Snowmass, CO, 1997.
212. Scherle P, Behrens T, Staudt LM. Ly-GDI, a GDP-dissociation inhibitor of the RhoA GTP-binding protein, is expressed preferentially in lymphocytes. Proc Natl Acad Sci USA 1993; 90:7568–7572.
213. Schleifer LS, Kahn RA, Hanski E, Northup JK, Sternweis PC, Gilman AG. Requirements for cholera toxin-dependent ADP-ribosylation of the purified regulatory component of adenylate cyclase. J Biol Chem 1982; 257:20–23.
214. Schweins T, Wittinghofer A. Structures, interactions and relationships. Curr Biol 1994; 4:547–550.

215. Seabra MC, Brown MS, Goldstein JL. CAAX farnesyltransferase. In: Zerial M, Huber LA, eds. Guidebook to the Small GTPases. New York: Oxford University Press Inc., 1995:41–43.
216. Seabra MC, Goldstein JL. Brown MS. CAAX geranylgeranyltransferase. In: Zerial M, Huber LA, eds. Guidebook to the Small GTPases. New York: Oxford University Press Inc., 1995:43–45.
217. Seabra MC, Reiss Y, Casey PJ, Brown MS, Goldstein JL. Protein farnesyltransferase and geranylgeranyltransferase share a common a-subunit. Cell 1991; 65:429–434.
218. Serafini T, Orci L, Amherdt M, Brunner M, Kahn RA, Rothman JE. ADP-ribosylation factor is a subunit of the coat of Golgi-derived COP-coated vesicles: a novel role for a GTP-binding protein. Cell 1991; 67:239–253.
219. Settleman J, Albright CF, Foster LC, Weinberg RA. Association between GTPase activators for Rho and Ras families. Nature 1992; 359:153–154.
220. Settleman J, Narahimhan V, Foster LC, Weinberg RA. Molecular cloning of cDNAs encoding the GAP-associated protein p190: implications for a signaling pathway from ras to the nucleus. Cell 1992; 69:539–549.
221. Sewell JL, Kahn RA. Sequences of the bovine and yeast ADP-ribosylation factor and comparison to other GTP-binding proteins. Proc Natl Acad Sci USA 1988; 85:4620–4624.
222. Shimooku K, Akisue T, Jinnai H, Hitomi T, Ogino C, Yoshida K, Nakamura S-I, Nishizuka Y. Reconstitution of GTP S-dependent phospholipase D activity with ARF, RhoA, and a soluble 36-kDa protein. FEBS Lett 1996; 387:141–144.
223. Shiritaki H, Kaibuchi K, Sakoda T, Kishida S, Yamaguchi T, Wada K, Miyazaki M, Takai Y. Rabphilin-3a, a putative target protein for smg p25a/Rab3a p25 small GTP-binding protein related to synaptotagmin. Mol Cell Biol 1993; 13:2061–2068.
224. Shiritaki H, Kaibuchi K, Yamaguchi T, Wada K, Horiuchi H, Takai Y. A possible target for the smg-25a/rab3a small GTP-binding protein. J Biol Chem 1992; 267:10946–10949.
225. Siddiqi AR, Smith JL, Ross AH, Qiu RG, Symons M, Exton JH. Regulation of phospholipase D in HL60 cells. Evidence for a cytosolic phospholipase D. J Biol Chem 1995; 270:8466–8473.
226. Singer WD, Brown HA, Bokoch GM, Sternweis PC. Resolved phospholipase D activity is modulated by cytosolic factors other than Arf. J Biol Chem 1995; 270:14944–14950.
227. Singer WD, Brown HA, Jiang X, Sternweis PC. Regulation of phospholipase D by protein kinase C is synergistic with ADP-ribosylation factor and independent of protein kinase activity. J Biol Chem 1996; 271:4504-2-4510.
228. Sogaard M, Tani K, Ruby Ye R, Geromanos S, Tempst P, Kirchhausen T, Rothman JE, Sollner T. A Rab protein is required for the assembly of SNARE complexes in the docking of transport vesicles. Cell 1994; 78:937–948.
229. Soldati T, Shapiro AD, Dirac Svejstrup AB, Pfeffer SR. Membrane targeting of the small GTPase Rab9 is accompanied by nucleotide exchange. Nature 1994; 369:76–78.
230. Sollner T, Whiteheart SW, Brunner M, Erdjument-Bromage H, Geromanos S,

Tempst, Rothman JE. SNAP receptors implicated in vesicle targeting and fusion. Nature 1993; 362:318–324.

231. Spaargaren M, Bischoff JR. Identification of the guanine nucleotide dissociation stimulator ral1 as a putative effector molecule of R-Ras, H-Ras, K-Ras and Rap. Proc Natl Acad Sci USA 1994; 91:12609–12613.

232. Spiro DJ, Taylor TC, Melançon P, Wessling-Resnick M. Cytosolic ADP-ribosylation factors are not required for endosome-endosome fusion but are necessary for GTPγS inhibition of fusion. J Biol Chem 1995; 270:13696–13697.

233. Stearns T, Kahn RA, Botstein D, Hoyt MA. ADP-ribosylation factor is an essential protein in *Saccharomyces cerevisiae* and is encoded by two genes. Mol Cell Biol 1990; 10:6690–6699.

234. Stearns T, Willingham MC, Botstein D, Kahn RA. ADP-ribosylation factor is functionally and physically associated with the Golgi complex. Proc Natl Acad Sci USA 1990; 87:1238–1242.

235. Stenmark H, Parton RG, Steele-Mortimer O, Lutcke A, Gruenberg J, Zerial M. Inhibition of Rab5 GTPase activity stimulates membrane fusion in endocytosis. EMBO J 1994; 13:1287–1296.

236. Stenmark H, Vitale G, Ullrich O, Zerial M. Rabaptin-5 is a direct effector of the small GTPase Rab5 in endocytic membrane fusion. Cell 1995; 83:423–432.

237. Stowers L, Yelon D, Berg LJ, Chant J. Regulation of the polarization of T cells toward antigen-presenting cells by Ras-related GTPase CDC42. Proc Natl Acad Sci USA 1995; 92:5027–5031.

238. Symons M. Rho family GTPases: the cytoskeleton and beyond. Trends Biochem Sci 1996; 21:178–181.

239. Takai Y, Sasaki T, Tanaka K, Nakanishi H. Rho as a regulator of the cytoskeleton. Trends Biochem Sci 1995; 20:227–231.

240. Tanigawa G, Orci L, Amherdt M, Ravazzola M, Helms J, Rothman J. Hydrolysis of bound GTP by ARF protein triggers uncoating of Golgi-derived COP-coated vesicles. J Cell Biol 1993; 123:1365–1371.

241. Taylor JR, Ryu J, T.V. C, Raffin TV. Lymphangioleiomyomatosis: clinical course in 32 patients. N Engl J Med 1990; 323:1254–1260.

242. Teal S, Hsu V, Peters P, Klausner R, Donaldson J. An activating mutation in ARF1 stabilizes coatomer binding to Golgi membranes. J Biol Chem 1994; 269:3135–3138.

243. Terui T, Kahn R, Randazzo P. Effects of acid phospholipids on nucleotide exchange properties of ADP-ribosylation factor 1. J Biol Chem 1994; 269:28130–28135.

244. Tisdale EJ, Bourne HR, Khosravi-Far R, Der CJ, Balch WE. GTP-binding mutants of Rab1 and Rab2 are potent inhibitors of vesicular transport from the endoplasmic reticulum to the Golgi complex. J Cell Biol 1992; 119:749–761.

245. Torres VE, Bjornsson J, King BF, Kumar R, Zincke H, Edell ES, Wilson TO, Hattery RR, Gomez MR. Extrapulmonary lymphangioleiomyomatosis and lymphangiomatous cysts in tuberous sclerosis complex. Mayo Clin Proc 1995; 70:641–648.

246. Torti M, Ramaschi G, Sinigaglia F, Lapetina EG, Balduini C. Association of the

low molecular weight GTP-binding protein rap2b with the cytoskeleton during platelet aggregation. Proc Natl Acad Sci USA 1993; 90:7553-7557.

247. Treisman R. Regulation of transcription by MAP kinase cascades. Curr Opin Cell Biol 1996; 8:205–215.

248. Tsai S-C, Adamik R, Haun RS, Moss J, Vaughan M. Differential interaction of ADP-ribosylation factors 1, 3, and 5 with rat brain Golgi membranes. Proc Natl Acad Sci USA 1992; 89:9272–9276.

249. Tsai S-C, Adamik R, Huan RS, Moss J, Vaughan M. Effects of brefeldin A and accessory proteins on association of ADP-ribosylation factors 1, 3, and 5 with Golgi. J Biol Chem 1993; 268:10820–10825.

250. Tsai S-C, Adamik R, Moss J, Vaughan M. Identification of a brefeldin A-insensitive guanine nucleotide-exchange protein for ADP-ribosylation factor in bovine brain. Proc Natl Acad Sci USA 1994; 91:3063–3066.

251. Tsai S-C, Adamik R, Moss J, Vaughan M. Purification and characterization of a guanine nucleotide-exchange protein for ADP-ribosylation factor from spleen cytosol. Proc Natl Acad Sci USA 1996; 93:305–309.

252. Tsai S-C, Noda M, Adamik R, Chang PP, Chen H-C, Moss J, Vaughan M. Stimulation of choleragen enzymatic activities by GTP and two soluble proteins purified from bovine brain. J Biol Chem 1988; 263:1768–1772.

253. Tsai S-C, Noda M, Adamik R, Moss J, Vaughan M. Enhancement of choleragen ADP-ribosyltransferase activities by guanyl nucleotides and a 19-kDa membrane protein. Proc Natl Acad Sci USA 1987; 84:5139–5142.

254. Tsuchiya M, Price SR, Tsai S-C, Moss J, Vaughan M. Molecular identification of ADP-ribosylation factor mRNAs and their expression in mammalian cells. J Biol Chem 1991; 266:2772—2777.

255. Ullrich O, Horiuchi H, Bucci C, Zerial M. Membrane association of rab5 mediated by GDI-dissociation inhibitor and accompanied by GDP/GTP exchange. Nature 1994; 367:157–160.

256. Van Blesen T, Hawes BE, Luttrell DK, Krueger KM, Touhara K, Porfiri E, Sakaue M, Luttrell LM, Lefkowitz RJ. Receptor-tyrosine-kinase- and GBG-mediated MAP kinase activation by a common signalling pathway. Nature 1995; 376:781–784.

257. van der Sluijs P, Hull M, Huber LA, Male P, Goud B, Mellman I. Reversible phosphorylation-dephosphorylation determines the localization of rab4 during the cell cycle. EMBO J 1992; 11:4379–4389.

258. Vanhove B, Hofer-Warbinek R, Kapetanopoulos A, Hofer E, Bach FH, de Martin R. Gem, a GTP-binding protein from mitogen-stimulated T cells, is induced in endothelial cells upon activation by inflammatory cytokines. Endothelium 1997; 5:51–61.

259. Vojtek AB, Cooper JA. Rho family members: activators of MAP kinase cascades. Cell 1995; 82:527–529.

260. Vojtek AB, Hollenber SM, Cooper JA. Mammalian Ras interacts directly with the serine/threonine kinase Raf. Cell 1993; 74:205–214.

261. Walker MW, Bobak DA, Tsai S-C, Moss J, Vaughan M. GTP but not GDP analogues promote association of ADP-ribosylation factors, 20-kDa protein activators of cholera toxin, with phospholipids and PC-12 cell membranes. J Biol Chem 1992; 267:3230–3235.

262. Walworth NC, Brennwald P, Kabcennell AK, Garrett M, Novick P. Hydrolysis of GTP by Sec4 protein plays an important role in vesicular transport and is stimulated by a GTPase-activating protein in Saccharomyces cerevisiae. Mol Cell Biol 1992; 12:2017–2028.
263. Watanabe G, Saito Y, Madaule P, Ishizaki T, Fujisawa K, Morii N, Mukai H, Ono Y, Kakizuka A, Narumiya S. Protein kinase N (PKN) and PKN-related protein Rhophilin as targets of small GTPase Rho. Science 1996; 271:
264. Watkins PA, Moss J, Vaughan M. Effects of GTP on choleragen-catalyzed ADP-ribosylation of membrane and soluble proteins. J Biol Chem 1980; 255:3959–3963.
265. Weber E, Berta G, Tousson A, St. John P, Weaver Green M, Gopalokrishnan U, Jilling T, Sorscher EJ, Elton TS, Abrahamson DR, Kirk KL. Expression and polarized targeting of a Rab3 isoform in epithelial cells. J Cell Biol 1994; 125:
266. Weiss O, Holden J, Rulka C, Kahn RA. Nucleotide binding and cofactor activities of purified bovine brain and bacterially expressed ADP-ribosylation factor. J Biol Chem 1989; 264:21066–21072.
267. Wittinghofer A. Three-dimensional structure of p21 and its implications. In: Lacal JC, McCormick F, eds. The ras Superfamily of GTPases. Boca Raton, FL: CRC Press, 1993:37–63.
268. Wittinghofer A, Valencia A. Three-dimensional structure of Ras and Ras-related proteins. In: Zerial M, Huber LA, eds. Guidebook to the Small GTPases, New York: Oxford University Press, 1995;20–29.
269. Xu GF, Lin B, Tanaka K, Dunn D, Wood D, Gesteland R, White R, Weiss R, Tamanoi F. The catalytic domain of the neurofibromatosis type I gene product stimulates ras GTPase and complements ira mutants of S. cerevisiae. Cell 1990; 63:835–841.
270. Xu GF, P OC, Viskochil D, Cawthon R, Robertson M, Culver M, Dunn D, Stevens J, Gesteland R, White R, et al. The neurofibromatosis type 1 gene encodes a protein related to GAP. Cell 1990; 62:599–608.
271. Yamaguchi T, Shirataki H, Kishida S, Miyazaki M, Nishikawa J, Wada K, Numata SI, Kaibuchi K, Takai Y. Two functionally different domains of Rabphilin-3a, Rab3a p25/smg p25A-binding and phospholipid, and Ca2+-binding domains. J Biol Chem 1993; 268:27164–27170.
272. Yokoyama N, Hayashi N, Seki T, Pante N, Ohba T, Bishii K, et al. A giant nucleopore protein that binds Ran/TC4. Nature 1995; 376:184–188.
273. Zahraoui A, Joberty G, Arpin M, Fontaine JJ, Hellio R, Tavitian A, Louvard D. A small rab GTPase is distributed in cytoplasmic vesicles in non-polarized cells but colocalizes with the tight junction marker ZO-1 in polarized epithelial cells. J Cell Biol 1994; 124:101–105.
274. Zalcman G, Closson V, Linares-Cruz G, Lerebours F, Honore N, Tavitian A, Olofsson B. Regulation of Ras-related RhoB protein expression during the cell cycle. Oncogene 1995; 10:1935–1945.
275. Zerial M. Rab proteins. In: Zerial M, Huber LA, eds. Guidebook to the GTPases. New York: Oxford University Press Inc., 1995:295–306.
276. Zerial M, Stenmark H. Rab GTPases in vesicular transport. Curr Opin Cell Biol 1993; 5:613–620.
277. Zhang C-J, Rosenwald AG, Willingham MC, Skuntz S, Clark J, Kahn R. Expres-

sion of a dominant allele of human ARF1 inhibits membrane traffic in vivo. J Cell Biol 1994; 124:289–300.

278. Zheng Y, Bagrodia S, Cerione RA. Activation of phosphoinositide 3-kinase activity by Cdc42Hs binding to p85. J Biol Chem 1994; 269:18727–18730.
279. Zheng Y, Olson MF, Hall A, Cerione RA, Toksoz D. Direct involvement of the small GTP-binding protein Rho in lbc oncogene function. J Biol Chem 1995; 270:9031–9034.
280. Zhu J, Bilan PJ, Moyers JS, Antonetti DA, Kahn CR. Rad, a novel Ras-related GTPase, interacts with skeletal muscle beta-tropomyosin. J Biol Chem 1996; 271:768–773.
281. Zhu J, Reynet C, Caldwell JS, Kahn CR. Characterization of Rad, a new member of Ras/GTPase superfamily, and its regulation by a unique GTPase-activating protein (GAP)-like activity. J Biol Chem 1995; 270:4805–4812.
282. Zigmond SH. Signal transduction and actin filament organization. Curr Opin Cell Biol 1996; 8:66–73.

24

Molecular and Immunological Characterization of Melanocyte Lineage-Specific Antigens

MARCO W. J. SCHREURS, GOSSE J. ADEMA, and CARL G. FIGDOR

University Hospital Nijmegen
Nijmegen, The Netherlands

I. Introduction

Pigmentation is one of the most remarkable characteristics that distinguishes species in nature. In mammals, the pigment system is comprised of a single specialized cell type, the melanocyte. Melanocytes constitute only a small part of the cells present in the skin and eyes of mammals, but are solely responsible for the production of the pigment melanin. The production of melanin accounts for virtually all the visible pigmentation in skin and eyes. The significance of melanin lies in the biological utility of the many physicochemical properties of this compound: absorption of solar ultraviolet (UV) radiation, absorption of light and radiant heat, scavenging of free radicals, and chelation of heavy metal ions. Furthermore, in the animal kingdom the light-absorbing properties of melanin are used in adaptive coloration, display, and various aspects of camouflage and mimicry (1).

During embryonic development, mammalian melanocytes originate from two distinct sites. The melanocytes that constitute the retinal pigment epithelium (RPE), which lies behind the retina of the eye, differentiate from the posterior layer of the infolded neuroectoderm which has developed into the optic cup. Dermal melanocytes originate in, and migrate from, the neural crest. Upon completion of the process of neurulation, the ectodermal cells constituting the ridges of the neural folds will become the neural crest. Progenitor melanocytes, melanoblasts, subsequently migrate to three principal locations: the epidermal/dermal border of the skin, the hair bulbs in the dermis of the skin, and the iris, choroid, and retina of the eyes. Within the melanocyte, the process of pigment biosynthesis is restricted to specialized organelles, melanosomes. Premelanosomes are derived from the smooth endoplasmic reticulum (SER) and become immature melanosomes upon fusion with Golgi apparatus-derived coated vesicles containing the enzymes and structural elements required for pigment synthesis. The onset of melanogenesis results in melanosome maturation, characterized by a gradual increase in melanosome electron density as a result of melanin deposition, which ultimately gives rise to a mature melanosome. Mature melanosomes migrate from the perinuclear and endoplasmic regions into the dendritic processes of the melanocyte and are subsequently translocated to surrounding keratinocytes. Within keratinocytes the translocated melanosomes occur either as nonaggregated particles or as aggregates of two or more particles within membrane-enclosed vesicles. Once redistributed in keratinocytes, the melanosomes are subject to lysosomal degradation and are ultimately removed from the skin through loss of the stratum corneum (2–5).

The epidermal melanin unit, the three-dimensional association of one melanocyte with approximately 35 viable keratinocytes, serves as the integrated cellular structure that habitats the events described above. Human skin contains a large number of these units, and its color is the visual impact of melanin within them. For pigmentation to proceed normally, the many complex events and interactions briefly outlined above must occur with precision during development and differentiation of melanocytes. Mutations affecting these events and interactions may result in altered or defective pigmentation. A large number of such mutations has been identified in humans as well as in the mouse, and these have been mapped to a substantial number of distinct genetic loci (6–8). A number of these genes have been cloned, which has resulted in the identification of different enzymes and structural elements involved in the process of pigment synthesis.

Here we will review and discuss the characterization of a number of these gene products. We shall focus on those gene products that are shared between normal and transformed melanocytes and have been implicated in the immune response against melanoma, a tumor resulting from the malignant transformation melanocytes.

II. Melanocyte Lineage-Specific Antigens

The most striking characteristic of melanocyte differentiation resides in its ability to synthesize the pigment melanin from the amino acid tyrosine in a highly

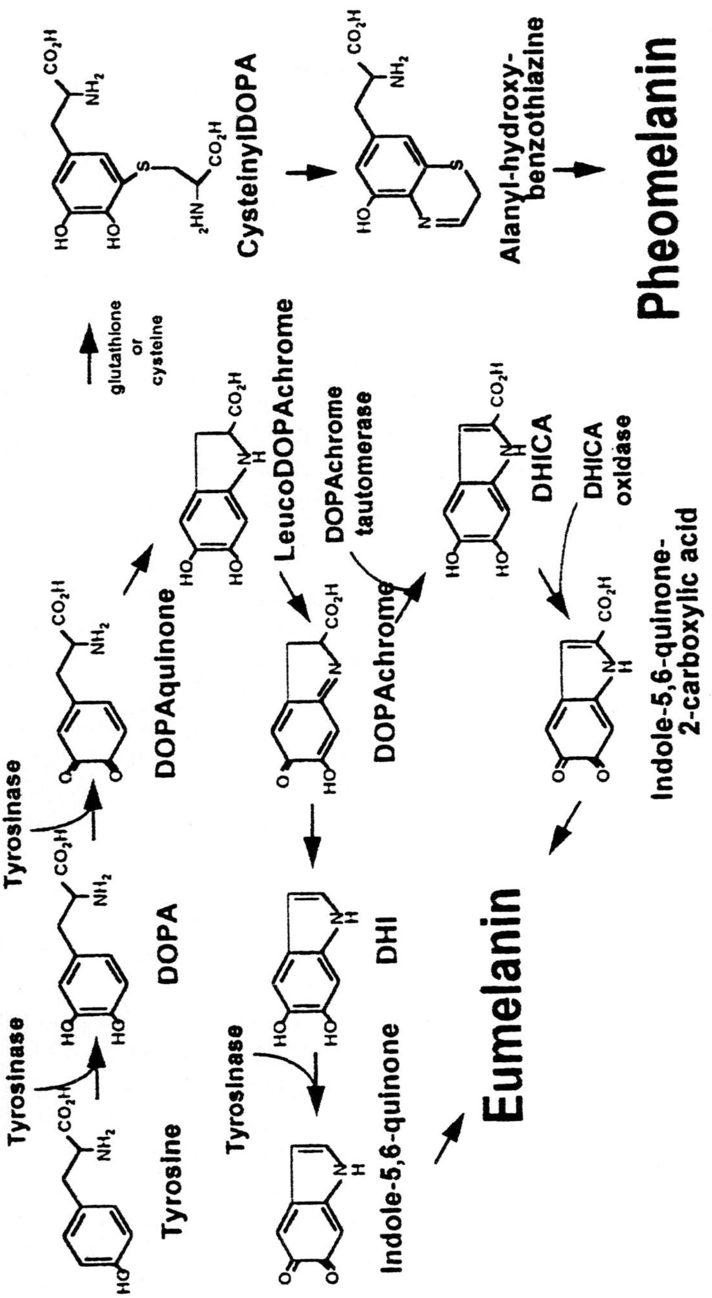

Figure 1 Schematic representation of the biochemical conversion of the amino acid tyrosine to the pigment melanin. The molecular interactions involved in the melanin biosynthetic pathway are depicted as originally proposed by Lerner and Fitzpatrick (9) and later modified by Korner and Pawelek (10). DOPA: 3,4-Dihydroxyphenylalanine; DHI: 5,6-dihydroxyindole; DHICA: 5,6-dihydroxyindole-2-carboxylic acid. (From Ref. 7.)

specialized organelle, the melanosome. The biosynthesis of melanin and the enzymes involved in this process are depicted in Figure 1 (7,9,10). Consequently, melanocyte differentiation is characterized by the specific expression of gene products involved in the biochemical conversion of tyrosine to melanin. Among these gene products are the enzymes shown in Figure 1 as well as structural elements of the melanosome.

The melanoma cell is the malignant counterpart of the melanocyte. As such, it is characterized by anaplasia, rapid growth rate, invasion of local tissue, and the ability to metastasize (11). In spite of the general tendency of tumor cells to dedifferentiate, a substantial part of melanoma tumors remains pigmented (12). This indicates that the biochemical machinery, including enzymes and structural elements, responsible for pigment synthesis is retained upon malignant transformation of melanocytes. As a result, a number of gene products responsible for pigment synthesis are shared between normal and transformed cells of the melanocyte lineage and thus are collectively referred to as melanocyte lineage–specific or differentiation antigens. Malignant melanoma is one of the most immunogenic tumors in humans, characterized by the observed spontaneous tumor regression and the presence of cytotoxic T lymphocytes (CTL) as well as antibodies reacting with melanoma cells in patients (13,14). The isolation and subsequent analysis of tumor-infiltrating lymphocytes (TIL) has indicated that the immune system of a melanoma patient preferentially reacts against melanocyte lineage-specific antigens (15).

The molecular cloning of the genes involved in pigment synthesis, combined with the immunogenicity of melanocyte lineage-specific antigens, has resulted in extensive molecular and immunological characterization of these antigens. A number of these antigens, including the enzymes tyrosinase and tyrosinase-related proteins 1 and 2 as well as the proteins with suspected or yet unknown function Pmel17/gp100 and Melan A/MART-1 will be discussed below in more detail.

A. Tyrosinase

The best characterized genetic locus involved in mouse coat color mutations is the albino locus (*c*-locus) on chromosome 7 (6,8). Mice homozygous for the *albino* mutation (*c*/*c*) all lack pigment in both neural crest–derived melanocytes and in the RPE, resulting in white coat color and pink eyes. Albino mice possess a full complement of pigment cells (designated amelanotic melanocytes), which are, however, incapable of any melanin synthesis (16,17). Since it has long been appreciated that the enzyme tyrosinase acts as a key regulator in melanin biosynthesis (9,10), it was presumed that the albino phenotype resulted from the lack of functional tyrosinase activity.

Different putative murine tyrosinase cDNA clones, pMT4 (18) and Tyrs33 (19), were isolated, but did not provide direct evidence for this assumption. The first indication that the *c*-locus indeed encodes tyrosinase was provided by Kwon et al. (20), who isolated a putative human tyrosinase cDNA clone (Pmel34) by screening a human melanocyte cDNA expression library with a polyclonal antibody directed against purified hamster tyrosinase. The isolated cDNA clone was shown to hybridize to genomic fragments at or around the mouse *c*-locus, thus representing a likely candidate for human tyrosinase. The same cDNA clone was subsequently used as a probe to isolate the corresponding cDNA clone from a B16 murine melanoma cDNA library (21). This resulted in the cloning and isolation of several independent putative mouse tyrosinase cDNA clones (pmcTyr1-4). Analysis of corresponding genomic clones demonstrated that the various tyrosinase cDNAs arose from alternative splicing, alternate promoter usage, and possibly alternate polyadenylation site usage (21). Functional analysis of the isolated mouse tyrosinase cDNA clones revealed that the most abundantly expressed clone (pmcTyr1) encoded enzymatically active tyrosinase upon expression in tyrosinase-negative cells (22). The structural gene encoding mouse tyrosinase was shown to map near or at the albino locus on chromosome 7, spanning approximately 70 kb, and is comprised of five exons which are separated by large introns (21,22). A full-length cDNA clone encoding human tyrosinase was subsequently isolated from a human melanoma cDNA library and was shown to confer tyrosinase-mediated melanin synthesis upon expression in tyrosinase-negative L cell mouse fibroblasts (23). Cloning of the genomic structure of the human tyrosinase (*TYR*) gene revealed the presence of five exons spanning more than 50 kb on the long arm of human chromosome 11 (24,25). Furthermore, the human equivalent of mouse albinism (type 1), oculocutaneous albinism (OCA), was shown to be genetically liked to the *TYR* structural gene (26). The ultimate evidence that the albino phenotype resulted from the lack of functional tyrosinase activity was provided by Beermann et al. (27). The albino phenotype could be rescued in transgenic mice by introduction of a minigene encoding functional tyrosinase into the germline of albino mice, resulting in pigmentation of both skin and eyes (27).

The tyrosinase protein consists of 529 amino acids from which a hydrophobic signal peptide of 18 amino acids is cleaved, giving rise to the mature tyrosinase protein (20). An apparant transmembrane domain near the carboxyl terminus and the presence of potential N-linked glycosylation sites indicate that tyrosinase is a transmembrane glycoprotein, which locates on the inner surface of the melanosome. The presence of histidine- and cysteine-rich sequences have been implicated as copper-binding sites and in the formation of multimeric protein complexes, respectively (28,29).

B. Tyrosinase-Related Proteins

The search for the gene encoding tyrosinase resulted, next to the cloning of tyrosinase itself, in the isolation and cloning of two other genes with approximately

40% homology to tyrosinase and to each other (30,31). These isolated genes were subsequently designated tyrosinase-related proteins (TRP).

The gene encoding TRP-1, previously isolated as the putative mouse tyrosinase cDNA pMT4 (18), was shown to map to the *brown* (*b*) locus on mouse chromosome 4 (30) and genetically linked to coat color mutations at this locus, which result in the production of brown instead of black melanin (6,8). The human homolog of TRP-1 was identified as the previously isolated gp75 antigen, an abundantly expressed melanosomal glycoprotein (32). The human *b*-locus gene was mapped to human chromosome 9 and was initially designated CAS2 locus (33) but was later renamed the *TYRP1* locus (34). Structural analysis of the gene revealed over 90% sequence homology between human and mouse and the existance of 1 noncoding followed by 7 coding exons in total, separated by 7 introns, spreading over 24 kb of genomic DNA (34). There has been no human TRP-1 mutation conclusively identified thus far. However, recently an individual with brown OCA was identified that lacked expression of TRP-1, possibly due to a mutation found in the individual's TRP-1 gene (35).

The overall primary protein structure of TRP-1 is very similar as described for tyrosinase, including a carboxy-terminal transmembrane domain, putative N-linked glycosylation sites, and domains rich in cysteins and histidines (28,29). The function of TRP-1 in the biosynthesis of melanin is not yet clear and remains in general dispute. Evidence exists that TRP-1 expression in fibroblasts results in stereospecific DOPAchrome tautomerase (Fig. 1) activity, not observed in nontransfected fibroblasts (36). In contrast, other data, generated by expression of TRP-1 in fibroblasts and by immunoaffinity purification of TRP-1 from melanocytes, indicated that TRP-1 functions as DHICA oxidase (Fig. 1), downstream of DOPAchrome tautomerase in melanin synthesis (37).

Molecular cloning of TRP-2 confirmed the existence of a third member of the tyrosinase related gene family (31). TRP-2 was shown to map to the *slaty* (*slt*) locus on mouse chromosome 14, mutation of which results in slight dilution of coat pigmentation (6,8,31). The human homolog of TRP-2 was subsequently isolated and shown to map to human chromosome 13 (38). Characterization of the genomic structure of the human (*TYRP2* locus) and mouse TRP-2 genes has indicated the presence of 8 exons encompassing 55 kb of genomic DNA (34,39). Human pigmentation disorders genetically linked to the *TYRP2* locus have not been identified yet. The TRP-2 gene has a different structure compared to the genes of the other tyrosinase gene family members with respect to the number and position of coding exons, consistent with the suggestion that this gene family resulted from gene duplication (39).

The primary protein structure of TRP-2 is similar to its family members with respect to the presence of the conserved domains described above (29) and was shown to function enzymatically in pigment synthesis (Fig. 1) as DOPAchrome tautomerase (40).

C. Pmel17/gp100

The coat color of mice homozygous for the silver (*si*) mutation is characterized by variable hypopigmentation, resulting from a reduced number of melanosomes present in hair-bulb melanocytes (6,8). Furthermore, melanocytes isolated from silver mutant mice exhibit a reduced proliferative capacity, associated with reduced in vivo survival (41).

As described above, the screening of a human melanocyte cDNA library with antityrosinase antibodies resulted in the isolation of a human tyrosinase cDNA clone (20). The same screening resulted in the cloning of a cDNA species that did not share homology with the isolated tyrosinase cDNA and was subsequently designated Pmel17-1 (20). The human Pmel17 cDNA was shown to map near the *silver* locus on mouse chromosome 10 and in a syntenic region on human chromosome 12 (42). To investigate whether the silver coat color mutation of mice was genetically linked to a putative Pmel17 mutation, Pmel17 cDNA clones were isolated from normal and *silver* mouse melanocytes (43). Sequence comparison of both isolated mouse Pmel17 cDNAs indeed revealed a defect in *silver* Pmel17, providing evidence for the assumed genetic linkage (43,44). The DNA sequence and genomic structure of the human Pmel17 gene on chromosome 12 have been determined recently (45). The human Pmel17 gene was found to consist of 11 exons, ranging in size from 85 to 723 bp, and to span approximately 9.1 kb of genomic DNA. Pmel17 has been implicated as a likely candidate gene for some cases of human OCA not associated with known albinism loci (45).

Recently, a cDNA clone was isolated from a human melanoma cDNA library, which encodes a protein recognized by different melanocyte lineage-specific monoclonal antibodies (46). The isolated cDNA clone, gp100-cl, appeared to be almost identical to the human Pmel17 cDNA with an in-frame deletion of 21 bp in gp100-cl as the most striking difference (47). Analysis of the genomic organization of part of the gene encoding gp100 revealed that both gp100 and Pmel17 are encoded by a single gene via alternative splicing of a single precursor RNA (47). In addition to Pmel17, the gp100-cl cDNA was found to be 80% homologous to the putative protein (RPE1) product encoded by a partial bovine cDNA isolated from RPE (48). Furthermore, significant homology exists (42%) between gp100-cl and a melanosomal matrix glycoprotein MMP115 isolated from chicken RPE (49). Recently, the murine gp100 cDNA has been isolated independently from a mouse melanocyte cDNA library (50) as well as from a B16 mouse melanoma cDNA library (51) and was shown to be approximately 80% homologous to human gp100, similar to human and mouse Pmel17 (43).

The proteins encoded by the human Pmel17/gp100 gene consist of 668 amino acids (Pmel17) and 661 amino acids (gp100). Cleaving off of an amino-terminal signal peptide gives rise to the mature proteins. Both Pmel17 and gp100 are characterized by the presence of a carboxy-terminal transmembrane region, five putative N-linked glycosylation sites, histidine-, threonine-, and cystein-rich domains, and three repeats of a 26-amino-acid motif in the middle of the molecule (28,42,47). The expression pattern of Pmel17/gp100 in melanosomes is similar to that of the tyrosinase family and suggests that this protein functions somewhere in melanin biosynthesis (46). Given its homology with the melanosomal matrix protein MMP115, Pmel17/gp100 might constitute a structural component of the melanosome rather than an enzymatic component. Indeed, evidence exists for this hypothesis since Pmel17/gp100 was shown to be present in premelanosomes, but not in coated vesicles known to deliver the enzymes to premelanosomes (52). In contrast, recent data have indicated that Pmel17/gp100 catalyzes the polymerization of DHICA to melanin (Fig. 1), suggesting that Pmel17/gp100 is a component of the complex of membrane-bound melanogenic oxidoreductive enzymes and cofactors (53,54).

D. Melan-A/MART-1

The most recent addition to the family of melanocyte lineage–specific antigens is Melan-A/MART-1. Two identical cDNA species encoding Melan-A/MART-1 were isolated independently from human melanoma cDNA libraries by cDNA expression cloning using antimelanoma CTL isolated from melanoma patients (55,56). The isolated cDNAs were subsequently referred to as Melan-A (55) and MART-1 (56) and failed to show significant homology with any gene recorded in the databases. Expression of Melan-A/MART-1 was shown to be restricted to normal and transformed cells of the melanocyte lineage (55–57). At the protein level Melan-A/MART-1 expression was characterized by a uniform cytoplasmic staining pattern as determined by serological analysis (57). The gene corresponding to the Melan-A/MART-1 cDNA was isolated from a human genomic library and comprises 5 exons, separated by 4 introns, spanning approximately 18.5 kb of genomic DNA (55). The chromosomal localization of the Melan-A/MART-1 gene has not been identified yet. Murine Melan-A/MART-1 has been cloned recently from a mouse melanocyte cDNA library (50).

The putative Melan-A/MART-1 protein consists of 118 amino acids, is devoid of a signal sequence, is rich in proline residues, and contains an amino-terminal transmembrane region (55,56). Whether Melan-A/MART-1 functions at all as a structural or enzymatic component in melanin biosynthesis remains to be established as does genetic linkage to any of the known human or mouse pigmentation defects.

The loci and chromosomal locations of the human and mouse melanocyte lineage-specific antigens discussed above are summarized in Table 1.

Table 1 Loci and Chromosomal Locations of Human and Mouse Genes Encoding the Melanocyte Lineage–Specific Antigens

	Human		Mouse	
Gene product	Locus	Location	Locus	Location
Tyrosinase	*TYR*	Chr. 11	*albino* (*c*)	Chr. 7
TRP-1	*TYRP1*	Chr. 9	*brown*(*b*)	Chr. 4
TRP-2	*TYRP2*	Chr. 13	*slaty* (*slt*)	Chr. 14
Pmel17	*Pmel17l*	Chr. 12	*silver* (*si*)	Chr. 10
Gp100	*gp100*	Chr. 12	*silver* (*si*)	Chr. 10
Melan A/MART-1	Unknown		Unknown	

III. Control of Melanocyte Lineage-Specific Expression

Within the minigene encoding wild-type tyrosinase, used to rescue the albino phenotype in transgenic mice, 5.5 kb of 5'-flanking sequence derived from the mouse tyrosinase gene was included as promoter (27). The transgenic mice generated using this minigene showed wild-type tyrosinase expression precisely overlapping the expression of the endogenous gene, restricted to melanocytic cells present in the skin and in the eyes. This indicates that all elements required for melanocyte-specific expression were included in the 5.5 kb of 5' flanking tyrosinase sequence. To define the regulatory elements within this tyrosinase promoter sequence dictating melanocyte-specific expression, a series of deletion mutants was constructed and fused to a reporter gene (58). Expression of these constructs in melanocytic and nonmelanocytic cells revealed that only 270 bp of 5'-flanking sequence were sufficient to dictate melanocyte-specific expression, indicating the presence of all required *cis*-regulatory elements within this part of the tyrosinase promoter. Furthermore, transgenic mice generated using these 270 bp of tyrosinase promoter sequence showed a similar transgene expression pattern as compared to the use of 5.5 kb of tyrosinase promoter (58,59).

Similar experiments using a series of deletion mutants constructed from the mouse TRP-1 promoter revealed that as little as 44 bp of 5'-flanking promoter sequence conferred melanocyte-specific expression (60). Within this part of the TRP-1 promoter an 11 bp motif, designated M-box, was found to be completely conserved between the TRP-1 and tyrosinase promoters and thus would represent a likely candidate *cis*-regulatory element. However, positive regulation of transcription by the M-box could also be detected in nonmelanocytic cells, consistent with the finding that the M-box binds the basic-helix-loop-helix-leucine zipper (bHLH-LZ) transcription factor USF (61).

Besides the M-box, additional *cis*-regulatory elements involved in melanocyte-specific transcription have been found in the TRP-1 as well as in the tyrosinase promoter, including the TATA region, a second positive regulatory element, and two negative regulatory, repressor elements (60–62). A melanocyte-specific factor, MSF, was shown to bind to the identified repressor elements and thus might serve as an antirepressor that allows TRP-1 expression in a melanocyte-restricted fashion (61). In addition, the mouse microphthalmia (*mi*) locus has been shown to encode a novel member of the bHLH-LZ family of transcription factors (63). Since mutations at the *mi* locus have been implicated in some pigmentation defects (6–8), this locus might encode melanocyte-specific M-box binding factor involved in melanocyte lineage-restricted expression (62). Indeed, recent date have indicated that the human homolog of the mouse *mi* locus product, microphthalmia-associated transcription factor (MITF), regulates melanocyte-specific expression of human tyrosinase (64).

The exact factors that control melanocyte lineage-specific expression still remain to be elucidated. In addition, there is evidence that restricted expression of melanocyte lineage-specific antigens is not absolute. Using a sensitive RT-PCR–based approach, transcripts derived from the tyrosinase gene as well as from the Pmel17/gp100 gene could detected in nonmelanocytic cells and normal tissues (51,65,66).

IV. Immune Responses Against Melanocyte Lineage-Specific Antigens

During the past few decades it has become possible to generate tumor-specific CTL in vitro from peripheral blood, draining lymph nodes, and (metastatic) tumor deposits of human cancer patients. The isolation of tumor-specific CTL as well as tumor-reactive antibodies has indicated that the immune system of a cancer patient is able to recognize an array of different tumor-associated antigens.

A number of CTL isolated from melanoma patients were shown to recognize not only melanoma cells, but also major histocompatibility complex (MHC) class I matched normal melanocytes (67). This suggested that at least some of the melanoma-reactive CTL recognize antigens shared between normal and neoplastic melanocytes, possibly members of the melanocyte lineage-specific family of antigens. The first evidence for this assumption was the identification of tyrosinase as target for antimelanoma $CD8^+$ CTL (68). Specific investigation of the tyrosinase-derived epitopes recognized by MHC class I restricted CTL revealed two HLA-A2 presented epitopes (69), an epitope presented by HLA-A24 (70), and an epitope presented by HLA-B44 (71). Recent studies have indicated that one of the two HLA-A2 presented epitopes, present at position 369–377 in the tyrosinase protein, is naturally processed with an aspartic acid as a third residue instead of a tyrosinase gene–encoded asparagine (72). The aspartic acid residue results from a deamination of the asparagine residue, which represents the first example of posttranslational modification of a naturally processed MHC class I presented epitope. In addition, two tyrosinase-derived MHC class II (HLA-DR4) binding epitopes were identified (73), indicating the involvement of $CD4^+$ helper T cells in the antimelanoma immune response as well. Besides the antityrosinase cellular immune response described above, humoral immunity has also been shown to participate in the antimelanoma immune response. Significant amounts of antityrosinase antibodies could be detected in sera of patients with malignant melanoma with either metastatic disease or no evidence of disease (74).

Prior to the cloning and characterization of the TRP-1 gene, the antigen it encodes, gp75, had been identified as a melanoma differentiation antigen recognized by serum IgG antibodies in melanoma patients (14,32). Cloning of the gene encoding an antigen recognized by HLA-A31–restricted CTL isolated from a melanoma patient revealed that the nucleotide sequence of this antigen was almost identical to TRP-1 (75). This indicated that TRP-1 constitutes an immune target for antimelanoma CTL. Interestingly, the antigenic peptide presented by HLA-A31 was not derived from the normal TRP-1 protein, but instead resulted from translation of an alternative open reading frame (ORF) of the same gene (76). The usage of an alternative ORF to produce an antigenic protein product represents a novel mechanism for generating tumor antigens.

The gp100 antigen was identified as a target for antimelanoma CTL through reconstitution of CTL reactivity following expression of the cDNA encoding gp100 in a gp100-negative MHC class I matched melanoma cell line (77). Independently, the gp100 antigen was identified as target for antimelanoma CTL using a strategy involving the isolation of peptides directly from MHC class I molecules present at the cell surface of melanoma cells (78–80). Peptide pools generated by HPLC-mediated fractionation of peptides eluted from MHC class I molecules were loaded back on MHC class I matched target cells and used in CTL reconstitution assays. Further fractionation and purification steps allowed the isolation of putative antigenic epitopes and resulted in the identification of a HLA-A2 presented gp100-derived epitope (81). In addition, four other gp100-derived epitopes were found to be recognized by antimelanoma CTL in the context of HLA-A2 (82–84). Recently, the gp100 antigen has also been shown to be involved in HLA-A3–restricted CTL responses against melanoma cells, which resulted in the identification of a HLA-A3 presented epitope (85). Given the high homology between gp100 and Pmel17, due to the alternative splicing of a single precursor RNA (47), the antigenic epitopes present in the gp100 protein are fully conserved in the Pmel17 protein. Consequently, expression of the cDNA encoding Pmel17 in MHC class I matched target cells confers similar sensitivity to gp100-reactive CTL-mediated lysis as compared to expression of the cDNA encoding gp100 (86). Investigation of a substantial number of CTL clones generated from peripheral blood of a melanoma patient indicated that the majority of these clones is directed against HLA-A2 presented Pmel17/gp100-derived epitopes, suggesting some preference for this antigen in the antimelanoma CTL response (87). However, a larger number of melanoma patient-derived CTL must be investigated to provide more conclusive evidence for this assumption.

As described above, the most recent addition to the family of melanocyte lineage–specific antigens, Melan A/MART-1, was first identified as a melanoma-associated antigen rather than a component involved in melanin biosynthesis (55,56). Similar to gp100, Melan A/MART-1 is recognized by a high percentage of melanoma TILs as well as in vitro generated melanoma-reactive CTLs. Two overlapping epitopes derived from Melan A/MART-1 have been identified that are recognized by antimelanoma CTL in the context of HLA-A2, one of which was isolated using peptide elution from surface MHC class I molecules (88,89).

The antigenic peptides derived from melanocyte lineage-specific antigens identified thus far are summarized in Table 2.

V. Specific Immunotherapy of Malignant Melanoma

The array of CTL-defined epitopes derived from melanocyte lineage-specific antigens has certainly indicated the immunogenicity of these antigens. However,

Table 2 The Presenting MHC Restriction Element, Sequence, and Position Within the Protein of Antigenic Peptides Derived from Melanocyte Lineage-Specific Antigens

Antigen	MHC	Epitope[a]	Position
Tyrosinase	HLA-A2	MLLAVLYCL	1–9
	HLA-A2	YMDGTMSQV	369–377
	HLA-A24	AFLPWHRLF	206–214
	HLA-B44	SEIWRDIDF	192–200
	HLA-DR4	QNILLSNAPLGPQFP	56–70
	HLA-DR4	SYLQDSDPDSFQD	450–462
TRP-1	HLA-A31	MSLQRQFLR	Alternate ORF
Pmel17/gp100	HLA-A2	KTWGQYWQV	154–162
	HLA-A2	ITDQVPGSV	209–217
	HLA-A2	YLEPGPVTA	280–288
	HLA-A2	LLDGTATLRL	457–466
	HLA-A2	VLYRYGSFSV	476–485
	HLA-A3	ALLAVGATK	17–25
Melan A/MART-1	HLA-A2	AAGIGILTV	27–35
	HLA-A2	ILTVILGVL	32–40

[a]Single letter amino acid code.

the role of this immunogenicity in in vivo tumor rejection remains elusive since the majority of melanoma tumors grow progressively in spite of the presence of tumor-reactive CTL. The fact that most CTL epitopes identified are derived from "self"-antigens and are presented by "nonprofessional" antigen-presenting cells suggests the induction of a certain state of T-cell tolerance allowing the observed progressive tumor growth. Indeed, TIL isolated from melanoma tumors usually require much higher amounts of growth factors (IL-2) for in vitro propagation as compared to, for instance, virus-reactive T cells. Enhancing the in vivo immune response directed against melanoma-derived epitopes using defined immunization/vaccination strategies might result in more effective tumor eradication. During the past few years substantial effort has been put in designing such immunotherapeutical strategies and investigating their feasibility in mouse model systems (90,91). Moreover, a number of clinical vaccine trials have been initiated with melanoma patients using the identified melanoma-associated antigens (92). In particular, novel vaccination strategies, including the use of dendritic cells, recombinant viruses, and naked DNA, may be used to induce or enhance antimelanoma tumor immunity (93–95).

Potential drawbacks of immune responses directed against melanocyte lineage-specific antigens include the immunoselection of antigen-loss variants in vivo. Recent data have shown that the CTL response directed against melanocyte lineage-specific antigens mediated the regression of antigen-positive tumors, but selects for antigen-loss variants (96). This indicates that genetic drift of melanoma cells resulting in a loss of the expression of some or even all melanocyte lineage-specific antigens could induce selective immune escape and allow progressive tumor growth. Furthermore, autoimmune destruction of normal melanocytes present in skin and eyes may represent an adverse effect resulting from immune responses directed against melanocyte lineage-specific antigens. Passive immunization of mice with TRP-1–specific antibodies was shown to induce protection and rejection of both subcutaneous melanoma tumors and lung metastases, but also resulted in in vivo destruction of melanocytes (97). This phenomenon has already been appreciated in the pathogenesis of the autoimmune pigmentation disorder vitiligo due to the isolation of melanocyte-reactive serum antibodies, including antityrosinase IgG (98,99). Occurrence of vitiligo has been observed in approximately 30% of melanoma patients responding to antimelanoma immunotherapy and has been shown to be associated with improved survival of melanoma patients (100,101). This indicates that melanocyte destruction indeed could occur in response to antimelanoma immunotherapy, but may turn out to become a welcome adverse effect during treatment of a lethal disease.

VI. Concluding Remarks

The molecular characterization of melanocyte lineage-specific antigens has provided substantial insight in the pathogenesis of several pigmentation disorders allowing more detailed diagnosis of a given defect within the biosynthesis of melanin. The complex mechanisms controlling melanocyte lineage-restricted expression of the pigmentation-associated gene products are becoming less unclear, but still require further study.

Involvement of melanocyte lineage-specific antigens in the immune response against malignant melanoma has boosted the development of novel strategies to treat this type of cancer, which is characterized by aggressive behavior, high metastatic potential, and relative resistance to conventional radio- and chemotherapy.

The optimal ways to induce or enhance antitumor immune responses and the severity of potential adverse effects upon using melanocyte lineage-specific antigens as tumor targets will be evaluated in the next several years.

References

1. Jimbow K, Fitzpatrick TB, Quevedo WC Jr. Formation, chemical compositions and functions of melanin pigments in mammals. In: Matolsky, ed. Biology of the Integument. Vol. 2. New York: Springer-Verlag, 1986:278–296.
2. Kawamura K, Fitzpatrick TB, Seiji M. Biology of Normal and Abnormal Melanocytes. Baltimore: University Park Press, 1971.
3. Montagna W, Parakkal PF. The Structure and Function of Skin. New York: Academic Press, 1974.
4. Fitzpatrick TB. Biology and Diseases of Dermal Pigmentation. Tokyo: University of Tokyo Press, 1981.
5. Hearing VJ, Kind RA. Determinants of skin color: melanocytes and melanization. In: Levine N, ed. Pigmentation and Pigmentary Abnormalities. New York: CRC Press, 1994:3–18.
6. Silvers WK. The Coat Colors of Mice: A Model for Mammalian Gene Action and Interaction. New York: Springer-Verlag, 1979.
7. Spritz RA, Hearing VJ Jr. Genetic disorders of pigmentation. Adv Hum Genet 1994; 22:1–45.
8. Jackson IJ. Molecular and developmental genetics of mouse coat color. Annu Rev Genet 1994; 28:189–217.
9. Lerner AB, Fitzpatrick TB. Biochemistry of melanin formation. Physiol Rev 1950; 30:91–126.
10. Korner AM, Pawelek J. Mammalian tyrosinase catalyzes three reactions in the biosynthesis of melanin. Science 1982; 217:1163–1165.
11. Clark WH, Elder DE, Guerry DI V, Epstein MN, Greene MH, van Horn M. The development and subsequent cellular evolution of the primary human cutaneous malignant melanomas. Hum Pathol 1984; 15:1147–1165.
12. Jimbow K, Lee SK, King MG, Hara H, Chen H, Dakour J, Marusyk H. Melanin pigments and melanosomal proteins as differentiation markers unique to normal and neoplastic melanocytes. J Invest Dermatol 1993; 100:259S–268S.

13. Knuth A, Wolfel T, Meyer zum Buschenfelde KH. T cell responses to human malignant tumours. Cancer Surv 1992; 13:39–52.
14. Mattes MJ, Thomson TM, Old LJ, Lloyd KO. A pigmentation-associated, differentiation antigen of human melanoma defined by a precipitating antibody in human serum. Int J Cancer 1983; 32:717–721.
15. Robbins PF, Kawakami Y. Human tumor antigens recognized by T cells. Curr Opin Immunol 1996; 8:628–636.
16. Halaban R, Moellmann G, Tamura A, Kwon BS, Kuklinska E, Pomerantz S, Lerner AB. Tyrosinases of murine melanocytes with mutations at the *albino* locus. Proc Natl Acad Sci USA 1988; 85:7241–7245.
17. Bennett DC, Cooper PJ, Dexter TJ, Devlin LM, Heasman J, Nester B. Cloned mouse melanocyte lines carrying the germline mutations albino and brown: complementation in culture. Development 1989; 105:379–385.
18. Shibahara S, Tomita Y, Sakakura T, Nager C, Chaudhuri B, Muller R. Cloning and expression of cDNA encoding mouse tyrosinase. Nucleic Acids Res 1986; 14:2413–2427.
19. Yamamoto H, Takeuchi S, Kudo T, Makino K, Nakata A, Shinoda T, Takeuchi T. Cloning and sequencing of mouse tyrosinase cDNA. Jpn J Genet 1987; 62:271–274.
20. Kwon BS, Haq AK, Pomerantz SH, Halaban R. Isolation and sequence of a putative cDNA clone for human tyrosinase that maps at the mouse c-albino locus. Proc Natl Acad Sci USA 1987; 84:7473–7477.
21. Ruppert S, Müller G, Kwon B, Schütz G. Multiple transcripts of the mouse tyrosinase gene are generated by alternative splicing. EMBO J 1988; 7:2715–2722.
22. Müller G, Ruppert S, Schmid E, Schütz G. Functional analysis of alternatively spliced tyrosinase gene transcripts. EMBO J 1988; 7:2723–2730.
23. Bouchard B, Fuller BB, Vijayasaradhi S, Houghton AN. Induction of pigmentation in mouse fibroblasts by expression of human tyrosinase cDNA. J Exp Med 1989; 169:2029–2042.
24. Barton DE, Kwon BS, Francke U. Human tyrosinase gene, mapped to chromosome 11 (q14->q21), defines second region of homology with mouse chromosome 7. Genomics 1988; 3:17–24.
25. Giebel LB, Strunk KM, Spritz RA. Organization and nucleotide sequences of the human tyrosinase gene and a truncated tyrosinase-related segment. Genomics 1991; 9:435–445.
26. Giebel LB, Strunk KM, King RA, Hanifin JM, Spritz RH. A frequent tyrosinase gene mutation in classic, tyrosinase-negative (type IA) oculocutaneous albinism. Proc Natl Acad Sci USA 1990; 87:3255–3258.
27. Beermann F, Ruppert S, Hummler E, Bosch FX, Müller G, Rüther U, Schütz G. Rescue of the albino phenotype by introduction of a functional tyrosinase gene into mice. EMBO J 1990; 9:2819–2826.
28. Kwon BS. Pigmentation genes: the tyrosinase gene family and the Pmel17 gene family. J Invest Dermatol 1993; 100:134S–140S.
29. del Marmol V, Beermann F. Tyrosinase and related proteins in mammalian pigmentation. FEBS Lett 1996; 381:165–168.

30. Jackson IJ. A cDNA encoding tyrosinase-related protein maps to the mouse brown locus. Proc Natl Acad Sci USA 1988; 85:3492–3496.
31. Jackson IJ, Chambers DM, Tsukamoto K, Copeland NG, Gilbert DJ, Jenkins NA, Hearing VJ. A second tyrosinase-related protein, TRP2, maps to and is mutated at the mouse slaty locus. EMBO J 1992; 11:527–535.
32. Vijayasaradhi S, Bouchard B, Houghton AN. The melanoma antigen gp75 is the human homologue of the mouse b (brown) locus gene product. J Exp Med 1990; 171:1375–1380.
33. Chintamaneni C, Ramsay M, Colman MA, Fox MF, Pickard RT, Kwon BS. Mapping the human CAS2 gene, the homologue of the mouse brown (*b*) locus, to human chromosome qp22-ptr. Biochem Biophys Res Commun 1991; 178:227–235.
34. Sturm RA, O'Sullivan BJ, Box NF, Smith AG, Smit SE, Puttick ER, Parsons PG, Dunn IS. Chromosomal structure of the human TYRP1 and TYRP2 loci and comparison of the tyrosinase-related protein gene family. Genomics 1995; 29:24–34.
35. Boissy RE, Zhao H, Oetting WS, Austin LM, Wildenberg C, Boissy YL, Zhao Y, Sturm RA, Hearing VJ, King RA, Nordlund JJ. Mutation in and lack of expression of tyrosinase-related protein-1 (TRP-1) in melanocytes from an individual with brown oculocutaneous albinism: a new subtype of albinism classified as "OCA3". Am J Hum Genet 1996; 58:1145–1156.
36. Winder AJ, Wittbjer A, Odh G, Rosengren E, Rorsman H. The mouse brown (b) locus protein functions as a dopachrome tautomerase. Pigment Cell Res 1994; 7:305–310.
37. Kobayashi T, Urabe K, Winder A, Jimenez-Cervantes C, Imokawa G, Brewington T, Solano F, Garcia-Borron JC, Hearing VJ. Tyrosinase related protein 1 (TRP1) functions as a DHIC oxidase in melanin biosynthesis. EMBO J 1994; 13:5818–5825.
38. Yokoyama K, Suzuki H, Yasumoto K, Tomita Y, Shibahara S. Molecular cloning and functional analysis of a cDNA coding for human DOPAchrome tautomerase/tyrosinase-related protein-2. Biochim Biophys Acta 1994; 121:317–321.
39. Budd PS, Jackson IJ. Structure of the mouse tyrosinase-related protein-2/dopachrome tautomerase (Tyrp2/Dct) gene and sequence of two novel slaty alleles. Genomics 1995; 29:35–43.
40. Tuskamoto K, Jackson IJ, Urabe K, Montague PM, Hearing VJ. A second tyrosinase-related protein, TrP-2, is a melanogenic enzyme termed DOPAchrome tautomerase. EMBO J 1991; 11:519–526.
41. Spanakis E, Lamina P, Bennett DC. Effects of the developmental colour mutations silver and recessive spotting on proliferation of diploid and immortal mouse melanocytes in culture. Development 1992; 114:675–680.
42. Kwon BS, Chintamaneni C, Kozak CA, Copeland NG, Gilbert DJ, Jenkins N, Barton D, Francke U, Kobayashi Y, Kim KK. A melanocyte-specific gene, Pmel17, maps near the silver coat color locus on mouse chromosome 10 and is in a syntenic region on human chromosome 12. Proc Natl Acad Sci USA 1991; 88:9228–9232.
43. Kwon BS, Kim KK, Halaban R, Pickard RT. Characterization of mouse Pmel17 gene and silver locus. Pigment Cell Res 1994; 7:394–397.
44. Kwon BS, Halaban R, Ponnazhagan S, Kim K, Chintamaneni C, Bennett D,

Pickard RT. Mouse silver mutation is caused by a single base insertion in the putative cytoplasmic domain of Pmel17. Nucleic Acids Res 1995; 23:154–158.

45. Bailin T, Lee ST, Spritz RA. Genomic organization and sequence of D12S53E (Pmel17), the human homologue of the mouse silver (si) locus. J Invest Dermatol 1996; 106:24–27.
46. Adema GJ, de Boer AJ, van 't Hullenaar R, Denijn M, Ruiter DJ, Vogel AM, Figdor CG. Melanocyte lineage-specific antigens recognized by monoclonal antibodies NKI-beteb, HMB-50, and HMB-45 are encoded by a single cDNA. Am J Pathol 1993; 143:1579–1585.
47. Adema GJ, de Boer AJ, Vogel AM, Loenen WAM, Figdor CG. Molecular characterization of the melanocyte lineage-specific antigen gp100. J Biol Chem 1994; 269:20126–20133.
48. Kim RY, Wistow GJ. The cDNA REP1 and monoclonal antibody HMB-50 define gene products preferentially expressed in retinal pigment epithelium. Exp Eye Res 1992; 55:657–662.
49. Mochii M, Agata K, Eguchi G. Complete sequence and expression of a cDNA encoding a chicken 115-kDa melanosomal matrix protein. Pigment Cell Res 1991; 4:41–47.
50. Zhai Y, Yang JC, Spiess P, Nishimura MI, Overwijk W, Carrol MW, Roberts B, Restifo NP, Rosenberg SA. Cloning and characterization of the genes encoding the murine homologues of the human melanoma antigens MART1 and gp100. J Immunother. 1997; 20:15–25.
51. Schreurs MWJ, de Boer AJ, Schmidt A, Figdor CG, Adema GJ. Cloning, expression and tissue distribution of the murine homologue of the melanocyte lineage-specific antigen gp100. Melanoma Res 1997; 7:463–470.
52. Kobayashi T, Urabe K, Orlow SJ, Higashi K, Imokawa G, Kwon BS, Potterf B, Hearing VJ. The Pmel17/silver locus protein—characterization and investigation of its melanogenic function. J Biol Chem 1994; 269:29198–29205.
53. Chakraborty AK, Platt JT, Kim KK, Kwon BS, Bennett DC, Pawelek JM. Polymeryzation of 5,6-dihydroxyindole-2-carboxylic acid to melanin by the Pmel17/silver locus protein. Eur J Biochem 1996; 236:180–188.
54. Lee ZH, Hou L, Moellmann G, Antol K, Fraser M, Halaban R, Kwon BS. Characterization and subcellular localization of human Pmel17/silver, a 110-kDa (pre)melanosomal membrane protein associated with 5,6-dihydroxyindole-2-carboxylic acid (DHICA) converting activity. J Invest Dermatol 1996; 106:605–610.
55. Coulie PG, Brichard V, Vanpel A, Wolfel T, Schneider J, Traversari C, Mattei S, Deplaen E, Lurquin C, Szikora JP, Renauld JC, Boon T. A new gene coding for a differentiation antigen recognized by autologous cytolytic T lymphocytes on HLA-A2 melanomas. J Exp Med 1994; 180:35–42.
56. Kawakami Y, Eliyahu S, Delgado CH, Robbins PF, Rivoltini L, Topalian SL, Miki T, Rosenberg SA. Cloning of the gene coding for a shared human melanoma antigen recognized by autologous T cells infiltrating into tumor. Proc Natl Acad Sci USA 1994; 91:3515–3519.
57. Chen YT, Stockert E, Jungbluth A, Tsang S, Coplan KA, Scanlan MJ, Old LJ. Serological analysis of Melan-A/MART-1, a melanocyte-specific protein

homogenously expressed in human melanomas. Proc Natl Acad Sci USA 1996; 93:5915–5919.

58. Kluppel M, Beermann F, Ruppert S, Schmid E, Hummler E, Schütz G. The mouse tyrosinase promoter is sufficient for expression in melanocytes and in the pigmented epithelium of the retina. Proc Natl Acad Sci USA 1991; 88:3777–3781.
59. Beermann F, Schmid E, Ganss R, Schütz G, Ruppert S. Molecular characterization of the mouse tyrosinase gene: pigment cell-specific expression in transgenic mice. Pigment Cell Res 1992; 5:295–299.
60. Lowings P, Yavuzer U, Goding CR. Positive and negative elements regulate a melanocyte-specific promoter. Mol Cell Biol 1992; 12:3653–3662.
61. Yavuzer U, Goding CR. Melanocyte-specific gene expression: role of repression and identification of a melanocyte-specific factor, MSF. Mol Cell Biol 1994; 14:3494–3503.
62. Ganss R, Schütz G, Beermann F. The mouse tyrosinase gene. Promoter modulation by positive and negative regulatory elements. J Biol Chem 1994; 269:29808–29816.
63. Hodgkinson CA, Moore KJ, Nakayama A, Steingrimmson E, Copeland MG, Jenkins NA, Arnheiter H. Mutations at the mouse microphthalmia locus are associated with defects in a gene encoding a novel basic-helix-loop-helix-zipper protein. Cell 1993; 74:395–404.
64. Yasumoto K, Yokoyama K, Shibata K, Tomita Y, Shibahara S. Microphthalmia-associated transcription factor as a regulator for melanocyte-specific transcription of the human tyrosinase gene. Mol Cell Biol 1994; 14:8058–8070.
65. Battyani Z, Xerri L, Hassoun J, Bonerandi JJ, Grob JJ. Tyrosinase gene expression in human tissues. Pigment Cell Res 1993; 6:400–405.
66. Brouwenstijin N, Slager EH, Bakker ABH, Schreurs MWJ, van der Spek CW, Adema GJ, Schrier PI, Figdor CG. Transcription of the gene encoding melanoma-associated antigen gp100 in tissues and cell lines other than those of the melanocyte lineage. Br J Cancer 1997; 76:1562–1566.
67. Anichini A, Maccalli C, Mortarini R, Salvi S, Mazzocchi A, Squarcina P, Herlyn M, Parmiani G. Melanoma cells and normal melanocytes share antigens recognized by HLA-A2-restricted cytotoxic T cell clones from melanoma patients. J Exp Med 1993; 177:989–998.
68. Brichard V, van Pel A, Wölfel T, Wölfel C, de Plaen E, Lethe B, Coulie P, Boon T. The tyrosinase gene codes for an antigen recognized by autologous cytolytic T lymphocytes on HLA-A2 melanomas. J Exp Med 1993; 178:489–495.
69. Wölfel T, van Pel A, Brichard V, Schneider J, Seliger B, Zumbuschenfelde KHM, Boon T. Two tyrosinase nonapeptides recognized on HLA-A2 melanomas by autologous cytolytic T lymphocytes. Eur J Immunol 1994; 24:759–764.
70. Kang X-Q, Kawakami Y, Sakaguchi IK, El-Gamil M, Wang R-F, Yanelly JR, Apella E, Rosenbers SA, Robbins PF. Identification of a tyrosinase epitope recognized by HLA-A24 restricted tumor-infiltrating lymphocytes. J Immunol 1995; 155:1343–1348.
71. Brichard VG, Herman J, Vanpel A, Wildmann C, Gaugler B, Wölfel T, Boon T, Lethe B. A tyrosinase nonapeptide presented by HLA-B44 is recognized on a hu-

man melanoma by autologous cytolytic T lymphocytes. Eur J Immunol 1996; 26:224–230.

72. Skipper JC, Hendrickson RC, Gulden PH, Brichard V, van Pel A, Chen Y, Shabanowitz J, Wölfel T, Slingluff CLJr, Boon T, Hunt DF, Engelhard VH. An HLA-A2-restricted tyrosinase antigen on melanoma cells results from posttranslational modification and suggests a novel pathway for processing membrane proteins. J Exp Med 1996; 183:527–534.
73. Topalian SL, Gonzales MI, Parkhurst M, Li YF, Southwood S, Sette A, Rosenberg SA, Robbins PF. Melanoma-specific CD4(+) T cells recognize nonmutated HLA-DR-restricted tyrosinase epitopes. J Exp Med 1996; 183:1965–1971.
74. Merimsky O, Beharav E, Shoenfeld Y, Chaitchik S, Tsigelman R, Cohen-Aloro D, Fishman P. Anti-tyrosinase antibodies in malignant melanoma. Cancer Immunol Immunother 1996; 42:297–302.
75. Wang R-F, Robbins PF, Kawakami Y, Kang X-Q, Rosenberg SA. Identification of a gene encoding a melanoma tumor antigen recognized by HLA-A31-restricted tumor-infiltrating lymphocytes. J Exp Med 1995; 181:799–804.
76. Wang R-F, Pakhurst M, Kawakami Y, Robbins PF, Rosenberg SA. Utilization of an alternative open reading frame of a normal gene in generating a novel human cancer antigen. J Exp Med 1996; 183:1131–1140.
77. Bakker ABH, Schreurs MWJ, de Boer AJ, Kawakami Y, Rosenberg SA, Adema GJ, Figdor CG. Melanocyte lineage-specific antigen gp100 is recognized by melanoma-derived tumor-infiltrating lymphocytes. J Exp Med 1994; 179:1005–1009.
78. Henderson RA, Cox AL, Sakaguchi K, Appella E, Shabanowitz J, Hunt DF, Engelhard VH. Direct identification of an endogenous peptide recognized by multiple HLA-A2.1-specific cytotoxic T cells. Proc Natl Acad Sci USA 1993; 90:10275–10279.
79. Slingluff CL,Jr., Cox AL, Henderson RA, Hunt DF, Engelhard VH. Recognition of human melanoma cells by HLA-A2.1-restricted cytotoxic T lymphocytes is mediated by at least six shared peptide epitopes. J Immunol 1993; 150:2955–2963.
80. Storkus WJ, Zeh HJ, Maeurer MJ, Salter RD, Lotze MT. Identification of human melanoma peptides recognized by class I restricted tumor infiltrating T lymphocytes. J Immunol 1993; 151:3719–3727.
81. Cox AL, Skipper J, Chen Y, Henderson RA, Darrow TL, Shabanowitz J, Engelhard VH, Hunt DF, Slingluff CLJ. Identification of a peptide recognized by five melanoma-specific human cytotoxic T cell lines. Science 1994; 264:716–719.
82. Kawakami Y, Eliyahu S, Delgado CH, Robbins PF, Sakaguchi K, Appella E, Yannelli JR, Adema GJ, Miki T, Rosenberg SA. Identification of a human melanoma antigen recognized by tumor-infiltrating lymphocytes associated with in vivo tumor rejection. Proc Natl Acad Sci USA 1994; 91:6458–6462.
83. Bakker ABH, Schreurs MWJ, Tafazzul G, de Boer AJ, Kawakami Y, Adema GJ, Figdor CG. Identification of a novel peptide derived from the melanocyte-specific gp100 antigen as the dominant epitope recognized by an HLA-A2.1-restricted anti-melanoma CTL line. Int J Cancer 1995; 62:97–102.
84. Kawakami Y, Eliyahu S, Jennings C, Sakaguchi K, Kang X, Southwood S, Robbins PF, Sette A, Appella E, Rosenberg SA. Recognition of multiple epitopes in the

human melanoma antigen gp100 by tumor-infiltrating T lymphocytes associated with in vivo tumor regression. J Immunol 1995; 154:3961–3968.
85. Skipper JC, Kittlesen DJ, Hendrickson RC, Deacon DD, Harthun NL, Wagner SN, Hunt DF, Engelhard VH,, Slingluff CLJr. Shared epitopes for HLH-A3-restricted melanoma-reactive human CTL include a naturally processed epitope from Pmel-17/gp100. J Immunol 1996; 157:5027–5033.
86. Adema GJ, Bakker ABH, De Boer AJ, Hohenstein P, Figdor CG. Pmel17 is recognized by monoclonal antibodies NKI-beteb, HMB-45 and HBM-50 and by anti-melanoma CTL. Br J Cancer 1996; 73:1044–1048.
87. Zarour H, De Smet C, Lehman F, Marchand M, Lethé B, Romero P, Boon T, Renauld J-C. The majority of autologous cytolytic T-lymphocyte clones derived from peripheral blood lymphocytes of a melanoma patient recognize an antigenic peptide derived from gene Pmel17/gp100. J Invest Dermatol 1996; 107:63–67.
88. Kawakami Y, Eliyahu S, Sakaguchi K, Robbins PF, Rivoltini L, Yannelli JR, Appella E, Rosenberg SA. Identification of the immunodominant peptides of the MART-1 human melanoma antigen recognized by the majority of HLA-A2-restricted tumor infiltrating lymphocytes. J Exp Med 1994; 180:347–352.
89. Castelli C, Storkus WJ, Maeurer MJ, Martin DM, Huang EC, Parmanik BN, Nagabhushan TL, Parmiani G, Lotze MT. Mass spectrometric identification of a naturally processed melanoma peptide recognized by CD8(+) cytotoxic T lymphocytes. J Exp Med 1995; 181:363–368.
90. Melief CJM, Offringa R, Toes REM, Kast WM. Peptide-based cancer vaccines. Curr Opin Immunol 1996; 8:651–657.
91. Restifo NP. The new vaccines: building viruses that elicit antitumor immunity. Curr Opin Immunol 1996; 8:658–663.
92. Jaeger E, Bernhard H, Romero P, Ringhoffer M, Arand M, Karbach J, Ilsemann C, Hagedorn M, Knuth A. Generation of cytotoxic T-cell responses with synthetic melanoma-associated peptides in vivo: implications for tumor vaccines with melanoma-associated antigens. Int J Cancer 1996; 66:162–169.
93. Bakker ABH, Marland G, de Boer AJ, Huijbens RJ, Danen EH, Adema GJ, Figdor CG. Generation of antimelanoma cytotoxic T lymphocytes from healthy donors after presentation of melanoma-associated antigen-derived epitopes by dendritic cells in vitro. Cancer Res 1995; 55:5330–5334.
94. Zhai Y, Yang JC, Kawakami Y, Spiess P, Wadsworth SC, Cardoza LM, Couture LA, Smith AE, Rosenberg SA. Antigen-specific tumor vaccines: development and characterization of recombinant adenoviruses encoding MART-1 or gp100 for cancer therapy. J Immunol 1996; 156:700–710.
95. Schreurs MWJ, de Boer AJ, Adema GJ, Figdor CG. Genetic vaccination against the melanocyte lineage-specific gp100 antigen induces CTL-mediated tumor protection. Cancer Res, in press.
96. Jager E, Ringhoffer M, Karbach J, Arand M, Oesch F, Knuth A. Inverse relationship of melanocyte differentiation antigen expression in melanoma tissues and CD8+ cytotoxic-T-cell responses: evidence for immunoselection of antigen-loss variants in vivo. Int J Cancer 1996; 66:470–476.
97. Hara I, Takechi Y, Houghton AN. Implicating a role for immune recognition of

self in tumor rejection: passive immunization against the *brown* locus protein. J Exp Med 1995; 182:1609–1614.

98. Gilhar A, Zelickson B, Ulman Y, Etzioni A. In vivo destruction of melanocytes by the IgG fraction of serum from patients with vitiligo. J Invest Dermatol 1996; 105:683–686.
99. Baharav E, Merimski O, Shoenfeld Y, Zigelman R, Gilbrud B, Yecheskel G, Youinou P, Fishman P. Tyrosinase as an autoantigen in patients with vitiligo. Clin Exp Immunol 1996; 105:84–88.
100. Rosenberg SA, White DE. Vitiligo in patients with melanoma: Normal tissue antigens can be targets for cancer immunotherapy. J Immunother 1996; 19:81–84.
101. Nordlund JJ, Kirkwood JM, Forget BM, Milton G, Albert DM, Lerner AB. Vitiligo in patients with metastatic melanoma: a good prognostic sign. J Am Acad Dermatol 1983; 9:689–696.

25

Cellular Heterogeneity in Lymphangioleiomyomatosis

JOHN A. KELLY, SHAN C. CHU, and JOEL MOSS

National Heart, Lung, and Blood Institute
National Institutes of Health
Bethesda, Maryland

Lymphangioleiomyomatosis (LAM) is a rare disorder of unknown etiology that occurs almost exclusively in women of childbearing years (1–7). LAM is characterized microscopically by abnormal smooth muscle proliferation along the thoracic and abdominal lymphatics and in lymph nodes (8–10). These smooth muscle cells display considerable morphological heterogeneity (6,11,12–16). Characterization of the proliferating cells in LAM is pivotal to understanding this perplexing disease.

It is possible to relate the clinical features of LAM to the anatomical sequelae of abnormal smooth muscle proliferation (6). It has been proposed that abnormal smooth muscle proliferation may obstruct bronchioles, causing airflow obstruction and air trapping, possibly leading to formation of bullae and pneumothoraces. Obstruction of lymph nodes may lead to chylous effusions and ascites, findings common in this disease. Likewise, obstruction of pulmonary venules may result in hemosiderosis and hemoptysis (6). Because of the possible role of abnormal smooth muscle cells in the pathogenesis of LAM, the origin and nature of these cells have been of interest. In view of the characteristic abnormal appearance of these "smooth muscle cells," they have been termed "LAM cells."

I. Cellular Heterogeneity in Lymphangioleiomyomatosis

A. Historical and Microscopic Aspects

Enterline and Roberts were the first to recognize LAM as an entity (17), noting a proliferation of cells with smooth muscle characteristics. Because of the close association of these abnormal smooth muscle cells with lymphatics, they were felt to be pericytes, giving rise to the term lymphangiopericytoma for the disease (17). Corning and Enterline noted heterogeneity among the cells (18), describing both round cells with pleomorphic nuclei containing distinct nucleoli and spindle-shaped cells with elongated nuclei. Both cell types were interspersed in all lesions and blended with each other. Although agreeing that the cells resembled smooth muscle, these investigators did not feel that they originated from pericytes, using the term lymphangiomyoma to describe the benign, hamartomatous smooth muscle proliferation and lymphatic elements. The terminology for the disease has evolved with lymphangiomyomatosis (19), and subsequently lymphangioleiomyomatosis (20), being used to describe the widespread smooth muscle proliferation.

B. Ultrastructural Features

Ultrastructural studies were undertaken to understand better the subcellular organization of LAM cells. The first ultrastructural examination of LAM tissue was of a mediastinal lesion (21). The predominant cell type was described as fusiform. The cells were closely packed in parallel, with elongated nuclei aligned along the long axis of the cell. Myofilaments were seen in the cytoplasm, running parallel to the nuclei; they tended to concentrate near the nuclear membrane, forming marginal densities (21). These characteristics were consistent with smooth muscle cells. Granules of various densities were also noted, especially near the nucleus. Similar findings were subsequently obtained with tissue from LAM lung (22). The cells were predominantly spindle shaped, with densely packed myofilaments situated below the plasma membrane. Later reports, however, noted, in addition to the smooth muscle cells with abundant myofilaments, other cells. These cells varied in size and amount of myofibril and displayed abundant granular endoplasmic reticulum and large glycogen stores (11,12,23). The cellular heterogeneity has been interpreted as due to either differences in extent of differentiation of the same cell line or the involvement of different cell types in the disease process (14). In agreement with the smooth muscle appearance of LAM cells, α-smooth muscle actin and desmin were detected by immunohistochemistry in the cytoplasm of LAM cells, from both the lung and lymph nodes (23–25).

II. Reactivity with HMB-45 Monoclonal Antibody

LAM cells react with monoclonal antibody HMB-45 (*H*uman *M*elanoma, *B*lack) (13–16,26), an antibody generated against an extract of melanoma (27). This antibody recognizes a cytoplasmic antigen in junctional nevi but not intradermal nevi and reacts with fetal and neonatal melanocytes but not normal adult melanocytes (27). Renal angiomyolipoma (26,28–30), hepatic angiomyolipoma (31,32), clear cell tumor of the lung (33–35), cardiac rhabdomyoma, and tuberous sclerosis-associated brain lesions (36) also react with HMB-45. Unlike other tuberous sclerosis-associated lesions, subependymal giant cell astrocytomas do not stain with HMB-45 (37).

Ultrastructural studies of melanomas have shown that HMB-45 immunoreactivity is localized to melanosomes (38). HMB-45 reactivity was seen in stage 1 and 2 melanosomes (immature melanosomes without melanin) and in the nonmelanized portion of stage 3 melanosomes (38,39). In melanotic lesions, HMB-45 reactivity correlates with melanosome formation and may correlate best with factors that stimulate the formation of melanosomes such as systemic hormones and cytokines (40). HMB-45 has also been shown to react with immature melanosomes in fetal retinal pigmented epithelial cells (41). HMB-45 staining thus may be a marker of melanogenesis as opposed to a marker of melanocyte lineage (14,16,41). As Bonetti et al. (14) noted, many of the cells that demonstrate HMB-45 immunoreactivity have intracytoplasmic, membrane-bound granules; these have been noted in LAM cells (11,42), renal angiomyolipoma (30,43), hepatic angiomyolipoma (32), and clear cell tumor of the lung (34). In several clear cell tumors, Gaffey et al. (34) noted the full spectrum of melanosomes. Recent immunoelectron microscopic observations have demonstrated that the reactivity with HMB-45 in LAM cells is localized to structures with the morphological characteristics of stage 1 and 2 melanosomes (15).

Clearly, identification of antigens recognized by HMB-45 is important in understanding the biology of LAM cells. HMB-45 has been shown to react with peptides of various sizes. On Western blots, HMB-45 reacted with a 10 kDa protein from both a pigmented human cell line Mel-1 and an unpigmented metastatic melanoma cell line HM 919 (44). HMB-45 reacted with a 7 kDa peptide from Mel-57 cells and a 100 kDa protein from conditioned medium of melanoma cells (45). Among proteins from melanoma and fetal retinal pigmented epithelium, HMB-45 identified, on immunoblot analysis, a family of proteins ranging from 25 to 70 kDa, with a prominent triplet at 25 to 28 kDa (41). HMB-45 recognized antigen(s) in the range of 30–35 kDa from the human melanoma cell line HU-214 (46). Kapur et al. (41) demonstrated that pretreatment of retinal pigment epithelium paraffin sections with neuraminidase abolished HMB-45 reactivity, suggesting that the epitope is a sialylated glycoconjugate. Subsequent work with melanoma cells has supported this conclusion (46). In addition, pretreatment of renal angiomyolipoma with neuraminidase abolished staining with HMB-45 (47). Immunoprecipitation and immunoblotting studies established that an antigen recognized by HMB45 is a 100 kDa glycoprotein, termed gpl00 (48,49). An RNA species of 2.5 kb was the major product detected by a cDNA probe, which is consistent with the size of gpl00 cDNA (48). The smaller proteins may be derived from the larger 100 kDa (gp100) protein by degradation (49). gp100 mRNA was recently been detected by Northern analysis in LAM, but not in control, lung (15), consistent with the view that HMB-45 staining in LAM lung is due to the presence of gp100.

gp100 is a type-1 transmembrane glycoprotein, which is almost identical to another melanocyte-specific protein Pmel 17 (50). gp100 and Pmel 17 cDNAs originate via alternative splicing of a single transcript (49). In all normal and malignant cells expressing the gp100/Pmel 17 gene, gp100 and Pmel are expressed simultaneously (49,50). In addition, Pmel 17, like gpl00, is recognized by the monoclonal antibodies NKI-beteb, HMB-45, and HMB-50 (50). The human Pmel gene maps to chromosome 12 in the region of 12pter-ql2 (51). A linkage analysis of 15 tuberous sclerosis (TSC) families suggested the existence of a third locus for TSC (TSC3) on chromosome 12q22-24.1 (52). This is close to the phenylalanine hydroxylase (PAH) gene locus 12q22-24. In the liver, PAH catalyzes the first step in the conversion of phenylalanine to tyrosine. In addition, the structural gene for dopamine beta-hydroxylase (DBH) has been localized to 9q34 (53), the same area to which TSC1 has been mapped (54). DBH is an enzyme in the catecholamine neurotransmitter pathway, a pathway related to that of melanin synthesis (52). Thus, there may be a link between TSC and a defect in melanogenesis, as suggested by immunohistochemical and genetic studies. However, a large linkage analysis involving 1622 members of 128 families with tuberous sclerosis did not support the existence of major loci on 12q (55). TSC-determining loci have been mapped to chromosomes 9q34(TSCl) and 16pl3(TSC2), both of which have been identified (54,65) and are believed each to account for 50% of TSC families (57).

III. Immunophenotypical Heterogeneity in LAM

A. HMB-45

Immunophenotypical heterogeneity with HMB-45 has been described in human melanomas, with high-intensity staining in hypertrophied melanocytes, and lesser staining in spindle and epitheloid melanoma cells (58). Likewise, heterogeneity in HMB-45 staining has been noted in LAM; most LAM cells with strongly positive HMB-45 reactivity have epitheloid features, whereas only rare spindle cells are HMB-45 positive (13–15). This immunophenotypical heterogeneity has also been described in renal angiomyolipoma, in that HMB-45-positive cells tended to be large and epitheloid with abundant cytoplasm and a round nucleus, whereas spindle-shaped cells stained less intensely (47). Smoller et al. examined HMB-45 expression under a range of growth conditions (59); the presence of HMB-45 reactivity within melanocytes did not correlate with proliferation but was associated with activation by specific growth factors.

B. Cell Cycle

Techniques for examining cellular proliferation utilize our understanding of the cell cycle (60). Following cell division, the cell enters the Gl phase, which is of variable duration. Toward the end of this phase, in late Gl, the cell becomes committed to replication. The S, or synthetic phase, is characterized by DNA synthesis for replication of the cellular genome. DNA synthesis may occur during other phases of the cycle, however, this unscheduled synthesis, as opposed to programmed S-chase synthesis, is for repair purposes. The S-phase is relatively constant in duration and is followed by G2. After a relatively short G2 phase, mitosis (M phase) occurs. This involves breakdown of the nuclear envelope, condensation of nuclear components into visible chromosomes, formation of the mitotic spindle, alignment of the chromatids to form a metaphase plate, and subsequent migration of duplicated chromosomes to the poles of the spindle where they reconstitute intact nuclei. Cytokinesis then occurs with the formation of two cells, which are now in a new Gl stage. Mitosis is a short phase, the only part that can be examined by simple morphological examination (60–62). Most techniques for evaluating proliferation quantify cells at a specified stage of the cell cycle (state measurements). Rate measurements, which actually measure proliferation of new cells, require multiple samples over time and hence are used less often (60,62).

C. Proliferating Cell Nuclear Antigen

Proliferating cell nuclear antigen (PCNA) is a nonhistone, 37 kDa auxiliary nuclear protein (63–65). PCNA, which serves as a cofactor (processitivity factor) for DNA polymerase delta (63,66–68), is important in DNA replication and in cell-cycle progression (69–73). PCNA is also involved in DNA repair (63,74,75). There is a cyclic increase in PCNA synthesis with a peak in early S phase of the cell cycle (76). In addition, the distribution of PCNA changes with the stage of the cell cycle. Cells in Gl, G2, and mitosis stain weakly with anti-PCNA antibodies, whereas cells in S phase demonstrate variability in intensity and distribution of reactivity as they progress through the stage (77). In early S phase, PCNA is found throughout the nucleoplasm with the exception of the nucleoli. As the cell progresses through S phase, the staining becomes more intense and redistributes to the nucleoli. Based on these and other data, it is believed that monoclonal antibodies to PCNA (78,79) can serve as S phase markers (79–81). Confocal laser scanning microscopy, after simultaneous immunofluorescent labeling with bromodeoxyuridine (BrdUrd) and anti-PCNA antibodies, demonstrated that PCNA colocalizes with newly replicated DNA during the S phase (82). In addition, studies suggest that PCNA activation at sites of DNA synthesis is secondary to a phosphorylation reaction (83). Immunofluorescence studies have revealed two populations of PCNA (84). A soluble form, which is lost after fixation with organic solvents, is felt not to be related to DNA synthesis. This form, which can be seen after formaldehyde fixation, is responsible for nuclear staining throughout the cell cycle. After methanol fixation, only the insoluble PCNA, which is associated with DNA replication (S phase), reacts with anti-PCNA antibodies. PCNA immunolocalization with monoclonal antibodies has been shown to be useful in assessing cell proliferation when the histological specimens have been prepared correctly (85–88).

Dual labeling for HMB-45 and PCNA, in melanoma cells and LAM cells, was performed to determine the relationship between HMB-45 expression and cell proliferation (15). In both cell types, an inverse relationship was observed between reactivity for PCNA and HMB-45. LAM cells that were strongly reactive with HMB-45 were negative or only weakly positive for PCNA, and cells strongly positive for PCNA were negative or only weakly positive for HMB-45. Few cells reacted with both antibodies. A similar relationship was demonstrated in melanoma cells. Since LAM cells that did not react with HMB-45 were positive with anti-PCNA antibodies and may be in a more proliferative state, these cell populations may be more responsible for the progression of the disease than the characteristic HMB-45-positive cells.

IV. Importance of HMB-45

A. Diagnosis of LAM

HMB-45 staining in the lung is both specific and sensitive for the presence of LAM cells. When HMB-45 staining was examined in 52 transbronchial and 17 open lung biopsies, only the six specimens with microscopic features of LAM showed positive staining (14). Similar results were found in 72 open-lung biopsies obtained during procedures for treatment for recurrent spontaneous pneumothoraces (89). The five patients with clinical and histological features consistent with LAM had biopsies that reacted with HMB-45. Furthermore, HMB-45 immunoreactivity helped confirm the diagnosis of LAM in a patient with suggestive clinical features and only subtle smooth muscle proliferation. HMB-45 immunoreactivity was not observed in other conditions that can mimic LAM, such as primary spontaneous pneumothorax, eosinophilic granuloma, pulmonary emphysema, and idiopathic pulmonary fibrosis. Diagnosis of LAM has usually required an open or thoracoscopic lung biopsy, although the diagnosis has been made on transbronchial biopsy (90,91). The availability of HMB-45 as a sensitive and specific marker for LAM cells may help in confirming the diagnosis of LAM on tissue obtained by transbronchial biopsy (14,92,93).

B. Diagnosis of Angiomyolipoma

HMB-45 staining has also shown to be sensitive and specific for renal angiomyolipoma. Pea et al. (29) noted that HMB-45 reactivity was found in 10 angiomyolipomas, whereas 10 renal cell carcinomas, 12 retroperitoneal sarcomas, 10 Wilms' tumors, 20 normal kidneys and 5 normal adrenal glands did not react with the antibody. All of the renal angiomyolipomata demonstrated HMB-45 immunoreactivity, whereas the other lesions and the normal organs did not. In a similar study of 72 primary renal tumors and two retroperitoneal liposarcomas, HMB-45 immunoreactivity was present in 17 of 19 renal angiomyolipomata, whereas the other tumors (15 renal cell carcinomas, 8 Wilms' tumors, 6 transitional cell carcinomas, 6 mesoblastic nephromas, 4 leiomyomas, 3 leiomyosarcomas, 3 oncocytomas, 2 renal cortical adenomas, 1 squamous cell carcinoma, 1 rhabdoid tumor, 4 cystic partially differentiated nephroblastomas) were all negative (94). HMB-45 may thus help distinguish renal angiomyolipoma from other tumors of the kidney and retroperitoneum. When fine needle aspiration cytology samples from renal angiomyolipoma were tested against HMB-45, 7 of 8 cases were reactive (95). None of the control samples, including 13 renal cell carcinomas, 2 transitional cell carcinoma, and 1 squamous carcinoma, were positive for HMB-45. Since a conservative approach to management is advocated for renal angiomyolipoma, the ability to differentiate renal angiomyolipoma from other renal and retroperitoneal lesions is crucial (96,97). However, the clinical context in which the renal lesion occurs may be important in interpreting the significance of positive HMB-45 immunoreactivity. Whereas sporadic renal cell carcinoma may not demonstrate HMB-45 immunoreactivity (29,98), tuberous sclerosis–associated renal carcinoma may react with HMB-45 (98,99). Like renal angiomyolipoma, hepatic angiomyolipoma may be difficult to differentiate from other liver lesions if the fat content is low; HMB-45 staining may be useful confirming the diagnosis (31).

C. Tuberous Sclerosis and LAM

Tuberous sclerosis complex (TSC) is an autosomal dominant disorder characterized by hamartomas that involve multiple organ systems (100). Pulmonary involvement in this condition occurs in 2.3%, and although TSC occurs in both sexes, the lung disease is manifest in females (101). The pulmonary manifestations of TSC and LAM include dyspnea, pneumothorax, hemoptysis, and chylothorax. The latter is more common in LAM (102,103). The lungs in both conditions have similar appearances by CT (104,105), and histologically they are essentially identical (106). Renal angiomyolipomata are common in both LAM and TSC (2,107). The reactivity of the lesions of both LAM and TSC, with HMB-45, further supports a link between these conditions.

D. Tumor Vaccines

Intracellular proteins, like gp100, can be processed and presented as peptide targets for cytotoxic T lymphocytes (CTL) (108,109). Bakker et al. (109) demonstrated that gp100 is recognized by melanoma-derived tumor-infiltrating lymphocytes (TIL). The adoptive transfer of TILs that recognize gp100 produced objective regression of melanoma metastases (110). Immunization with tumor-associated gpl00 peptides can produce an antitumor immune response in patients with metastatic melanoma (111). Vaccines using recombinant viruses encoding gp100 have been developed (112,113). As immunotherapies are developed for the treatment of malignant melanomas, other conditions, such as LAM, that express this antigen, may also benefit.

V. Summary

LAM cells display morphological and immunophenotypical heterogeneity (Table 1). LAM cells react with HMB-45, a marker of melanogenesis, due to the expression of gp100. HMB-45 has been localized to immature melanosomes in melanocytes and to structures with the morphological characteristics of immature melanosomes in LAM. The interesting observation of an inverse relationship between HMB-45 reactivity and PCNA immunoreactivity raises issues regarding the proliferating cell in LAM. Whereas attention has been paid to HMB-45–positive cells, these may not be the determinants of prognosis in LAM. More attention

Table 1 Heterogeneity of LAM cells

	Type 1	Type 2
Microscopic	Epitheloid features Pleomorphic nuclei	Spindle shaped Elongated nuclei
E.M.	Abundant ER	Abundant myofibrils
HMB-45	Commonly positive	Rarely positive
PCNA	Rarely	Commonly positive

PCNA = Proliferating cell nuclear antigen.

needs to be paid to the PCNA-positive cells or the ratio of PCNA/HMB-45 positive cells, for this may have mechanistic and prognostic implications.

References

1. Kalassian KG, Doyle RG, Kao P, Ruoss S, Raffin T. Lymphangioleiomyomatosis: new insights. Am J Respir Crit Care Med 1997; 155:1183–1186.
2. Chu SC, Horiba K, Usuki J, Avila NA, Chen CC, Travis WD, Ferrans VJ, Moss J. Comprehensive evaluation of 25 patients with lymphangioleiomyomatosis. Am J Respir Crit Care Med 1997; 155:A330.
3. Kitaichi M, Nishimura K, Itoh H, Izumi T. Pulmonary lymphangioleiomyomatosis: a report of 46 patients including a clinicopathologic study of prognostic factors. Am J Respir Crit Care Med 1995; 151:527–533.
4. Taylor JR, Ryu J, Colby T, Raffin T. Lymphangioleiomyomatosis: clinical course in 32 patients. N Engl J Med 1990; 323:1254–1260.
5. Bradley SL, Dines DE, Soule EH, Muhm JR. Pulmonary lymphangiomyomatosis. Lung 1980; 158:69–80.
6. Corrin B, Liebow AA, Friedman PJ. Pulmonary lymphangiomyomatosis. A review. Am J Pathol 1975; 79:347–382.
7. Silverstein EF, Ellis K, Wolff M, Jaretzki A. Pulmonary lymphangiomyomatosis. Am J Roentgenol 1974; 120:832–850.
8. Hasleton PS. Pulmonary lymphangioleiomyomatosis. In: Hasleton PS, ed. Spencer's Pathology of the Lung. 5th ed. New York: McGraw-Hill, 1996:939–983.
9. Carrington CB, Cugell DW, Gaensler EA, Marks A, Redding RA, Schaff JT, Tomasian A. lymphangioleiomyomatosis. Physiologic-pathologic-radiologic correlations. Am Rev Respir Dis 1977; 116:977–995.
10. Joliat G, Stalder H, Kapanci Y. Lymphangiomyomatosis: a clinico-anatomical entity. Cancer 1972; 31:455–461.
11. Basset F, Soler P, Marsac J, Corrin B. Pulmonary lymphangiomyomatosis. Three new cases studied with electron microscopy. Cancer 1976; 38:2357–2366.
12. Kane PB, Lane BP, Cordice JWV, Greenberg GM. Ultrastructure of the proliferating cells in pulmonary lymphangiomyomatosis. Arch Pathol Lab Med 1978; 102:618–622.
13. Bonetti F, Pea M, Martignoni G, Zamboni G, Iuzzolino P. Cellular heterogeneity in lymphangiomyomatosis of the lung. Hum Pathol 1991; 22:727–728.
14. Bonetti F, Chiodera PL, Pea M, Martignoni G, Bosi F, Zamboni G, Mariuzzi GM. Transbronchial biopsy in lymphangiomyomatosis of the lung. HMB45 for diagnosis. Am J Surg Pathol 1993; 17:1092–1102.
15. Usuki J, Horiba K, Matsumoto Y, Chu SC, Ferrans VJ, Moss J. Inverse correlation between markers of cell proliferation and expression of melanosomal antigens in smooth muscle cells in lymphangioleiomyomatosis (LAM) and in cultured melanoma cell lines. Am J Respir Crit Care Med 1998; 157:806A.
16. Bacci CE, Bonetti F, Pea M, Martignoni G, Gown AM. HMB-45: a review. Appl Immunohistochem 1996; 4:73–85.

17. Enterline HT, Roberts B. Lymphangiopericytoma. Case report of a previously undescribed tumor type. Cancer 1955; 8:582–587.
18. Corning JL, Jr., Enterline HT. Lymphangiomyoma, a benign lesion of chyliferous lymphatics synonymous with lymphangiopericytoma. Cancer 1966; 19:1909–1930.
19. Frack MD, Simon L, Dawson BH. The lymphangiomyomatosis syndrome. Cancer 1968; 22:428–437.
20. Basset F, Soler P, Marsac J, Corrin B. Pulmonary lymphangiomyomatosis. Three new cases studied with electron microscopy. Cancer 1976; 38:2357–2366.
21. Wolff M. Lymphangiomyoma: clinicopathologic study and ultrastructural confirmation of its histogenesis. Cancer 1972; 31:988–1007.
22. Vázquez JJ, Fernández-Cuervo L, Fidalgo B. Lymphangiomyomatsis. Morphogenetic study and ultrastructure confirmation of the histogenesis of the lung lesion. Cancer 1976; 37:2321–2328.
23. Peyrol S, Gindre D, Cordier JF, Loire R, Grimaud A. Characterization of the smooth muscle cell infiltrate and associated connective matrix of lymphangiomyomatosis. Immunohistochemical and ultrastructural study of two cases. J Pathol 1992; 168:387–395.
24. Matthews TJ, Hornall D, Sheppard MN. Comparison of the use of antibodies to α smooth muscle actin and desmin in pulmonary lymphangioleiomyomatosis. J Clin Path 1993; 46:497–480.
25. Õsterborg A, Christensson B, Silfverswärd C, Biberfeld P, Collins VP, Sunblad R, Mellstedt H. Lymphangiomyomatosis-immunohistochemical analysis of a case presenting with enlarged inguinal lymph nodes and without pulmonary involvement. Acta Oncol 1988; 28:287–289.
26. Hoon V, Thung SN, Kaneko M, Unger PD. HMB-45 reactivity in renal angiomyolipoma and lymphangioleiomyomatosis. Arch Pathol Lab Med 1994; 118:732–734.
27. Gown AM, Vogel AM, Hoak D, Gough F, McNutt MA. Monoclonal antibodies specific for melanocytic tumors distinguish subpopulations of melanocytes. Am J Pathol 1986; 123:195–203.
28. Chan JKC, Tsang WYW, Pau MY, Tang MC, Pang SW, Fletcher CDM. Lymphangiomyomatosis and angiomyolipoma: closely related entities characterized by hamartomatous proliferation of HMB-45-positive smooth muscle. Histopathology 1993; 22:445–455.
29. Pea M, Bonetti F, Zamboni G, Martignoni G, Riva M, Colombari R, Mombelli A, Bonzanini M, Scarpa A, Ghimenton C, Donati LF. Melanocyte-marker-HMB-45 is regularly expressed in angiomyolipoma of the kidney. Pathology 1991; 23:185–188.
30. Kaiserling E, Kröber S, Xiao J-C, Schaumburg-Lever G. Angiomyolipoma of the kidney. Immunoreactivity with HMB-45. Light-and electron-microscopic findings. Histopathology 1994; 25:41–48.
31. Terris B, Fléjou J-F, Picot R, Belghiti J, Hénin D. Hepatic angiomyolipoma. A report of four cases with immunohistochemical and DNA-flow cytometric studies. Arch Pathol Lab Med 1996; 120:68–72.
32. Weeks DA, Malott RL, Arneson M, Zuppan C, Aitken D, Mierau G. Hepatic

angiomyolipoma with striated granules and positivity with melanoma-specific antibody (HMB-45): a report of two cases. Ultrastruct Pathol 1991; 15:563–571.
33. Bonetti F, Pea M, Martignoni G, Doglioni C, Zamboni G, Capelli P, Rimondi P, Andrion A. Clear cell ("sugar") tumor of the lung is a lesion strictly related to angiomyolipoma—the concept of a family of lesions characterized by the presence of perivascular epitheloid cells (PEC). Pathology 1994; 26:230–236.
34. Gaffey MJ, Mills SE, Zarbo RJ, Weiss LM, Gown AM. Clear cell tumor of the lung. Immunohistochemical and ultrastructural evidence of melanogenesis. Am J Surg Pathol 1991; 15:644–653.
35. Gal AA, Koss MN, Hochholzer L, Cheifec G. An immunohistochemical study of benign clear cell ('Sugar') tumor of the lung. Arch Pathol Lab Med 1991; 115:1034–1038.
36. Weeks DA, Chase DR, Malott RL, Chase RL, Zuppan CW, Beckwith JB, Mierau GW. HMB-45 staining in angiomyolipoma, cardiac rhabdomyoma, other mesenchymal processes, and tuberous sclerosis-associated brain lesions. Int J Surg Pathol 1994; 1:191–198.
37. Gyure KA, Prayson RA. Subependymal giant cell astrocytoma: a clinicopathological study with HMB-45 and MIB-1 immunohistochemical analysis. Mod Pathol 10:313–317.
38. Schaumburg-Lever G, Metzler G, Kaiserling E. Ultrastructural localization of HMB-45 binding sites. J Cutan Pathol 1991; 18:432–435.
39. Taatjes DJ, Arendash-Durand B, von Turkovich M, Trainer TD. HMB-45 antibody demonstrates melanosome specificity by immunoelectron microscopy. Arch Pathol Lab Med 1993; 117:264–268.
40. Skelton III HG, Smith KJ, Barrett TL, Lupton GP, Graham JH. HMB-45 staining in benign and malignant melanocytic lesions. A reflection of cellular activation. Am J Dermatopathol 1991; 13:543–550.
41. Kapur RP, Bigler SA, Skelly M, Gown AM. Anti-melanoma monoclonal antibody HMB45 identifies an oncofetal glycoconjugate associated with immature melanosomes. J Histochem Cytochem 1992; 40:207–212.
42. Fukuda Y, Kawamoto M, Yamamoto A, Ishizaki M, Basset F, Masugi Y. Role of elastic fiber degradation in emphysema-like lesions of pulmonary lymphangiomyomatosis. Hum Pathol 1990; 21:1252–1261.
43. Mukai M, Torikata C, Ira H, Tamai S, Sugiura H, Tanaka Y, Sakamoto M, Hirohashi S. Crystalloids in angiomyolipoma. A previously unnoticed phenomenon of renal angiomyolipoma occurring at a high frequency. Am J Surg Pathol 1992; 16:1–10.
44. Esclamado RM, Gown AM, Vogel AM. Unique proteins defined by monoclonal antibodies specific for human melanoma. Some potential clinical applications. Am J Surg 1986; 152:376–385.
45. Vennegoor C, Hageman P, van Nouhijs H, Ruiter DJ, Calafat J, Ringens PJ, Rümke P. A monoclonal antibody specific for cells of the melanocyte lineage. Am J Pathol 1988; 130:179–192.
46. Chiamenti AM, Vella F, Bonnetti F, Pea M, Ferrari S, Martignoni G, Benedetti A, Suzuki H. Anti-melanoma monoclonal antibody HMB-45 on enhanced chemi-

luminescence-western blotting recognizes a 30-35 kDa melanosome-associated sialated glycoprotein. Melanoma Res 1996; 6:291–298.
47. Sturtz CL, Dabbs DJ. Angiomyolipomas: the nature and expression of the HMB-45 antigen. Mod Pathol 1994; 7:842–845.
48. Adema GJ, de Boer AJ, van't Hullenaar R, Denijin M, Ruiter DJ, Vogel AM, Figdor CG. Melanocyte lineage-specific antigens recognized by monoclonal antibodies NK1-beteb, HMB-50 and HMB-45 are encoded by a single cDNA. Am J Pathol 1993; 143:1579–1585.
49. Adema GJ, de Boer AJ, Vogel AM, Loenen WA, Figdor CG. Molecular characterization of the melanocytic lineage-specific antigen gp100. J Biol Chem 1994; 269:20126–20133.
50. Adema GJ, Bakker ABH, de Boer AJ, Hohenstein P, Figdor CG. pMel 17 is recognized by monoclonal antibodies NK1-beteb, HMB-45 and HMB-50 and by anti-melanoma CTL. Br J Cancer 1996; 73:1044–1048.
51. Kwon BS, Chintamaneni C, Kozak A, Copeland G, Gilbert DJ, Jenkins N, Barton D, Francke U, Kobayashi Y, Kim KK. A melanocyte-specific gene, Pmel 17, maps near the silver coat color locus on mouse chromosome 10 and is in a syntenic region on human chromosome 12. Proc Natl Acad Sci 1991; 88:9228–9232.
52. Fahsold R, Rott H-D, Lorenz P. A third gene locus for tuberous sclerosis is closely linked to the phenylalanine hydroxylase gene locus. Hum Genet 1991; 88:85–90.
53. Craig SP, Buckle VJ, Lamouroux A, Mallet J, Craig IW. Localization of the human dopamine beta hydroxylase (DBH) gene to chromosome 9q34. Cytogenet Cell Genet 1988; 48:48–50.
54. TSC1 consortium. Identification of the tuberous sclerosis gene TSC1 on chromosome 9q34. Science 1997; 277:805–808.
55. Sampson JR, Janssen AJ, Sandkuijl, and the Tuberous Sclerosis Collaborative Group. Linkage investigation of three putative tuberous sclerosis determining loci on chromosomes 9q, 11q, and 12q. J Med Genet 1992; 29:861–866.
56. The European Chromosome 16 Tuberous Sclerosis Consortium. Identification and characterization of the tuberous sclerosis gene on chromosome 16. Cell 1993; 75:1305–1315.
57. Sampson JR, Harris PC. The molecular genetics of tuberous sclerosis. Hum Mol Genet 1994; 3:1477–1480.
58. Bodey B, Kaiser HE, Goldfarb R. Immunophenotypically varied cell subpopulations in primary and metastatic human melanomas. Monoclonal antibodies for diagnosis detection of neoplastic progression and receptor directed immunotherapy. Anticancer Res 1996; 16:517–532.
59. Smoller BR, Hsu A, Kruger J. HMB-45 monoclonal antibody recognizes an inducible and reversible melanocyte cytoplasmic protein. J Cutan Pathol 1991; 18:315–322.
60. Dover R. An overview of methodologies for assessing proliferation and cell death. In: Jankowski JAZ, Polak JM, eds. Clinical Gene Analysis and Manipulation: Tools, Techniques and Troubleshooting. Cambridge: Cambridge University Press, 1995:151–163.
61. The cell division cycle. In: Alberts B, Bray D, Lewis J, Raff M, Roberts K, Watson

JD, eds. Molecular Biology of the Cell. 3d ed. Garland Publishing, Inc., 1994:864–870.

62. Hall PA, Levison DA. Review: assessment of cell proliferation in histological material. J Clin Pathol 1990; 43:184–192.
63. Kelman Z. PCNA: structure, functions and interactions. Oncogene 1997; 14:629–40.
64. Elias JM. Cell proliferation indexes: a biomarker in solid tumors. Biotech Histochem 1997; 72:78–85.
65. Hyde-Dunn J, Jones GE. Visualization of cell replication using antibody to proliferating cell nuclear antigen. Methods Mol Biol 1997; 75:341–347.
66. Fairman MP. DNA polymerase ∂/PCNA: actions and interactions. J Cell Sci 1990; 95:1–4.
67. Bravo R, Frank R, Blundell PA, Macdonald-Bravo H. Cyclin/PCNA is the auxiliary protein of DNA polymerase-∂. Nature 1987; 326:515–517.
68. Prelich G, Tan C-K, Kostura M, Mathews MB, So AG, Downey KM, Stillman B. Functional identity of proliferating cell nuclear antigen and a DNA polymerase-∂ auxiliary protein. Nature 1987; 326:517–520.
69. Wold MS, Weinberg DH, Virshup DM, Li JJ, Kelly TJ. Identification of cellular proteins required for simian virus 40 DNA replication. J Biol Chem 1989; 264:2801–2809.
70. Prelich G, Stillman B. Coordinated leading and lagging strand synthesis during SV40 DNA replication in vitro requires PCNA. Cell 1988; 53:117–126.
71. Prelich G, Kostura M, Marshak DR, Mathews MB, Stillman B. The cell-cycle regulated proliferating cell nuclear antigen is required for SV40 DNA replication in vitro. Nature 1987; 326:471–475.
72. Jaskulski D, DeRiel JK, Mercer WE, Calabretta B, Baserga R. Inhibition of cellular proliferation by antisense oligodeoxynucleotides to PCNA cyclin. Science 1988; 240:1544–1546.
73. Celis JE, Madsen P, Cellis A, Nielsen HV, Gesser B. Cyclin (PCNA, auxiliary protein of DNA polymerase ∂) is a central component of the pathway(s) leading to DNA replication and cell division. FEBS Lett 1987; 220:1–7.
74. Toschi L, Bravo R. Changes in cyclin/proliferating cell nuclear antigen distribution during DNA repair synthesis. J Cell Biol 1988; 107:1623–1628.
75. Celis JE, Madsen P. Increased nuclear cyclin?PCNA antigen staining of non S-phase transformed human amnion cells engaged in nucleotide excision DNA repair. FEBS Lett 1986; 209:277–283.
76. Morris GF, Mathews MB. Regulation of proliferating cell nuclear antigen during the cell cycle. J Biol Chem 1989; 264:13856–13864.
77. Celis JE, Celis A. Cell cycle-dependent variations in the distribution of the nuclear protein cyclin proliferating cell nuclear antigen in cultured cell: subdivision of S phase. Proc Natl Acad Sci USA 1985; 82:3262–3266.
78. Ogata K, Kurki P, Celis J, Nakumura RM, Tan EM. Monoclonal antibodies to a nuclear protein (PCNA/cyclin) associated with DNA replication. Exp Cell Res 1987; 168:475–486.
79. Waseem NH, Lane DP. Monoclonal antibody analysis of the proliferating cell

nuclear antigen (PCNA). Structural conservation and the detection of a nuclear form. J Cell Sci 1990; 96:121–129.
80. Beppu T, Ishida Y, Detection of S phase cells with an antibody to proliferating cell nuclear antigen (PCNA). J Histotechnol 1994; 17:325–328.
81. Landberg G, Roos G. Antibodies to proliferating cell nuclear antigen as S phase probes in flow cytometric cell cycle analysis. Cancer Res 1991; 51:4570–4574.
82. Humbert C, Santisteban MS, Usson Y, Robert-Nicoud M. Intranuclear co-localization of newly replicated DNA and PCNA by simultaneous immunofluorescent labelling and confocal microscopy in MCF-7 cells. J Cell Sci 1992; 103:97–103.
83. Prosperi E, Scovassi I, Stivala LA, Bianchi L. Proliferating cell nuclear antigen bound to DNA synthesis sites: phosphorylation and association with cyclin D1 and cylin A. Exp Cell Res 1994; 215:257–262.
84. Bravo R, Macdonald-Bravo H. Existence of two populations of cyclin/proliferating cell nuclear antigen during the cell cycle: association with DNA replication sites. J Cell Biol 1987; 105:1549–1554.
85. Kurki P, Ogata K, Tan EM. Monoclonal antibodies to proliferating cell nuclear antigen (PCNA)/cyclin as probes for proliferating cells by immunofluorescence microscopy and flow cytometry. J Immunol Methods 1988; 109:49–59.
86. Garcia RL, Coltrera MD, Gown AM. Analysis of proliferative grade using anti-PCNA/cyclin monoclonal antibodies in fixed, embedded tissues. Am J Pathol 1989; 134:733–739.
87. Hall PA, Levison DA, Woods AL, et al. Proliferating cell nuclear antigen (PCNA) immunolocalization in paraffin sections: an index of cell proliferation with evidence of deregulated expression in some neoplasms. J Pathol 1990; 162:285–294.
88. Shin DM, Varavud N, Ro JY, Lee JS, Hong WK, Hittelman WN. Sequential increases in proliferating cell nuclear antigen expression in head and neck tumorigenesis: a potential biomarker. J Natl Cancer Inst 1993; 85:971–978.
89. Tanaka H, Imada A, Morikawa T, Shibusa T, Satoh M, Sekina K, Abe S. Diagnosis of pulmonary lymphangioleiomyomatosis by HMB45 in surgically treated spontaneous pneumothorax. Eur Respir J 1995; 8:1879–1882.
90. Delgrande E, Delgrande B, Wallon J, Rosoux P. Diagnostic approach to pulmonary lymphangioleiomyomatosis. J Int Med 1994; 236:461–464.
91. Kuwabara H, Biyazima S, Osaka T, Yasuhara F, Chizimiatsu Y, Inatomi K, Washizaki M, Homma H, Saeki S, Yamanaka A. A case of pulmonary lymphangiomyomatosis diagnosed by TBLB and treated with progesterone and oophorectomy. Nippon Kyobu Shikkan Gakkai Zasshi 1984; 22:795–799.
92. Guinee DG, Feuerstein I, Koss MN, Travis WD. Pulmonary lymphangioleiomyomatosis. Diagnosis based on results of transbronchial biopsy and immunohistochemical studies and correlation with high-resolution computed tomography findings. Arch Pathol Lab Med 1994; 118:846–849.
93. Chiodera F, Pea M, Martignoni G, Zamboni G, Maran M, Montresor C, Mombello A, Bonetti F. Transbronchial biopsies in lymphangioleiomyomatosis of the lung: Moab HMB-45 is helpful for the diagnosis. Mod Pathol 1993; 6:129A.
94. Ashfaq R, Weinberg AG, Albores-Saavedra. J. Renal angiomyolipoma and HMB-45 reactivity. Cancer 1993; 71:3091–3097.

95. Bonzanini M, Pea M, Martignoni G, Zamboni G, Capelli P, Bernardello F, Bonetti F. Preoperative diagnosis of renal angiomyolipoma: fine needle aspiration cytology and immunocytochemical characterization. Pathology 1994; 26:170–175.
96. Steiner MS, Goldman SM, Fishman EK, Marshall FF. The natural history of renal angiomyolipma. J Urol 1993; 1782–1786.
97. Oesterling JE, Fishman EK, Goldman SM, Marshall FF. The management of renal angiomyolipoma. J Urol 1986; 135:1121–1124.
98. Bjornsson J, Nasimento AG, Gulino S. The expression of neural crest-associated markers in normal kidney and renal angiomyolipomas and carcinomas in patients with and without tuberous sclerosis. Mod Pathol 1995; 8:73A.
99. Bjornsson J, Short MP, Kwiatkowski DJ, Henske EP. Tuberous sclerosis-associated renal cell carcinoma. Clinical, pathological, and genetic features. Am J Pathol 1996; 149:1201–1208.
100. Kwiatkowski DJ, Short MP. Tuberous sclerosis. Arch Dermatol 1994; 130:348–354.
101. Castro M, Shepherd CW, Gomez MR, Lie JT, Ryu JH. Pulmonary tuberous sclerosis. Chest 1995; 107:189–195.
102. Valensi QJ. Pulmonary lymphangiomyoma, a probable forme fruste of tuberous sclerosis. Am Rev Respir Dis 1973; 108:1411–1415.
103. Broughton RBK. Pulmonary tuberous sclerosis presenting with pleural effusion. Br Med J 1970; 1:477–478.
104. Lenoir S, Grenier P, Brauner MW, Frija J, Remy-Jardin M, Revel D, Cordier J-F. Pulmonary lymphangiomyomatosis and tuberous sclerosis: comparison of radiographic and thin-section CT findings. Radiology 1990; 175:329–334.
105. Peng S-F, Chang Y-C, Su C-T, Yang P-C, Yao Y-T, Huang K-M, Hsu JC-Y. High-resolution computed tomography in pulmonary lymphangio(leio)myomatosis and pulmonary tuberous sclerosis. J Formos Med Ass 1996; 95:399–402.
106. Carron F, Ameille J, Leclerc P, Mornet P, Barbagellata M, Reynes M, Rochemaure J. Pulmonary lymphangioleiomyomatosis and Bourneville's tuberous sclerosis with pulmonary involvement: the same disease? Cancer 1983; 52:851–852.
107. Gomez M. Phenotypes of the tuberous sclerosis complex with a revision of diagnostic criteria. Ann NY Acad Sci 1991; 615:1–7.
108. Townsend A, Bodmer H. Antigen recognition by class I-restricted T lymphocytes. Ann Rev Immunol 1989; 7:601–624.
109. Bakker ABH, Schreurs MWJ, de Boer AJ, Kawakami Y, Rosenberg SA, Adema GJ, Figdor CG. Melanocyte lineage-specific antigen gp100 is recognized by melanoma-derived tumor-infiltrating lymphocytes. J Exp Med 1994; 179:1005–1009.
110. Kawakami Y, Eliyahu S, Delgado CH, Robbins PF, Sakaguchi K, Appella E, Yannelli JR, Adema GJ, Miki T, Rosenberg SA. Identification of a human melanoma antigen recognized by tumor-infiltrating lymphocytes associated with in vivo tumor rejection. Proc Natl Acad Sci 1994; 91:6458–6462.
111. Salgaller ML, Marincola FM, Cormier JN, Rosenberg SA. Immunization against epitopes in the human melanoma antigen gp100 following patient immunization with synthetic peptides. Cancer Res 1996; 56:4749–4757.
112. Zhai Y, Yang JC, Kawakami Y, Spiess P, Wadsworth SC, Cardoza LM, Couture

LA, Smith AE, Rosenberg SA. Antigen-specific tumor vaccines. Development and characterization of recombinant adenoviruses encoding MART1 or gp100 for cancer therapy. J Immunol 1996; 156:700–710.

113. Sakai C, Kawakami Y, Law LW, Furumura M, Hearing Jr., VJ. Melanosomal proteins as melanoma-specific immune targets. Rev Melanoma Res 1997; 7:83–95.

26

Oxidants and Antioxidants in Lung Injury
Potential Links with LAM

ANDRÉ M. CANTIN and BENOIT PAQUETTE

University of Sherbrooke
Sherbrooke, Quebec, Canada

I. Introduction

Lymphangioleiomyomatosis (LAM) is an uncommon lung disease (incidence < 1:100,000/year) affecting almost exclusively women in their child-bearing years (1). It is a disease of unknown etiology for which there is no cure. Kaplan-Meier plots of actuarial survival from several, but not all studies, would suggest that LAM is often associated with a fatal outcome within 10 years of diagnosis (2–5). One of the remarkable aspects of research in LAM is that despite the rarity of this condition, considerable information has been gathered (for review, see Ref. 1), which now allows us to predict that oxygen radicals are likely to play a major role not only in the pathophysiology, but possibly also in the etiology of LAM. The evidence leading to this assertion is summarized in this chapter.

II. Oxidants, Antioxidants, and Lung Disease

A. Oxidants

Oxygen is one of the most abundant elements in our world, comprising 47% of the earth's crust and 21% of the air we breathe (6). It is an essential molecule to support the combustion of organic compounds, a process by which mammalian cells generate the energy needed to sustain life (7). Although 90% of the oxygen consumed by cells undergoes a four-electron reduction to water by the cytochrome oxidase system without generating toxic species, the other 10% of oxygen utilized by cells undergoes single electron reductions, thus generating highly reactive, toxic oxidants (6). Many of these oxidants are free radicals, however, one of the oxidants of major biological importance is hydrogen peroxide (H_2O_2), which is not a free radical. We will therefore refer to these reactive oxygen species as oxidants rather than radicals. The major oxidant species derived from oxygen are summarized in Figure 1.

Single electron reduction of oxygen results in the formation of superoxide ($O_2^{\cdot-}$). Several enzymes, known as oxidases, are capable of reducing oxygen to form superoxide. One of the better known enzyme systems relevant to superoxide synthesis in the lung is NADPH oxidase, which is a membrane-bound enzyme complex particularly important in enabling phagocytes to kill bacteria (8). Deficiency of the NADPH oxidase system is the cause of chronic granulomatous disease (CGD), a condition characterized by recurrent bacterial infections, ultimately leading to death (8). In contrast to CGD, excess NADPH oxidase activity is observed in patients with interstitial lung diseases such as idiopathic pulmonary fibrosis. NADPH oxidase–dependent oxidant release is thought to play a significant role in the development of lung injury associated with pulmonary fibrosis (9).

In addition to oxidases, superoxide can be formed by nonezymatic oxidation-reduction cycling of specific compounds known as quinones and semiquinones (Fig. 2). Quinones and semiquinones are derived from the oxidation of various hydroxyphenols, which may be either exogenous (e.g., environmental pollutants such as benzene, benzo[*a*]pyrene, and 1-naphthol or chemotherapeutic agents such as diaziquones, anthracyclines, and mitomycin) or endogenous (e.g., cathechols, DOPA, or hydroxyestrones) (10–14). The role of the latter compounds may be critically important in the disease process of LAM, as will be discussed below.

Because superoxide is a very reactive species, it can directly attack targets, such as polyunsaturated fatty acids, as well as follow one of the two pathways that lead to the formation of the highly toxic hydroxyl radical (·OH). In the first pathway, superoxide can dismutate through a one-electron reduction to hydrogen peroxide (H_2O_2). Dismutation is catalyzed by the enzymes CuZn superoxide dismutase (SOD) in the cytoplasm and MnSOD in the mitochondria (15). Once H_2O_2 is formed, it is a stable species capable of diffusing through membranes and reacting with ferrous ions present even at remote sites to form ·OH (Fenton reaction) (6). The formation of ·OH is markedly accelerated when superoxide follows a second pathway, reducing ferric to ferrous ions, which subsequently catalyze the synthesis of ·OH from H_2O_2 (the iron-catalyzed Haber-Weiss reaction) (16).

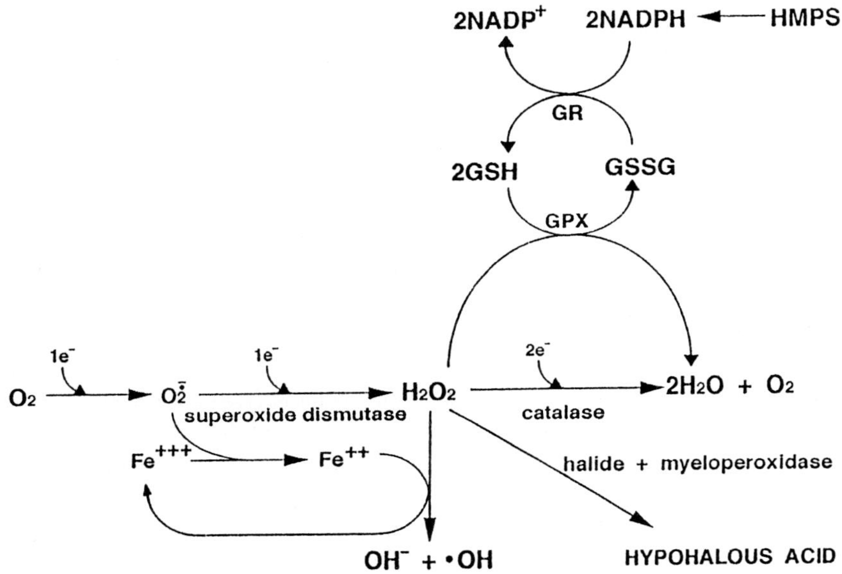

Figure 1 Oxidant synthesis and antioxidant enzymes in mammalian cells. O_2: Oxygen; O_2^-: superoxide; H_2O_2: hydrogen peroxide; Fe^{3+}: ferric ion; Fe^{2+}: ferrous ion; ·OH: hydroxyl radical; GSH: glutathione; GSSG: glutathione disulfide; GPX: glutathione peroxidase; GR: glutathione reductase; NADP+: nicotinamide adenine dinucleotide; HMPS: hexose monophosphate shunt system.

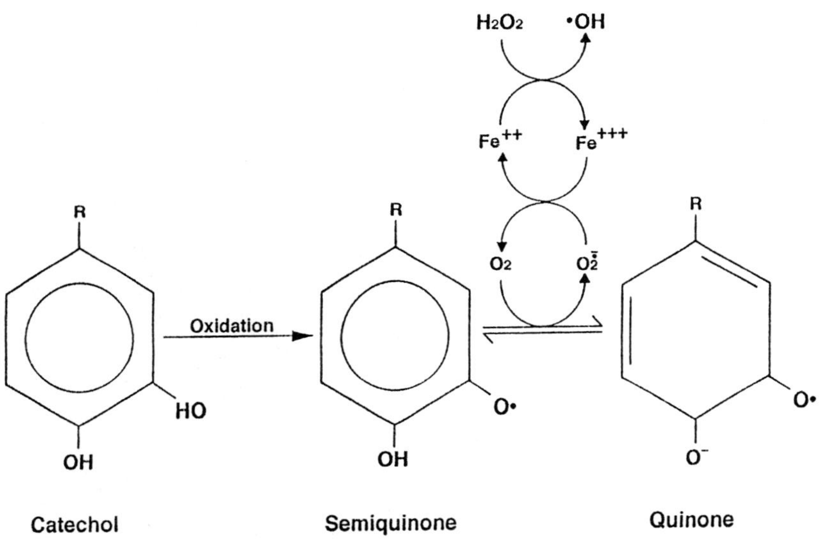

Figure 2 Structure-relation of catechols, semiquinones, and quinones. The two hydroxyl group locations are not specific and could be elsewhere on the aromatic ring.

Hydrogen peroxide is also capable of reacting with halides such as chloride in the presence of neutrophil-derived myeloperoxidase or eosinophil-derived peroxidase to form the potent oxidant hypohalous acid (HOCl) (17). Hypohalous acid (or hypohalide; OCl^- ionization is dependent upon the pH of the milieu) is highly toxic for cells and oxidatively inactivates alpha[1]-proteinase inhibitor (α1PI) (18). Oxidation of α1PI leads to a loss of the lung's major protective mechanism against neutrophil elastase–mediated tissue destruction and is thought to play a major role in the pathophysiology of emphysema (19). Hypohalous acid can also react with various primary and secondary amines to form stable chloramines. One of the most abundant sources of amines is the sulfonic amino acid taurine derived from neutrophils. Taurine oxidation by HOCl leads to the formation of taurine mono- or dichloramines in neutral and low pH, respectively (20). The taurine chloramines are organic anions that can enter lung epithelial cells through the DIDS-sensitive anion exchanger. Taurine dichloramines are approximately 100-fold more toxic than monochloramines. Once in the cell, taurine monochloramines are reduced through the glutathione system. However, at an acid pH, the much more toxic taurine dichloramines are formed, and once in the cells they induce cytotoxicity (21).

In addition to their potential for modulating protein function and inducing cytotoxicity, oxidants have recently been shown to play a major role in activating the transcription of several inflammatory genes (22). Hydrogen peroxide can diffuse through cell membranes and activate the transcription factor protein complex, NFκB (23). Once activated, NFκB binds to specific nucleotide sequences of several pro-inflammatory genes such as those of the proteins interleukin-8, immunoglobulins, tumor necrosis factor alpha, interleukin-l, and others. The binding of NFκB to nucleotide sequences in the 5′-flanking region of these genes activates their transcription, thus enhancing the inflammatory response.

B. Antioxidants

The lung is potentially exposed to many sources of toxic oxidants. Since inhaled air is 21% oxygen, the lung oxygen tensions are the highest of all tissues in the body. The lung is also often directly exposed to other inhaled oxidant gases, such as cigarette smoke and ozone, as well as to oxidant-generating inorganic particles, such as silica and asbestos (24). In addition to being exposed to inhaled oxidants, the vital gas-exchange function of the lung results in the pulmonary vasculature being exposed to the entire volume of the body's blood at least 1500 times a day. Any potential bloodborne oxidant sources such as metabolic products and xenobiotics will therefore have recurrent access to the lower respiratory tract. The only way the lung survives this massive exposure to numerous oxidant sources is through an elaborate and effective antioxidant system.

In addition to superoxide dismutases (discussed above), which detoxify superoxide, lung cells, particularly type II epithelial cells and macrophages, are rich in catalase. Catalase is a 240 kDa enzyme comprised of four polypeptide chains each containing a prosthetic group (protoporphyrin IX) at the active site allowing the catalytic two-electron reduction of H_2O_2 to water (25). Catalase is most effective in the presence of high H_2O_2 concentrations. In the presence of either low concentrations of H_2O_2 or of other peroxides, the glutathione (GSH) system plays a critical detoxification role (26). Glutathione-mediated reduction of peroxides is catalyzed by glutathione peroxidase. The glutathione disulfide (GSSG) formed during this reaction is restored to GSH through glutathione reductase, which utilizes NADPH generated from the hexose monophosphate shunt system as an electron donor.

Several of the cell's antioxidant systems are highly regulated, allowing the lung to adapt to a sustained oxidant stress. This is the case when the lung is chronically exposed to hyperoxia (27). Another example of antioxidant adaptation is that of subjects who chronically expose their lung epithelial cells to the high oxidant burden of cigarette smoke. These individuals have increased GSH in their lungs (28). The 5′-flanking region of the gene encoding the rat limiting enzyme in GSH synthesis, γ-glutamylcysteinyl synthetase (γGCS), contains an antioxidant response element (ARE), which increases transcription upon exposure to peroxides (29). Oxidant interaction with the ARE of the γ-GCS gene may lead to the increased lung epithelial lining fluid GSH levels observed in cigarette smokers.

Antoxidant systems can also be downregulated by certain mediators relevant to lung injury particularly transforming growth factor beta (TGF-β). Alveolar macrophages and lung epithelial cells have been shown to express TGF-β in a variety of lung diseases associated with tissue destruction and interstitial fibrosis (30–32). Liver cells exposed to TGF-β decrease their expression of catalase and glutathione reductase, two key enzymes in the detoxification of H_2O_2 (33). We have recently observed a similar effect of TGF-β on lung epithelial cells (34). In addition, we found that TGF-β1 markedly depletes lung epithelial cell GSH in vitro by suppressing the transcription of the γ-GCS gene (34).

Although each of the antioxidant systems discussed above is located within cells, it is clear that the lung is also uniquely protected against oxidants by catalase, GSH, and other low molecular weight antioxidants present in the extracellular milieu of the alveolar epithelial lining fluid (28,35). It is possible that extracellular antioxidants in the lung may play a role as a first line of defense against oxidants derived from inflammatory cells recruited to the alveolar surface.

C. Lung Disease

The list of lung diseases in which oxidants are thought to play a major pathophysiological or etiological role is long and growing (9,18,19,24,27,30–32,36–40). A partial list of major lung diseases associated with oxidants is presented in Table 1. In several of these lung diseases, such as hyperoxic lung injury, bleomycin-

Table 1 Lung Diseases Associated with Oxygen Radicals

Disease	Mechanism	Ref.
Emphysema	Tissue injury by oxidants in cigarette smoke Tissue injury by inflammatory cell oxidants α1PI inactivation by cigarette smoke α1PI inactivation by inflammatory cells	18,19
Adult respiratory distress syndrome	Inflammatory cell release of oxidants α1PI oxidative inactivation by inflammatory cells	37
Hyperoxia	Hyperoxia-mediated oxygen radical synthesis in cells	27
Idiopathic pulmonary fibrosis	Inflammatory cell oxidant release Glutathione deficiency	9,36
Inorganic dust disease	Inflammatory cell oxidant release Particle-mediated hydroxyl radical formation	24
Bleomycin	Iron-catalyzed superoxide and ·OH synthesis	30–32
BCNU	Inhibition of glutathione reductase	38
Paraquat	NADPH/cytochrome P450 reductase superoxide formation	39
Ionizing radiation	Hydroxyl radical production	40

associated fibrosis, paraquat injury, and ionizing radiation fibrosis, oxidants have been shown to cause the disease process. In addition to an association with an oxidant excess, it is interesting to note that some of these diseases such as IPF and BCNU toxicity are associated with antioxidant deficiencies. Patients with IPF express high levels of TGF-β1 in their lung epithelial cells (30,31). Expression of TGF-β may explain the low alveolar epithelial lining fluid GSH observed in patients with IPF (34). Clearly, the normal lung survives in a delicate balance between oxidant stress and antioxidant protection. A significant shift in this balance, through either an increased oxidant burden or an antioxidant deficiency, has the potential to result in tissue destruction and in mesenchymal cell proliferation with fibrosis.

III. Potential Role of Oxidants in LAM

A. Lung Histopathology of LAM

One of the prominent features in the LAM lung is the presence of cystic changes associated with hyperplastic type II cells and hemosiderin-laden macrophages (41). The extent of cystic changes has been found to indicate a poor prognosis (2). Elastic fiber degradation reminiscent of changes observed in lungs with an elastase/β1PI imbalance have also been reported, raising the possibility of oxidative inactivation of α1PI (1). However, the key histopathological feature observed in the lungs of patients with LAM is abnormal HMB-45 antigen-positive smooth muscle cell proliferation along the lymphatics, with discrete micronodular proliferation affecting lung parenchyma diffusely in the more advanced stages (42). While several growth factors have been identified as potent mitogens for mesenchymal cells, it is most interesting to note two recent observations indicating that oxidants can mediate mesenchymal cell proliferation. First, H_2O_2 has been shown to be required for vascular smooth muscle cell proliferation in response to platelet-derived growth factor (43). Second, a recent study by Irani et al. suggests that superoxide acts as a mediator of Ras-induced cell cycle progression in fibroblasts (44,45). In light of these studies, oxidant release may be a major factor in the induction of smooth muscle cell proliferation associated with LAM.

The abnormal cells in LAM lung tissues are distinctive in that their cytoplasm stains positively with the monoclonal antibody HMB-45 (42). The HMB-45–reactive antigen has been well characterized, and studies have shown it has full homology with the protein encoded by cDNA of Pmel 17, a protein thought to play a critical role in the conversion of indole-5,6-quinone and indole-5,6-quinone-2-carboxylic acid to eumelanin (Fig. 3) (1,13). Eumelanin, a black-brown pigment, is one of two major classes of cutaneous melanin, the other being the yellow-red pheomelanin (13,46). Since the precursors of eumelanin are quinones with the potential to generate superoxide and hydroxyl radicals and since HMB-45–reactive antigen is homologous to the Pmel gene product, this raises the possibility that quinone-derived oxidants may be directly involved in the pathophysiology of LAM.

B. Catechol Compounds and LAM

Catechol compounds are molecules comprising an aromatic ring which is hydroxylated at two sites (Fig. 2). This unique structure results in a compound which, when oxidatively metabolized, generates semiquinones and quinones (13,47). Patients with LAM have two striking characteristics that may at first seem unrelated but present a common catechol link: (1) the associations of LAM with phenylalanine-derived catechol metabolism and (2) the association of LAM with premenopausal women, pointing to a potential hormonal factor such as estrogens, which can be metabolized to catechols.

As noted above, the HMB-45–positive LAM cells express high levels of a protein homologous to Pmel 17/gp 100, which is involved in the conversion of catechol-derived quinones to eumelanin (13). In addition, patients with tuberous sclerosis, a disorder characterized by neurological involvement with epilepsy and mental retardation, is associated in less than 1% of cases with LAM (41). Whereas tuberous sclerosis affects males and females equally, only women with tuberous

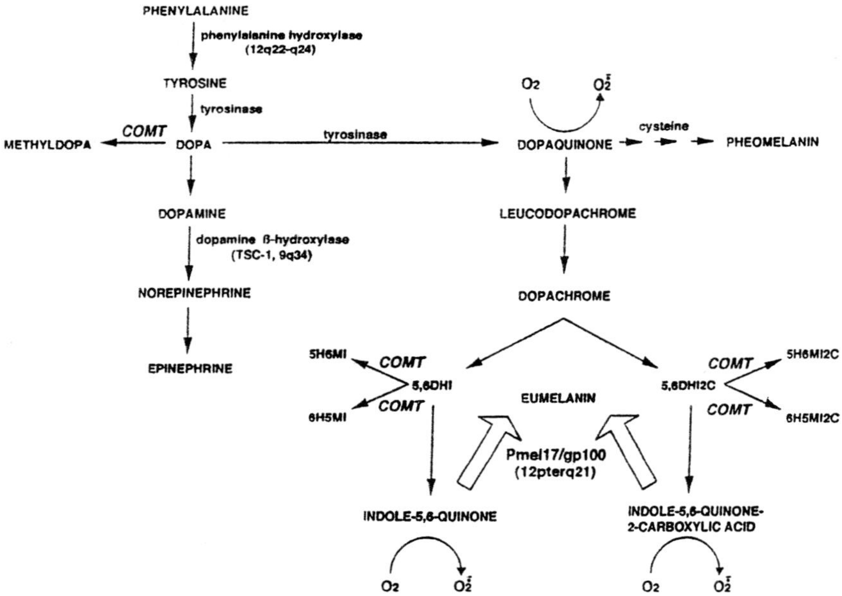

Figure 3 Phenylalanine-dependent catechol metabolic pathways. Chromosome mapping of tuberous sclerosis–determining loci (12q22-q24; TSC-1, 9q34) and the locus of the Pmel17/gp100 antigen are within parentheses. The locus at position 12q22-24 contains the gene encoding phenylalanine hydroxylase, and the TSC1 locus contains the gene for dopamine β-hydroxylase. The TSC1 gene at locus 9q34 has recently been cloned, and although its product, hamartin, is distinct from dopamine β-hydroxylase, the function of hamartin remains unknown (63). Pmel17/gp100 represents the antigen recognized by the monoclonal antibody HMB-45 in LAM cells. COMT: Catechol-O-methyltransferase; DOPA: dihydroxyphenylalanine; 5,6-DHI: 5,6-dihydroxyindole; 5H6MI, 6H5MI: 5,6- or 6,5-methoxyindole; 5,6-DH12C: 5,6-dihydroxyindole-2-carboxylic acid; 5H6M12C, 6H5M12C: 5,6- or 6,5-methoxyindole-2-carboxylic acid.

sclerosis have developed LAM. While 1% may seem like a low incidence, considering the much lower incidence of LAM in the general population, these data suggest that tuberous sclerosis is a risk factor for developing LAM. Interestingly, of the three loci associated with tuberous sclerosis, two (12q22-q24 and 9q34) are near the loci of genes encoding key enzymes in the metabolic pathway of phenylalanine and its catechol metabolites (Fig. 3) (1).

The second striking characteristic pointing to the possibility of defective catechol metabolism in LAM is the link to estrogens. LAM is a disease found exclusively in women, and almost exclusively in women of child-bearing years (2–5). These observations invite us to take a closer look at estrogen metabolism (Fig. 4). Estrone derived from estradiol is converted to either 16α-hydroxyestrone

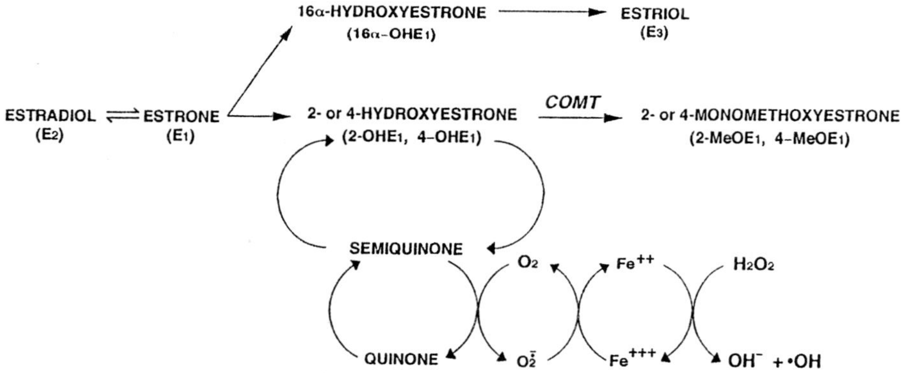

Figure 4 Catechol estrogen metabolism. 2- and 4-hydroxyestrone are catechol estrogens, which, when oxidized, form semiquinones and quinones. Semiquinone/quinone synthesis is prevented by catechol-O-methyltransferase (COMT).

or one of two catechol estrogens, 2- or 4-hydroxyestrone. As would be expected, both of these catechol estrogens can be oxidized to form semiquinones and quinones, which can subsequently react with oxygen and iron to produce toxic oxidants. The synthesis of catechol estrogens has been shown to play a role in renal tumorigenesis and in the enhancement of genomic instability (48–50).

C. Catechol Quinone Metabolism

Since DOPA catechols and estrogen catechols have the potential to produce superoxide and ·OH, one would expect that cells have safety mechanisms to keep the catechol and catechol-derived quinone levels as low as possible. These systems exist in the form of (1) catechol-O-methyltransferase or COMT, (2) DT-diaphorase, and (3) GSH conjugation.

The enzyme catechol-O-methyltransferase (COMT, EC 2.1.1.6) is thought to play a critical role in the prevention of catechol quinone formation, with subsequent oxidant synthesis (51,52). The COMT gene has been mapped on the human chomosome 22 to position 22ql1 (53,54). The COMT gene product can be one of two proteins—a soluble (S-COMT) or a membrane-bound (MB-COMT) form (55). Both proteins are encoded by the same mRNA, which is differentially translated to produce either the S-COMT or MB-COMT enzyme. The S-COMT predominates in most tissues, although the human brain is a notable exception. The MB-COMT has a higher affinity for dopamine, whereas the S-COMT favors other catechol substrates. Methylation of hydroxylated sites on the aromatic ring of catechol compounds by COMT prevents their conversion to semiquinones and quinones and, therefore, prevents the formation of toxic radicals. While kidney and liver cells are major sources of COMT, red blood cells are also rich in COMT and can convert significant amounts of catechol estrogens to their inoffensive monomethoxy-derivatives. Red blood cell COMT has been shown to play an important role in the detoxification of estrogen catechols, as low RBC COMT levels are thought to contribute to estrogen carcinogenicity in hamster kidneys (56).

In addition to COMT, at least two other systems are involved in the detoxification of quinones. First, DT-diaphorase or NAD(P)H:quinone acceptor oxidoreductase (EC 1.6.99.2) is a cytosolic enzyme which uses either NADH or NADPH as electron donors to induce a two-electron reduction of several different quinones to hydroxyquinones without the formation of the free intermediate semiquinone (57). Second, glutathione can react with quinones, including those derived from estrogen catechols, to form a glutathionyl-hydroquinone molecule. It is thought that the glutathionyl-hydroquinone molecule may be conjugated with UDP-glucoronate, a process that would contribute to detoxify electrophilic quinones (57).

IV. Conclusions and Future Directions

In the context of the above, let us now go out on a limb. We speculate that LAM may be caused by altered catechol metabolism. One possibility could be that LAM patients have defective COMT activity in their red blood cells. Such a defect would result in the accumulation of melanin and/or estrogen catechols with the potential of generating superoxide and ·OH. These oxidants could then induce tissue destruction and smooth cell proliferation. Why would the damage be more important in the lung than in other tissues? First, pulmonary endothelial cells are equipped with the nonneuronal transporter uptake I (58). This transporter was shown to be responsible for the pulmonary endothelial cell uptake of dopamine and to allow its metabolism through COMT at a 10-fold greater rate than noradrenaline (59). The lung vasculature can therefore take up circulating phenylalanine-derived catechols, which are potential sources of oxidants. The degree to which the lung vasculature can also take up other circulating catechols and catechol quinones is unknown. Second, the lung is exposed to the highest oxygen tensions of any tissue in the body and therefore any lung tissue quinones could react with oxygen and generate toxic oxidants.

Why do we believe the red blood cell may be important in LAM? At least three different lung transplantation groups have reported that LAM can recur in the transplanted lung (60–62). This points to a circulating factor causing LAM. In addition to a potential primary defect of COMT, it is possible that a humoral substance capable of inhibiting COMT activity may play a role in the pathogenesis of LAM. Finally, changes in other catechol quinone metabolic pathways such as DT-diaphorase, GSH conjugation, or the Pmel/gp100 protein itself may contribute to the lung changes charateristic of LAM.

What does the future hold? First, the hypothesis linking COMT and other catechol or quinone metabolic pathways to LAM can be readily verified. If COMT and other pathways are not involved in the pathogenesis or etiology of LAM, then we will be a little wiser and this information will allow us to focus our attention on some of the many other facets of an extremely complex disease. If quinone/semiquinone-derived oxidants are increased due to defective blood COMT activity, or other catechol metabolic pathways, then we may finally be able to develop rational strategies for the treatment of this devastating disease. The options would include approaches spanning the spectrum from the administration of exogenous antioxidants to the use of gene therapy. Whatever the outcome, future research into this disease is likely to produce important results not only for patients with LAM, but also for many patients with other lung diseases in which oxidants are involved.

References

1. Kalassian KG, Foyle R, Kao P, Ruoss S, Raffin TA. Lymphangioleiomyomatosis: new insights. Am J Respir Crit Care Med 1997; 155:1183–1186.
2. Kitaichi M, Nishimura K, Itoh H, Izumi T. Pulmonary lymphangioleiomyomatosis: a report of 46 patients including a clinicopathologic study of prognostic factors. Am J Respir Crit Care Med 1995; 151:527–533.
3. Silverstein E, Ellis K, Wolff M, Jaretzeki A III. Pulmonary lymphangioleiomyomatosis. Am J Roentgenol 1974; 120:12–50.
4. Corrin B, Liebow AA, Friedman PJ. Pulmonary lymphangioleiomyomatosis. A review. Am J Pathol 1975; 79:347–382.
5. Taylor JR, Ryu J, Colby TV, Raffin TA. Lymphangioleiomyomatosis. Clinical course in 32 patients. N Engl J Med 1990; 323 (18):1254–1260.
6. Halliwell B, Gutteridge JMC. Oxygen is poisonous—an introduction to oxygen toxicity and free radicals. In: Halliwell B, Gutteridge JMC, eds. Free Radicals in Biology and Medicine. New York. Oxford Science Publications, 1985:1–19.
7. Weibel ER. Cell respiration. In: Weibel ER, ed. The Pathway for Oxygen. Structure and Function in the Mammalian Respiratory System. Cambridge, MA: Harvard University Press, 1984:80–105.
8. Babior BM. Oxygen-dependent microbial killing by phagocytes (parts I and II). N Engl J Med 1978; 298:659–668.
9. Cantin AM, North SL, Fells GA, Hubbard RC, Crystal RG. Oxidant-mediated epithelial cell injury in idiopathic pulmonary fibrosis. J Clin Invest 1987; 79:1665–1673.
10. Powis G. Metabolism and reactions of quinoid anticancer agents. Pharmacol Ther 1987; 35:57–162.
11. Powis G. Free radical formation by antitumor quinones. Free Rad Biol Med 1989; 6:63–101.

12. Gutierrez PL. Mechanism(s) of bioreductive activation. The example of diaziquone (AZQ). Free Rad Biol Med 1989; 6:405–445.
13. Kwon BS. Pigmentation genes: the tyrosinase gene family and the pmel 17 gene family. J Inv Derm 1993; 100:134S–140S.
14. Martucci CP, Fishman J. P450 enzymes of estrogen metabolism. Pharmacol Ther 1993; 57:237–257.
15. McCord JM, Fridovich I. Superoxide dismutase. An enzymic function for erythrocuprein (hemocuprein). J Biol Chem 1969; 244:6049–6055.
16. Halliwell B, Gutteridge JMC. Protection against oxygen radicals in biological systems: the superoxide theory of oxygen toxicity In: Halliwell B, Gutteridge JMC, eds. Free Radicals in Biology and Medicine. New York: Oxford Science Publications, 1985:67–138.
17. Klebanoff SJ, Hamon CB. Role of myeloperoxidase-mediated antimicrobial systems in intact leukocytes. J Reticuloendothel Soc 1972; 12:170–196.
18. Johnson D, Travis J. The oxidative inactivation of human α1-proteinase inhibitor. Further evidence for methionine at the reactive center. J Biol Chem 1979; 254:4022–4026.
19. Carp H, Miller F, Hoidal JR, Janoff A. Potential mechanism of emphysema-α1-proteinase inhibitor recovered from lungs of cigarette smokers contains oxidized methionine and has decreased elastase inhibitor capacity. Proc Natl Acad Sci USA 1982; 79:2041–2045.
20. Thomas EL, Grisham MB, Melton DF, Jefferson MM. Evidence for a role of taurine in the in vitro oxidative toxicity of neutrophils toward erythrocytes. J Biol Chem 1985; 260:3321–3329.
21. Cantin AM. Taurine modulation of hypochlorous acid-induced lung epithelial cell injury in vitro. Role of anion transport. J Clin Invest 1994; 93:606–614.
22. Schreck R, Albermann K, Baeuerle PA. Nuclear factor kB: an oxidative stress-responsive transcription factor of eukaryotic cells (a review). Free Rad Res Commun 1992; 17: 221–237.
23. Schreck R, Rieber P, Baeuerle PA. Reactive oxygen intermediates as apparently widely used messengers in the activation of the NF-kB transcription factor and HIV-1. EMBO J 1991; 10:2247–2256.
24. Vallyathan V, Shi X. The role of oxygen free radicals in occupational and environmental lung diseases. Environ Health Perspect 1997; 105:165–177.
25. Deisseroth A, Dounce AL. Catalase: physical and chemical properties, mechanisms of catalysis and physiological role. Physiol Rev 1970; 50:319–375.
26. Cantin AM, Bégin R. Glutathione and inflammatory disorders of the lung. Lung 1991; 169:123–138.
27. Crapo JD, Barry BE, Foscue HA, Shelburne J. Structural and biochemical changes in rat lungs occuring during exposure to lethal and adaptive doses of oxygen. Am Rev Respir Dis 1980; 122:123–143.
28. Cantin AM, North SL, Hubbard RC, Crystal RG. Normal alveolar epithelial lining fluid contains high levels of glutathione. J Appl Physiol 1987; 63:152–157.
29. Mulcahy RT, Gipp JJ. Identification of a putative antioxidant response element in the 5′-flanking region of the human γ-glutamylcysteine synthetase heavy subunit gene. Biochem Biophys Res Commun 1995; 209:227–233.

30. Khalil N, O'Connor RN, Unruh HW, Warren PW, Flanders KC, Kemp A, Bereznay OH, Greenberg AH. Increased production an immunohistochemical localization of transforming growth factor-β in idiopathic pulmonary fibrosis. Am J Respir Cell Mol Biol 1991; 5:155–162.
31. Broekelmann TJ, Limper AH, Colby TV, McDonald JA. Transforming growth factor β1 is present at sites of extracellular matrix gene expression in human pulmonary fibrosis. Proc Natl Acad Sci USA 1991; 88:6642–6646.
32. Khalil N, Whitman C, Zuo L, Daniel pour D, Greenberg A. Regulation of alveolar macrophage transforming growth factor β secretion by corticosteroids in bleomycin-induced pulmonary inflammation in the rat. J Clin Invest 1993, 92:1812–1818.
33. Kayanoki Y, Fujii J, Suzuki K, Kawata S, Matsuzawa Y, Taniguchi N. Suppression of antioxidative enzyme expression by transforming growth factor βl in rat hepatocytes. J Biol Chem 1994; 269:15488–15492.
34. Arsalane K, Dubois CM, Muanza T, Bégin R, Boudreau F, Asselin C, Cantin AM. Transforming growth factor βl (TGFβl) is a potent inhibitor of glutathione (GSH) synthesis in the rat lung epithelial cell line A549: transcriptional effect on the GSH rate-limiting enzyme, γ-glutamylcysteine synthetase. Am J Respir Cell Mol Biol in press.
35. Davis WB, Pacht ER. Extracellular antioxidant defenses. In: Crystal RG, West JB, eds. Lung Injury. Raven Press, 1991:61–67.
36. Cantin AM, Hubbard RC, Crystal RG. Glutathione deficiency in the epithelial lining fluid of the lower respiratory tract in idiopathic pulmonary fibrosis. Am Rev Respir Dis 1989; 139:370–372.
37. Cochrane CG, Spragg RG, Revak SD. Pathogenesis of the adult respiratory distress syndrome: evidence of oxidant activity in bronchoalveolar lavage fluid. J Clin Invest 1983; 71:754–761.
38. O'Driscoll BR, Hasleton PS, Taylor PM, Poulter LW, Gattamaneni HR, Woodcock AA. Active lung fibrosis up to 17 years after chemotherapy with carmustine (BCNU) in childhood. N Engl J Med 1990; 323:378–382.
39. Smith LL. Paraquat toxicity. Phil Trans R Soc London B Biol Sci 1985; 311:647–657.
40. Rosiello RA, Merrill WW. Radiation-induced lung injury. In: Cooper JAD Jr, ed. Clinics in Chest Medicine. Drug-Induced Pulmonary Disease. Philadelphia: W.B. Saunders Company, 1990:65–71.
41. Colby TV, Carrington CB. Lymphangioleiomyomatosis and tuberous sclerosis. In: Thurlbeck WM, Churg AM, eds. Pathology of the Lung. Theme Medical Publishers Inc, 1995:589–737.
42. Bonetti F, Chiodera PL, Pea M, Martignoni G, Bosi F, Zamboni G, Mariuzzi GM. Transbronchial biopsy in lymphangiomyomatosis of the lung. HMB45 for diagnosis. Am J Surg Pathol 1993; 17:1092–1102.
43. Sundaresan M, Yu Z, Ferrans VJ, Irani K, Finkel T. Requirement for generation of H_2O_2 for platelet-derived growth factor signal transduction. Science 1995; 270:296–299.
44. Irani K, Xia Y, Zweier JL, Sollott SJ, Der CJ, Fearon ER, Sundaresan M, Finkel T,

Goldschmidt-Clermont PJ. Mitogenic signaling mediated by oxidants in ras-transformed fibroblasts. Science 1997; 275:1649–1652.
45. Pennisi E. Superoxides relay ras protein's oncogenic message. Science 1997; 275:1567–1568.
46. Jimbow K, Lee SK, King MG, Hara H, Chen H, Dakour J, Marusyk H. Melanin pigments and melanosomal proteins as differentiation markers unique to normal and neoplastic melanocytes. J Invest Dermatol 1993; 100:259S-268S.
47. Han X, Liehr JG. Microsome-mediated 8-hydroxylation of guanine bases of DNA by steroid estrogens: correlation of DNA damage by free radicals with metabolic activation to quinones. Carcinogenesis 1995; 16:2571–2574.
48. Zhu BT, Liehr JG. Quercetin increases the severity of estradiol-induced tumorigenesis in hamster kidney. Toxicol Appl Pharmacol 1994; 125:149–158.
49. Paquette B. Enhancement of genomic instability by 17 beta-estradiol in minisatellite sequences of X-ray-transformed mouse 1OT1/2 cells. Carcinogenesis 1996; 17:1221–1225.
50. Thibodeau P, Paquette B. Enhancement by estrogens of methotrexate resistance in breast cancer cells MCF-7. Submitted for publication.
51. Shibata T, Pavel S, Smit NPM, Mishima Y. Differences in subcellular distribution of catechol-O-methyltransferase and tyrosinase in malignant melanoma. J Invest Dermatol 1993; 100:222S–225S.
52. Butterworth M, Lau SS, Monks TJ. 17 beta-estradiol metabolism by hamster hepatic microsomes. Implications for the catechol-O-methyl transferase-mediated detoxication of catechol estrogens. Drug Metab Dispos 1996; 24:588–594.
53. Grossman MH, Emanuel BS, Budarf ML. Chromosomal mapping of the human catechol-O-methyltransferase gene to 22q11.1–q11.2. Genomics 1992; 12:822–825.
54. Winqvist R, Lundstrom K, Salminen M, Laatikainen M, Ulmanen I. The human catechol-O-methyltransferase (COMT) gene maps to band ql1.2 of chromosome 22 and shows a frequent RFLP with Bgll. Cytogen Cell Gen 1992; 59:253–257.
55. Lundstrom K, Tenhunen J, Tilgmann C, Karhunen T, Panula P, Ulmanen I. Cloning, expression and structure of catechol-O-methyltransferase. Biochim Biophys Acta 1995; 1251:1–10.
56. Li SA, Purdy RH, Li JJ. Variations in catechol O-methyltransferase activity in rodent tissues, possible role in estrogen carcinogenicity. Carcinogenesis 1989; 10:63–67.
57. Cadenas E, Hochstein P. Pro- and antioxidant functions of quinones and quinone reductases in mammalian cells. Adv Enzymol 1992; 65:97–146.
58. Bryan-Lluka LJ, Westwood NN, O'Donnell SR. Vascular uptake of catecholamines in perfused lungs of the rat occurs by the same process as uptake$_1$ in noradrenergic neurones. Naunyn-Schmiedeberg's Arch Pharmacol 1992; 345:319–326.
59. Bryan-Lluka LJ, O'Donnell SR. Dopamine and adrenaline but not isoprenaline, are substrates for uptake and metabolism in isolated perfused lungs of the rat. Naunyn-Schmiedeberg's Arch Pharmacol 1992; 346:20–26.
60. Nine SJ, Yousem SA, Paradis IL, Keenan R, Griffith BP. Lymphangioleiomyomatosis: recurrence after lung transplantation. J Heart Lung Transplant 1994; 13:714–719.

61. O'Brien JD, Lium JH, Parosa JF, Deyoung BR, Wick MR, Trulock EP. Lymphangiomyomatosis recurrence in the allograft after single-lung transplantation. Am J Respir Crit Care Med 1995; 151:2033–2036.
62. Boehler A, Speich R, Russi EW, Weder W. Lung transplantation for lymphangioleiomyomatosis. N Engl J Med 1996; 335:1275–1280.
63. Van Slegtenhorst and the TSC1 consortium. Identification of the tuberous sclerosis geneTSC1 on chromosome 9q34. Science 1997; 277:805–808.

27

Extracellular Matrix Turnover in Pathologic Conditions

The Role of Matrix Metalloproteinases and Their Inhibitors

WILLIAM G. STETLER-STEVENSON and SUSAN E. HOEGY

National Cancer Institute
National Institutes of Health
Bethesda, Maryland

I. Introduction to Extracellular Matrix Turnover

The extracellular matrix (ECM) functions as a scaffolding to support the cellular elements of most tissues and organs. It is now well recognized that in addition to this structural function, there are components of the ECM that function to modulate cell growth and tissue differentiation (1,2). As such processes occur, they can in turn influence the composition of the extracellular matrix and result in the formation of specialized extracellular barriers between tissue compartments, such as basement membranes. Tissue differentiation is the result of a changing dynamic between epithelial and stromal cellular elements that is mediated by alteration in the matrix composition and formation. Changes in the composition of the extracellular matrix require removal of the existing matrix along with the synthesis of new matrix components. Removal of matrix components is accomplished through the action of proteases that can selectively degrade matrix macromolecules. This process may also result in the liberation of matrix-bound materials that can influence cellular proliferation and alteration of cell-matrix contacts that may be required for cell survival under nonpathologic conditions (3,4). As this process continues, new extracellular matrix is synthesized and assembled. Both matrix turnover and replacement occurs simultaneously in an orderly and progressive fashion, to establish a new homeostatic endpoint consistent with the differentiated state of the tissue. This occurs in a balanced and progressive fashion such that there is preservation of tissue boundaries and matrix functions of structural integrity and growth regulation. These processes are examples of necessary physiological roles matrix metalloproteinases (MMPs) may have in normal cellular maintenance and growth of certain cells and tissues.

Pathologic conditions result in alterations in both the cellular and extracellular matrix elements that disrupt the balance achieved in the differentiated tissue. This results in alterations in the distribution, composition, and/or function of the extracellular matrix that may further contribute to the progression of a disease state. Understanding the processes of extracellular matrix turnover may allow identification of targets for directed therapeutic intervention.

Turnover of the extracellular matrix is a unique biological problem because of the high collagen content of most extracellular matrix structures and the resistance of these triple helical molecules to the action of most proteases. We now know that connective tissue remodeling, either physiologic or pathologic, is in most cases a highly organized process that involves the selective action of a group of related proteases that are active at neutral pH and can collectively degrade most, if not all, components of the extracellular matrix, including collagen. These proteases are the matrix metalloproteases, also known as the matrixins. These are zinc-dependent endopeptidases that are a subgroup of a larger, more diverse superfamily of enzymes known as the metzincins, which include proteases such as astacin and adamalysin (5,6).

II. Overview of the Matrixin Family

Matrix metalloproteinases are zinc atom–containing endopeptidases with optimal activity at neutral pH. Most of these enzymes are secreted as zymogens by a variety of connective tissue cells, including fibroblasts, osteoblasts, chondrocytes, and endothelial cells, as well as inflammatory cells such as macrophages, neutrophils, and lymphocytes. The synthesis and activation of these proteases are tightly regulated at several levels. With the exception of RXKR sequence–containing members (stromelysin-3 and MT-MMPs), all are secreted as inactive proenzymes and activated extracellularly by either a plasminogen cascade system or by another member of the MMP family (Sec. III). Once activated, the proteinases are further regulated by their endogenous inhibitors, the tissue inhibitors of metalloproteinases (TIMPS) in the extracellular environment, or by α_2 macroglobulin in the plasma (7).

The matrixin family currently has 20 members that can be subdivided into six groups based on their substrate specificities and structural homologies (Table 1): collagenases, gelatinases, stromelysins, elastases, RXKR secreted, and RXKR

Table 1 Matrix Metalloproteinase Types and Their Substrates

Subgroup	Enzyme	MMP number	MW (kDa)	Substrate(s)
Interstitial collagenases	Interstitial collagenase	MMP-1	52,57	Collagens I, II, III, VII, VIII, and X, gelatin, PG core protein
	Neutrophil collagenase	MMP-8	75	Fibrillar collagens
	Collagenase-3	MMP-13	54	Fibrillar collagens
Gelatinases	Gelatinase-A	MMP-2	72	Gelatin, collagens, I, IV, V, VII, and X, elastin, laminin-5, FBN, PG core protein, VN galectin-3, bFGF receptor
	Gelatinase-B	MMP-9	92	
Stromelysins	Stromelysin-1	MMP-3	52,58	FBN, PG core protein,
	Stromelysin-2	MMP-10	58	Laminin, collagens IV, V, IX, and X
	Matrilysin	MMP-7	28	Elastin, pro-interstitial collagenase
Elastases	Metalloelastase	MMP-12	53	Elastin, plasminogen (angiostatin precursor)
RXKR, secreted type	Stromelysin-3	MMP-11	29	α_1-Antitrypsin
RXKR, membrane type	MTI-MMP	MMP-14	66	proGEL A, gelatin, collagens I, II, and III, FBN, VN, laminin-$_1$, α_2M
	MT2-MMP	MMP-15	76	proGEL A
	MT3-MMP	MMP-16	70	proGEL A, gelatin
	MT4-MMP	MMP-17	—	proGEL A

proGEL A = Pro-gelatinase A; bFGF = basic fibroblast growth factor; PG = proteoglycans; FBN = fibronectin; VN = vitronectin; α_2M = alpha$_2$-macroglobulin.

membrane. The first group includes MMP-1 (interstitial) and MMP-8 (neutrophil) collagenase, which degrade collagen types I, II, and III. Group 2 contains two forms of gelatinases/type IV collagenases: gelatinase A (MMP-2) and gelatinase B (MMP-9). Both gelatinases cleave collagen types IV, V, VII, X, and XI and denatured collagens (gelatins). Recently, gelatinases have been shown to degrade fibrillar type I collagen and cell surface components such as galectin-3 and bFGF receptor (4,8). The third group is made of stromelysins, which have a broad substrate specificity and degrade proteoglycans, laminin, fibronectin, and some collagens. The fourth group of MMPs includes the elastases, which are referred to as the metalloelastases and are responsible for degrading elastins and generation of the plasminogen fragment angiostatin, a potent inhibitor of tumor angiogenesis. The fifth group includes the secreted, soluble MMPs that contain a furin recognition sequence exemplified by stromelysin-3, and the sixth group consists of the membrane-bound (or membrane type, MT-) MMPs that contain a furin recognition sequence (9–13). The furin recognition motif, RXKR, is thought to be the site of proenzyme activation for these family members, and this may occur prior to secretion (14). A recent report demonstrates that MT1-MMP possesses gelatinolytic activity and is secreted in a complex with TIMP-2 (15). Additionally, MT1-MMP was shown to cleave the propeptide sequence of pro-MMP-2 in a sequence-specific manner (16). This processing was blocked by TIMP-2 or BB-94, but not by TIMP-1. The substrate specificity of other MT-MMPs is still poorly understood, but they are believed to be involved in the cellular activation of proMMP-2 (gelatinase A).

III. Domain Structure of the Matrixins

Comparison and alignment of the amino acid sequences for the human MMPs reveals a high degree of homology between these enzymes. This sequence comparison also shows that MMPs have distinct domains that are conserved between subgroups. The minimal structure comprises a signal peptide, a pro-domain, and a catalytic domain (Fig. 1). This is reflected in the smallest member of the matrixin family known as matrilysin (MMP-7). The signal peptide domain directs the translational product to the endoplasmic reticulum. The pro-peptide is involved in the maintenance of enzyme latency and is removed during activation of the enzyme (17). The catalytic domain contains a highly conserved site in which three histidine residues coordinate the zinc ion binding in the activated protease.

Except for matrilysin, all MMPs contain a C-terminal domain that is homologous to both hemopexin and vitronectin (18). The C-terminal domain of the collagenases (MMPs 1 and 8) binds the enzymes to the collagens of types I–III

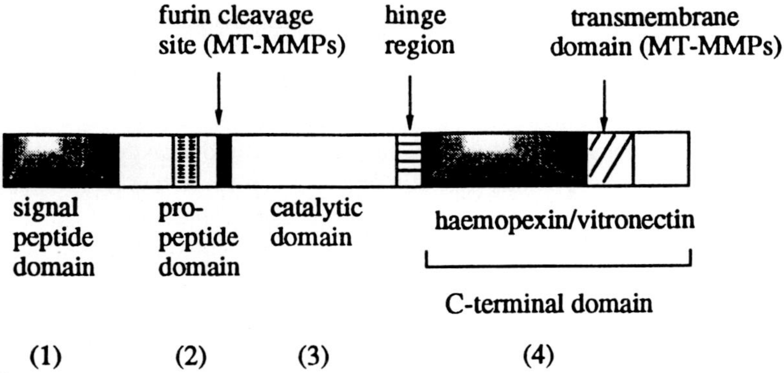

Figure 1 Structural characteristics of matrix metalloproteinases. Four domains are found in all members of the MMP family: (1) signal peptide domain; (2) propeptide domain; (3) catalytic domain; and (4) C-terminal domain (sequence homology with hemopexin and vitronectin). MT-MMPs contain one or both of the following structural features: the furin cleavage site and the transmembrane domain.

(19), thereby positioning the substrate for cleavage at the active site (20). However, this collagen cleavage specificity does not reside solely in the C-terminal domain of collagenase, and the catalytic domain also contributes to specificity. Stromelysin does not cleave collagen, but it does bind to it through its C-terminal domain (19).

Gelatinases also bind macromolecular substrates such as collagen, but do so using three fibronectin-related type II modules, which are inserted into their catalytic domains (21). Their substrate-degrading activity is not lost upon removal of the C-terminal domain (22). For MMP-2 (gelatinase A), however, the C-terminal domain serves three important functions: (1) cell surface binding, that in turn leads to (2) proenzyme activation (23–25), and (3) binding of the proenzyme to the endogenous inhibitor, TIMP-2 (22,26).

Membrane-type matrix metalloproteinases (MT-MMPs) have a transmembrane domain that results in cell surface localization of these proteases. MT-MMPs, as well as stromelysin-3, possess a basic amino acid–rich sequence that corresponds to a furin enzyme recognition site, RXKR. This sequence seems to account for the activation of stromelysin-3 before secretion of the enzyme from the cell and may also be important in cell-mediated activation of MT-MMPs (13,27). Before the identification of these new features, MMPs were thought to be secreted as soluble zymogens requiring activation in the extracellular compartment. While this still applies to most members of the MMP family, recent discovery of novel members broadens our definition of the MMPs.

IV. Multilevel Regulation of MMP-2 (Gelatinase A)

Many members of the matrixin family are regulated principally at the transcriptional level. Examples include MMP-1 and MMP-3. These genes contain classic transcriptional regulator elements, such as AP-1 and PEA-3 sites. MMP-2 (gelatinase-A) is unique among matrixin family members in that it represents an example of multilevel regulation that involves cellular regulation of enzyme activation. Synthesis of MMP-2 (gelatinase A) appears to be regulated at both the transcriptional and posttranscriptional levels in fibroblasts studied in vitro. However, the constitutive high levels of MMP-2 (gelatinase A) mRNA expression seen in many tissues suggest that regulation of proenzyme activation is more relevant for the control and induction of MMP-2 (gelatinase A) action than other members of the matrixin family in which transcriptional control is more important. Following activation, enzyme activity is then downregulated by TIMPs.

Unlike other MMPS, proMMP-2 (gelatinase A) is constitutively expressed by many cell types, and its transcription is not readily induced by agents such as TPA or IL-1α, which have been shown to increase transcription of other MMPs (i.e., interstitial collagenase and gelatinase B) as much as 100-fold (28–30). Inducers of MMP expression are generally thought to act at the level of transcriptional activation of the gene and promoter elements. Analysis of the MMP-2 (gelatinase A) promoter regions shows marked differences between this protease and other MMPs (31) The MMP-2 (gelatinase A) promoter is distinguished by the lack of known *trans*-activator sequences (AP-1, PEA-3), the presence of a unique noncanonical TATA box as well as a putative enhancer element (AP-2) located at nucleotides -223 to -422 relative to the translational start site (32,33). The TATA site is usually located ~30 bp from the transcriptional start site and plays a pivotal role in the transcriptional regulation of most promoters, whereas the AP-2 enhancer plays a role in cell-type specific expression. Other distinctive features of the MMP-2 (gelatinase A) promoter include an SP-1 consensus sequence located 120 base pairs from the start site and an adenovirus ElA repressor element (34). Unlike other MMPs, the MMP-2 (gelatinase A) promoter also lacks an upstream TGF-β inhibitory element (TIE) (31). Consistent with this sequence information is the observation that MMP-2 (gelatinase A) transcription is not suppressed but slightly upregulated by TGF-β (28,35). Presence of the AP-2 element (5′-GCCCCAGGC-3′) contributes to cell-type specific expression of at least two MMPs: MMP-2 (gelatinase A) and gelatinase B (36). An AP-2 enhancer element (–1650 bp) is indispensable for transcription of the human MMP-2 (gelatinase A) gene in HT1080 cells (34). Similarly, in the rabbit gelatinase B promoter, the AP-1 site at –56 bp and an AP-2-1-like element located between –432 and –330 bp have been shown to be essential for PMA inducibility in primary epithelial cells (37). The unique transcriptional regulation of MMP-2 (gelatinase A), and the fact that MMP-2 (gelatinase A) is constitutively expressed and not transcriptionally regulated, has led to the suggestion that MMP-2 (gelatinase A) acts as a "housekeeping" gene (35). However, this incorrectly implies that transcriptional activation of the MMP-2 (gelatinase A) gene results in a direct increase in MMP-2 (gelatinase A) activity. The proenzyme form of MMP-2 (gelatinase A) is stable and does not undergo spontaneous activation under physiologic conditions (38). The cellular regulation of proMMP-2 (gelatinase A) activation plays a pivotal role in the initiation of ECM turnover.

There is evidence for posttranscriptional regulation of MMP-2 (gelatinase A) expression (35). While TGF-β1 suppresses overall proteolytic activity through reduced proteinase synthesis and by increased TIMP expression, it increases the levels of MMP-2 (gelatinase A) secreted by human fibroblasts and rat bone cells (35). The total cellular abundance of MMP-2 (gelatinase A) mRNA was found to increase 1.5- to 2.2-fold, an amount similar to the increase seen in the synthesis of MMP-2 (gelatinase A) protein. In human fibroblasts treated with TGF-β1, the half-life ($t_{1/2}$) of MMP-2 (gelatinase A) mRNA increased from 46 to 150 hours, but the stability of TIMP-1 mRNA was unaffected (35). This approximately threefold increase in the stability of the MMP-2 (gelatinase A) mRNA induced by TGF-β1 would augment the elevated levels of MMP-2 (gelatinase A) mRNA produced by increased MMP-2 (gelatinase A) transcription. These data indicate that TGF-β1 acts both transcriptionally and posttranscriptionally to elevate MMP-2 (gelatinase A) expression, however, the mechanism of these effects have not been studied in detail.

ProMMP-2 (gelatinase A) is also unique among MMP family members in that it is usually found complexed with the endogenous inhibitor TIMP-2 (Table 2). While, in general, active MMPs are inhibited by TIMPs binding to the active site, proMMP-2 (gelatinase A) interacts selectively to TIMP-2, but not TIMP-1 (39–43). By deletion mutagenesis, it has been shown that interactions between the C-terminal domains of TIMPs and MMPs influence the rate of complex formation. Ionic interactions involving the negatively charged C-terminus of TIMP-2 are thought to be important in the rapid binding to the C-terminus of proMMP-2 (gelatinase A) (44). Evidence from studies involving truncated enzymes and cross-linking methods suggests the following model: the N-terminal domain of TIMP is inhibitory, while the C-terminal domain confers binding specificity. So, while the N-terminal domain of TIMP-1 and -2 bind to the N-terminal domain of active MMP-2 (gelatinase A), only the C-terminal domain of TIMP-2 will bind specifically to the C-terminal domain of proMMP-2 (gelatinase A). As evidence to support this model, C-terminally truncated forms of proMMP-2 (gelatinase A) will not bind TIMP-2, but activated C-terminally truncated MMP-2 (gelatinase A) is inhibited by TIMP-2 (22,44–46). In addition, cross-linked proMMP-2 (gelatinase A)/TIMP-2 complex can still be activated and show MMP-2 (gela-

Table 2 Tissue Inhibitors of Matrix Metalloproteinases

TIMP #	MW (kDa)	mRNA (kb)	Associated proteins	Sites of expression[a]	Pro-MMP complex	MT-MMP inhibition	Gelatinase inhibitor
1	28	0.9	proGELB	Ovary, bone	MMP-9	No	Yes
2	21	1.1,	proGELA	Lung, placenta, brain	MMP-2	Yes	Yes
3	24	4.5-	ECM	Kidney, brain	MMP-2	Yes	Yes
4	22	1.4	?	Heart, brain	?	?	Yes

[a]The sites of expression listed in this table include the major areas of TIMP localization. proGELA = Pro-gelatinase A; proGELB = pro-gelatinase B; ECM = extracellular matrix; MT-MMP = membrane-type matrix metalloproteinase.

tinase A) activity, which suggests that the TIMP-2 is not entirely bound to the active site (26). However, this gelatinase/TIMP-2 complex retains 10% of the proteolytic activity of the enzyme that is free of TIMP-2. Upon the cleavage of the profragment, the active site of MMP-2 (gelatinase A)/TIMP-2 complex becomes available for binding the second domain of TIMP-2. This site is not specific for TIMP-2 and the active enzyme is inhibited by all TIMPs. It has also been found that the latent proMMP-2 (gelatinase A)/TIMP-2 complex is capable of binding activated gelatinase B to form a ternary complex devoid of MMP-2 (gelatinase A) activity (47,48). This evidence suggests that when TIMP-2 is complexed to proMMP-2 (gelatinase A), the inhibitory N-terminal domain of TIMP-2 is available for interaction with gelatinase B. Recently, the newest member of the TIMP family, TIMP-4, is also found to bind to the C-terminus of MMP-2 (gelatinase A) (49). The interaction of proMMP-2 (gelatinase A) with any TIMP-4 has not been observed in cell cultures or tissues to date, so the physiological significance of these in vitro interactions remains to be clarified.

Recent data suggest that TIMP-2 may mediate the cell surface activation of proMMP-2 (gelatinase A) by binding to a MT1-MMP–containing complex on the cell surface. Thus, TIMP-2 may play a dual role in its interaction with MMP-2 (gelatinase A). Interaction of TIMP-2 with proMMP-2 (gelatinase A) may facilitate cell surface–mediated activation, whereas interaction with active MMP-2 (gelatinase A) results in inhibition. In summary, much progress has been made recently in explaining the interactions between TIMPs and the gelatinases. However, the question remains whether the two TIMP domains interact with the two gelatinase-binding sites simultaneously or whether the TIMP molecule can only interact with one binding site at a time.

V. Regulation of Proenzyme Activation

The latency of MMPs is thought to be maintained by coordination between the unpaired cysteine residue in the prodomain and the zinc atom at the active site. Disruption of this zinc atom interaction with the sulfhydryl functionality of the cysteine residue and coordination with H_2O is necessary to obtain catalytic activity. The unpaired cysteine residue in proMMP-2 (gelatinase A) remains cryptic in the holo-proenzyme but is exposed upon removal of divalent cations by chelating agents (42). Upon dissociation of this Cys-Zn interaction, MMP-2 (gelatinase A) undergoes an autolytic cleavage, which removes an 8 kDa peptide by hydrolysis at the Asn90-Tyr91 bond at a site homologous (Phe>Tyr) to that cleaved in other MMPs eight residues downstream from the conserved Cys residue in the propeptide activation locus (42). This processing appears to occur in two steps, with an initial cleavage at Asn37-Leu38 that generates an obligatory 65 kDa intermediate similar to that observed in the cell surface activation of proMMP-2 (gelatinase A) (Kleiner and Stetler-Stevenson, unpublished observations) (50).

Physiologic activation of proMMP-2 (gelatinase A) is regulated at the level of the cell surface by a membrane-associated activator as first proposed in 1990 by Brown et al. (28). Activation of proMMP-2 (gelatinase A) involves interaction of proMMP-2 (gelatinase A), TIMP-2, and the activator protein and requires an intact proMMP-2 (gelatinase A) C-terminal domain. A membrane-associated specific activator of MMP-2 (gelatinase A) can be induced in a range of cell types by agents such as concanavalin A, cytochalasin D, phorbol esters, and TGF-β1 (30,51,52). Activation of proMMP-2 (gelatinase A) by membrane preparations from cells treated with these agents is blocked by MMP inhibitors, including 1,10-phenanthroline, synthetic peptide inhibitors, and the TIMPs (21,52). This membrane-dependent activation of proMMP-2 (gelatinase A) results in initial cleavage of the pro-peptide at Asn37-Leu38 to give a 65 kDa intermediate, followed by cleavage at Asn80-Phe81 to give the final 62 kDa active enzyme (53,54). Cleavage at Asn80-Phe81 also occurs during autoactivation in the presence of an organomercurial reagent (42), and this observation suggests that the association of MMP-2 (gelatinase A) with membrane component(s) may initiate the eventual autoactivation of the enzyme (53–55).

Sato et al. (13) cloned a novel MMP with a transmembrane domain (MT1-MMP), which they propose represents the cell membrane-associated activator of proMMP-2 (gelatinase A). MT1-MMP is also proposed to act as a receptor for TIMP-2. The MT1-MMP-TIMP-2 complex can bind proMMP-2 (gelatinase A) to form a trimeric complex through the carboxyl-terminus of proMMP-2 (gelatinase A) (24). Formation of this complex may lead to subsequent activation of proMMP-2 (gelatinase A). MT1-MMP has a transmembrane (TM) domain, and truncation of this domain was initially reported to abolish MMP-2 (gelatinase A) activation (56). This suggests that the TM domain serves to anchor and localize MT1-MMP at a position on the cell surface that facilitates proMMP-2 (gelatinase A)/TIMP-2 complex activation. Binding, localization, and activation of proMMP-2 (gelatinase A) on the cell surface depends on cooperative interactions between a number of different molecules, including MT1-MMP and TIMP-2. The role of TIMP-2 in these interactions is a controversial matter, and while some results indicate that TIMP-2 inhibits the cell surface activation of proMMP-2 (gelatinase A), others suggest it may enhance activation through formation of proMMP-2 (gelatinase A)/TIMP-2 complex, which facilitates binding of the proMMP-2 (gelatinase A) to the cell surface. TIMP-2 may achieve this effect either by binding to MT1-MMP or to another TIMP-2-binding protein (T2BP), thus localizing proMMP-2 (gelatinase A) in close proximity to MT1-MMP.

Interestingly, some tumor cell lines have been shown to bind proMMP-2 (gelatinase A) without concomitantly activating the enzyme (57), which suggests that there is a receptor for proMMP-2 (gelatinase A) that may be distinct from MT1-MMP. There is evidence that the integrin $\alpha_v\beta_3$ is involved in binding proMMP-2 (gelatinase A) to the cell surface (58). MMP-2 and $\alpha_v\beta_3$ form an SDS-stable complex in vitro that involves binding of $\alpha_v\beta_3$ to the noncatalytic C-terminal domain of MMP-2 (gelatinase A). Expression of $\alpha_v\beta_3$ on the surface of cultured melanoma cells enables them to bind MMP-2 (gelatinase A) in a proteolytically active form that allowed cell-mediated degradation of collagen. It has not yet been reported what effect TIMP-2 may have in this interaction or if proMMP-2 (gelatinase A) binding to $\alpha_v\beta_3$ results in autoproteolytic activation. It would also be interesting to know if this integrin receptor is proteolytically modified by MMP-2 (gelatinase A) activity and if this may influence cell attachment.

It has also been reported that thrombin and urokinase facilitate the cell surface activation of proMMP-2 (gelatinase A). This suggests that multiple mechanisms may be evoked for the cellular control of proMMP-2 (gelatinase A) activation. The exact details of these multiple activation mechanisms and their relative significance in various physiologic processes and pathologic states remain to be elucidated. However, the redundancy of possible mechanisms for the cellular control of proMMP-2 (gelatinase A) activation hints at the significance of this level of regulation in controlling matrix turnover.

The fact that processing and activation of MMP-2 (gelatinase A) appears to be restricted to the cell surface is likely to have important implications in vivo. Cell surface activation allows migrating and invading cells to focus MMP-2 (gelatinase A) activity immediately adjacent to areas of the extracellular matrix that are in the cell path and thus limits the amount of matrix that needs to be turned over (51,59,60). Consistent with this idea, active MMP-2 (gelatinase A) appears to be localized to the invadopodia of malignant cells (61).

VI. Substrate Specificity

MMP-2 [MMP-2 (gelatinase A)] regulates the turnover of a number of ECM components (Table 1). MMP-2 (gelatinase A) cleaves a number of peptide bonds in denatured collagen (gelatin) such as Gly-Val, Gly-Leu, Gly-Glu, Gly-Asn, and Gly-Ser to produce small peptides (62,63). Besides gelatin and types IV and V collagen, MMP-2 (gelatinase A) also cleaves type VII collagen, found in anchoring fibrils (64), cartilage type X collagen (65,66), and elastin (67). It is interesting to note that pepsin-solubilized type IV collagen is degraded by both MMP-2 (gelatinase A) and MMP-9 (gelatinase B) (68), whereas the full-length type IV collagen apparently is resistant to proteolysis by both gelatinases (69). These findings raised concerns as to whether gelatinases actually function as true "type IV collagenase" in vivo. While the initial cleavage site of soluble type IV collagen by MMP-2 (gelatinase A) has been found to be located one quarter of the distance from the NH_2-terminus (70,71), the cleavage site of the full length native type IV collagen remains to be determined.

While both MMP-2 (gelatinase A) and MMP-9 (gelatinase B) bind to type I collagen, only MMP-2 (gelatinase A) has been shown to cleave soluble, triple helical type I collagen generating 3/4 N-terminal and 1/4 C-terminal fragments characteristic of vertebrate interstitial collagenases (72). MMP-2 (gelatinase A) cleaves type I collagen at the same Gly-Ile/Leu bond in the collagen alpha chains as interstitial collagenases. MMP-2 (gelatinase A) is also capable of degrading reconstituted type I collagen fibrils. The closely related gelatinase B is unable to cleave soluble or fibrillar collagen under identical conditions, indicating that type I collagenolytic activity of MMP-2 (gelatinase A) is not a general property of the gelatinase subgroup of MMPs. In addition to fibrillar and nonfibrillar collagen, MMP-2 (gelatinase A) has been shown to degrade elastin (67,73). These findings suggest that the name MMP-2 (gelatinase A) is a misnomer and that this protease may have a much greater role in turnover of a variety of extracellular matrix components than previously appreciated. This should emphasize the importance of determining the critical substrates for these proteases in vivo.

To date, very little is known about the in vivo substrate specificity of MMP-2 (gelatinase A). Aside from its ability to degrade various components of ECM, MMP-2 (gelatinase A) has been shown to possess a β-secretase activity. In HeLa cells transfected with an amyloid protein precursor (APP) 695 expression plasmid, MMP-2 (gelatinase A) cleaves the 110 kDa cell surface APP, releasing a 100 kDa form of the protein. While a peptide homologous to the β-secretase site is cleaved by MMP-2 (gelatinase A), a peptide homologous to the α-secretase site is not cleaved (74,75). This recent finding may represent one of many in vivo substrates of MMP-2 (gelatinase A). Additional potential substrates identified in vitro include vitronectin and laminin-5 (15,76).

VII. MMP-2 [MMP-2 (Gelatinase A)] in LAM

Descriptive studies suggest a role for MMPs in many physiologic processes including intrahepatic bile duct formation (77), small bowel development (78), mammary gland branching morphogenesis (79), salivary gland morphogenesis (80), wound healing and cycling endometrium (81,82). Particularly interesting is the demonstration that stromelysin-mediated dissociation of breast epithelial cells from their underlying basement membrane is concomitant with the induction of programmed cell death (83). Recent studies from several laboratories also suggest that MMP-2 (gelatinase A) activity may play an important role in T lymphocyte transmigration across subendothelial cell basement membranes (84,85). These are self-limited processes that preserve matrix integrity and function.

Lymphangiomyomatosis (LAM) is a disease that exists in women of reproductive age and is characterized by the proliferation of smooth muscle cells derived from lymphatic vessels and the formation of air-filled cysts. Most of the studies conducted thus far have focused on the effects of hormone control. These studies, however, do not explain the mechanism for formation of the cystic lesions characteristic of this disease. Development of these cysts has been attributed to the degeneration of collagen and elastic fibers (86). Since much has been studied about the degeneration of extracellular matrix components such as collagens by MMPs in tumor cells, it is also of interest to examine the relationship between MMPs and TIMPs in LAM.

MMPs and TIMPs may play direct roles in the structural damage and cystic lesions that develop in the pathological condition known as LAM (87). Increased MMP-2 (gelatinase A) activity appears to be responsible for the cystic destruction of the lung parenchyma in LAM. MMP-9 and MMP-1 are also expressed at an increased level compared with normal bronchiolar and vascular smooth muscle, but to a lesser extent. Elastic fibers found in LAM lesions showed immunohistochemical reactivity for MMP-2. TIMP-1 and TIMP-2 levels were not increased in LAM cells. These findings suggest that proliferating cells in patients with LAM (referred to as LAM cells) serve as a primary source for MMP-2 and that these elevated levels are responsible for the cystic destruction of lung parenchyma in LAM. An important observation in these studies is no detectable infiltration of the lung tissue by other cell types, such as neutrophils, eosinophils, and macrophages, that could otherwise provide lytic activity against connective tissue in lesions of LAM. Therefore, it is an imbalance of MMPs and TIMPs, produced by proliferating LAM cells, that appears responsible for the cystic destruction that is a major histopathologic feature of this disease.

VIII. Summary

During the evolution of many pathologic conditions the alterations in extracellular matrix are more extreme and result in changes in matrix distribution, composition, and function. Interstitial lung diseases, as exemplified by the recent findings in LAM, illustrate how this imbalance contributes to evolution of the disease process. These alterations can provide useful insights into the dynamics of stromal matrix turnover as well as the function and significance of matrix components. The expression of matrixin family proteases are also linked with other pathologic processes involving extracellular matrix turnover, such as tumor cell invasion and rheumatoid arthritis (88–90). A number of correlative studies have clearly demonstrated that several members of the MMP family may be overexpressed in either the malignant cells of the tumor or adjacent reactive stromal fibroblasts. Overexpression of MMPs is associated with the malignant progression in human lung, prostate, gastric, colon, breast, ovary, thyroid, as well as head and neck squamous carcinomas (reviewed in Refs. 88,89). These descriptive studies are supported by the demonstration of a functional role for MMP activity in tumor cell invasion through the use of MMP inhibitors (88,89,91). It would be useful to demonstrate a functional role for MMP activity in neoplastic conditions using a similar approach. This would also explore the possible clinical utility of MMP inhibitors for the treatment of these conditions. However, many of these pathologic conditions, such as LAM, await the development of a suitable animal model.

References

1. Lochter A, Bissell MJ. Involvement of extracellular matrix constituents in breast cancer. Semin Cancer Biol 1995; 66:165–173.
2. Ruoslathi E, Yamaguchi Y. Proteoglycans as modulators of growth factor activities. Cell 1991; 64:867–869.
3. Frisch SM, Vuori K, Ruoslahti E, Chan-Hui PY. Control of adhesion-dependent cell survival by focal adhesion kinase. J Cell Biol 1996; 134:793–799.
4. Levi E, Fridman R, Miao HQ, Ma YS, Yayon A, Vlodavsky I. Matrix metalloproteinase 2 releases active soluble ectodomain of fibroblast growth factor receptor 1. Proc Natl Acad Sci USA 1996; 93:7069–7074.
5. Hooper NM. Families of zinc metalloproteinases. FEBS Lett 1994; 354:1–6.
6. Stocker W, Grams F, Baumann U, et al. The metzincins–topological and sequential relations between the astacins, adamalysins, seralysins, and matrixins (collagenases) define a superfamily of zinc-peptidases. Protein Sci 1995; 4:823–840.
7. Ray JM, Stetler-Stevenson WG. TIMP-2 expression modulates human melanoma cell adhesion and motility. Ann NY Acad Sci 1994; 732:233–247.
8. Ochieng J, Fridman R, Nangia-Makker P, et al. Galectin-3 is a novel substrate for human matrix metalloproteinases-2 and -9. Biochemistry 1994; 33:14109–14114.
9. Rouyer N, Wolf C, Chenard MP, et al. Stromelysin-3 gene expression in human cancer: an overview. Invasion Metastasis 1995; 14:269–275.
10. Wolf C, Rouyer N, Lutz Y, et al. Stromelysin 3 belongs to a subgroup of proteinases expressed in breast carcinoma fibroblastic cells and possibly implicated in tumor progression. Proc Natl Acad Sci USA 1993; 90:1843–1847.
11. Wolf C, Chenard MP, Durand de Grossouvre P, Bellocq JP, Chambon P, Basset P. Breast-cancer-associated stromelysin-3 gene is expressed in basal cell carcinoma and during cutaneous wound healing. J Invest Dermatol 1992; 99:870–872.
12. Will H, Hinzmann B. cDNA sequence and mRNA tissue distribution of a novel human matrix metalloproteinase with a potential transmembrane segment. Eur J Biochem 1995; 231:602–608.
13. Sato H, Takino T, Okada Y, et al. A matrix metalloproteinase expressed on the surface of invasive tumour cells. Nature 1994; 370:61–65.
14. Pei D, Weiss SJ. Furin-dependent intracellular activation of the human stromelysin-3 zymogen. Nature 1995; 375:244–247.

15. Imai K, Ohuchi E, Aoki T, et al. Membrane-type matrix metalloproteinase 1 is a gelatinolytic enzyme and is secreted in a complex with tissue inhibitor of metalloproteinases 2. Cancer Res 1996; 56:2707–2710.
16. Kinoshita T, Sato H, Takino T, Itoh M, Akizawa T, Seiki M. Processing of a precursor of 72-kilodalton type IV collagenase/MMP-2 (gelatinase A) by a recombinant membrane-type 1 matrix metalloproteinase. Cancer Res 1996; 56:2535–2538.
17. Van Wart HE, Birkedal-Hansen H. The cysteine switch: a principle of regulation of metalloproteinase activity with potential applicability to the entire matrix metalloproteinase gene family. Proc Natl Acad Sci USA 1990; 87:5578–5582.
18. Libson AM, Gittis AG, Collier IE, Marmer BL, Goldberg GI, Lattman EE. Crystal structure of the haemopexin-like C-terminal domain of MMP-2 (gelatinase A). Nat Struct Biol 1995; 2:938–942.
19. Murphy G, Allan JA, Willenbrock F, Cockett MI, O'Connell JP, Docherty AJ. The role of the C-terminal domain in collagenase and stromelysin specificity. J Biol Chem 1992; 267:9612–9618.
20. Bode W. A helping hand for collagenases: the haemopexin-like domain. Structure 1995; 3:527–530.
21. Murphy G, Nguyen Q, Cockett MI, et al. Assessment of the role of the fibronectin-like domain of MMP-2 (gelatinase A) by analysis of a deletion mutant. J Biol Chem 1994; 269:6632–6636.
22. Murphy G, Willenbrock F, Ward RV, Cockett MI, Eaton D, Docherty AJ. The terminal domain of 72 kDa MMP-2 (gelatinase A) is not required for catalysis, but is essential for membrane activation and modulates interactions with tissue inhibitors of metalloproteinases. Biochem J 1992; 283:637–641.
23. Emmert-Buck MR, Emonard HP, Corcoran ML, Krutzsch HC, Foidart JM, Stetler-Stevenson WG. Cell surface binding of TIMP-2 and pro-MMP-2/TIMP-2 complex. FEBS Lett 1995; 364:28–32.
24. Strongin AY, Collier I, Bannikov G, Marmer BL, Grant GA, Goldberg GI. Mechanism of cell surface activation of 72-kDa type IV collagenase. Isolation of the activated form of the membrane metalloprotease. J Biol Chem 1995; 270:5331–5338.
25. Ward RV, Atkinson SJ, Reynolds JJ, Murphy G. Cell surface-mediated activation of proMMP-2 (gelatinase A): demonstration of the involvement of the C-terminal domain of proMMP-2 (gelatinase A) in cell surface binding and activation of proMMP-2 (gelatinase A) by primary fibroblasts. Biochem J 1994; 304:263–269.
26. Kleiner DE, Jr., Unsworth EJ, Krutzsch HC, Stetler-Stevenson WG. Higher-order complex formation between the 72-kilodalton type IV collagenase and tissue inhibitor of metalloproteinases-2. Biochemistry 1992; 31:1665–1672.
27. Seiki M. Membrane type-matrix metalloproteinase and tumor invasion. Curr Top Microbiol Immunol 1996; 213:23–32.
28. Brown PD, Levy AT, Margulies IM, Liotta LA, Stetler-Stevenson WG. Independent expression and cellular processing of Mr 72,000 type IV collagenase and interstitial collagenase in human tumorigenic cell lines. Cancer Res 1990; 50:6184–6191.
29. Collier IE, Smith J, Kronberger A, et al. The structure of the human skin fibroblast collagenase gene. J Biol Chem 1988; 263:10711–10713.
30. Overall CM, Sodek J. Concanavalin A produces a matrix-degradative phenotype in

human fibroblasts. Induction and endogenous activation of collagenase, 72-kDa gelatinase, and Pump-1 is accompanied by the suppression of the tissue inhibitor of matrix metalloproteinases. J Biol Chem 1990; 265:21141–21151.

31. Matrisian LM. Matrix metalloproteinase gene expression. Ann NY Acad Sci 1994; 732:42–50.
32. Huhtala P, Chow LT, Tryggvason K. Structure of the human type IV collagenase gene. J Biol Chem 1990; 265:11077–11082.
33. Templeton NS, Stetler-Stevenson WG. Identification of a basal promoter for the human Mr 72,000 type IV collagenase gene and enhanced expression in a highly metastatic cell line. Cancer Res 1991; 51:6190–6193.
34. Frisch SM, Reich R, Collier IE, Genrich LT, Martin G, Goldberg GI. Adenovirus ElA represses protease gene expression and inhibits metastasis of human tumor cells. Oncogene 1990; 5:75–83.
35. Overall CM, Wrana JL, Sodek J. Transcriptional and post-transcriptional regulation of 72-kDa gelatinase/type IV collagenase by transforming growth factor-beta 1 in human fibroblasts. Comparisons with collagenase and tissue inhibitor of matrix metalloproteinase gene expression. J Biol Chem 1991; 266:14064–14071.
36. Benbow U, Brinckerkoff CE. The AP-1 site and MMP gene regulation: What is all the fuss about? Matrix Biol 1997; 15:519–526.
37. Fini ME, Bartlett JD, Matsubara M, Rinehart WB, Mody MK, Girard MT, Rainville M. The rabbit gene for 92-kDa matrix metalloproteinase. Role of AP1 and AP2 in cell type-specific transcription. J Biol Chem 1994; 269:28620–28628.
38. Kleiner DE, Jr., Tuuttila A, Tryggvason K, Stetler-Stevenson WG. Stability analysis of latent and active 72-kDa type IV collagenase: the role of tissue inhibitor of metalloproteinases-2 (TIMP-2). Biochemistry 1993; 32:1583–1592.
39. Goldberg GI, Manner BL, Grant GA, Eisen AZ, Wilhelm S, He CS. Human 72-kilodalton type IV collagenase forms a complex with a tissue inhibitor of metalloproteases designated TIMP-2. Proc Natl Acad Sci USA 1989; 86:8207-8211.
40. Goldberg GI, Collier IE, Eisen AZ, Grant GA, Marmer BL, Wilhelm SM. Mosaic structure of the secreted ECM metalloproteases and interaction of the type IV collagenases with inhibitors. Matrix Suppl 1992; 1:25–30.
41. Goldberg GI, Strongin A, Collier IE, Genrich LT, Marmer BL. Interaction of 92-kDa type IV collagenase with the tissue inhibitor of metalloproteinases prevents dimerization, complex formation with interstitial collagenase, and activation of the proenzyme with stromelysin. J Biol Chem 1992; 267:4583–4591.
42. Stetler-Stevenson WG, Krutzsch HC, Wacher MP, Margulies IM, Liotta LA. The activation of human type IV collagenase proenzyme. Sequence identification of the major conversion product following organomercurial activation. J Biol Chem 1989; 264:1353-1356.
43. Wilhelm SM, Collier IE, Marmer BL, Eisen AZ, Grant GA, Goldberg GI. SV40-transformed human lung fibroblasts secrete a 92-kDa type IV collagenase which is identical to that secreted by normal human macrophages [published erratum appears in J Biol Chem 1990; 265(36):22570]. J Biol Chem 1989; 264:17213–17221.
44. Willenbrock F, Crabbe T, Slocombe PM, et al. The activity of the tissue inhibitors of metalloproteinases is regulated by C-terminal domain interactions: a kinetic analysis of the inhibition of MMP-2 (gelatinase A). Biochemistry 1993; 32:4330–4337.

45. Fridman R, Fuerst TR, Bird RE, et al. Domain structure of human 72-kDa gelatinase/type IV collagenase. Characterization of proteolytic activity and identification of the tissue inhibitor of metalloproteinase-2 (TIMP-2) binding regions. J Biol Chem 1992; 267:15398–15405.
46. Nguyen Q, Willenbrock F, Cockett MI, O'Shea M, Docherty AJ, Murphy G. Different domain interactions are involved in the binding of tissue inhibitors of metalloproteinases to stromelysin-1 and MMP-2 (gelatinase A). Biochemistry 1994; 33:2089–2095.
47. Curry VA, Clark IM, Bigg H, Cawston TE. Large inhibitor of metalloproteinases (LIMP) contains tissue inhibitor of metalloproteinases (TIMP)-2 bound to 72,000-M(r) progelatinase. Biochem J 1992; 285:143–147.
48. Kolkenbrock H, Orgel D, Hecker-Kia A, Noack W, Ulbrich N. The complex between a tissue inhibitor of metalloproteinases (TIMP-2) and 72kDa progelatinase is a metalloproteinase inhibitor. Eur J Biochem 1991; 198:775–781.
49. Bigg HF, Shi YE, Liu YE, Steffensen B, Overall CM. Specific, High affinity binding of tissue inhibitor of metalloproteinase-4 (TIMP-4) to the COOH-terminal hemopexin-like domain of human MMP-2 (gelatinase A). J Biol Chem 1997; 272:15496–15500.
50. Ito A, Nakajima S, Sasaguri Y, Nagase H, Mori Y. Co-culture of human breast adenocarcinoma MCF-7 cells and human dermal fibroblasts enhances the production of matrix metalloproteinases 1, 2 and 3 in fibroblasts. Br J Cancer 1995; 71:1039–1045.
51. Brown PD, Bloxidge RE, Anderson E, Howell A. Expression of activated gelatinase in human invasive breast carcinoma. Clin Exp Metastasis 1993; 11: 183–189.
52. Ward RV, Atkinson SJ, Slocombe PM, Docherty AJ, Reynolds JJ, Murphy G. Tissue inhibitor of metalloproteinases-2 inhibits the activation of 72 kDa progelatinase by fibroblast membranes. Biochim Biophys Acta 1991; 1079:242-246.
53. Strongin AY, Marmer BL, Grant GA, Goldberg GI. Plasma membrane-dependent activation of the 72-kDa type IV collagenase is prevented by complex formation with TIMP-2. J Biol Chem 1993; 268:14033–14039.
54. Strongin AY, Collier IE, Krasnov PA, Genrich LT, Marmer BL, Goldberg GI. Human 92 kDa type IV collagenase: functional analysis of fibronectin and carboxyl-end domains. Kidney Int 1993; 43:158–162.
55. Bergmann U, Tuuttila A, Stetler-Stevenson WG, Tryggvason K. Autolytic activation of recombinant human 72 kilodalton type IV collagenase. Biochemistry 1995; 34:2819–2825.
56. Cao J, Sato H, Takino T, Seiki M. The C-terminal region of membrane type matrix metalloproteinase is a functional transmembrane domain required for pro-gelatinase A activation. J Biol Chem 1995; 270:801–805.
57. Emonard HP, Remacle AG, Noel AC, Grimaud JA, Stetler-Stevenson WG, Foidart JM. Tumor cell surface-associated binding site for the M(r) 72,000 type IV collagenase. Cancer Res 1992; 52:5845–5849.
58. Brooks PC, Stromblad S, Sanders LC, et al. Localization of matrix metalloproteinase MMP-2 to the surface of invasive cells by interaction with integrin alpha v beta 3. Cell 1996; 85:683–693.
59. Brown PD, Bloxidge RE, Stuart NS, Gatter KC, Carmichael J. Association between

expression of activated 72-kilodalton MMP-2 (gelatinase A)nd tumor spread in non-small-cell lung carcinoma. J Natl Cancer Inst 1993; 85:574–578.
60. Brown PD, Kleiner DE, Unsworth EJ, Stetler-Stevenson WG. Cellular activation of the 72 kDa type IV procollagenase/TIMP-2 complex. Kidney Int 1993; 43:163–170.
61. Monsky WL, Kelly T, Lin CY, et al. Binding and localization of M(r) 72,000 matrix metalloproteinase at cell surface invadopodia. Cancer Res 1993; 53:3159–3164.
62. Seltzer JL, Adams SA, Grant GA, Eisen AZ. Purification and properties of a gelatin-specific neutral protease from human skin. J Biol Chem 1981;256:4662–4668.
63. Seltzer JL, Akers KT, Weingarten H, Grant GA, McCourt DW, Eisen AZ. Cleavage specificity of human skin type IV collagenase (gelatinase). J Biol Chem 1990; 265:20409–20413.
64. Seltzer JL, Eisen AZ, Bauer EA, Morris NP, Glanville RW, Burgeson RE. Cleavage of type VII collagen by interstitial collagenase and type IV collagenase (gelatinase) derived from human skin. J Biol Chem 1989; 264:3822–3826.
65. Gadher SJ, Schmid TM, Heck LW, Woolley DE. Cleavage of collagen type X by human synovial collagenase and neutrophil elastase. Matrix 1989; 9:109–115.
66. Welgus HG, Fliszar CJ, Seltzer JL, Schmid TM, Jeffrey JJ. Differential susceptibility of type X collagen to cleavage by two mammalian interstitial collagenases and 72-kDa type IV collagenase. J Biol Chem 1990; 265:13521–13527.
67. Senior RM, Griffin GL, Fliszar CJ, Shapiro SD, Goldberg GI, Welgus HG. Human 92- and 72-kilodalton type IV collagenases are elastases. J Biol Chem 1991; 266:7870–7875.
68. Mainardi CL, Dixit SL, Kang AH. Degradation of type-IV (basement membrane) collagen by a proteinase isolated from human polymorphonuclear leukocyte granules. J Biol Chem 1980; 255:5435–5441.
69. MacKay AR, Hartzler JL, Pelina MD, Thorgeirsson UP. Studies on the ability of 65kDa and 92kDa tumour cell gelatinases to degrade type-IV collagen. J Biol Chem 1990; 265:21929–21934.
70. Fessler LI, Duncan KG, Fessler JH, Salot T, Tryggvason K. Characterization of procollagen IV cleavage products produced by a specific tumor collagenase. J Biol Chem 1984; 259:9783–9789.
71. Murphy G, Ward R, Hembry RM, Reynolds JJ, Kuhn K, Tryggvason K. Characterization of gelatinase from pig polymorphonuclear leukocytes. Biochem J 1989; 258:463–452.
72. Aimes RT, Quigley JP. Matrix metalloproteinase-2 is an interstitial collagenase. Inhibitor-free enzyme catalyzes the cleavage of collagen fibrils and soluble native type I collagen generating the specific 3/4- and 1/4-length fragments. J Biol Chem 1995; 270:5872–5876.
73. Murphy G, Houbrechts A, Cockett MI, Williamson RA, O'Shea M, Docherty AJ. The N-terminal domain of tissue inhibitor of metalloproteinases retains metalloproteinase inhibitory activity [published erratum appears in Biochemistry 1991; 30(42):10362]. Biochemistry 1991; 30:8097-8102.
74. LePage RN, Fosang AJ, Fuller SJ, et al. MMP-2 (gelatinase A) possesses a beta-secretase-like activity in cleaving the amyloid protein precursor of Alzheimer's disease. FEBS Lett 1995; 377:267–270.

75. Roher AE, Kasunic TC, Woods AS, Cotter RJ, Ball MJ, Fridman R. Proteolysis of A beta peptide from Alzheimer disease brain by MMP-2 (gelatinase A). Biochem Biophys Res Commun 1994; 205:1755–1761.
76. Giannelli G, Falk-Marzillier J, Schiraldi O, Stetler-Stevenson WG, Quaranta V. Induction of cell migration by matrix metalloproteinase-2 cleavage of laminin-5. Science 1997; 277:225–228.
77. Terada T, Okada Y, Nakanuma Y. Expression of matrix proteinases during human intrahepatic bile duct development. A possible role in biliary cell migration. Am J Pathol 1995; 147:1207–1213.
78. Patterton E, Hayes WP, Shi YB. Transcriptional activation of the matrix metalloproteinase gene stromelysin-3 coincides with thyroid hormone-induced cell death during frog metamorphosis. Dev Bio 1995; 167.
79. Sympson CJ, Talhouk RS, Alexander CM, et al. Targeted expression of stromelysin-1 in mammary gland provides evidence for a role of proteinases in branching morphogenesis and the requirement for an intact basement membrane for tissue-specific gene expression. J Cell Biol 1994; 125:681–693.
80. Hayakawa T, Kishi J-I, Nakanishi Y. Salivary gland morphogenesis: possible involvement of collagenase. In: Birkedal-Hansen H, Werb Z, Welgus H, VanWart H, eds. Matrix Metalloproteinases and Inhibitors. New York: Gustav Fischer, 1992:344-351.
81. Rodgers WH, Matrisian LM, Giudice LC, et al. Patterns of matrix metalloproteinase expression in cycling endometrium imply differential functions and regulation by steroid hormones. J Clin Invest 1994; 94:946–953.
82. Saarialho-Kere UK, Pentland AP, Birkedal-Hansen H, Parks WC, Welgus HG. Distinct populations of basal keratinocytes express stromelysin-1 and stromelysin-2 in chronic wounds. J Clin Invest 1994; 94:79–88.
83. Boudreau N, Sympson CJ, Werb Z, Bissell MJ. Suppression of ICE and apoptosis in mammary epithelial cells by extracellular matrix. Science 1995; 267:891–893.
84. Romanic AM, Madri JA. The induction of 72-kD gelatinase in T cells upon adhesion to endothelial cells is VCAM-1 dependent. J Cell Biol 1994; 125:1165-1178.
85. Leppert D, Waubant E, Galardy R, Bunnett NW, Hauser SL. T cell gelatinases mediate basement membrane transmigration *in vitro*. J Immunol 1995; 154:4379-4389.
86. Fukuda YK, Yamamoto A, Ishizaki M, Bassett F, Masugi Y. Role of elastic fiber degradation in emphysema-like lesions of pulmonary lymphangiomyomatosis. Hum Pathol 1990; 21:1252-1261.
87. Hayashi TF, Stetler-Stevenson WG, Liotta LA, Moss J, Ferrans VJ, Travis WD. Immunohistochemical study of matrix metalloproteinases (MMPS) and their tissue inhibitors (TIMPs) in pulmonary lymphangioleiomyomatosis (LAM). Human Pathol 1997; 28: 1071–1078.
88. Stetler-Stevenson WG, Aznavoorian S, Liotta LA. Tumor cell interactions with the extracellular matrix during invasion and metastasis. Annu Rev Cell Biol 1993; 9:541–573.
89. Stetler-Stevenson WG, Liotta LA, Kleiner D, Jr. Extracellular matrix 6: role of

matrix metalloproteinases in tumor invasion and metastasis. FASEB J 1993; 7:1434–1441.

90. Birkedal-Hansen H, Moore WG, Bodden MK, et al. Matrix metalloproteinases: a review. Crit Rev Oral Biol Med 1993; 4:4197–4250.
91. MacDougall JR, Matrisian LM. Contributions of tumor and stromal matrix metalloproteinases to tumor progression, invasion and metastasis. Cancer Metast Rev 1995; 14:351–362.

28

Surrogate Markers of Lung Destruction

CLIFFORD TAGGART, RAY COAKLEY, PATRICIA GLYNN, SHANE O'NEILL, and NOEL G. McELVANEY

Royal College of Surgeons in Ireland/Beaumont Hospital
Dublin, Ireland

I. Introduction

Much of the lung damage associated with pathological states is mediated through the actions of proteases and oxidants on the various elements of the lung matrix. This damage is not detectable early in its course by currently available diagnostic modalities such as chest roentgenograms, computed tomography (CT) scan, blood gas estimations, or pulmonary function tests. By the time abnormalities have been detected using these tests, lung damage, often irreversible, has already occurred. This has led to the search for "surrogate markers" of lung destruction similar to "liver function tests," which ideally would give an indication of lung disease at its earliest onset and also measure its progression and response to treatment.

In the process of respiration, the large surface area of the lung is repeatedly exposed to microorganisms, particulates, gases, and aerosols, all of which can cause damage (1). Furthermore, the lung is also exposed to damage from within, often by the very mechanisms developed to protect against external attack. Cigarette smoke, a mixture of gas and particulate matter rich in oxidants, is a classic example of external attack. Other potentially damaging inhaled gases include nitrogen dioxide, sulfur dioxide, and ozone. Exposure to high oxygen concentrations is also associated with significant lung injury mediated in large part through the generation of reactive oxidant species. Inhalation of particulates such as asbestos fibers and silicates is associated with a wide variety of lung diseases including fibrosis, pleural disease, and cancer. Potential mechanisms for these conditions include release of oxidants and proteases by lower respiratory tract macrophages in the process of ingestion of these particulates. In addition to these inhaled agents, a wide variety of drugs can also mediate injury to lung cells, often via different mechanisms. Bleomycin induces DNA strand breakage by chelating metal, with the resulting drug-metal complex generating a single electron transfer to oxygen to generate superoxide (2), whereas nitrofurantoin is oxidized directly under aerobic conditions, to liberate a free electron, thus generating hydrogen peroxide, hydroxyl radical, and superoxide. In this regard it is noteworthy that high inspired oxygen concentrations in patients with prior bleomycin therapy enhance the development of bleomycin-induced lung injury (3).

"Internal attack" may occur in the lungs as a consequence of overburdened or uncontrolled lung defense mechanisms. The lung has many defense systems located throughout the upper and lower airways. Large particulates and most microbes impact against the mucosa and are removed by sneezing, coughing, and mucociliary clearance. Smaller particles and bacteria may escape clearance and reach the alveolar ducts, but here they undergo phagocytosis by macrophages and other inflammatory cells, particularly neutrophils. There are estimated to be 15–30 × 10^9 macrophages in the human lung (4) with approximately 50–100 macrophages per alveolus. Macrophages engulf foreign particles through surface receptors resulting in a marked change in the cellular metabolism of these cells, referred to as the respiratory burst. During this respiratory burst, large amounts of superoxide and hydroxyl radicals are released along with hydrogen peroxide. The generation of these highly reactive oxygen species plays a central role in the killing of microorganisms by phagocytes but extracellular release of oxidants can also cause lung damage. Other potential sources of lung damage by macrophages include proteases such as collagenases and gelatinases as well as the mediators, LTB4 and IL-8, that attract and activate neutrophils at sites of inflammation in the lung.

Neutrophils are another important part of the lung defense armamentarium, but they also serve as a major source of potentially damaging proteases (5). Proteases stored in the neutrophil are released extracellularly depending on the cellular response to various stimuli. During phagocytosis of foreign material, proteases can "leak" into the extracellular space (6), while directed release of azurophilic granules can also occur as part of the inflammatory response, a process that also includes the respiratory burst and myeloperoxidase-mediated oxidant production. Neutrophil proteases are also released from granules following damage or death of the cell. The actions of neutrophil elastase (NE), the major protease contained within the azurophilic granules of neutrophils, have been particularly well characterized. Neutrophil elastase is capable of degrading elastin, collagen (types I–IV), fibronectin, laminin, and proteoglycans (7,8) as well as a wide variety of coagulation and complement factors. As a result of its high concentration and broad range of activity, NE is thought to play a major role in the pathogenesis of a variety of lung diseases including emphysema, bronchitis, cystic fibrosis, asthma, bronchopulmonary pneumonia, and adult respiratory distress syndrome. In this regard, NE has been found in association with lung elastin and connective tissue following intratracheal administration with concomitant reduction in elastin content (9,10) and evidence of lung destruction. Other serine proteases found within the azurophilic granules of neutrophils include cathepsin G and proteinase 3. Although they can act on a wide range of substrates, their role in lung disease is still unclear. Neutrophils also store metalloproteases, which are elevated in the sputum of individuals with cystic fibrosis suggesting that a metalloprotease/antimetalloprotease imbalance may also play a role in the lung disease associated with this condition (11).

As noted earlier, leukocytes attracted to the lungs during inflammation undergo respiratory burst. This results in the formation of a variety of oxidizing species including superoxide radicals (O_2^-), hydroxyl radicals (OH·), hydrogen peroxide (H_2O_2), hypochlorous acid (HOC1), and nitric oxide (NO). Superoxide anion is degraded to H_2O_2 by superoxide dismutase (SOD) (12), while H_2O_2 may be converted to HOC1 by myeloperoxidase or to H_2O by catalase. Metal-catalyzed oxidation can result in the formation of OH· from H_2O_2. The role of NO in lung disease is unclear, but it can be induced by inflammatory stimuli in macrophages (13) and has been shown to have cytotoxic effects and serve as a regulator of cellular responses such as vasodilation. NO also reacts with superoxide anion to form peroxynitrite ($ONOO^-$), which has been implicated in a number of pulmonary disorders (14). Against this oxidant burden the lung has evolved a sophisticated set of antioxidant defenses, but in chronic disorders such as cystic fibrosis (CF) or idiopathic pulmonary fibrosis (IPF) the antioxidant protective screen is reduced rendering the lung more susceptible to oxidant-induced injury.

Apart from direct toxic effects, oxidants also cause pulmonary injury by interfering with other host defense mechanisms. Inactivation, by oxidation, of the serpin α^1-antitrypsin (α_1AT), which inhibits a variety of serine proteases, is thought responsible for much of the lung damage associated with adult respiratory distress syndrome (ARDS) (15) and cigarette smoking (16). Oxidatively inactivated α_1AT is incapable of inhibiting NE, thus leading to unopposed proteolytic damage by this enzyme. Oxidants are also responsible for the activation of collagenase secreted by neutrophils (17), and studies have also indicated the involvement of oxidant-producing enzymes such as glucose oxidase (18) and xanthine oxidase (19) in increased permeability and attraction of neutrophils.

In addition to its effects on protein, oxidant stress can also affect lipid and DNA. In lung injury induced by thermal skin trauma, complement activation leads to neutrophil-mediated lung injury followed by the appearance of conjugated dienes, lipid hydroperoxides, and N,N′-iminopropenes in lung homogenates and plasma (20). Various oxidant stresses, including H_2O_2, induce DNA strand breaks in a variety of target cells. The repair processes invoked by this oxidative stress can become overburdened leading to misrepair, chromosomal aberrations, and mutations.

Early detection of these proteolytic and oxidant-induced insults to the lung may enable timely recognition of disease onset and appropriate therapeutic intervention before irreversible damage has occurred. With this as background the remainder of this chapter will focus on surrogate markers of proteolytic and oxidative lung injury and the various sites at which these markers can be sampled (Table 1). These sites include (1) bronchial secretions including bronchoalveolar lavage (BAL), tracheal aspirates, and induced sputum, (2) epithelial cells, (3) plasma or serum, and (4) urine.

II. Markers of Lung Destruction

A. Bronchial Secretions

Bronchial secretions are composed of cellular and noncellular components. Normal bronchoalveolar lavage (BAL) contains 85–90% macrophages, 7–12% lymphocytes, 0–2% neutrophils, and <1% eosinophils and basophils. In certain disease states these numbers can can alter dramatically, and this may be one of the earliest indicators of ongoing pathology in conditions such as cystic fibrosis (CF) (21), sarcoidosis (22), and idiopathic pulmonary fibrosis (IPF) (23). Neutrophil numbers are increased in CF (21), IPF (23), and bronchopulmonary dysplasia (BPD) (21,23,24). Interestingly, increased neutrophil numbers may precede evidence of acute infection or obvious lung destruction as assayed by standard methodologies (21). Lymphocytes predominate in sarcoidosis (22) and berylliosis (25,26). High lymphocyte counts may be present in relatively asymptomatic individuals with sarcoidosis and may give an indication of response to standard therapy. An increase in lymphocyte proliferation in response to beryllium is seen in individuals with berylliosis, a response that helps differentiate this condition from sarcoidosis (26). Abnormalities in BAL macrophages may result from ingestion of particles such as asbestos, silica, and coal dust in exposed individuals.

The noncellular component of BAL contains cytokines and chemoattractants in certain inflammatory conditions, e.g., IL-2 released by T lymphocytes in active sarcoidosis (27) and IL-8 in individuals with IPF (28) and CF (29).

Table 1 Detectable Substances Indicative of Lung Destruction and Associated Disease States

Marker	Degradation product	Sampling site	Disease state (Ref.)
Lipid			
Content		Lavage	Cystic fibrosis (44)
			Bronchiectasis (44)
Peroxidation products	Malondialdehyde	Lung homogenates and plasma	Trauma-induced lung injury (19)
	Lipid hydroperoxide		
	Conjugated dienes		
	N,N′-Iminopropenes		
Protein oxidation			
All proteins	Methionine sulfoxide	Lavage	Cigarette smoking (15)
			Hyperoxia (31)
	Carbonyl groups	Lavage/liver (rat)	Infant respiratory distress (41,42)
Specific proteins	α_1-Antitrypsin	Lavage	
Proteolytic degradation			
Elastolytic activity	Free elastase		Cystic fibrosis (29),
	Increased α_1-N.E complexes	Lavage	COPD (30), ARDS (53),
	Reduced anti-NE capacity		asthma (55)
Elastin	Elastin-derived peptides	Plasma	COPD (56)
	Desmosine	Urine	Cigarette smoking (57)
	Isodesmosine		Cystic fibrosis (72)
Collagen	Hydroxylysylpyridinoline	Urine	Emphysema (73)
	Lysylpyridinoline		
Fibrinogen	Aα-21 peptide	Plasma	Cigarette smoking (61)
DNA	Sister chromatid exchange	Bronchial brushing and lavage cells	(48–50)
	Chromosome aberration		
	Strand breaks		

In many cases these cytokines may be elevated prior to the onset of clinically active disease. The noncellular component of bronchial secretions may also contain active NE indicating that the normal anti-NE capacity of the epithelial lining fluid (ELF) (2–4 μM) has been overwhelmed and the epithelial surface is now exposed to the unopposed attack of NE (30). This is almost invariably found in adults with CF and also in those with asthma (31). The complete loss of anti-NE activity in bronchial secretions may be preceded by decreasing anti-NE capacity as seen in young children with CF, cigarette smokers, individuals exposed to hyperoxia, and premature neonates requiring ventilatory support. In this regard, analysis of bronchial secretions from cigarette smokers (16) and normals exposed to hyperoxia (32) has shown increased methionine sulfoxide content (Fig. 1). This is consistent with oxidation of the active site methionines in α_1AT to methionine sulfoxide. However, the methionine sulfoxide measured in bronchial secretions represents all oxidized methionine, not only the oxidized active site methionine in α_1AT. In order to improve the usefulness of this analysis, methodologies

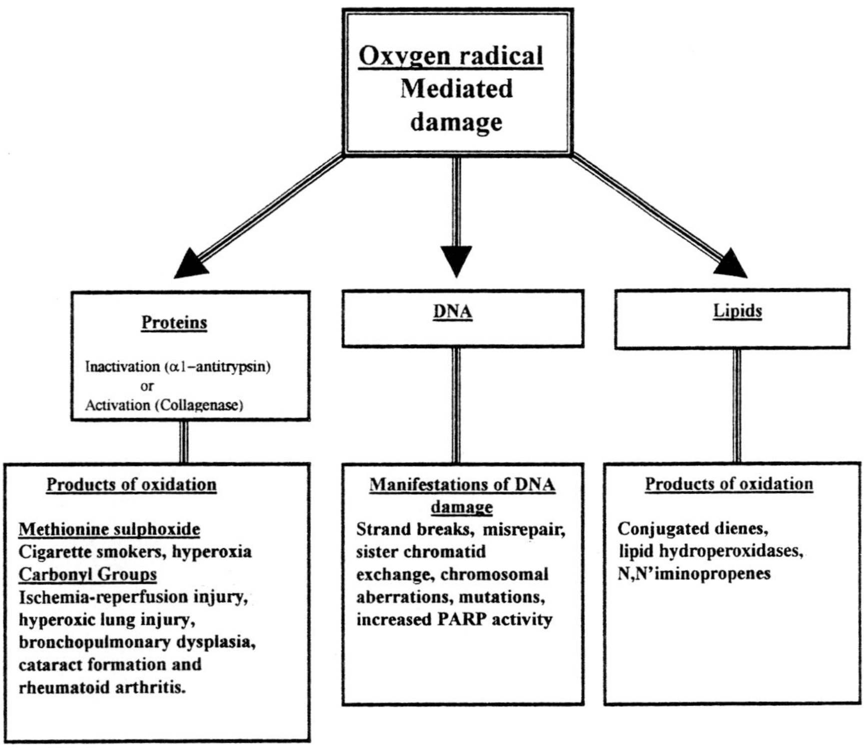

Figure 1 Mechanisms of oxygen radical–mediated molecular damage in protein, DNA, and lipids.

have been developed to determine which methionines on the α_1AT molecule have been oxidized. The basis of these new techniques lies in the ability of cyanogen bromide to cleave after methionine residues but not after methionine sulfoxide residues. Cleaved fragments are then separated and quantified by HPLC and those fragments containing methionine sulfoxide identified by the Edman degradation method of peptide sequencing (33). These techniques have been used to evaluate the oxidative inactivation of α_1AT by H_2O_2 in vitro and can be modified to evaluate α_1AT purified from bronchial secretions to determine the number, sequence, and degree of methionine oxidation with particular emphasis on the methionines at 358 and 351, which are felt to represent the active site (34).

Another methodology to assess oxidative stress in proteins from bronchial secretions is measurement of carbonyl content. Oxidation of proteins by mixed function oxidation (MFO) reactions leads to conversion of some amino acid side chains to carbonyl derivatives, and the levels of protein-bound carbonyl provide a measure of the extent of oxidative modification. Carbonyl groups can be detected by reaction with 2,4-dinitrophenylhydrazine (DNPH) followed by analysis by HPLC, which detects the resulting hydrazone formed in the reaction between the carbonyl group and DNPH (35). This is used to quantify carbonyl groups present in the sample. Carbonyl groups can also be detected by Western blot analysis using an antidinitrophenyl antibody following reaction with DNPH (36). Increases in protein carbonyl content have been shown in the lung (37) and brain (38) following ischemia-reperfusion, in human cataracts (39), in synovial fluid from individuals with rheumatoid arthritis (40), in animals (41) exposed to hyperoxia and in ventilated preterm neonates (42) (Fig. 1). In animals exposed to hyperoxia, increased protein carbonyl content was not limited to the lung but was also found in the liver, suggesting a systemic effect of hyperoxia (41). More recently, increased carbonyl content has been demonstrated in the tracheal aspirates of neonates requiring ventilation (43) and in normal adults undergoing short-duration exposure to hyperoxia. In both neonates and adults the increased carbonyl content was associated with decreased anti-NE protection indicative of an increased oxidant stress. Furthermore, the data indicated that elevated carbonyl content of tracheal aspirates in the first 3 days of life predicted the need for continued ventilatory support. Oxidation of lipids in bronchial secretions is less well defined (44) despite the fact that it has been shown in disease states such as CF and bronchiectasis that levels of lipid are increased in bronchial secretions (45).

B. Bronchial Brushing

Early injury to bronchial epithelial cells in disease states may show detectable functional and histological changes. Bronchial epithelial cells can be obtained with a cytology brush during bronchoscopy (46) and may be assessed for cell number and type, as well as occult evidence of infection (47).

Oxidant-mediated DNA damage may be measured in bronchial epithelial cells. Oxidized DNA bases from epithelial cells can be measured by gas chromatography (48), whereas DNA strand breaks can be quantified by the addition of ethidium bromide to cell lysates followed by fluorimetry to detect the amount of residual double-stranded DNA (49). Additionally, sister chromatid exchange, chromosome aberrations, and mutation frequency (50,51) can also be used to determine DNA damage in lung cells (Fig. 1). DNA repair can act as an indicator of DNA damage. Recent work has demonstrated that peroxynitrite ($ONOO^-$), a potent oxidant which triggers DNA strand breakage, results in the activation of poly (ADP-ribose) synthetase (PARP), an enzyme essential for DNA repair, in human pulmonary epithelial cells and increases epithelial paracellular permeability (52).

However, whereas bronchial secretions and brushings may give some important indications of early lung disease, along with its extent and amenability to treatment they involve relatively invasive techniques which has led to increased interest in blood and urine evaluations in the evaluation of lung disease.

C. Blood

A surrogate marker in blood reflecting NE-mediated proteolysis in the lung has for long been the "holy grail" of those interested in surrogate markers of lung destruction. A number of studies have shown that some NE from the epithelial surface can cross into the blood stream, where it is rapidly neutralized by the large antiprotease protection provided by circulating α_1AT. High levels of NE-α_1AT complexes in blood have been used as a marker of lung inflammation in conditions such as CF (53), ARDS (54,55), and asthma (56) (Fig.2). However, this measurement, of necessity, reflects not only the NE burden but also the anti-NE protection and as such may give misleading information, as in the case of α_1AT deficiency, a condition where the markedly reduced α_1AT in blood and on the respiratory epithelial surface leads to increased susceptibility to NE-induced damage. Here the low NE-α_1AT complex levels (secondary to the low α_1AT) would not reflect an increased NE burden on the respiratory epithelial surface.

A more direct methodology involves measurement of elastin-derived peptides (EDP) (Fig. 2). EDPs are derived from the proteolytic breakdown of mature, cross-linked elastin. An ELISA has been developed for the detection of EDPs in the blood and is based on the use of antibodies to EDP (57). These antibodies are raised in experimental rabbits by digesting elastin with purified human NE followed by injection into rabbits to raise antibodies to EDP. Kucich et al. showed that EDP levels are higher in chronic obstructive pulmonary disease (COPD) patients compared to normals, with non-COPD smokers having intermediate levels of EDPs (57). These results were confirmed by Schriver et al. (58), who also demonstrated elevated levels of EDP in COPD patients compared to

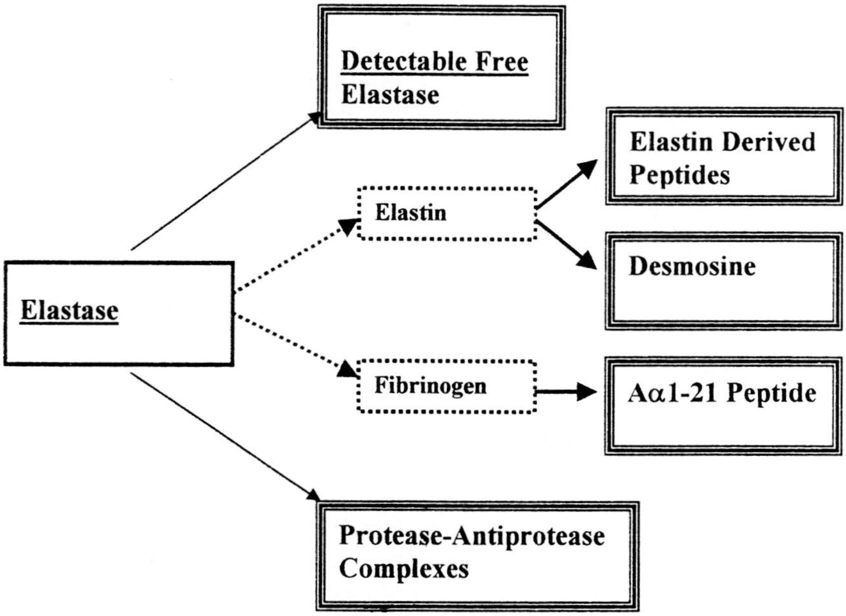

Figure 2 Surrogate markers of elastolytic lung destruction measured in urine and plasma.

normals. This study also showed elevated levels of EDP in some smokers, raising the question as to whether or not these individuals are at higher risk for emphysema over time than smokers with normal EDP levels. However, other studies have shown conflicting results (59,60).

Another plasma-based measurement which shows some promise is that developed by Weitz et al. (60), which makes use of the fact that NE cleaves the Val(Aα21)-Glu(Aα22) bond at the terminal NH_2-region of the Aα chain of fibrinogen. This leads to the release of the fibrinopeptide A–containing fragment Aα1-21, which can be measured using an RIA (Fig. 2). In individuals with α_1AT deficiency, plasma levels of Aα1-21 are higher than those in normals or in smokers (61). The levels of Aα1-21 are also higher in the plasma of cigarette smokers than nonsmokers (62).

Interestingly, Aα1-21 levels are detectable in nonsmoking individuals with normal levels of α_1AT and no obvious illnesses. These observations may be explained by the fact that NE from stimulated neutrophils can cleave substrates even in the presence of plasma containing α_1AT (63). In contrast, MeO-Suc-Ala-Ala-Pro-ValCH_2C1, a low molecular weight inhibitor of NE, blocks >99% of the fibrinogenolysis mediated by similarly stimulated neutrophils. This suggests that

NE escapes antiprotease inhibition in vivo because of the close contact between migrating neutrophils and fibrinogen giving rise to the ongoing low-level fibrinogenolysis and circulating Aα1-21 levels in these normal individuals. Secretory leukoprotease inhibitor (SLPI), an antiprotease with a smaller molecular weight than α_1AT (12 kDa vs. 52 kDa), can effectively inhibit the fibrinogenolysis mediated by stimulated neutrophils adherent to matrices (64). This observation suggests that in certain environments small molecular weight protease inhibitors may be more effective than the larger natural inhibitor α_1AT in inhibiting NE.

Oxidants have the ability to directly oxidize proteins and lipids and are also capable of mediating DNA damage. Many of the methodologies previously applied to BAL can also be applied to serum and plasma samples to evaluate oxidative damage.

Increases in carbonyl formation have been reported in rats exposed to hyperoxia with changes not confined to the lung but also associated with increases in liver carbonyl levels (41). DNA strand breakage has been observed in a number of cell types including macrophages, neutrophils, human embryo lung fibroblasts, and a murine leukocytic tumor cell line (65). The potential exists for analysis of DNA scission in peripheral blood cells as an in vivo method of determination of oxidant damage to lung tissue. Hydrogen peroxide can also cause lipid peroxidation in the presence of metal ions, and a number of these products including fatty acid hydroperoxides and aldehydes are potential mutagens (Fig.1). Pulmonary dysfunction in CF has been correlated with elevated plasma levels of malondialdehyde, an indicator of lipid peroxidation, but not with lipid hydroperoxide or protein carbonyl concentrations (66).

D. Urine

One of the earliest surrogate markers of lung destruction to be measured was desmosine (DES), a cross-linking amino acid unique to elastin (Fig. 2). Its use followed the discovery that intratracheal administration of elastase to laboratory animals resulted in the appearance of large amounts of elastin peptide fragments containing desmosine (67) and the related molecule isodesmosine (IDES) (68) in the urine.

The data from individuals with α_1AT deficiency is contradictory. In one study urine DES was not found to be elevated in α_1AT-deficient individuals or individuals with IPF compared to controls (69), while another more recent study has shown that urinary DES is increased in α_1AT deficiency to about the same level as in nonhereditary COPD (70). These discordant results may be partly explained by the problems inherent in all studies requiring analysis of molecules in 24-hour collections of urine or by the different methodologies used to measure DES and IDES. The first methods employed to measure DES involved a radio immunoassay which used ^{125}I-desmosine and a rabbit antidesmosine antibody (71). This was subsequently replaced by the methodology of Laurent et al. who developed an avidin-biotin ELISA for measuring DES, which also used a rabbit antidesmosine antibody (72). While this method was more sensitive and eliminated the need to use radiolabeled compounds, the ELISA technique appeared to give spuriously elevated DES values due to interfering substances in the urine. The more recent methodologies for measuring DES and the IDES involve separating contaminants in urine from the DES and IDES fractions by gel filtration and spiking the samples beforehand with radiolabeled DES and IDES to ensure that no significant loss of urinary DES or IDES occurred during filtration (68). DES and IDES are then quantified by HPLC as well as by amino acid analysis. This method has been applied successfully to multiple measurements of urinary DES/IDES including the measurement of elevated levels of both in CF (73). Other urinary markers of lung destruction include hydroxylysylpyridinoline (HP) and lysylpyridinoline (LP), which are markers for the degradation of collagen. These are raised significantly in individuals with COPD and smokers compared to normals (74).

III. Conclusion

Lung destruction is mediated by a variety of different mechanisms, which because of the lungs large functional reserve may progress unnoticed until irreversible destruction has occurred. The presently available methodologies to detect lung injury are relatively insensitive, with the result that by the time lung injury has been detected, substantial damage has already occurred. Ongoing research has led to the discovery of a number of potential surrogate markers of early lung injury. These markers may not only enable detection of lung disease at its earliest stage before irreversible damage, but may also provide a means of following response to therapeutic regimens.

References

1. Weibel ER. Design of airways and blood vessels considered as branching trees. In: The Lung: Scientific Foundations. 2d ed. Philadelphia: Lippincott-Raven, 1996:
2. Burger RM, Kent TA, Howitz SB, Munck E, Peisach J. Mossbauer study of iron bleomycin and its activation intermediates. J Biol Chem 1983; 258:1559–1564.
3. Gilson AJ, Sahn SA. Reactivation of bleomycin lung toxicity following oxygen administration. Chest 1985; 88:304–306.
4. Crapo JD, Barry BE, Gehr P, Bachofen M, Weibel ER. Cell number and characteristics of the normal human lung. Am Rev Respir Dis 1982; 125:332—337.
5. Weissman G, Zurier RB, Hoffstein S. Leucocytes as secretary organs of inflammation. Agents/Actions 1973; 3:370-379.

6. Falloon J, Gallin JI. Neutrophil granules in health and disease. J Allergy Clin Immunol 1986; 77:653–662.
7. Gadek JE, Fells GA, Wright DG, Crytal RG. Human neutrophil elastase functions as a type III collagen "collagenase." Biochem Biophys Res Commun 1980; 95:1815–1822.
8. McElvaney NG, Crystal RG. Proteases and lung injury. In: Crystal RG, West JB, Barnes PF, Weibel ER, Cherniack NS, eds. The Lung: Scientific Foundation. New York: Raven Press, Inc., 1997:2205–2219.
9. Karlinsky JB, Snider GL. Animal models of emphysema. Am Rev Respir Dis 1978; 117:1109–1133.
10. Kuhn C, Yu SY, Chraplyvy M, Linder HE, Senior RM. The induction of emphysema with elastase, II: Changes in connective tissue. Lab Invest 1976; 34:372–380.
11. Power C, O'Connor CM, MacFarlane D, O'Mahoney S, Gaffney K, Hayes J, Fitzgerald MX. Neutrophil collagenase in sputum from patients with cystic fibrosis. Am J Respir Crit Care Med 1994; 150:818–822.
12. Klebanoff SJ. Oxygen metabolism and the toxic properties of phagocytes. Ann Intern Med 1980; 93:480–489.
13. Sandy MS, Moldeus P, Ross D, Smith MT. Role of redox cycling and lipid peroxidation in biperidyl herbicide toxicity. Biochem Pharmacol 1986; 35:3095–3100.
14. Royall JA, Kooy NW, Beckman JS. Nitric oxide-related oxidants in acute lung injury. N Horizons 1995; 3:113–122.
15. Cochrane CG, Spragg RG, Revak SD. Pathogenesis of adult respiratory distress syndrome. J Clin Invest 1983; 71:754–761.
16. Carp H, Miller F, Hoidal JR, Janoff A. Potential mechanism of emphysema: alphal-proteinase inhibitor recovered from lungs of cigarette smokers contains oxidised methionine and has decreased elastase inhibitory capacity. Proc Natl Acad Sci USA 1982; 79:2041–2045.
17. Weiss SJ. Tissue destruction by neutrophils. N Engl J Med 1989; 32:365–368.
18. Schraufstatter IU, Revak SD, Cochrane CG. Proteases and oxidants in pulmonary inflammation injury. J Clin Invest 1984; 73:1175–1184.
19. Johnson KJ, Fantone JC, Kaplan J, Ward PA. In vivo damage of rat lungs by oxygen metabolites. J Clin Invest 198l; 67:983–993.
20. Till GO, Hatherill JR, Tourtellotte WW, Lutz MJ, Ward PA. Lipid peroxidation and acute lung injury after thermal trauma to skin. Evidence for a role for hydroxyl radical. Am J Pathol 1985; 119:376–384.
21. Birrer P, McElvaney NG, Rudeberg A, Wirz Sommer C, Liechti-Gallati S, Kraemer R, Hubbard R, Crystal RG. Neutrophil elastase-anti-neutrophil elastase imbalance on the respiratory epithelial surface in children with cystic fibrosis. Am Rev Respir Dis 1994; 150:207–213.
22. Hunninghake GW, Fullmer JD, Young RC Jr, Gadek JE, Crystal RG. Localization of the immune response in sarcoidosis. Am Rev Respir Dis 1979; 120:49–57.
23. Crystal RG, Fulmer JD, Roberts WC, Moss ML, Line BR, Reynolds HY. Idiopathic pulmonary fibrosis. Clinical, histological, radiographic, physiologic, scintigraphic, cytologic and biochemical aspects. Ann Intern Med 1976; 85:769–788.

24. Ogden BE, Murphy SA, Saunders GC, Pathak D, Johnson JD. Neonatal lung neutrophils and elastase/proteinase inhibitor imbalance. Am Rev Respir Dis 1984; 130:817–821.
25. Epstein PE, Dauber JH, Rossman MD, Daniele RP. Bronchoalveolar lavage in a patient with chronic berylliosis: evidence for hypersensitivity pneumonitis. Ann Intern Med 1982; 97:213–216.
26. Saltini C, Winestock K, Kirby M, Pinkston P, Crystal RG. Maintenance of alveolitis in patients with chronic beryllium disease by beryllium-specific helper T cells. N Engl J Med 1989; 320:1103–1109.
27. Pinkston P, Bitterman RB, Crystal RG. Spontaneous release of interleukin-2 by lung T lymphocytes in active pulmonary sarcoidosis. N Engl J Med 1983; 308:793–800.
28. Carre PC, Mortenson RL, King TE Jr, Noble PW, Sable CL, Riches DW. Increased expression of the interleukin-8 gene by alveolar macrophages in idiopathic pulmonary fibrosis. A potential mechanism for the recruitment and activation of neutrophils in lung fibrosis. J Clin Invest 1991; 88:1802–1810.
29. McElvaney NG, Nakamura H, Birrer P, Herbert CA, Wong WL, Alhonso M, Baker JB, Catalano MA, Crystal RG. Modulation of airway inflammation in cystic fibrosis: In vivo suppression of interleukin-8 on the respiratory epithelial surface by aerosolization of recombinant secretory leucoprotease inhibitor. J Clin Invest 1992; 90:1296–1301.
30. McElvaney NG, Hubbard RC, Birrer P, Chernick M, Caplan D, Frank MM, Crystal RG. Aerosol α1-antitrypsin treatment for cystic fibrosis. Lancet 1991; 26:392–394.
31. Bonanno A, Mirabella A, Vignola AM, Riccobono L. Mirabella F, Bellia V, Bonsignore G. Increased levels of elastase and alphal-antitrypsin in sputum of asthmatic patients. Am J Respir Crit Care Med 1997; 155:A66.
32. McElvaney NG, Cervantes-Laurean D, Wehr N, Gabrielle K, Barnes P, Robinson W, Moss J, Levine RL. Short-duration hyperoxia in normal subjects is associated with increased oxidation of bronchoalveolar lavage proteins and decreased antiprotease protection screen. Am J Respir Crit Care Med 1996; 153:A737.
33. Levine RL, Mosoni L, Berlett BS, Stadtman ER. Methionine residues as endogenous antioxidants in proteins. Proc Natl Acad Sci USA 1996; 93:15036–15040.
34. Cervantes-Laurean D, Levine RL, McElvaney NG, Moss J. Preferential oxidation of methionine 358 and methionine 351 in alphal-antitrypsin correlates with loss of anti-elastase activity. Am J Respir Crit Care Med 1997; 155:A186.
35. Levine RL, Garland D, Oliver CN, Amici A, Climent I, Lenz A-G, Ahn B-W, Shaltiel S, Stadtman ER. Determination of carbonyl content in oxidatively modified proteins. Methods Enzymol 1990; 186:464–478.
36. Levine RL, Williams JA, Stadtman ER, Shacter E. Carbonyl assays for determination of oxidatively modified proteins. Methods Enzymol 1994; 233:346–357.
37. Ayene IS, Al-Medhi AB, Fisher AB, Inhibition of lung tissue oxidation during ischemia/reperfusion by 2-mercaptopropionylglycine. Arch Biochem Biophys 1993; 303:307–312.
38. Oliver CN, Starke-Reed PE, Stadtman ER, Liu GJ, Carney JM, Floyd RA. Oxidative damage to brain proteins, loss of glutamine synthetase activity, and production

of free radicals during ischemia/reperfusion-induced injury to gerbil brain. Proc Natl Acad Sci USA 1990; 87:5144–5147.
39. Garland D. Role of site-specific, metal-catalyzed oxidation in lens-aging and cataract: a hypothesis. Exp Eye Res 1990; 50:677–682.
40. Chapman ML, Rubin BR, Gracy RW. Increased carbonyl content of proteins in synovial fluid from patients with rheumatoid arthritis. J Rheumatol 1989; 16:15–18.
41. Starke PE, Oliver CN, Stadtman ER. Modification of hepatic proteins in rats exposed to high oxygen concentration. FASEB J 1987; 1:36–39.
42. Taggart C, Coakley R, Byrne A, Allen K, O'Reilly D, O'Neill G, Murphy J, O'Neill S, McElvaney NG. Increased alpha1-antitrypsin on the respiratory epithelial surface of ventilated pre-term neonates helps protect against proteolytic damage. Am J Respir Crit Care Med 1997; 155:A262.
43. Gladstone IM, Levine RL. Oxidation of proteins in neonatal lungs. Pediatrics 1994; 93:764–768.
44. Widdicombe JG. Role of lipids in airway function. Eur J Respir Dis 1987; 71 (suppl 153):197–204.
45. Matthews LR, Spector S, Lemm J, Potter JL. Studies on pulmonary secretions. Am Rev Respir Dis 1963; 88:199–204.
46. Danel C, Erzurum SC, McElvaney NG, Crystal RG. Quantitative assessment of the epithelial and inflammatory cell populations in large airways of normals and individuals with cystic fibrosis. Am J Respir Crit Care Med 1996; 153:363–368.
47. Eissa NT, Chu CS, Danel C, Crystal RG. Evaluation of the respiratory epithelium of normals and individuals with cystic fibrosis for the presence of adenovirus E1a sequences relevant to the use of E1a-adenovirus vectors for gene therapy for the respiratory manifestations of cystic fibrosis. Hum Gene Ther 1994; 5:1105–1114.
48. Djuric Z, Luongo DA, Harper DA. Quantitation of 5-(hydroxymethyl) uracil in DNA by gas chromatography with mass spectral detection. Chem Res Toxicol 1991; 4:687–691.
49. Birnboim HC, Jevcak JJ. Fluorometric method for rapid detection of DNA strand breaks in human white blood cells produced by low doses of radiation. Cancer Res 1981; 41:1889–1892.
50. Chatteerjee S, Petzold SJ, Berger SJ, Berger NA. Strategy for selection of cell variants deficient in poly(ADP-ribose) polymerase. Exp Cell Res 1987; 172:245–257.
51. Albertine RJ, Niklas JA, O'Neill JP. Somatic cell gene mutations in humans: biomarkers for genotoxicity. Environ Health Pers (suppl) 1993; 101:193–201.
52. Szabo C, saunders C, O'Connor M, Salzman AL. Peroxynitrite causes energy depletion and increases permeability via activation of poly (ADP-ribose) synthetase in pulmonary epithelial cells. Am J Respir Cell Mol Biol 1997; 16:105–109.
53. Meyer KC, Lewandoski JR, Zimmerman JJ, Nunley D, Calhoun WJ, Dopico GA. Human neutrophil elastase and elastase-alpha l-antiprotease complex in cystic fibrosis. Comparison with interstitial lung disease and evaluation of the effect of intravenously administered antibiotic therapy. Am Rev Respir Dis 1991; 144:580–585.
54. Lee CT, Fein AM, Lippmann M, Holtzman H, Kimbel P, Weinbaum G. Elastolytic activity in pulmonary lavage fluid from patients with adult respiratory distress syndrome. N Engl J Med 1981; 304:192–196.

55. McGuire WW, Spragg RG, Cohen AB, Cochrane CG. Studies on the pathogenesis of the adult respiratory distress syndrome. J Clin Invest 1982; 69:543–553.
56. Suaaya F, Tanaka H, Yinagishi M, Yokogawa K, Honma S, Uno E, Sekine K, Abe S. Plasma elastase: alpha l-protease inhibitor complex level is elevated during severe asthma attack in adults. Am J Respir Crit Care Med 1994; 149:
57. Kucich U, Christner P, Lippman M, Kimbel P, Williams G, Rosenbloom J, Weinbaum G. Utilization of a peroxidase antiperoxidase complex in an enzyme-linked immunosorbent assay of elastin-derived peptides in human plasma. Am Rev Respir Dis 1985; 131:709–713.
58. Schriver EE, Davidson JM, Sutcliffe MC, Swindell BB, Bernard GR. Comparison of elastin peptide concentrations in body fluids from healthy volunteers, smokers, and patients with chronic obstructive pulmonary disease. Am Rev Respir Dis 1992; 145:762–766.
59. Frette C, Wei SM, Jacob MP, Kauffmann F, Pham QT. Factors related to serum elastin peptide level in French coal miners. Am Rev Respir Dis 1992; 145:A535.
60. Frette C, Wei SM, Neukirch F, Sesboue R, Martin JP, Jacob MP, Kauffmann F. Relationships of serum elastin peptide level to age, FEV1, smoking habits, alcohol consumption and PI phenotype. An epidemiological study in working men. Thorax 1992; 47:937–942.
61. Weitz JI, Landman SL, Crowley KA, Birken S, Morgan FJ. Development of an assay for in vivo neutrophil elastase activity. Increased elastase activity in patients with alpha-l-proteinase inhibitor deficiency. J Clin Invest 1986; 78:155–163.
62. Weitz JI, Crowley KA, Landman SL, Lipman BI, Yu J. Increased human neutrophil elastase activity in cigarette smokers. Ann Intern Med 1987; 107:680–682.
63. Weitz JI, Huang SL, Landman SC, Nickolson SC, Silverstein SC. Elastase mediated fibrinogenolysis by chemoattractant-stimulated neutrophils occurs in the presence of physiologic concentrations of antiproteinases. J Exp Med 1988; 166:1838–1850.
64. Rice WG, Weiss SJ. Regulation of proteolysis at the neutrophil-substrate interface by secretary leucoprotease inhibitor. Science 1990; 249:178–181.
65. Schraufstatter IU, Hyslop PA, Jackson JH, Cochrane CG. Oxidant-induced DNA damage of target cells. J Clin Invest 1988; 82:1040–1050.
66. Brown RK, Wyatt H, Price JF, Kelly FJ. Pulmonary dysfunction in cystic fibrosis associated with oxidative stress. Eur Respir J 1996; 9:334–339.
67. Goldstein RA, Starcher BC. Urinary excretion of elastin peptides containing desmosine after intratracheal injections of elastase in hamsters. J Clin Invest 1978; 61:1286–1290.
68. Stone PJ, Bryan-Rhadfi J, Lucey EC, Ciccolella DE, Crombie G, Faris B, Snider GL, Franzblau C. Measurement of urinary desmosine by isotope dilution and high performance liquid chromatography. Am Rev Respir Dis 1991; 144:284–290.
69. Pelham F, Wewers M, Crystal R, Buist SA, Janoff A. Urinary excretion of desmosine (elastin cross-links) in subjects with PiZZ alpha-1-antitrypsin deficiency, a phenotype associated with hereditary predisposition to pulmonary emphysema. Am Rev Respir Dis 1985; 132:821–823.
70. Stone PJ, Morris TA, Franzblau C, Snider GL. Preliminary evidence that augmen-

tation therapy diminishes degradation of cross-linked elastin in alpha-1-antitrypsin deficient humans. Respiration 1995; 62:76–79.
71. Davies SF, Offord KP, Brown MG, Campe H, Niewoehner D. Urine desmosine is unrelated to cigarette smoking or to spirometric function. Am Rev Respir Dis 1983; 128:473–475.
72. Laurent P, Magne L, De Palmas J, Bignon J, Jaurand M-C. Quantitation of elastin in human urine and rat pleural mesothelial cell matrix by a sensitive avidin-biotin ELISA for desmosine. J Immunol Meth 1988; 107:1–11.
73. Stone PJ, Konstan MW, Berger M, Dorkin HL, Franzblau C, Snider GL. Elastin and collagen degradation products in urine of patients with cystic fibrosis. Am J Respir Crit Care Med 1995; 152:157–162.
74. Stone PJ, Gottlieb DJ, O'Connor GT, Ciccolella DE, Breuer R, Bryan-Rhadfi J, Shaw HA, Franzblau C, Snider GL. Elastin and collagen degradation products in urine of smokers with and without chronic obstructive pulmonary disease. Am J Respir Crit Care Med 1995; 151:952–959.

29

Cell Adhesion Molecules in the Pathogenesis of Lung Disease

JOHN R. SPURZEM and STEPHEN I. RENNARD

University of Nebraska Medical Center
Omaha, Nebraska

I. Introduction

Lymphangiomyomatosis (LAM) of the lung is characterized by irregular proliferations of smooth muscle cells as well as areas of fibrosis and cystic changes (1,2). Current concepts regarding the origins of the proliferating smooth muscle cells are discussed in other chapters of this text. There is evidence that abnormalities of matrix biology are involved in disorders such as lymphangiomyomatosis. Studies of Alport's syndrome and diffuse leiomyomatosis (3) have shown linkage to mutations in collagen genes. In Alport's syndrome mutations in the COL4A3 and COL4A4 genes are found. In diffuse leiomyomatosis, a disorder with diffuse proliferation of smooth muscle cells in the esophagus and respiratory tract, mutations in the COL4A5 and COL4A6 genes are found. The concepts of the pathogenesis of LAM also include the idea that the nodular and laminar infiltrates of smooth muscle cells lead to disruption of airways, alveoli, vascular structures, and lymph flow. Disruption of normal architecture likely leads to damage, inflammation, and stimulation of repair. Thus, the later pathologic features of LAM such as the characteristic cystic lesions share pathogenetic mechanisms with other interstitial lung diseases. Clinicopathologic studies suggest that prognosis in LAM is related to the degree of lung disruption, cystic changes, and fibrosis (4). In some respects, then, processes in the pathogenesis of LAM overlap with the pathogenesis of other fibrotic, interstitial lung diseases (5).

Processes of inflammation and repair are a complex interplay of cell proliferation, migration, and modification of the extracellular matrix. In order for cells to proliferate and migrate into areas of inflammation and damage, the cells must interact with the surrounding matrix. It has been known for some time that matrix proteins are necessary for the proliferation of mesenchymal cells (6). When cells migrate they must alter their relationship to the surrounding matrix proteins. Migrating cells must strike a balance between adhesion and mobility. In recent years there has been an explosion of knowledge regarding cell surface receptors that are specific for matrix proteins. It is now known that the family of receptors known as integrins can bind to extracellular matrix components providing signal into cells and provide adhesion capability (7).

The ability of cells to adhere to each other and extracellular matrix is influenced by growth factors and cytokines. The signaling systems of growth factors interact with signaling pathways that control the activation of integrins (7). The accumulation of integrins into focal adhesion complexes with connections to the cytoskeleton is also controlled by signaling pathways (8). The fact that growth factors and peptides important in development also influence repair processes reinforces the concept that development and repair share many features (9). Fibrosis and disordered repair leading to loss of alveolar structure might be viewed as inadequate repetition of development. The rest of this chapter will discuss cell-cell and cell-matrix interactions as they relate to inflammation and repair of the lung. As noted, some of the concepts, particularly those of the growth factors, will overlap with development.

II. Cell-Matrix Adhesion Molecules

It is now known that cells interact with specific matrix elements such as collagen using an assortment of cell surface molecules. Families of receptors have been described with the family of integrins being the best characterized (Table 1). Integrins are heterodimers of alpha and beta chains. Some beta chains are promiscuous and can associate with more than one alpha chain to make different receptors. Similarly, some alpha chains can associate with several different beta chains. The $\beta 1$-containing receptors have also been called the very late activation (VLA) subfamily after their early descripton as late activation markers on lymphocytes (10). Integrins can be formed into subfamilies based on common use of an alpha or beta chain. Profiles of integrin expression on lung cells have been described (11). Some integrins are expressed on many cell types, while others are more restricted in expression. Pulmonary epithelial cells express $av\beta 6$,

Table 1 Extracellular Matrix Receptors

Integrin receptor families	
α1/β1	Laminin, collagen
α2/β1	Collagen, laminin
α3/β1	Laminin, collagen, fibronectin
α6/β1	Laminin
α7/β1	Laminin
α4/β1	Fibronectin
α5/β1	Fibronectin
α8/β1	Tenascin, fibronectin, vitronectin
α9/β1	Tenascin
αv/β1	Fibronectin
α6/β4	Laminin
α4/β7	Fibronectin
αIIbβ3	Fibronectin, fibrinogen, thrombospondin
αv/β3	Vitronectin, fibrinogen, VWF
αv/β5	Vitronectin
αv/β6	Fibronectin
αv/β8	Vitronectin
Nonintegrins	
69 kD	Laminin
CD44	Hyaluronic acid
Syndecan	Collagen, fibronectin
SLIPS	Fibronectin, vitronectin, thrombospondin, collagens, laminin
GRIPS	Fibronectin

SLIPS = Syndecan-like intercalated proteoglycans; GRIPS = glypican-related integral membrane proteoglycans.
Source: Adapted from Refs. 7,68,111,126,127.

which is relatively specific for epithelial cells and likely serves important functions during development and repair (12).

Binding sites on matrix molecules have been described for many of the integrins. The first described integrin recognition site was the Arg-Gly-Asp (RGD) peptide sequence that is common to collagens, laminin, fibronectin, fibrinogen, and vitronectin. The first described fibronectin receptor, α5β1, binds to this recognition site (13). The αv-containing integrins also appear to bind to this peptide sequence (14). Other binding sites include the Glu-Ile-Leu-Asp-Val (EILDV) peptide sequence that is found in the alternatively spliced region of fibronectin that is recognized by α4β1 (15,16). Several integrin-binding sites have been described in laminin. The RGD sequence is found in the Pl fragment of the

A chain of laminin. The α3β1 and α6β1 integrins, however, bind to different regions in the carboxy-terminal region of the laminin A chain (17,18).

An important feature of integrin function is that they combine on the cell surface to form assemblies of receptors that have been called focal contacts or adhesions (19). Focal adhesions provide an important connection between the extracellular matrix and the cytoskeleton. Although integrins have small cytoplasmic tails, there is interaction with cytoplasmic proteins, which collect in focal adhesions. These proteins both strengthen the connections with actin filaments and participate in signaling processes (7,8,20) (Fig. 1). Talin, vinculin, α-actinin, fimbrin, filamin, and gelsolin are found in focal adhesions and participate in these connections (21). The ability of cells to form focal adhesions is important in the context that integrins themselves have fairly low affinity for their ligands (22,23).

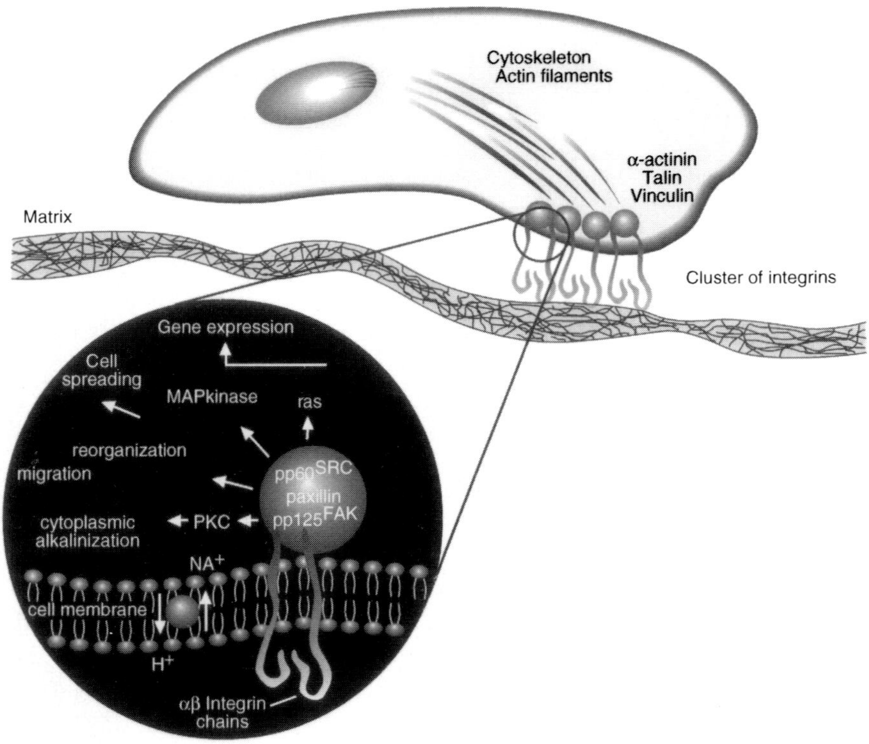

Figure 1 Focal contacts are sites where cytoskeletal elements interact with a cluster of transmembrane receptors—integrins. It is now known that important molecules with signaling activity are also located in focal contacts (inset). Various signal transduction systems can be modulated that influence diverse cellular activities. (Courtesy of Thorax, BMJ Publishing Group.)

Focal adhesions provide a mechanism for the strengthening of cell-matrix attachments.

Integrins themselves do not have kinase or other enzymatic activity in their cytoplasmic domains. However, as noted above, integrins aggregate in focal adhesions in association with other proteins capable of signaling activity. Proteins found in focal adhesions with enzymatic activity include paxillin, tensin, and $pp125^{FAK}$ (FAK) (20,24). Binding of fibronectin to cells can lead to tyrosine phosphorylation of FAK and increased kinase activity of FAK (25). Tyrosine phosphorylation events are triggered in fibroblasts by cross-linking of integrins, similar to the phosphorylation events seen after transformation by the oncogene $pp60^{src}$. Recent studies directly link integrin-mediated signaling to the Ras signal pathway through phosphorylation of FAK (26) and to the mitogen-activated protein (MAP) kinases (27). Activated FAK is thought to interact with a number of signaling molecules including Src, Crk, Grb2, Ras, MAPkinase, and Rho (28). Adhesion of many cell types to fibronection leads to cytoplasmic alkalinization. Cytoplasmic alkalinization is also seen in oncogene transformed cells with anchorage-independent growth. When integrins bind to matrix proteins and signaling is initiated within the cell, the flow of information into the cell is sometimes termed "outside-in" signaling (7). It is also apparent that signals derived from attachment to matrix intersect with signals from oncogenes and growth factors. Information from the matrix environment is thus intimately involved in development and repair of tissues.

In a way that might be termed "inside-out signaling" (7), activation of cells by cytokines and growth factors can influence the assembly of focal contacts and thus control the ability of cells to attach to matrix proteins. The assembly of focal contacts is a complex procedure that has an ordered, sequential process. The subject of signals involved in focal adhesion assembly has been recently reviewed (28). It is apparent that signals derived from growth factors such as platelet-derived growth factor (PDGF) and epidermal growth factor (EGF) activate Rac and Rho GTPases, which influence the recruitment of focal adhesion proteins such as talin, vinculin, FAK, and paxillin. Interestingly, stimuli from diverse mediators such as lysophosphatidic acid (LPA), bradykinin, and bombesin also activate the same GTPases and have similar effects on focal adhesion assembly and cell attachment (29,30). The idea that a mediator of development like bombesin is also active in processes controlling cell attachment is attractive as tissue repair and regeneration are analogous to development (29).

In the studies described by Ridley and Hall (29), activated RhoA is required for focal adhesion assembly in Swiss 3T3 cells. It is not clear whether this is true for all cell types and for all matrix proteins. In studies performed by Yamada and Miyamoto (30) with primary fibroblasts, focal adhesion assembly can be initiated without growth factor stimulation. Cell types may thus vary in the role of growth factor stimulation in focal adhesion assembly. Studies with airway epithelial cells suggest that different matrix substrates also influence the need for growth factor stimulation. Primary cultures of airway epithelial cells do not require growth factor stimulation to adhere to fibronectin, but do require the addition of growth factors to the culture medium in order to adhere to collagens (31,32). The ability of the bronchial epithelial cells to attach correlated with the formation of focal contacts. The ability to form focal adhesions and the influence of growth factors may be dependent on the matrix substrate and integrins involved. The fact that the dominant matrix proteins in fresh airway wounds are fibronectin and fibrin (33,34) suggests that these matrix proteins have specialized roles in wound repair. These components of the provisional matrix might therefore be crucial in support of cell attachment and cell migration into an airway wound.

The discussion so far has focused on integrins that participate in focal adhesions. Integrins expressed by epithelial cells with affinity for laminin can participate in hemidesmosomes. The integrin $\alpha6\beta4$ localizes to hemidesmosomes, which function to link the intermediate filament network with extracellular matrix (35). Similar to focal adhesions, a cytoplasmic, multiprotein complex is also thought to be necessary for the formation of the hemidesmosome as well as signaling. The cytoplasmic domain of $\beta4$ can be phosphorylated after clustering of the integrins. The complex appears to be linked to the Ras pathway. The integrin $\alpha6\beta1$ also binds to laminin but does not appear to participate in hemidesmosomes. The role of laminins in development and morphogenesis is being explored (36,37). Turnover and new expression of laminins may be important in lung disease. Altraja et al. (38) have examined the expression of laminin chains in asthmatic airways. The $\alpha2$ and $\alpha3$ laminin chains are associated with morphogenesis but have increased expression in severe asthmatic airways. Thus, laminin receptors also may play a role in injury and repair processes.

Other cell surface molecules have an affinity for matrix besides integrins. These include CD44, syndecans, and a nonintegrin laminin receptor. The roles of these molecules in cell-matrix interactions is also being explored. The cell surface proteoglycan CD44 has been called the Hermes antigen, pgp-1, ECMRIII, and the hyaluronate receptor. Originally described as a homing receptor for lymphocytes with a molecular weight of 90 kDa (39), larger sized CD44 molecules have been described due to splice variants and variable addition of glycosaminoglycan side chains (40,41). CD44 has significant affinity for hyaluronic acid and is important for the migration of certain tumor cells. One of the larger splice variants has been called CD44E, the epidermal" variant (41). CD44, as identified by monoclonal antibodies, has a wide tissue distribution, including pulmonary epithelial cells (42). It has recently been demonstrated that CD44 can interact with actin filaments (43). The cytosolic protein ezrin provides the link between CD44 and the cytoskeleton (44,45).

Several other proteoglycans (peptide core chains with one or more glycosaminoglycan side chains) have been described that are important in the adhesion and migration of cells. Syndecan is an integral membrane proteoglycan that can bind to fibrillar collagens and fibronectin through its heparan sulfate side chains (46,47). Similar proteoglycans with heparan sulfate side chains have been grouped as syndecan-like intercalated proteoglycans (SLIPS) (47). Dystroglycan is a cell surface glycoprotein complex that binds to the E3 domain of laminin (48,49). The complex is made up of an α and a β subunit, which are derived from the same mRNA transcript. The dystroglycan complex links laminin adhesion to dystrophin of the cytoskeleton. Abnormalities of the dystroglycan complex are thought to underlie many of the muscular dystrophies (48,50). Thus, adhesion to laminin is critical for normal functioning of muscle cells. Recent studies have shown that dystroglycan has roles in other cell types. The dystroglycan complex is thought to be important in epithelial morphogenesis (49,51).

Another nonintegrin cell surface protein with affinity for matrix is the 67–69 kDa receptor for laminin. This receptor binds to the Tyr-Ile-Gly-Ser-Arg (YIGSR) peptide sequence in the laminin B1 chain. The role of this receptor in tumor cell invasion and metastasis is an area of active investigation (52,53), but its role in adhesion and migration of normal cells is less well studied.

III. Cell-Matrix Interactions in Fibrosis and Repair

A. Adhesion and Migration of Cells

Several models of lung injury have been used to examine the process of repair in the lung. Wounding of the airway has been used to demonstrate the migration of airway epithelial cells into a wounded area, which is followed by reepithelialization (33,34,54). These careful studies demonstrate that epithelial cells at the edge of the wound flatten out and begin to migrate over the provisional matrix in the wound. Other cells including fibroblasts and endothelial cells obviously must respond as well, depending on the depth and severity of the wound.

In vitro studies of the ability of normal bovine and human airway epithelial cells to adhere to different matrix substrates relate to the ability of epithelial cells to intiate the reepithelialization process. Primary cultures of normal airway epithelial cells readily adhere to collagens, fibronectin, and vitronectin over a 1- to 2-hour time period (11,55). Interestingly, normal human bronchial epithelial cells do not adhere to fibrinogen, consistent with their lack of expression of the avβ3 integrin, the integrin with described affinity for fibrinogen (11). Bronchial epithelial cells which had been cultured for several days showed increased adhesion to some matrix coatings compared to freshly isolated cells, suggesting that some aspect of adhesion mechanisms could be modulated by the in vitro environment (55). One possible explanation for an increase in adhesion during culture could be autocrine or paracrine effects of TGF-β. TGF-β is produced by normal bovine bronchial epithelial cells during culture (56). When TGF-β is added exogenously to early primary cultures of bronchial epithelial cells, adhesion for matrix is increased (57). TGF-β modulates the spectrum of integrins expressed by bronchial epithelial cells (57–60). Increased expression of α5β1 could be important in the ability to adhere to provisional matrix containing fibronectin (33,34).

An important function of integrins during attachment to matrix proteins is the formation of focal adhesions. As described above, focal adhesions strengthen the links to the cytoskeleton. Not all of the integrins known to be expressed by cells such as airway epithelial cells may be used in focal adhesions. Immunofluorescence studies have confirmed that some but not all integrins appear in focal adhesions when bronchial epithelial cells are allowed to attach for 2 hours to various matrix proteins. When bronchial epithelial cells were adherent to collagens, α2 but not α3 was found in focal adhesions (61) (Fig. 2). Thus, while both the α2β1 and α3β1 integrins have affinity for collagens, they appear to function in different capacities. Similarly, when bronchial epithelial cells were adherent to fibronectin, αv but not α5 was found in focal adhesions (Fig 3). This was consistent with observations that new primary cultures of bronchial epithelial cells have low expression of the α5β1 integrin (60). If passaged cells were used in the studies, α5β1 did appear in focal adhesions, consistent with new expression in in vitro cultures. The ability to increase expression of α5β1 may be important in injury and repair.

Some matrix adhesion molecules do not function in stable focal adhesions. CD44 is a cell surface glycoprotein (see above). CD44 has been studied in regard to migration and invasion of tumor cells (41,42). CD44 may be involved in deadhesion, enabling cells to mobilize lamellipodia. Expression of CD44 is increased in areas of airway damage in asthma (62). CD44 may play a role in repair processes through facilitation of cell migration.

The ability of cells to migrate over or through matrix would seem related to but not completely overlapping with the ability to adhere to matrix. Migration requires a balance between adhesion/anchoring and deadhesion/mobility. DiMilla and colleagues have evaluated the relationship between adhesion strength and migration of smooth muscle cells. They found that maximal migration occurred when the cells had moderate adhesion strength (63). Alterations in the expression of integrins may alter adhesion strength and thus alter migration. Integrins may also be "activated" in certain circumstances (7) so that growth factors and cytokines may alter the ability of cells to migrate (57,64).

The ability of matrix molecules to directly modulate fibroblast and bronchial epithelial cell migration has been studied using the modified Boyden cham-

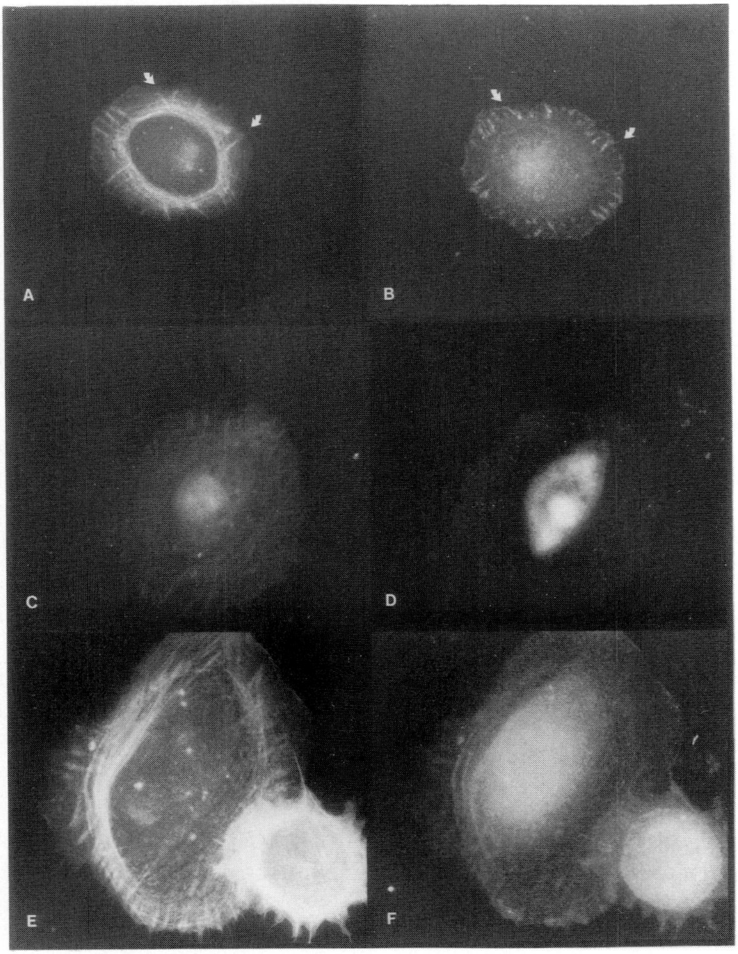

Figure 2 Localization of α2-integrin chains in focal contacts in bronchial epithelial cells adherent to type I collagen. Cells were allowed to adhere to collagen-coated coverslips for 2 hours, fixed with paraformaldehyde, permeabilized with triton X-100, and stained with FITC-conjugated phalloidin (to identify actin filaments) and a monoclonal antibodies to integrin chains. The antibody binding was identified with TRITC-conjugated goat anti-mouse IgG antibody. Two-color epifluorescence microscopy was used to examine the cells. Actin filament staining is shown in panels A, C, and E. Examples of stains for α2 (panel B), α3 (panel D), and α5 (panel F) are shown. Only the antibody to α2 localized to focal contacts as shown with arrows in panels A and B. (1000×)

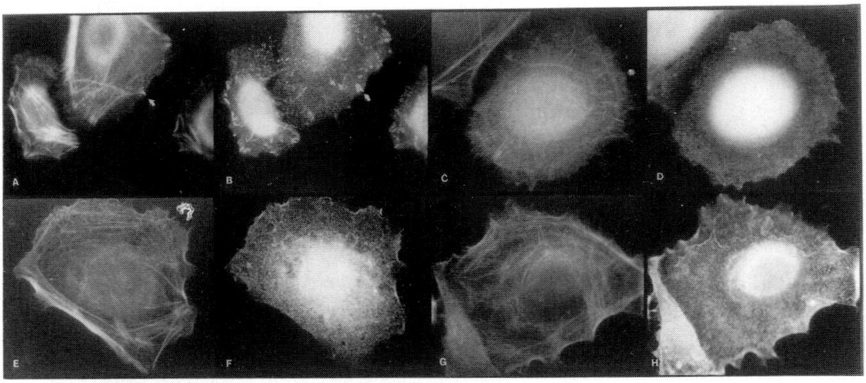

Figure 3 Localization of integrin chains in bronchial epithelial cells adherent to fibronectin. Cells were cultured for 2 hours on fibronectin-coated coverslips and stained as in Figure 2. Panels A, C, E, and G show actin stains. Panel B shows αv staining in focal contacts (arrow) that correspond to actin filaments in the same cell in panel A (arrow). Antibodies to αvβ5 (D), β3 (F), and β1 (H) did not similarly demonstrate localization of staining in focal contacts.

ber technique. Fibronectin, vitronectin, and collagens readily stimulate bovine bronchial epithelial cell migraion in these assays. Laminin does not appear to support epithelial cell migration (65). Fibroblast migration is also stimulated by fibronectin (66,67). The role of fibronectin in cell recruitment is emphasized by the finding that fibronectin is the major stimulant for fibroblast migration in supernatants of cultured epithelial cells (66). "Checkerboard" analyses with varying concentrations of the matrix proteins both above and below the chamber membranes demonstrate that the stimulatory effect is not just an increase in chemokinesis but that the migration is directed towards increasing gradients of the matrix proteins, "haptotaxis." The ability of matrix proteins, particularly the matrix proteins of inflammation such as fibronectin, to stimulate bronchial epithelial cell migration, either through gradients in the substrata or in soluble form, would seem to be an important aspect of morphologic changes that occur during development and repair.

Smooth muscle cell attachment and migration have also been evaluated to some extent (63). Interestingly, smooth muscle cells express an integrin, α8β1, that is expressed only on smooth muscle cells (68,69). This integrin is a receptor for fibronectin, vitronectin, and tenascin, a matrix protein found in the subepithelial/basement membrane region as well as in pulmonary arteries (70). The reason for the unique expression of α8β1 is not yet clear.

B. Cell Survival and Apoptosis

In addition to strengthening cell attachment mechanisms, focal adhesions also serve as intersections for signaling to the cell. Signals from the extracellular matrix to the cell are likely important in the survival of cells. The ability of the underlying substrata to alter growth and morphologic characteristics of cultured airway epithelial cells has been noted since the early reports of epithelial cell culture. Precoating culture dishes with fibronectin improved plating efficiency and growth rates of human bronchial epithelial cells (71). Matrix attachments have been thought to be essential as an important mechanism preventing dysplastic growth (72). Culture of fetal bovine tracheal epithelial cells on Engelbreth-Holm-Swarm (EHS) substrate induces a more cuboidal cell shape and more cells per dish than when collagen alone is used (73), suggesting that a number of matrix proteins are required for the normal differentiation of cells. Signals from matrix have long been known to be essential for the growth of mesenchymal cells as well. Fibronectin has been characterized as a growth factor for fibroblasts (6).

In addition to effects on cell proliferation, recent reports describe effects of cell-matrix interactions on programmed cell death (apoptosis.) Disruption of cell-matrix interactions of Madin-Darby canine kidney (MDCK) epithelial cells or immortalized keratinocytes induced apoptosis (74). Frisch and Francis have coined a new name for apoptosis induced by lack of matrix adhesion, "anoikis" (74). Anoikis may be a feature of epithelial cells more than mesenchymal cells. Unlike the epithelial cell that were studied, normal fibroblasts enter growth arrest when in cell suspension but not apoptosis. Frisch and Francis hypothesize that epithelial or endothelial cells undergo cell death after losing contact with matrix in order to prevent inappropriate location or growth (74,75). Specific integrins have been investigated in regard to apoptosis. Antibodies to the integrin chain αv have been shown to induce apoptosis in a tumor cell line (76). The αv integrins are also important in preventing apoptosis of normal bronchial epithelial cells (77). αv containing integrins involved in both cell-matrix adhesion and cell-cell adhesion modulated apoptosis of bronchial epithelial cells. In conditions that promoted cell-cell aggregation, but not adhesion to matrix, there was less apoptosis than when there was less aggregation. Signals from cell-cell adhesion may cross-react with signals from cell-matrix adhesion.

The discussion of matrix effects on bronchial epithelial cells is not meant to discount the effects of matrix components on other cells types. The importance of extracellular matrix to the differentiation of alveolar epithelial cells has been reviewed (78). Culturing alveolar type II cells on varying matrix components has profound effects on cytoskeletal organization and transepithelial resistance (79). Shannon et al. have shown that matrix composition is critical for expression of surfactant components, SP-A, SP-B, and SP-C (80). The differentiated function of expression of surfactant-associated proteins is thus likely dependent on cell-matrix interactions as well as cell-cell interactions (80).

The profound effects of cell-matrix interactions on the growth, survival, and function of lung mesenchymal and epithelial cells suggests that there may be opportunities for intervention. The effects of cytokines on cell attachment and migration imply that modulation of inflammatory processes should affect repair processes. Integrin function may be a target for intervention. Examples of anti-integrins in nature confirm that disruption of integrin function is a feasible approach. Snake venoms contain kistrin, an anti-integrin (81). Peptides that inhibit $\alpha v\beta 3$ function have been used in animal studies of cancer (82,83). $\alpha v\beta 3$ function is critical for angiogenesis, a process necessary for tumor growth. Antagonists of $\alpha v\beta 3$ induce tumor regression in the animal models. The ability to modulate cell-matrix interactions would seem to be a powerful tool.

IV. Cell-Cell Adhesion Molecules

A number of specialized molecules and structures have been described that are involved in cell-cell adhesion (Table 2). The three largest families of receptors are the integrins, the immunoglobulin (Ig) superfamily, and the cadherin superfamily. Many integrins are described above, mainly those integrins functioning in cell-matrix interactions. A subfamily of integrins, the $\beta 2$-containing integrins, are primarily cell-cell adhesion molecules. Some integrins such as those containing $\alpha 2$ and $\alpha 3$, best known as cell-matrix adhesion molecules, may also have roles in cell-cell adhesion (84). The Ig superfamily is diverse, containing molecules such as the leukocyte adhesion molecules, CD2, LFA-3, PECAM-1, and ICAM-1. The Ig superfamily also contains neural cell adhesion molecule (NCAM). The cadherin family of cell-cell adhesion molecules have been considered a separate family but have recently been shown to have structural similarities with the Ig structures (85). Unlike most members of the Ig superfamily, cadherins are dependent on calcium, a property they share with integrins. A family of molecules that are expressed on endothelial molecules and function during early adhesion of leukocytes to endothelial cells is the selectin family. In order to lend some organization to a discussion of such a diverse array of adhesion molecules, the rest of this discussion will be divided into sections on cell-cell adhesion in morphogenesis and repair and cell-cell adhesion in inflammatory processes.

A. Cell-Cell Adhesion in Morphogenesis and Repair

Cadherins are thought to be critical to the development of all solid tissues. The roles of cadherins during development have been recently reviewed (86–88). The best-described cadherins are E-cadherin (epithelial), N-cadherin (neural), P-cadherin (placental), and L-CAM (liver cell adhesion molecule). E-cadherin is

Table 2 Cell-Cell Adhesion Molecules in the Lung

	Other names	Ligands
Integrins		
αLβ2	CD11a/CD18, LFA-1	ICAM-1, ICAM-2, ICAM-3
αMβ2	CD11b/CD18, Mac-1	ICAM-1, C3bi
αxβ2	CD11c/CD18, p150,95	C3bi, fibrinogen
Immunoglobulin superfamily		
PECAM-1	CD31	PECAM-1
ICAM-1, ICAM-2		αLβ2, αMβ2
VAM-1	Vascular-CAM	α4β1
CD2	LFA-2	LFA-3
LFA-3		CD2
N-CAM	Neural-CAM	N-CAM
Selectins		
L-Selectin		E-Selectin, P-selectin
E-Selectin	ELAM-1	L-Selectin
P-Selectin	GMP-140	L-Selectin
Cadherins		
E-Cadherin	Epithelial-cadherin	E-Cadherin
P-Cadherin	Placental-cadherin	P-Cadherin
V-Cadherin	Vascular cell-cadherin	
N-Cadherin	Neural cell-cadherin	N-Cadherin
Desmocollins		Desmocollins, desmogleins
Desmogleins		Desmogleins, desmocollins

Source: Adapted from Refs. 108, 111, 116.

expressed very early in in embryonic development and is primarily expressed on epithelial cells in adult tissues. In the human bronchus and alveolus, E-cadherin is expressed at intercellular contacts of epithelial cells and particularly at the lateral aspects of columnar cells (89). This location of E-cadherin is consistent with the location of intermediate/adherens junctions that interact with actin filaments of the cytoskeleton. P-cadherin has been identified in bronchial epithelium but not in alveolar epithelium (90,91).

The expression of cadherins is modulated in disease states. Differential epression of cadherins has been described for different lung cancers. Loss of expression of E-cadherin has been described for non–small-cell lung cancers (92) and poorly differentiated squamous cell cancers (93). E-cadherin expression was more prominent in well-differentiated squamous cell cancers. The expression of cadherins may therefore relate to ability of tumor cells to invade and demonstrate malignant behavior. Kasper and colleagues have described cadherin expression in several animal models of lung injury. Using a pan-cadherin antibody, they found that radiation injury of the lung caused increased cadherin expression in bronchial epithelial cells, interstitial cells, and type II pneumocytes (94). Using an antibody to E-cadherin, Kasper et al. found that human lung specimens with fibrosis demonstrated spotty, cytoplasmic staining of alveolar epithelial cells rather than the normal basolateral membrane staining (95). In a rat model of radiation-induced fibrosis, Kasper et al. found enhanced expression of E-cadherin on the surface of type I alveolar epithelial cells (96). The results imply that modulation of cadherin expression and function is important during repair and remodeling of the epithelium. For example, decreased function might be necessary for cell migration or proliferation.

Desmosomal cadherins are another group of adhesion molecules involved in cell-cell adhesion. Desmosomal cadherins are transmembrane adhesion molecules that are found in desmosomes. Green and Jones have recently reviewed the structure and function of desmosomes (97). Similar to the other cadherins described above, desmosomal cadherins, including desmocollins and desmogleins, are calcium-dependent transmembrane adhesion molecules that participate in homotypic cell-cell adhesion. The exact role of desmosomal cadherins in the adhesion is not yet clear, however. Desmosomal cadherins apparently have a functional complexity that the classical cadherins such as E-cadherin do not have. Three desmocollin and three desmoglein genes have been identified (98,99). Each of the desmocollin genes also produces splice variants (100). It is not clear whether the individual desmogleins and desmocollins have homophilic adhesion in the same way as classical cadherins.

Similar to focal adhesions, desmosomes include a complex of cytoplasmic proteins that make possible connections to the cytoskeleton. Plakoglobin is related to β-catenin, which is present in adherens junctions with E-cadherin (97). Plakoglobin is present in other types of cell-cell junctions with or without the classic cadherins (101). Plakophilin is related to plakoglobin and may bind directly to intermediate filaments. Desmoplakin also functions to anchor intermediate filaments to desmosomes. Other proteins present in the plaque on the cytplasmic side of a desmosome include the bullous pemphigoid antigen (BPAG1), plectin, and IFAP300. Similar to focal adhesions, desmosomes may transduce signals (102). Perhaps more important to injury and repair, the function of desmosomes is modulated by several stimuli. Garrod et al. have reviewed data suggesting that stimuli such as wounding can revert stable desmosomes from calcium independence (102). The function of desmosomes is likely regulated by reversible protein phosphorylation. Growth factors induce tyrosine phosphorylation of plakoglobin (103). In this regard it interesting that activation of PKC is known to modulate desmosome function. As discussed earlier in this review, PKC activation is associated with increased mobility of epithelial cells. Modulation or disassembly of desmosomes may be necessary for cell migration.

The functions of adhesion complexes are different in different cell types. The differences relate to the usage of different intermediate filaments of the cytoskeleton (104). Epithelial cells express an assortment of keratins. Vimentin is expressed primarily in fibroblasts. Muscle cells express another intermediate filament protein, desmin. The role of desmin in the integrity of muscle cells has been explored in knockout mouse models. The lack of desmin expression does not affect development but does affect the function of actively contracting muscles shortly after birth (105,106). Smooth muscle cells were not affected as much as other cell types. Other intermediate filament proteins no doubt substitute for desmin to a certain extent during morphogenesis of muscle cells. The proliferating smooth muscle cells of lymphangiomyomatosis have been examined. They coexpress vimentin, desmin, and α-smooth muscle actin, similar to some smooth muscle cells found in normal arterial walls (1). This has been suggested to imply the origin of the proliferating smooth muscle cells.

B. Cell-Cell Adhesion in Inflammatory Processes

There has been an explosion of knowledge regarding the mechanisms of recruitment of inflammatory cells to sites of inflammation (107–110). Cell-cell adhesion and leukocytes in the lung has been reviewed (111–113). The subject is relevant to the study of interstitial lung diseases in that ongoing inflammation and injury are thought to be central to the pathogenesis of most interstitial disorders (5). Inflammatory processes have not recieved as much attention in relation to lymphangiomyomatosis. The disruption of alveolar walls in the cystic changes of lymphangiomyomatosis is associated with injured epithelium and disruption of elastin fibers (114). An imbalance of proteases and antiproteases was suggested as a mechanism, but specific inflammatory processes have not been investigated in lymphangiomyomatosis. The discussion of cell-cell adhesion in inflammatory processes will therefore be somewhat general in approach.

As Hogg and Doerschuk describe (113), an immense number of leukocytes traffic through the pulmonary vasculature. The stimuli that initiate adherence to endothelial cells has been the topic of many studies. Leukocytes must adhere to endothelial cells prior to emigration into tissue. The mechanisms of leukocyte adherence to endothelial cells are complex, but models have been proposed. Springer and others have proposed a multistep process in which both neutrophils and mononuclear leukocytes appear to follow traffic signals in a series of adhesive interactions (108). The selectin family of adhesion molecules are the first adhesion molecules to be engaged. The adhesion mediated by selectins has been termed rolling adhesion. L-Selectin is expressed on leukocytes, E-selectin and P-selectin on endothelial cells. The ligands for selectins are sialylated carbohydrates on specific mucin-like molecules. The next phase of adhesion is mediated by leukocyte integrins. The β2 family of integrins include the adhesion molecules known as LFA-1, Mac-1, CR3, and CD11/CD18 (Table 2). Ligands for integrins that are found on endothelial cells are members of the Ig superfamily, ICAM-1,

ICAM-2, ICAM-3, and VCAM-1. Additional integrins that function in lymphocyte-endothelial adhesion are α4β1 and α4β7. Ligands include fibronectin and VCAM-1 (115). The phase of adhesion mediated by integrin-ICAM adhesion is thought to be stronger than selectin-mediated adhesion, allowing migration of the cells through the endothelial barrier.

An important aspect of integrin-mediated leukocyte adhesion is that leukocyte chemoattractants increase expression of and activate integrins (116). β2 integrins undergo a conformational change after activation. Springer (108) puts these features together into a three-step model of leukocyte emigration. Selectins act first, chemoattractants activate leukocytes, followed by a strengthening of adhesion and transendothelial migration. Videomicroscopic studies of mesenteric microvessels support this paradigm (117). An initial loose adhesive interaction, rolling adhesion, is followed by stronger, more stable adhesive contacts.

While much attention is focused on leukocyte-endothelial cell adhesion, the inflammatory process also includes adhesion of leukocytes to mesenchyme and epithelial cells. The concept of an epithelial compartment of inflammation in which epithelial cells support leukocyte activation, survival and retention has been discussed by Gauldie and colleagues (118,119). Structural cells such as fibroblasts and epithelial cells produce important cytokines and chemoattractants (120–122). Epithelial cells express ICAM-1, and the expression of ICAM-1 is increased in vitro by a number of cytokines. Interferon-γ is perhaps the most potent in this regard (112). Viral infection will also increase ICAM-1 expression and neutrophil adherence (123–125). Animal models of pulmonary inflammation have also shown increases in ICAM-1 expression on endothelial cells and alveolar epithelial cells (112). Adhesion molecules appear to play important roles in the recruitment and retention of inflammatory cells in pulmonary inflammation. The localization of inflammatory cells facilitates elimination of pathogens but may also promote cellular injury and release of mesenchymal cell mitogens in fibrotic processes.

V. Conclusion

The explosion of knowledge of adhesion molecules has allowed investigators to formulate innovative hypotheses. Future studies will be able to address approaches to modulate cell-matrix interactions and cell-cell interactions. Already, anti-integrins have been studied in animal models of metastatic cancer. Anti-leukocyte integrins have been studied in models of pulmonary inflammation. The importance of cell-matrix and cell-cell interactions to the pathogenesis of pulmonary disorders would seem to bolster the idea that modulating these mechanisms will have powerful effects on disease processes. Clearly, cell-matrix and cell-cell adhesion biology holds many secrets to disease mechanisms.

References

1. Peyrol S, Gindre D, Cordier JF, Loire R, Grimaud JA. Characterization of the smooth muscle cell infiltrate and associated connective matrix of lymphangiomyomatosis. Immunohistochemical and ultrastructural study of two cases. J Pathol 1992; 168:387–395.
2. Kane PB, Lane BP, Cordice JWV, Greenberg GM. Ultrastructure of the proliferating cells in pulmonary lymphangiomyomatosis. Arch Pathol Lab Med 1978; 102:618–622.
3. Hudson BG, Reeders ST, Tryggvason K. Ty[e IV collagen: structure, gene organization, and role in human diseases. J Biol Chem 1993; 268:26033–26036.
4. Kitaichi M, Nishimura K, Itoh H. Izumi T. Pulmonary lymphangioleiomyomatosis: a report of 46 patients including a clinicopathologic study of prognostis factors. Am J Respir Crit Care Med 1995; 151:527–533.
5. Crystal RG, Bitterman PB, Rennard SI, Hance AJ, Keogh BA. Interstitial lung diseases of unknown cause. Disorders characterized by chronic inflammation of the lower respiratory tract (first of two parts). N Engl J Med 1984; 310:154–166.
6. Rennard SI, Hunninghake GW, Bitterman PB, Crystal RG. Production of fibronectin by the human alveolar macrophage: a mechanism for the recruitment of fibroblasts to sites of tissue injury in interstitial lung diseases. Proc Natl Acad Sci USA 1981; 78:7147–7151.
7. Hynes RO. Integrins: versatility, modulation, and signaling in cell adhesion. Cell 1992; 69:11–25.
8. Spurzem JR. Function at the junction: dynamic interactions between lung cells and extracellular matrix. Thorax 1996; 51:956–958.
9. Spurzem JR, Rennard SI, Romberger DJ. Bombesin-like peptides and airway repair: a recapitulation of lung development? Am J Respir Cell Mol Biol 1997; 16:209–211.
10. Hemler M. VLA proteins in the integrin family: structures, functions, and their role on leukocytes. Annu Rev Immunol 1990; 8:365–400.
11. Mette S, Pilewski J, Buck C, Albelda S. Distribution of integrin cell adhesion receptors on normal bronchial epithelial cells and lung cancer cells in vitro and in vivo. Am J Respir Cell Mol Biol 1993; 8:562–572.
12. Huang X, Chen A, Agrez M, Sheppard D. A point mutation in the integrin beta 6 subunit abolishes both alpha v beta 6 binding to fibronectin and receptor localization to focal contacts. Am J Respir Cell Mol Biol 1995; 13:245–251.
13. Pytela R, Pierschbacher MD, Ruoslahti E. Identification and isolation of a 140kd cell surface glycoprotein with properties expected of a fibronectin receptor. Cell 1985; 40:191–198.
14. Smith JW, Cheresh DA. Integrin (avb3)-ligand interaction. Identification of a heterodimeric RGD binding site on the vitronectin receptor. J Biol Chem 1990; 265:2168–2172.
15. Wayner E, Garcia-Pardo A, Humphries M, McDonald J, Carter W. Identification and characterization of the T lymphocyte adhesion receptor for an alternative cell attachment domain (CS-1) in plasma fibronectin. J Cell Biol 1989; 109:1321–1330.

16. Guan J-L, Hynes R. Lymphoid cells recognize an alternatively spliced segment of fibronectin via the integrin receptor a4β1. Cell 1990; 60:53–61.
17. Martin G, Timpl R. Laminin and other basement membrane components. Ann Rev Cell Biol 1987; 3:57–85.
18. Gehlsen KR, Sriramarao P, Furcht LT, Skubitz APN. A synthetic peptide derived from the carboxy terminus of the laminin A chain represents a binding site for the a3βl integrin. J Cell Biol 1992; 117:449–459.
19. Turner C, Burridge K. Transmembrane molecular assemblies in cell-extracellular matrix interactions. Curr Opin Cell Biol 1991; 3:849–53.
20. Dedhar S, Hannigan GE. Integrin cytoplasmic interactions and biderectional transmembrane signalling. Curr Opin Cell Biol 1996; 8:657–669.
21. Critchley DR, Gilmore A, Hemmings L, et al. Cytoskeletal proteins in adherens-type cell matrix junctions. Biochem Soc Trans 1991; 19:1028–1033.
22. Akiyama SK, Hasegawa E, Hasegawa T, Yamada K. The interaction of fibronectin fragments with fibroblastic cells. J Biol Chem 1985; 260:13256–13260.
23. Johansson S, Forsberg E, Lundgren B. Comparison of fibronectin receptors from rat hepatocytes and fibroblasts. J Biol Chem 1987; 262:7819–7824.
24. Clark EA, Brugge JS. Integrin and signal transduction pathways: the road taken. Science 1994; 268:233–239.
25. Juliano R, Haskill S. Signal transduction from the extracellular matrix. J Cell Biol 1993; 120:577–85.
26. Schlaepfer D, Hanks S, Hunter T, van der Geer P. Integrin-mediated signal transduction linked to Ras pathway by GRB2 binding to focal adhesion kinase. Nature 1994; 372:786–791.
27. Chen Q, Kinch M, Lin T, Burridge K, Juliano R. Integrin-mediated cell adhesion activates mitogen-activated protein kinases. J Biol Chem 1994; 269:26602–26605.
28. Craig SW, Johnson RP. Assembly of focal adhesions: progress, paradigms, and potents. Curr Opin Cell Biol 1996; 8:74–85.
29. Ridley AJ, Hall A. The small-GTP binding protein rho regulates the assembly of focal adhesions and actin stress fibers in response to growth factors. Cell 1992; 70:389–399.
30. Yamada KM, Miyamoto S. Integrin transmenbrane signaling and cytoskeletal control. Curr Opin Cell Biol 1995; 7:681–689.
31. Spurzem JR, Aoshiba K, Emanuel S, Wyatt T. Matrix dependence of focal contact formation by bronchial epithelial cells. Am J Respir Crit Care Med 1996; 153:A632.
32. Aoshiba K, Rennard SI, Spurzem JR. Biosynthesized matrix prevents apoptosis of bronchial cells in growth factor-deficient conditions. Am J Respir Crit Care Med 1996; 153:A536.
33. Erjefalt JS, Erjefalt I, Sundler F, Persson CG. Microcirculation-derived factors in airway epithelial repair in vivo. Microvasc Res 1994; 48:161–178.
34. Erjefalt JS, Erjefalt I, Sundler F, Persson CG. In vivo restitution of airway epithelium. Cell Tissue Res 1995; 281:305–316.
35. Borradori L, Sonnenberg A. Hemidesmosomes: roles in adhesion, signaling and human diseases. Curr Opin Cell Biol 1996; 8:647–656.

36. Ekblom P. Receptors for laminins during epithelial morphogenesis. Curr Opin Cell Biol 1996; 8:700–706.
37. Virtanen I, Laitinen A, Tani T, et al. Differential expression of laminins and their integrin receptors in developing and adult human lung. Am J Respir Cell Mol Biol 1996; 15:184–196.
38. Altraja A, Laitinen A, Virtanen I, et al. Expression of laminins in the airways in various types of asthmatic patients: a morphometric study. Am J Respir Cell Mol Biol 1996; 15:482–488.
39. Picker L, De Los Toyos J, Telen M, Haynes B, Butcher E. Monoclonal antibodies against the CD44 [In(lu)-related p80], and Pgp-1 antigens in man recognize the Hermes class of lymphocyte homing receptors. J Immunol 1989; 142:2046–2051.
40. Hofmann M, Rudy W, Zoller M, et al. CD44 splice variants confer metastatic behavior in rats: homologous sequences are expressed in human tumor cell lines. Cancer Res 1991; 51:5292–5297.
41. Brown T, Bouchard T, St. John T, Wayner E, Carter W. Human keratinocytes express a new CD44-core protein (CD44E) as a heparan sulfate intrinsic membrane proteoglycan with additional exons. J Cell Biol 1991; 113:207–221.
42. Alho A, Underhill C. The hyaluronate receptor is preferentially expressed on proliferating epithelial cells. J Cell Biol 1989; 108:1557–1565.
43. Tsukita S, Oishi k, Sato N, Sagara J, Kawai A, Tsukita SH. ERM family members as molecular linkers between the cell surface glycoprotein CD44 and actin-based cytoskeleton. J Cell Biol 1994; 126:391–401.
44. Gary R, Bretscher A. Ezrin self-association involves binding of an N-terminal domain to a normally masked C-terminal domain that includes the F-actin binding site. Mol Biol Cell 1995; 6:1061–1075.
45. Turunen 0, Wahlstrom T, Vaheri A. Ezrin has a COOH-terminal actin-binding site that is conserved in the ezrin protein family. J Cell Biol 1994; 126:1445–1453.
46. Elenius K, Salmivirta M, Inki P, Mali M, Jalkanen M. Binding of human syndecan to extracellular matrix proteins. J Biol Chem 1990; 265:17837–17843.
47. David G. Integral membrane heparan sulfate proteoglycans. FASEB J 1993; 7:1023–1030.
48. Deyst KA, Bowe MA, Leszyk JD, Fallon JR. The alpha-dystroglycan-beta-dystroglycan complex. Membrane organization and relationship to an agrin receptor. J Biol Chem 1995; 270:25956–25959.
49. Henry MD, Campbell KP. Dystroglycan: an extracellular matrix receptor linked to the cytoskeleton. Curr Opin Cell Biol 1996; 8:625–631.
50. Ozawa E, Yoshida M, Suzuki A, Mizuno Y, Hagiwara Y, Noguchi S. Dystrophin-associated proteins in muscular dystrophy. Hum Mol Genet 1995; 4:1711–1716.
51. Durbeej M, Larsson E, Ibraghimov-Beskrovnaya O, Roberds SL, Campbell KP, Ekblom P. Non-muscle alpha-dystroglycan is involved in epithelial development. J Cell Biol 1995; 130:79–91.
52. Iwamoto Y, Robey F, Graf J, et al. YIGSR, a synthetic laminin pentapeptide, inhibits experimental metastasis formation. Science 1987; 238:1132–1134.
53. Montuori N, Sobel ME. The 67-kDa laminin receptor and tumor progression. Curr Top Microbiol Immunol 1996; 213:205–214.

54. Keenan KP, Wilson TS, McDowell EM. Regeneration of hamster tracheal epithelium after mechanical injury. IV. Histochemical, immunocytochemical and ultrastructural studies. Virchows Arch (Cell Pathol) 1983; 43:213–240.
55. Rickard KA, Shoji S, Spurzem JR, Rennard SI. Attachment characteristics of bovine bronchial epithelial cells to extracellular matrix components. Am J Respir Cell Mol Biol 1991; 4:440–448.
56. Sacco O, Romberger D, Rizzino A, Beckmann JD, Rennard SI, Spurzem JR. Spontaneous production of transforming growth factor-β2 by primary cultures of bronchial epithelial cells: effects on cell behavior in vitro. J Clin Invest 1992; 90:1379–1385.
57. Spurzem JR, Sacco O, Rickard KA, Rennard SI. Transforming growth factor-β increases adhesion but not migration of bovine bronchial epithelial cells to matrix proteins. J Lab Clin Med 1993; 122:92–102.
58. Kumar NM, Sigurdson SL, Sheppard D, Lwebuga MJ. Differential modulation of integrin receptors and extracellular matrix laminin by transforming growth factor-beta 1 in rat alveolar epithelial cells. Exp Cell Res 1995; 221:385–94.
59. Sheppard D, Cohen DS, Wang A, Busk M. Transforming growth factor β differentially regulates expression of integrin subunits in guinea pig airway epithelial cells. J Biol Chem 1992; 267:17409–17414.
60. Wang A, Yokosaki Y, Ferrando R, Balmes J, Sheppard D. Differential regulation of airway epithelial integrins by growth factors. Am J Respir Cell Mol Biol 1996; 15:664–672.
61. Spurzem JR, Emanuel S, Rennard SI. Differential distribution of integrins to focal contact points during adhesion of bronchial epithelial cells to matrix proteins. Clin Res 1993; 41:647A.
62. Lackie PM, Baker JE, Gunther U, Holgate ST. Expresion of CD44 isoforms is increased in the airway epithelium of asthmatic subjects. Am J Respir Cell Mol Biol 1997; 16:14–22.
63. DiMilla PA, Stone JA, Quinn JA, Albelda SM, Lauffenburger DA. Maximal migration of human smooth muscle cells on fibronectin and type IV collagen occurs at an intermediate attachment strength. J Cell Biol 1993; 122:729–737.
64. Ito H, Rennard SI, Spurzem JR. Mononuclear cell conditioned medium enhances bronchial epithelial cell migraiton but inhibits attachment to fibronectin. J Lab Clin Med 1996; 127:494–503.
65. Rickard KA, Taylor J, Rennard SI, Spurzem JR. Migration of bovine bronchial epithelial cells to extracellular matrix components. Am J Respir Cell Mol Biol 1993; 8:63–68.
66. Shoji S, Rickard KA, Ertl RF, Robbins RA, Linder J, Rennard SI. Bronchial epithelial cells produce lung fibroblast chemotactic factor: fibronectin. Am J Respir Cell Mol Biol 1989; 1:13–20.
67. Lark MW, Laterra J, Culp LA. Close and focal contact adhesions of fibroblasts to a fibronectin-containing matrix. Fed Proc 1985; 44:394–403.
68. Schnapp LM, hatch N, Ramos DM, Klimanskaya IV, Sheppard D, Pytela R. The human integrin alpha 8 beta I functions as a receptor for tenascin, fibronecfin, vitronectin. J Biol Chem 1995; 270:23196-231202.

69. Schnapp LM, Breuss JM, Ramos DM, Sheppard D, Pytela R. Sequence and tissue distribhution of the human integrin alpha 8 subunit: a beta I -associated alpha subunit expressed in smooth muscle cells. J Cell Sci 1995; 108:537-544.
70. Weinacker A, Ferrando R, Elliott M, Hogg J, Balmes J, Sheppard D. Distribution of integrins alpha v beta 6 and alpha 9 beta 1 and their known ligands, fibronectin and tenascin, in human airways. Am J Respir Cell Mol Biol 1995; 12:547–557.
71. Lechner JF, Haugen A, Autrup H, McClendon IA, Trump BF, Harris CC. Clonal growth of epithelial cells from normal adult human bronchus. Cancer Res 1981; 41:2294–2304.
72. Stoker M, Gherards E, Perryman M, Gray J. Anchorage and growth regulation in normal and virus-transformed cells. Int J Cancer 1968; 3:683–693.
73. Schumann BL, Cody TE, Miller ML, Leikauf GD. Isolation, characterization, and long-term culture of fetal bovine tracheal epithelial cells. In Vitro Cell Dev Biol 1988; 24:211–216.
74. Frisch SM, Francis H. Disruption of epithelial cell-matrix interactions induces apoptosis. Cell Biol 1994; 124:619–626.
75. Ruoslahti E, Reed JC. Anchorage dependence, integrins, and apoptosis. Cell 1994; 77:477–478.
76. Bates RC, Buret A, van Helden DF, Horton MA, Bums GF. Apoptosis induced by inhibition of intercellular contact. J Cell Biol 1994; 125:403–415.
77. Aoshiba K, Rennard SI, Spurzem JR. Cell-matrix and cell-cell interactions modulated apoptosis fo bronchial epithelial cells. Am J Physiol 1997; 272 (Lung Cell Mol Physiol 16):L28–L37.
78. Sannes PL. Structural and functional relationships between type II pneumoncytes and components of extracellular matrix. Exp Lung Res 1991;17:639–659.
79. Sugahara K, Kiyota T, Clark RA, Mason RJ. The effect of fibronectin on cytoskeleton structure and transepithelial resistance of alveolar type II cells in primary culture. Virchows Arch B Cell Pathol Incl Mol Pathol 1993; 64:1151-122.
80. Shannon JM, Emrie A, Fisher JH, Kuroki Y, Jennings SD, Mason RJ. Effect of a reconstituted basement membrane on expression of surfactant apoproteins in cultured adult rat alveolar type II cells. Am J Respir Cell Mol Biol 1990; 2:183–192.
81. Handagama P, Bainton D, Jacques Y, Conn M, Lazarus R, Shuman M. Kistrin, an integrin antagonist, blocks endocytosis of fibrinogen into guinea pig megakaryocyte and platelet a-granules. J Clin Invest 1993; 91:193–200.
82. Brooks PC, Montgomery AM, Rosenfeld M, et al. Integrin alpha v beta 3 antagonists promote tumor regression by inducing apoptosis of angiogenic blood vessels. Cell 1994; 79:1157–1164.
83. Buck C. What's potentially more effective than a Roto-Rooter and less toxic than Drano? Anti-adhesion mimetics! J Clin Invest 1995; 95:2431–2432.
84. Carter WG, Wayner EA, Bouchard TS, Kaur P. The role of integrins a2βl and a3β1 in cell-cell and cell-substrate adhesion of human epidermal cells. J Cell Biol 1990; 110:1387–1404.
85. Wagner G. E-Cadherin: a distant member of the immunoglogulin superfamily. Science 1995; 267:342.

86. Takeichi M. Cadherin cell adhesion receptors as a morphogenetic regulator. Science 1991; 251:1451–1455.
87. Huber O, Bierkamp C, Kemler R. Cadherins and catenins in development. Curr Opin Cell Biol 1996; 1996:685–691.
88. Larue L, Antos C, Butz S, et al. A role for cadherins in tissue formation. Development 1996; 122:1491–1507.
89. Roche WR, Montefort S, Baker J, Holgate ST. Cell adhesion molecules and the bronchial epithelium. Am Rev Respir Dis 1993; 148:S79–S82.
90. Montefort S, A HE, Robinson C, Holgate ST. The bronchial epithelium as a target for inflammatory attack in asthma. Clin Exp Allergy 1992; 22:511–522.
91. Shimoyama Y, Hirohashi S, Hirano S, et al. Cadherin cell-adhesion molecules in human epithelial tissues and carcinomas. Cancer Res 1989; 49:2128–2133.
92. Sorscher SM, Rusack V, Graziano S, Cagle M, Feramisco JR, Green MR. Immunohistochemical evaluation of E-cadherin and epidermal growth factor receptor in non-small cell lung cancer. Mod Pathol 1995; 8:450–455.
93. BAohm M, Totzeck B, Birchmeier W, Wieland I. Differences of E-cadherin expression levels and patterns in primary and metastatic human lung cancer. Clin Exp Metastasis 1994; 12:55–62.
94. Kasper M, MAuller M. Modulation of pan-cadherin expression in alveolar epithelial cells of mini pigs with pulmonary fibrosis. Acta Histochem 1994; 96:439–444.
95. Kasper M, Behrens J, Schuh D, MAuller M. Distribution of E-cadherin and Ep-CAM in the human lung during development and after injury. Histochem Cell Biol 1995; 103:281–286.
96. Kasper M, Huber O, Grossmann H, Rudolph B, Trankner, C, Mauller M. Immunocytochemical distribution of E-cadherin in normal and injured lung tissue of the rat. Histochem Cell Biol 1995; 104:383–390.
97. Green KJ, Jones JCR. Desmosomes and hemidesmosomes: structure and function of molecular components. FASEB J 1996; 10:871–881.
98. King IA, Sullivan KH, Bennett R, Buxton RS. The desmocollins of human foreskin epidermis: identification and chromosomal assignment of a third gene and expression patterns of the three isoforms. J Invest Derm 1995; 105:314–321.
99. Koch PJ, Godlschmidt MD, Zimbelmann R, Troyanovsky R, Franke WW. Complexity and expression patterns of the desmosomal caderins. Proc Natl Acad Sci USA 1992; 89:353–357.
100. Troyanosvsky SM, Troyanovsky RB, Eshkind LG, Leube RE, Franke WW. Identification of amino acid sequence motifs in desmocollin, a desmosomal glycoprotein, that are required for plakoglobin binding and plaque formation. Proc Natl Acad Sci USA 1994; 91:10790–10794.
101. Franke WW, Kapprell H-P, Cowin P. Immunolocalization of plakoglobin in endothelial junctions: identification as a special type of *Zonulae adhaerentes.* Biol Cell 1987; 59:205–218.
102. Garrod D, Chidgey M, North A. Desmosomes: differentiation, development, dynamics and disease. Curr Opin Cell Biol 1996; 8:670–678.
103. Shibamoto S, Hayakawa M, Takeuchi K, et al. Tyrosine phosphorylation of β-

catenin and plakoglobin enhanced by hepatocyte growth factor and epidermal growth factor in human carcinoma cells. Cell Adher Commun 1994; 1:295–305.
104. Chou Y-H, Skalli O, Goldman D. Intermediate filaments and cytoplasmic networking: new connections and more functions. Curr Opin Cell Biol 1997; 9:49–63.
105. Milner Dj, Weitzer G, Tran D, Bradley A, Capetanaki Y. Disruption of muscle architecture and myocardial degeneration in mice lacking desmin. J Cell Biol 1996; 134:1255–1270.
106. Li Z, Colucci-Guyon E, Pincon-Raymond R, et al. Cardiovascular lesions and skeletal myopathy in mice lacking desmin. Dev Biol 1996; 175:362–366.
107. Schleiffenbaum B, Fehr J. Regulation and selectivity of leukocyte emigration. J Lab Clin Med 1996; 127:151–168.
108. Springer TA. Traffic signals for lymphocyte recirculation and leukocyte emigration: the multistep paradigm. Cell 1994; 76:301–314.
109. McEver RP, Moore KL, Cummings RD. Leukocyte trafficking mediated by selectin-carbohydrate interactions. J Biol Chem 1995; 270:11025–11028.
110. Carlos TM, Harlan JM. Leukocyte-endothelial adhesion molecules. Blood 1994; 84:2068–2101.
111. Pilewski JM, Albelda SM. Adhesion molecules in the lung. An overview. Am Rev Respir Dis 1993; 148:S31–S37.
112. Churchill L, Gundel RH, Letts LG, Wegner CD. Contribution of specific cell-adhesion glycoproteins to airway alveolar inflammation and dysfunction. Am Rev Respir Dis 1993; 148:S83–S87.
113. Hogg JC, Doerschuk CM. Leukocyte traffic in the lung. Annu Rev Physiol 1995; 57:97–114.
114. Fukuda Y, Kawamoto M, Yamamoto A, Ishizaki m, Basset F, Masugi Y. Role of elastic fiber degradation in emphysema-like lesions of pulmonary lymphangioleiomyomatosis. Human Pathol 1990; 21:1252–1261.
115. Chin JE, Hatfield CA, Winterrowd GE, et al. Airway recruitment of leukocytes in mice is dependent on a4-integrins and vascular cell adhesion molecule-1. Am J Physiol 1997; 272(Lung Cell Mol Physiol):L219–L229.
116. Wahl SM, Feldman GM, McCarthy JB. Regulation of leukocyte adhesion and signaling in inflammation and disease. J Leukoc Biol 1996; 59:789–796.
117. Lawerence MB, Springer TA. Leukocytes roll on a selectin at physiologic flow rates: distinction from and prerequisite for adhesion through integrins. Cell 1991; 65:859–873.
118. Gauldie J, Jordana M, Cox G, Ohtoshi T, Dolovich J, Denburg J. Fibroblasts and other structural cells in airway inflammation. Am Rev Respir Dis 1992; 145:S14–S17.
119. Denburg JA, Dolovich J, Ohtoshi T, Cox G, Gauldie J, Jordana M. The microenvironmental differentiation hypothesis of airway inflammation. Am J Rhinol 1990; 4:29–34.
120. Rolfe MW, Kunkel SL, Standiford TJ, et al. Expression and regulation of human pulmonary fibroblast-derived monocyte chemotactic peptide-1. Am J Physiol 1992; 263:L536–L545.

121. Denburg JA, Gauldie J, Dolovich J, Ohtoshi T, Cox G, Jordana M. Structural cell-derived cytokines in allergic inflammation. Arch Allergy Appl Immunol 1991; 94:127–132.
122. Smith RE, Stricter RM, Phan SH, Kunkel SL. C-C chemokines: novel mediators of the profibrotic inflammatory response to bleomycin challenge. Am J Respir Cell Mol Biol 1996; 15:693–702.
123. Tosi MF, Stark JM, Hamedani A, Smith CW, Gruenerts DC, Huang YT. Intercellular adhesion molecule-1 (ICAM- 1)-dependent and ICAM-1-independent adhesive interactions between polymorphonuclear leukocytes and human airway epithelial cells infected with parainfluenza virus type 2. J Immunol 1992; 149:3345–3349.
124. Robbins RA, Koyama S, Spurzem JR, et al. Modulation of neutrophil and mononuclear cell adherence to bronchial epithelial cells. Am J Respir Cell Mol Biol 1992; 7:19–29.
125. Raz M, Robbins RA, Kelling CL, et al. Viral infection of bovine bronchial epithelial cells induces increased neutrophil chemotactic activity and neutrophil adhesion. Clin Sci 1993; 85:753–760.
126. Yokosaki Y, Palmer EL, Prieto AL, et al. The integrin alpha 9 beta 1 mediates cell attachment to a non-RGD site in the third fibronectin type III repeat of tenascin. J Biol Chem 1994; 269:26691–26696.
127. Sheppard D. Identification and characterization of novel airway epithelial integrins. Am Rev Respir Dis 1992; 148:S38–S42.

AUTHOR INDEX

Italic numbers give the page on which the complete reference is listed.

A

B

C

E

F

J

K

M

N

P

Q

R

S

T

U

W

X

Y

Z

SUBJECT INDEX

D

E

F

G

H

I

P

Q

R

S

T

U

V

15

Airway Smooth Muscle in Asthma

STEWART J. LEVINE and JAMES H. SHELHAMER

National Heart, Lung and Blood Institute
National Institutes of Health
Bethesda, Maryland

Changes in the mass or responsiveness of airway smooth muscle may play an important role in the development of airway obstruction in patients with asthma. This chapter will address the role of airway smooth muscle abnormalities in asthma. Topics that will be reviewed include the pathology of airway smooth muscle in asthma, the contribution of increased airway smooth muscle mass and contractility versus impaired smooth muscle relaxation to excessive airway narrowing, and the mechanisms underlying smooth muscle hypertrophy and hyperplasia associated with asthmatic airway inflammation.

I. Pathologic Features of Airway Smooth Muscle in Asthma

Increased smooth muscle mass, airway wall thickening, and airway narrowing represent characteristic pathologic features of many asthmatic airways (1–3). Information regarding pathologic increases in airway smooth muscle thickening have mostly been derived from autopsy studies of patients either succumbing to status asthmaticus or patients with underlying asthma who have died from other causes (1,2,4–7). The mechanism responsible for increases in asthmatic airway smooth muscle thickening most likely involves both hyperplasia and hypertrophy. Early postmortem studies of asthma suggested that hyperplasia was predominantly responsible for the excess smooth muscle volume, which was increased approximately threefold in asthmatic airways as compared to controls (6,8). Recently, detailed morphometric analyses utilizing "unbiased" three-dimensional sampling methodology to assess the mean number of airway smooth muscle cells per unit length and the mean volume of single muscle cells have delineated two patterns of increased airway smooth muscle mass in patients with fatal asthma (5,9). In type I asthmatics, smooth muscle thickening was limited to only the larger bronchi (radius > 1–2 mm) and was attributed to increased smooth muscle number consistent with hyperplasia without coexistent hypertrophy. In contrast, type II asthmatics demonstrated airway smooth muscle thickening, which was present throughout both the central and peripheral airways and was predominantly a result of cellular hypertrophy with only mild coexistent hyperplasia in the larger bronchi. In addition, no hyperplasia was noted in smaller bronchioles (radius < 1 mm) in either type I or type II asthmatics. Although these findings demonstrate that both hypertrophy and hyperplasia contribute to the increased smooth muscle thickening present in asthma, neither the pathogenic mechanisms nor the clinical correlates associated with these two different patterns of airway smooth muscle thickening have been established. Last, when central bronchi (radius > 1 mm) of both type I and II asthmatics were combined, then airway smooth muscle cell numbers were increased 2.86 ± 0.38 times as compared to controls, which is similar to the estimate from the earlier postmortem study (5,6).

Differences in airway smooth muscle area have also been noted between cases of nonfatal and fatal asthma (1). In an autopsy study involving 35 patients, patients with fatal asthma were found to have a significantly larger smooth muscle area in large and small cartilaginous airways (basement membrane perimeter > 4 mm) as compared to those with nonfatal asthma. However, in large membranous bronchi (basement membrane perimeter 2–4 mm) there were no differences in smooth muscle area between cases of fatal and nonfatal asthma, although both were increased compared to controls without asthma. In addition, cases of fatal asthma had greater total wall, inner wall, outer wall, mucous gland, and cartilage areas than did controls and nonfatal cases. This suggests that airway structural changes may be present in both large and small airways in fatal asthma, but are mainly confined to the small airways in nonfatal cases.

II. Structure-Function Correlates in Airway Smooth Muscle Contraction in Asthma

Structural changes in the asthmatic airway, including smooth muscle thickening, may have important physiological consequences regarding airway narrowing and bronchial hyperresponsiveness (7,8). In an autopsy study of 18 asthmatic patients